Handbook of Antibiotics

Third Edition

Handbook of Antibiotics

Third Edition

Richard E. Reese, M.D.
Clinical Professor of Medicine
University of New England
    College of Osteopathic Medicine
Biddeford, Maine

Robert F. Betts, M.D.
Professor of Medicine
University of Rochester School of
    Medicine and Dentistry
Associate Physician
Department of Medicine
Strong Memorial Hospital
Rochester, New York

Bora Gumustop, M.D.
Gastroenterology Fellow
University of Wisconsin Medical School
University of Wisconsin Hospital and Clinics
Madison, Wisconsin

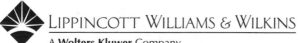
LIPPINCOTT WILLIAMS & WILKINS
A **Wolters Kluwer** Company
Philadelphia · Baltimore · New York · London
Buenos Aires · Hong Kong · Sydney · Tokyo

Acquisitions Editor: Jonathan Pine
Developmental Editor: Ellen DiFrancesco
Production Editor: Aureliano Vázquez, Jr.
Manufacturing Manager: Kevin Watt
Cover Illustration by: Kevin Kall
Compositor: Circle Graphics
Printer: R.R. Donnelley, Crawfordsville

QV
39
R329h
2000

© 2000 by Richard E. Reese and Robert F. Betts
Published by Lippincott Williams & Wilkins
530 Walnut Street
Philadelphia, PA 19106 USA
LWW.com

Printed in the USA

Library of Congress Cataloging-in-Publication Data

Reese, Richard E.
  Handbook of antibiotics / Richard E. Reese, Robert F. Betts, Bora
    Gumustop.—3rd ed.
    p. ; cm.
  Includes bibliographical references and index.
  ISBN 0-7817-1611-X
    1. Antibiotics—Handbooks, manuals, etc. I. Betts, Robert F. II.
      Gumustop, Bora. III
  Title.
    [DNLM: 1. Antibiotics—Handbooks. QV 39 R329h 2000]
RM267.R44 2000
615'.329—dc21   99-088572

10 9 8 7 6 5 4 3 2 1

This book is dedicated to Ann Sullivan Baker, M.D.
Ann was an Associate Professor of Medicine
at Harvard Medical School, Physician on
the Medical Services of the Massachusetts
General Hospital,
and Director of the Infectious Disease Service at
the Massachusetts Eye and Ear Infirmary in Boston,
a good friend and colleague.

Contents

Preface ix

PART I: Common Infections

1. Upper Respiratory Infections and Influenza 3
2. Pneumonia 39
3. Skin and Soft-Tissue Infections 73
4. Urinary Tract Infections (UTIs) 89
5. Acute Diarrhea, Gastroenteritis,
   and Food Poisoning 106
6. Intraabdominal Infections 132
7. Sepsis 157
8. Infective Endocarditis 171
9. Acute Joint and Bone Infections 183
10. Sexually Transmitted Diseases and Pelvic
    Inflammatory Disease 192
11. Fever and Apparent Acute CNS Infection 212
12. Approach to the Febrile Patient Without
    an Obvious Source 232
13. Miscellaneous 250
    Part A: Microbiology Lab Pointers 250
    Part B: Infection Control Issues 263

PART II: Antibiotic Use

14. Introduction to Antiobiotic Use 277
15. Prophylactic Antibiotics 309
16. Penicillin G and Penicillin-Resistant
    Streptococcus pneumoniae 326
17. Penicillinase-Resistant Penicillins 339
18. Broad-Spectrum Penicillins and
    Beta-lactam/Beta-lactamase Combinations 343
19. The Cephalosporins 365
20. Unique Beta-lactam Antibiotics: Monobactams
    and Carbapenems (Aztreonam, Imipenem,
    and Meropenem) 401
21. Aminoglycosides 415
22. Clindamycin 435
23. Chloramphenicol 441
24. Sulfonamides and
    Trimethoprim-Sulfamethoxazole 446
25. Trimethoprim 463
26. Macrolides: Erythromycin, Clarithromycin,
    and Azithromycin 468
27. Tetracyclines 493

28. Vancomycin, Linezolid, and
     Quinupristin/Dalfopristin 503
29. Metronidazole 521
30. Rifampin, Rifapentin, and Rifabutin 527
31. Spectinomycin 542
32. Fluoroquinolones 544
33. Urinary Antiseptics 564

Appendixes 575

Subject Index 591

Preface

This book is intended for medical students, house officers, practicing physicians, physician assistants, and other health professionals involved in evaluating patients and prescribing antibiotics.

It is estimated that up to 50% of antibiotics prescribed in the United States are inappropriately used. Frequently, the antibiotic is not indicated. Often when it is indicated, the incorrect antibiotic is chosen, the dose is incorrect, or the duration is inappropriate for the clinical situation.

The *Handbook of Antibiotics* provides a concise discussion—not just a series of tables—of virtually all of the antibiotics currently in use, including the new antibiotics that have been approved in the last year. It has become increasingly difficult for the clinician to stay abreast of these new agents, especially with respect to their pharmacokinetics and their side effects. This handbook provides that necessary information to the practitioner in an easy-to-use outline format.

An additional important feature of this handbook is that concise discussions of common infectious diseases are provided. These discussions emphasize clinical reasoning as to when to use a standard antibiotic, or whether a newer agent is recommended. We hope that this approach, which is unique for a handbook, will help the clinician reduce the figure of 50% inappropriate antibiotic usage.

We believe that this material will be practical and useful. This is because the recommendations therein are based on a combined 50 years of patient care, as well as answers to challenging questions posed by clinicians at all levels of training and experience. Furthermore, from these interactions we have modified this text in response to helpful suggestions, thus speaking to the needs of the users.

After the success of the first edition (1983) and second edition (1986) of *A Practical Approach to Infectious Diseases,* many suggested that we publish separately its section on antibiotic agents. The fourth edition of *A Practical Approach to Infectious Diseases* was published in 1996. This third edition of the *Handbook of Antibiotics* is, in part, a concise update of the antibiotic discussions of that text and a discussion of the initial considerations and management of common entities (e.g., sepsis, pneumonia, URI, UTI) in Part I. The discussion of specific antibiotics follows in Part II.

We thank Mary Muller and the personnel at the Text Processing Department at Bassett Healthcare, Cooperstown, New York, for their help in typing and preparing this text; Linda Muehl, librarian, for her tremendous help in doing multiple literature searches; and Joseph S. Bertino, Jr., Pharm.D., Michael A. Foltzer, M.D., and Alan J. Kozak, M.D., at Bassett Healthcare for their useful advice. One of the authors (R.E.R., who was at Bassett Healthcare until late 1999) thanks Walter A. Franck, M.D., Physician-in-Chief at Bassett Healthcare, for his encouragement and support of this writing project.

In addition, we thank all those at Lippincott Williams & Wilkins who aided in the fruition of this book. Finally, we thank our wives, Shirley, Sherrill, and Betsy, for their patience, encouragement, and support during the preparation of this text.

Richard E. Reese, M.D.
Robert F. Betts, M.D.
Bora Gumustop, M.D.

PART I

Common Infections

Upper Respiratory Infections and Influenza

Approximately 20 million office prescriptions per year in the United States are written for upper respiratory infections (1,2). The most common diagnoses are otitis media, nonspecific upper respiratory tract infections (URIs), bronchitis, pharyngitis, and sinusitis (1). These infectious accounted for more than 75% of prescriptions written annually in physicians' offices (1). Therefore a practical approach to these common problems is essential.

I.   **Clinically relevant pathophysiology of URIs.** The **"common cold"** usually involves the sinuses.

A.   **Computed tomographic (CT) changes.** An important study documented that rhinovirus-induced **common colds are associated with CT abnormalities of the sinuses in more than 85% of cases** and these abnormalities resolve without antibiotics! Therefore **the common cold is really a viral rhinosinusitis** (3), not just a rhinitis (4).

B.   **Mucopurulent rhinitis** (thick, opaque, or discolored nasal discharge) **frequently develops 1 to 3 days after the onset of the common cold** because nasal secretions contain desquamated epithelial cells, polymorphonuclear cells, and nonpathogenic bacteria that normally colonize the upper respiratory tract (4).

This is not an indication of bacterial infection and thus is not an indication for antimicrobial treatment (4).

II. **Excessive outpatient antibiotic use.** Even though antibiotics do not affect the clinical course of uncomplicated viral illness, recent studies have emphasized that **common viral respiratory tract infections** are **often inappropriately treated with antibiotics** in both adults and children. More than 40% to 50% of children and adults with common colds or URIs, and more than 60% to 70% of children and adults with bronchitis with no underlying lung disease receive unnecessary antibiotics (2,5). As discussed later in this chapter, antibiotics are also often unnecessarily prescribed for children with the common findings of asymptomatic otitis media with middle ear effusions (6).

III. **Problems from excessive antibiotic use.**

A.   **Increasing bacterial resistance.** Excessive use of antibiotics in ambulatory practice has contributed to the emergence of antibiotic-resistant bacteria in our communities (1,2,6,7). It is especially worrisome if antibiotics are often not even indicated, as in uncomplicated viral respiratory infections, and yet still used.

Now more than 30% of respiratory isolates of *Streptococcus pneumoniae* isolated are penicillin resistant. (See detailed discussion of this issue on pages 326–330.)

This has complicated the antibiotic decision-making process especially in acute otitis media (AOM) and community-acquired pneumonia (Chap. 2)

B. **Unwanted side effects.** Patients treated with antibiotics for viral infections "gain" only the side effects associated with those antibiotics along with the considerable out-of-pocket or out-of-insurance-fund expense. Many patients are now admitted with severe *Clostridium difficile* colitis or severe drug rash or drug fever that costs them time lost from work and the health care system excess expense. Once allergic to one class of antibiotics, alternative agents used in the future may be more expensive or broader in spectrum than clinically necessary.

IV. **Why do physicians overprescribe antibiotics,** especially in the ambulatory setting (7–9)?

A. **Insufficient time** to discuss with patients/families why an antibiotic is not really needed is a consequence of pressure to see patients in a shorter period of time. With pressures to see more patients, writing a prescription is easier than explaining why an antibiotic should not be used. See Sec. II.

B. **Lack of understanding of the natural history** of viral respiratory infections and acute otitis media (AOM) with effusion contributes.

C. **Clinician experience and patient experience and/or expectations.** When a clinician does not care for children as often as adults, the physician may be more inclined to use antibiotics for URIs. When a child or adult has received antibiotics for a similar illness in the past, that experience raises his or her expectations for antibiotics (8).

D. **Economic pressures** are poorly studied but are probably very important. Concerns about patient/parent satisfaction and retention are often cited as reasons for using antibiotics. In managed-care settings, physicians may believe antibiotics may reduce the likelihood of return visits for URIs.

V. **Possible approaches** (7,9)

A. **Physician education** about the pathogenesis of common URIs and the judicious use of antibiotics is essential.

1. **Education must begin in medical school/house staff training.**

a. Data on the pathogenesis of these infections and appropriate use of nonsteroidal antiinflammatory drugs (NSAIDs) and antihistamines should be provided (see later discussions).

b. Education must emphasize lack of efficiency in viral infections, frequency of side effects, and increasing incidence of bacterial resistance.

2. **In pediatrics,** an excellent series on important principles for judicious use of antibiotics has recently been published (6). Essential points of this

supplement are summarized in the discussions that follow.

3. **In adults,** fewer published guidelines are available but the pharyngitis guideline (10) is discussed below. More guidelines are needed.

B. **Education of the general public** is as important as physician education (7,9).

1. **Materials that** help **explain** the potential **harm** of **unnecessary** use of **antibiotics** are available for pediatric patients and **should be used regularly.** * Brochures are being developed for use in adults. One reviewer emphasizes: "Parents are busy and want their children well yesterday" (9).

2. **Physicians need to educate the public** about the appropriate use of antibiotics (e.g., at community meetings, with newspaper columns, etc.).

3. The media and medical community need to reach the general population about the benefits of anti-inflammatory drugs and first-generation antihistamines' role early in cold symptoms. See Sec. I.D. under "The Common Cold."

C. **Economic pressures must be refocused** to promote more judicious use of antibiotics (8). Managed-care administrators must be made aware that management policies that indirectly encourage antibiotic overuse are, in the long run, not cost-effective. Increased costs from unnecessary prescriptions, adverse drug reactions, and treatment failures in patients with antibiotic-resistant infections must be weighed against the perceived benefits of therapy (8). These topics need further clinical study and input from national organizations expert in antibiotic use.

Nasopharyngitis (the Common Cold)/ Upper Respiratory Infections (URI)

I. **Background.** As previously discussed, the common cold is really a rhinosinusitis (3,4).

A. **Acute illness** is characterized by rhinorrhea, sneezing, sore throat, cough, and in children, low-grade fever.

1. Children may have three to eight colds per year (4).
2. Adults typically have one to three colds per year.

B. **Etiology.** Rhinoviruses and coronaviruses account for the majority of infections in children; rhinoviruses are especially important in adults.

C. **Course**

1. The **usual duration is 3 to 7 days** with peak symptoms on the second and third days.

---

* See pamphlet "Your Child and Antibiotics: Unnecessary Antibiotics Can Be Harmful," prepared by the American Academy of Pediatrics, Centers for Disease Control and Prevention, and American Society for Microbiology.

2. **Mucopurulent rhinitis (thick, opaque, or dis-colored nasal discharge) frequently develops and is not an indication for antimicrobial treatment, as discussed earlier (4).**

D. **Therapy**
   1. **Antimicrobial agents should not be given for the common cold.** Controlled trials of anti-microbial treatment of the common cold have con-sistently failed to show that treatment changes the course or outcome (4).

      Antimicrobials should not be given "to prevent bacterial complications" of the common cold since this is not an effective strategy (4).
   2. **Symptomatic therapy**
      a. **Naproxen,** a NSAID, in a randomized, double-blind, controlled trial of experimental rhinovirus colds in young adults had a bene-ficial effect on the symptoms of headache, malaise, myalgia, and cough (11). Virus shed-ding was not altered. Prostaglandins may be among the inflammatory mediators that play a role in the pathogenesis of rhinovirus colds (11) and presumably other viral colds. Pre-sumably, other NSAID may have a similar effect.
      b. **First-generation antihistamines.** Al-though early studies suggested the role of antihistamines in the therapy of common colds was controversial (12), recent studies suggest a potential benefit of early initiation of first-generation antihistamines in adults. **Clemastine fumarate** reduces sneezing and rhinorrhea (13). Likewise, **brompheni-ramine maleate** (e.g., the antihistamine in Dimetapp) was efficacious in reducing sneez-ing, rhinorrhea, and cough associated with rhinovirus colds (14). Mild drowsiness, dry mouth, and dry throat are potential side effects in a minority of patients.

         The role of antihistamines in children awaits further study.
      c. **Intranasal ipratropium bromide (Atro-vent)** has been shown to provide specific relief of rhinorrhea and sneezing with com-mon colds in adults in a randomized, double-blind, placebo-controlled trial (15). These studies have been done in patients more than 12 years old, and the nasal spray was used for 4 days.
      d. **Pseudoephedrine plus acetaminophen** when given to subjects who had cold symp-toms for less than 48 hours caused improve-ment of "sinus" pain, pressure, and congestion when compared with controls in a prelimi-nary report. The combination was well toler-

ated, except that 4% of the pseudoephedrine-acetaminophen subjects complained of nervousness (15A).

e. **Symptomatic therapy.** Acetaminophen in children and acetaminophen or aspirin in adults has been used. If a NSAID is used (Sec. a), we would avoid also using aspirin. Cold water vaporization has been used.

f. The use of antihistamines and oral decongestants has been advocated for treating children in an attempt to prevent AOM. However, these agents were initiated too late to be effective, and at that point, such therapy has not been beneficial. Further studies need to be done in this area.

3. **Complications.** In children, **AOM** or **bacterial sinusitis** may follow a cold and merit antibiotics; this is also true in a small proportion of adults with bacterial sinusitis. See specific later discussions of these entities.

E. **Transmission** is from person to person, requires close contact, and probably involves transfer of the virus from the hands of an infected person to an intermediate surface or directly to the hands of a susceptible person. **Therefore good handwashing can help prevent the spread of these viral infections.**

Acute Pharyngitis and Tonsillitis

The management of acute pharyngitis is an area of ongoing discussion. At any age, **the majority of cases** of pharyngitis (usually >70%) are not exudative, and **usually are due to viruses.** Group A beta-hemolytic streptococci (*Streptococcus pyogenes*) are the major cause of bacterial pharyngitis (particularly exudative tonsillitis), which is the only commonly occurring form of acute pharyngitis for which antibiotic therapy is definitively indicated. **Antibiotic therapy is advised (10) for group A streptococcal (GAS) infection** to (a) prevent the suppurative complications (e.g., peritonsillar abscess); (b) prevent nonsuppurative complications (e.g., rheumatic fever); (c) decrease infectivity to reduce transmission to family members, classmates, and close contacts and allow the rapid assumption of normal activities; and (d) prevent rare cases of invasive streptococcal syndromes. Controlled studies have demonstrated a slightly shorter duration of clinical illness as well.

Antimicrobial therapy is not of proven benefit in the treatment of acute pharyngitis due to bacteria other than GAS infection, with the exception of very rare infections due to *Corynebacterium diptheriae* (diphtheria) and *Neisseria gonorrhoeae* (10).

I. **Clinical presentation. No reliable predictive model based on clinical signs and symptoms exists to identify all individuals with streptococcal pharyngitis (10).**

A. The **"classical" clinical features of acute strepto-coccal pharyngitis** are the following: onset in winter or spring; school-age child; abrupt onset of fever, sore throat, headache, abdominal pain; pharyngeal tonsil-lar inflammation, often (but only 50% of the time) with yellowish exudates, swollen uvula; tender anterior cervical lymph nodes; scarlatiniform rash.

B. **Viral illness is suggested by absence of fever, rhinorrhea, obstruction of the nasal passage(s), cough, conjunctivitis, hoarseness** (which have up to 80% negative predictive value), and **diarrhea**. Viral infection is especially common in children less than 3 years of age (16).

C. **Differential diagnosis.** Several experts have tried to summarize the clinical presentation of GAS versus viral infections (**Table 1.1**).

II. **Laboratory testing should be performed in patients with acute pharyngitis whose clinical and epidemi-ologic features suggest GAS infection.** See Sec. I.

A. **Throat culture.** For GAS infection, the accuracy of a single throat culture plated on sheep blood agar is approximately 95%. Plates that are negative at 24 hours should be reexamined at 48 hours (10).

Table 1-1.   Differentiating features of pharyngitis caused by group A streptococci and viruses

	"Classic" Streptococcal Pharyngitis	Viral Pharyngitis
Season	Late winter or early spring	All seasons
Age	Peak: 5–11 yr	All ages
Symptoms	Sudden onset Sore throat, may be severe Headache Abdominal pain, nausea, vomiting	Onset varies Sore throat, often mild Fever varies Myalgia, arthralgia Abdominal pain may occur with influenza A or EBV
Signs	Pharyngeal erythema and exudate Tender, enlarged anterior cervical nodes Palatal petechiae Tonsillar hypertrophy Scarlet fever rash Absence of cough, rhinitis, hoarseness, conjunctivitis, and diarrhea	Characteristic enanthems Characteristic exanthems **Often have cough, rhinitis, hoarseness, conjunctivitis, or diarrhea**

Source: Modified from Tanz RR, Shulman ST. Pharyngitis. In: Long SS, Pickering LK, Prober CG, eds. *Principles and practice of pediatric infectious diseases.* New York: Churchill/Livingstone, 1997:202.

Throat swab specimens should be obtained from the surface of both tonsils (or tonsillary fossae) and the posterior pharyngeal wall. Other areas of the oropharynx and mouth are unacceptable for sampling, and these sites should not be touched before or after the appropriate areas have been sampled (10).

Interpretation of a positive result is complicated by the fact that colonization with group A streptococci is common. Thirty percent to 35% of asymptomatic grade schoolers in the winter may be colonized with group A streptococci. If these carriers have a true superimposed viral pharyngitis, a throat culture will show GAS infection. Since the clinician does not culture for viruses, this type of patient is assumed to have GAS infection and is often treated. This is one reason those patients with a sore throat and characteristics of viral illness only (Sec. I.B) do not need to be cultured.

B. **Rapid streptococcal antigen test.** This test has excellent specificity (>95%), so a **positive test for clinical purposes establishes the diagnosis**. However, the sensitivity of the antigen test is between 80% to 90% or even lower, when compared with cultures, so a **negative antigen test should be confirmed with conventional blood agar plate culture (10,16).** An area of debate is whether those who are antigen negative and culture positive may simply be colonized. Rapid identification and treatment of GAS pharyngitis can reduce the risk of spread of GAS infection, allowing these patients to return to school, day care, or work sooner and can reduce morbidity associated with this illness (10,16). Rapid therapy is not essential to prevent acute rheumatic fever (16). See Sec. III.

C. **Antibody studies** (ASO, streptozyme) are **not advised.** This test is more helpful in confirming prior GAS infections in patients suspected of having acute rheumatic fever or acute glomerulonephritis. It is also helpful in prospective epidemiologic studies conducted to separate patients with acute infections from those who are carriers (10).

III. **Therapy. Prior studies have shown that therapy can be safely postponed up to 9 days after onset of symptoms and still prevent acute rheumatic fever (10,16).** GAS infection is usually a self-limited disease: fever and constitutional symptoms disappear spontaneously within 3 to 4 days of onset even without therapy (10), which has resulted in difficulty reaching statistical significance for penicillin therapy in small placebo-controlled studies. Therefore the clinician has considerable flexibility in initiating therapy.

A. **If the rapid antigen test is positive, treatment is indicated.** If a rapid diagnostic test is negative, treatment is based on potential risk (i.e., underlying rheumatic heart disease) and clinical suspicion until culture results are available. If risk is low, one can obtain a throat culture and wait for the culture results.

B. **If the rapid antigen test is unavailable:**
1. In patients with mild illness and without underlying rheumatic heart disease, the results of the culture can be awaited.
2. In those with signs and symptoms highly suggestive of GAS infection, empiric therapy can be started, and if the cultures are negative, therapy can be discontinued.

C. **Regimens.** Unless contraindicated, **penicillin remains the treatment of choice** for GAS pharyngitis (10,17), and bid regimens, if taken, are effective (10,18) and may help improve compliance. Amoxicillin is an acceptable alternative to penicillin and is often prescribed since it is more palatable and the cost is comparable. However, because of its broader antimicrobial spectrum, use of amoxicillin results in greater selective pressure for resistant bacteria (16). Family members are not usually treated unless they exhibit symptoms and have positive cultures or strep screens, or they have rheumatic heart disease.

Common regimens are shown in Tables 1.2 and 1.3. In the penicillin-allergic patient, erythromycin is the major alternative, but if these agents cannot be tolerated, a first-generation cephalosporin or clindamycin can be used. The more expensive second- and third-generation cephalosporins are 10 to 20 times more expensive than penicillin, excessively broad spectrum, and, although sometimes encouraged by the pharmaceutical industry, seldom indicated (19). Tetracycline and sulfonamides are not recommended since many strains are resistant to these agents.

D. **Recurrent pharyngitis or "failure of therapy"** is a complex issue that has been reviewed elsewhere (10,17,20). Often these patients have viral pharyngitis or just the carrier state of GAS infection. See Sec. IV.C.

IV. **Miscellaneous**
A. **Antimicrobial resistance** to GAS infection has **not been a problem in the United States.** Penicillin resistance has not occurred, and less than 5% of GAS infections in the United States are resistant to erythromycin (10).

B. **Follow-up throat cultures are not indicated** for asymptomatic patients who have received a complete course of antibiotics for GAS infection (10).

C. **Streptococcal carriers do not ordinarily require further antibiotic therapy.** They are unlikely to spread GAS infection to close contacts and are at low risk, if any, for developing suppurative complications or acute rheumatic fever (10).

D. Outbreaks of GAS infection and "ping-pong" spread within a family are discussed elsewhere (10).

**Table 1-2. Treatment regimens
for acute streptococcal pharyngitis in children**

Oral Agents	Regimen	Cost of Course[‡]
Penicillin V	125 mg (if <27 kg) to 250 mg[#] (if >27 kg) bid for 10 days	$3
Erythromycin Ethylsuccinate	40 mg/kg/day (to max. of 1,000 mg/day) in two to four divided doses for 10 days	$20
Estolate	20–40 mg/kg/day (to max. of 1,000 mg/day) in two to four divided doses for 10 days	$11–22[§]
Cephalexin or Cephradine (first-generation cephalosporin)	25–50 mg/kg/day in two or three divided doses for 10 days	$10–80[˙]
Clarithromycin	15 mg/kg/day (to max. of 500 mg/day) divided bid for 10 days	$30–55[§]
Azithromycin	12 mg/kg once daily (with max. 500 mg on first day, 250 mg subsequent days) for 5 days	$28
Clindamycin*	20 mg/kg day (max. 1.8 g/day) divided tid for 10 days	$17.50

Parenteral Agent	Regimen	Cost for course
Benzathine penicillin G[†]	600,000 units if <27 kg and 1.2 million units if >27 kg IM once only	$6

Source: Courtesy of Joseph S. Bertino, Jr. Pharm.D., Bassett Healthcare, Cooperstown, NY.

[#] 500 mg bid for adolescents. See Table 1-3.

* Clindamycin has been used in patients with multiple antibiotic allergies and to eradicate the GAS "carrier state."

[†] The single IM dose eliminates the problem of compliance, but the shot is painful.

[‡] Actual wholesale costs (rounded off). 1999 Redbook.

[§] Depending on weight.

[˙] Wide range depending upon weight and whether generic or trade.

Table 1-3.   Treatment regimens for acute streptococcal pharyngitis in adults

Oral Agent	Regimen	Cost for Course[‡]
Penicillin V	500 mg bid or tid for 10 days	$3–4
Erythromycin **Avoid estolate**		
Other preparation (base, stearate, ethylsuccinate)	500 mg bid or 250 mg qid for ten days	$5.50–9
Clarithromycin	250 mg bid for 10 days	$69
Azithromycin	500 mg once on day 1, then 250 mg once daily for 4 days (i.e., 5-day course)	$38
Cephalexin or cephradine	500 mg bid, or 250 mg qid, for 10 days	$36–60[§]
Clindamycin*	300 mg bid–tid for 10 days	$68 (bid)– 101 (tid)

Parenteral Agent	Regimen	Cost for Course
Benzathine penicillin G[†]	1.2 million units IM once only	$6

Source: Courtesy of Joseph S. Bertino, Jr. Pharm.D., Bassett Healthcare, Cooperstown, NY.
* Clindamycin has been used in patients with multiple allergies and to eradicate the GAS "carrier state."
[†] The single IM dose eliminates the problem of compliance, but the shot is painful.
[‡] Approximate (rounded off) wholesale prices/range, 1999 Red Book.
[§] Range involves generic versus trade name (more expensive).

Acute Otitis Media

Acute otitis media (AOM) **is the most commonly diagnosed infectious disease of childhood** and AOM is the most common indication for outpatient antibiotic use in the United States (1). Approximately 30% of all office prescriptions for children are for otitis media (5), and about 20% of all office prescriptions for antibiotics (children and adults) are for otitis media (1). A recent report indicates the average child in the United States consumes an astonishing 3 months' worth of antibiotics for AOM during the first 2 years of life (21)! Therefore any efforts to improve the rational use of antibiotics must address otitis media. **Principles of judicious use of antibiotics for AOM have recently been published (22).**

Bacteria have been isolated from 50% to 60% of cases, and in a recent report, respiratory viruses (especially respiratory syncytial virus [RSV], parainfluenza virus, and influenza virus) were isolated in 41% of children (23).

I. **Principles of therapy (22)**

A. **Episodes of otitis media should be classified as AOM or otitis media with effusion (OME). The natural history of** appropriately treated **AOM includes persistent middle ear effusions for several weeks in the majority of children.**

   1. **AOM** is defined as the presence of **fluid** in the middle ear **in association with signs or symptoms of acute local or systemic illness.** Focal signs of AOM are otalgia or otorrhea or nonspecific fever (22).

   2. **OME** is defined as the presence of **fluid** in the middle ear **in the absence of signs or symptoms of acute infection.**

B. **Antibiotics are usually indicated for the treatment of AOM (22), but even this is not universally accepted. See Sec. 2.** About 80% of untreated children have clinical resolution by 7 to 14 days, compared with 95% of those treated with antibiotics (22). Unfortunately, there is **no consensus** on how to establish the **clinical diagnosis of AOM**. Various sets of criteria have been used.

   1. **Findings in AOM** (a detailed discussion of this topic is beyond the scope of this handbook).

      a. **A middle ear effusion is present,** without which the diagnosis of AOM cannot be supported except in rare circumstances when the practitioner may observe signs of acute inflammation in the hours before fluid accumulates in the middle ear (22).

      Pneumatic otoscopy should be used to assess the tympanic membrane (TM) in terms of (a) position, (b) color, (c) translucency, and (d) mobility (22).

      b. Such **local signs** as (a) otorrhea with evidence of middle ear origin, (b) bulging TM with cloudy or yellow fluid behind it or if TM is distinctly red, or (c) local ear pain should be sought.

      c. **Fever** is presumably indicative of AOM **when there are associated local signs**; in the absence of these local signs, fever often may be unrelated to middle ear effusion.

      d. **Nonspecific signs and symptoms** that do not help make the diagnosis of AOM include rhinorrhea, cough, irritability, anorexia, headache, vomiting, or diarrhea.

   2. **The Dutch approach emphasizing watchful waiting** has recently been reviewed and supported by Hirschmann (24). In his commentary, Hirschmann notes, **the crucial issue in AOM is whether to use antibiotics at all** (24). The placebo-controlled trials reveal a largely unim-

pressive effect in normal hosts. AOM infection spontaneously resolves in 80% to 90% of cases, with most symptoms subsiding within 24 hours after presentation. Failures in the placebo recipients arose primarily from inadequate pain control rather than from persisting fever or worsening infection (24). **Often AOM is overtreated for fear of complications, which are exaggerated**; mastoiditis and intracranial suppuration are, in fact, very rare complications in industrialized nations. Among 4,860 patients in the **Dutch study** in which patients received nose drops and analgesics alone for AOM, there was no case of meningitis and only one of mastoiditis, which responded well to oral antibiotics (24,25). **Hirschmann emphasizes that those findings indicate watchful waiting is safe for most patients and will detect the few who may genuinely benefit from antibiotic therapy (24).**

The **guidelines that the Dutch College of General Practitioners** adopted in 1990 incorporate this viewpoint. They **recommended that patients** 2 years and older receive symptomatic treatment (paracetamol [i.e., an acetaminophen-like agent for analgesia], with or without decongestant nose drops) for the first 3 days; if symptoms persist, options at that point are antimicrobial therapy or further observation. Management for those less than 2 years of age is the same, except that contact by telephone or a return visit is mandatory at 24 hours to assess progress. Those failing to improve may either undergo another 24 hours of observation or receive antibiotics (24,26).

3. In a commentary on Hirschmann's review and the Dutch approach, Gorbach (27) supports the watchful waiting for AOM and other proposals of Hirschmann (24), hoping that individual physicians and national groups will also embrace these suggestions (24,27). Gorbach notes that **for children who have severe symptoms, toxicity, and/or acute perforation of the drum, antibiotics are clearly indicated (27).**

C. **Antibiotics are not indicated for initial treatment of OME** (i.e., middle ear effusion in the absence of AOM should not be treated, as summarized elsewhere) (22).

1. Prior published guidelines for the diagnosis and treatment of OME* (28) suggested in 1994 either observation with no therapy or therapy with antibiotics. **With the accumulation of evidence**

---

* The expert panel (28) defined a patient with OME as a child between 1 and 3 years of age with effusion present 6 weeks after an acute episode of otitis media, with no apparent symptoms and no underlying medical conditions.

that antibiotic use increases the risk for both colonization and invasive disease with penicillin-resistant *Streptococcus pneumoniae,* observation without antibiotic therapy now appears to be the preferred option (i.e., the concerns over resistance should take precedence over the sometimes marginal benefits of antibiotic therapy) (22).

2. **For chronic OME* (lasting >3 months) accompanied by significant bilateral hearing loss, prior guidelines recommended antibiotic therapy or bilateral myringotomy with insertion of tympanotomy tubes (28). This approach is still reasonable (22).**

D. **Uncomplicated AOM may be treated with short-course (5 to 7 days) antibiotics in selected patients (22).** A short course may help reduce the likelihood of selecting out for resistant pathogens. See Sec. III.D for detailed discussion.

E. **Persistent middle ear effusion 2–8 weeks after therapy is expected and does not require retreatment (22).**

1. The natural history of appropriately treated AOM is for the middle ear effusion to persist for weeks to months (i.e., 70% of children have fluid in the middle ear at 2 weeks; 50%, at 1 month; 20%, at 2 months; and 10%, at 3 months, despite appropriate therapy) (22).

2. Therefore **when middle ear fluid is detected in asymptomatic children at follow-up visits for AOM, additional antibiotics are unnecessary (22).** If the child has another episode of AOM with effusion and needs antibiotics, focal signs should be present. See Sec. B.1.

F. **Antibiotic prophylaxis should be reserved for control of recurrent AOM.** Because of the potential consequences of the emergence of penicillin-resistant pneumococci, experts now advise using prophylaxis only **in limited and special settings.**

1. **Other interventions** that may reduce the incidence of AOM without the risks of antibiotic exposure should be undertaken (22):
   - Eliminating smoking at home
   - Reducing daycare attendance if possible
   - Eliminating pacifiers
   - Using influenza vaccine
   - Using conjugated pneumococcal vaccines and RSV vaccines (23) in the future

2. **Candidates for prophylaxis are summarized in Sec. IV.**

II. **Pathogens**

A. Prior studies have shown that bacteria are isolated from 50% to 60% of cases and include **S. *pneumoniae***

* See footnote on page 14.

(25% to 50%), *Hemophilus influenzae* (15% to 30%), *Moraxella catarrhalis* (3% to 20%).

1. See general discussion of penicillin-resistant *S. pneumoniae* in Chap. 16. In the United States 30% to 35% of respiratory *S. pneumoniae* are penicillin resistant.

2. In otitis media, preliminary data continue to suggest penicillin-resistant *S. pneumoniae* rates may be significantly higher in young children, especially if they have had previous courses of antibiotics and/or are in daycare settings (29).

3. Some experts feel that **the pneumococcus not only is the most common pathogen in AOM, but also is the most likely to cause severe or persistent symptomatology or suppurative and systemic complications if treated inappropriately (29). Consequently, treatment regimens must be active against *S. pneumoniae*.** See later.

B. **Viruses.** As previously discussed, viruses may be isolated in about 40% of cases, especially RSV, influenza, and parainfluenza (23).

III. **Therapy. The precise role of antibiotics in AOM continues to be debated** since it is well established that many patients have resolution of signs and symptoms without antibiotics. (See the Dutch approach of watchful waiting in Sec. I.B.2.) Nevertheless, most clinicians will treat children with high fever, acute perforation of the drum, and signs of middle ear infection (**Sec. I.B.1.**) with empiric antibiotics, although children with low grade or no fever and minimal or early signs of middle ear involvement can be treated symptomatically with follow-up evaluation in 24 to 48 hours (24,27,30,31), as summarized under Sec. I.B.2.

A. **Amoxicillin remains the initial drug of choice** in the nonallergic patient (29,32). In addition, amoxicillin will cover intermediately resistant *S. pneumoniae*.

The conventional dose of amoxicillin for AOM has been 40 mg/ kg/day divided up into three doses. Some experts are suggesting a higher dose range (60 to 90 mg/kg/day). The rationale is that amoxicillin appears to be an optimal agent for *S. pneumoniae*, the most worrisome pathogen, and although amoxicillin does not have intrinsic activity against beta-lactamase-producing strains of *H. influenzae*, the commonly isolated nontypable organisms have little or no capacity to cause invasive or suppurative complications **and both *M. catarrhalis* and *H. influenzae* tend to clear spontaneously at a much higher rate than that of pneumococci (29).**

B. **For second-line therapy** (i.e., for those not responding to amoxicillin), amoxicillin-clavulanate and cefuroxime axetil are considerations, but cefuroxime axetil appears to be associated with failures against penicillin-resistant *S. pneumoniae*. One dose of intramuscular ceftriaxone has also been used. (See C.)

**Table 1-4.   Antibiotics for acute otitis media
in children (e.g., child weighing 18.5 kg)**

Drug	Daily Dosage[#]	Cost (10 Days Therapy)*
Amoxicillin	40 mg/kg in 3 doses	$7
Amoxicillin	60–90 mg/kg in 3 doses	$14[†]
Amoxicillin-clavulanate	40/10 mg/kg** in 3 doses	$64[†]
Cefprozil	30 mg/kg in 2 doses	$64
Erythromycin-sulfisoxazole	50/150 mg/kg in 4 doses	$25
Trimethoprim-sulfamethoxazole	8/40 mg/kg in 2 doses	$19
Clarithromycin[‡]	15 mg/kg in 2 doses	$30
Ceftriaxone	Single IM dose, 50 mg/kg (not to exceed 1 g)	$40

Source: Courtesy of Joseph S. Bertino, Jr. Pharm.D., Bassett Healthcare, Cooperstown, NY.
[#] Daily dose usually divided up into 2 or 3 doses each day.
* Actual wholesale costs (rounded off), 1999 Red Book.
** **Higher doses are now often used, see p. 351.**
[†] Actual costs will vary, depending on weight of child.
[‡] Azithromycin is used in AOM. See Chapter 26.

C. **Other options** are shown on **Table 1.4**, including options for patients who are allergic to penicillins. A single intramuscular dose of ceftriaxone* (maximum dose is 50 mg/kg) is comparable in clinical efficacy to 10 days of oral TMP-SMZ (33) and is especially useful if compliance is a major concern.

D. **Uncomplicated AOM may be treated with a 5- to 7-day course in selected patients.** In the United States, AOM traditionally has been treated with a 10-day course of antibiotics. There are few controlled data to support such a practice, which seems to have been carried over from the recommendations for 10 days of penicillin for streptococcal pharyngitis (22).

   1. **Recent data indicate that 5 days of appropriate short-acting antibiotics are effective in "uncomplicated" AOM in children (34,35).** Advantages of shorter courses include less emergence of resistant bacteria and better compliance. Prior studies have shown that tympanocentesis data suggest that susceptible bacteria usually will be eradicated within 3 to 5 days after initiation of proper antibiotics (34).

* How well this regimen works in penicillin-resistant *S. pneumoniae* infections is not entirely clear. One author has suggested three daily doses of ceftriaxone 50 mg/kg/day if highly resistant strains are a concern. (Congeni BL. Therapy of AOM in an era of antibiotic resistance. *Pediatr Infect Dis J* 1999;18:371).

2. **"Complicated patients" should still receive traditional 10 or more days of therapy** until more clinical data are available (35). These include the following:
    - Children less than **2 years of age**
    - Children with **tympanic membrane perforation**
    - Those at higher risk for treatment failure, such as **those with underlying medical conditions, those with chronic or recurrent otitis media** (since these patients were typically excluded from short-course trials).

E. **Tympanocentesis** is the most accurate way to verify the diagnosis of AOM. This drains the fluid and allows cultures for the causative pathogens. Some experts argue this procedure should be done more often by clinicians. A bacterial pathogen is usually isolated in two-thirds of children with AOM and in 50% of children with persistent AOM; the rest require no antibiotics (35).

IV. **Prophylaxis** should be used **sparingly.** See Sec. I.F.

A. **Indications.** Control of recurrent AOM among children with three or more well-documented and separate episodes in the preceding 6 months or four or more episodes in the preceding 12 months is the only indication for which evidence of the beneficial effects of antibiotic prophylaxis has been persistent and persuasive (22).

Because of the concerns for promoting bacterial resistance in both the patient and community, prophylaxis should not be initiated for other indications.

B. **Duration.** Prophylaxis should not be for longer than 6 months, since longer courses are less effective and may be more likely to promote colonization with resistant bacteria (22).

C. **Agents**
    1. **Sulfisoxazole** (75 mg/kg/day in one or two divided doses) **is the preferred agent** and may be less likely than amoxicillin to produce colonization with beta-lactamase-producing bacteria or resistant pneumococci (22).
    2. Amoxicillin (e.g., 20 mg/kg once daily) has been used.
    3. Cephalosporins have not been shown to be effective (22).

Acute Bronchitis in the Normal Host

Even though the vast majority of these cases are viral in origin, antibiotics are commonly and unnecessarily prescribed for 66% of adults and 75% of children with uncomplicated acute bronchitis (2,5).

I. **Definitions/clinical diagnosis.** Bronchitis is defined as inflammation of the bronchial respiratory mucosa, resulting in a productive cough. The **clinical definition** of bronchitis **in normal children** is not well established, but most clinicians who make the diagnosis do so for a child with **cough, with or without fever or sputum production, excluding pneumonia, bronchiolitis, and asthma (36).** Similarly, **in adults without underlying chronic lung disease,** the diagnosis is usually based on the history of an acute productive cough, no or low-grade temperature, and no evidence of pneumonia on physical examination or chest x-ray.

However, the lack of consensus regarding nomenclature and clinical definition of cough illnesses leads to difficulty in comparing patient populations and results in reported studies.

II. **Etiology. Viruses cause the great majority of cases. In adults,** rhinoviruses, influenza, parainfluenza, and adenoviruses are common. **In children** parainfluenza, RSV, and influenza virus are especially important.

In older children, adolescents, and adults nonviral causes include *Mycoplasma pneumoniae* and *Chlamydia pneumonia;* these are difficult to diagnose but may be especially important in protracted syndromes (>10 days). The role for *Bordetella pertussis* (whooping cough) as a cause of protracted cough in adults is undergoing study.

III. **Principles of therapy** have been published for children (36), and many of these principles also apply to adults.

A. **Nonspecific cough/bronchitis in normal children, and normal adults, rarely warrants antibiotics (36).**

1. Prior studies of acute bronchitis in adults and cough illness/bronchitis in children have shown no benefit of antibiotics. Furthermore, prophylactic use of antibiotics in these patients does not prevent or decrease the severity of bacterial complications after viral URI (36).

2. Neither the character nor the culture of sputum or nasopharyngeal secretions is helpful in determining the need for antibiotics (36).

a. **Virus- and bacteria-induced airway inflammatory changes can cause "purulent" sputum with leukocytes.**

b. Common sputum or nasopharynx colonizers (e.g., *S. pneumoniae, H. influenzae, S. aureus*) can be cultured and inappropriately taken to be pathogens when actually the underlying process is only viral in origin.

3. Fever is commonly seen in early viral bronchitis, especially when caused by influenza and RSV, and in and of itself does not predict the need for antibiotics (36).

B. **For protracted cough (>10 days) antibiotics may be indicated.**

1. Viruses can cause a protracted cough, but a protracted course is less likely to be viral in origin.

In the absence of purulent sputum, *M. pneumoniae* should also be considered in older children, teenagers, and adults.

    a. **In children** most prolonged-cough illnesses are allergic, postinfectious, or viral and do not require antibiotics. Since reactive airway disease is common, even in the absence of wheezing, many of these patients respond well to bronchodilator therapy (36).

    b. **In adults,** in culture confirmed rhinovirus colds, 20% of subjects continued to have cough more than 14 days after onset of symptoms (36).

2. **In adolescents, young adults, and adults exposed to those under 45 years of age with prolonged respiratory illnesses (i.e., >10 days), *M. pneumoniae* is a clinical concern and difficult to prove, or disprove, and an empiric course of antibiotics** with a macrolide or doxycycline (in children >8 years of age) is suggested. The role of *C. pneumoniae* in this setting continues to be evaluated.

3. In children, pertussis and *M. pneumoniae* (see Sec. 2) benefit from antibiotics.

4. Children with chronic cough (>4 weeks) should be evaluated for reactive airway disease, tuberculosis, pertussis, cystic fibrosis, aspiration of a foreign body, or sinusitis.

5. **In summary, in adults and children with prolonged cough (>10 days) consideration of empiric therapy for *M. pneumoniae* is reasonable and suggested.** However, this approach should not be used for a specific patient on repeated occasions; instead reactive airway disease secondary to viral infection should be evaluated.

C. **Patients with underlying lung disease.** In these patients, **empiric antibiotics are used more commonly.** See next discussion.

    1. **Children** with cystic fibrosis and other severe lung disease (e.g., bronchopulmonary dysplasia, lung hypoplasia, chronic aspiration) are more likely to benefit from antibiotics, and therapy must be individualized (36).

    2. **Adults** with structural lung disease (e.g., bronchiectasis or obstructive lung disease/emphysema) also may benefit from antibiotics. See the next section.

Acute Exacerbations of Chronic Bronchitis

Chronic bronchitis typically is defined as the production of sputum on most days for at least 3 months per year for more than 2 years.

I. **Clinical presentation.** An acute exacerbation of chronic bronchitis is a clinical syndrome associated with an increase in cough, an increase of sputum (both in terms of amount and purulence or a change in color), and increased breathlessness without evidence of pneumonia either clinically or by chest roentgenography. Wheezing is common. Most patients do not have systemic symptoms.

Causes of acute exacerbations include environmental factors, such as exposure to cigarette smoke, pollutants, fumes, pollens, and the like; these are important cofactors. Respiratory viruses appear to play a more important role in these acute illnesses than do *M. pneumoniae*. Many of these patients are chronically colonized with *S. pneumoniae* and *H. influenzae*. Presumably, these colonizing bacteria become minimally invasive, and therefore patients are more symptomatic, in the setting of reduced white blood cell (WBC) function caused by the virus infection. **Viral and bacterial etiologies cannot be distinguished clinically.**

II. **Laboratory. The role of sputum cultures in this setting is unclear. Often empiric antibiotics are used without a sputum culture.** If in selected patients, cultures may be desirable (e.g., the patient with multiple antibiotic allergies), a sputum culture should be obtained **before** starting antibiotics, since cultures obtained after antibiotics are difficult to interpret.

III. **Therapy. The precise role of antibiotics in acute flare-ups of chronic bronchitis is still unclear (37,38).** Since minimally invasive bacterial infections are treatable infections in a patient with chronic lung disease who presents with increased cough and with purulent sputum, and often increased dyspnea, antimicrobial therapy is often initiated. **Historically, many of these patients seem to respond clinically to antibiotics for such exacerbation,** and some studies have shown that in the most severely symptomatic patients, antibiotics seem to help (37,38). Therapy is directed primarily against *S. pneumoniae* and *H. influenzae*. Various regimens have been recommended for adults. **(See Table 1.5.)** Duration of therapy varies, but typically, **5 days of therapy** is sufficient to reestablish host bacteria "equilibrium." **With recurrent bouts, antibiotic regimens can be rotated** with the hope of minimizing the selection of resistant pathogens. We do not favor continuous antibiotic use in these patients.

Acute Sinusitis

I. **Problems with definitions and clinical diagnosis.**
   A. As previously discussed, recent data indicate that in adults, and presumably children, well-documented **"common colds" are associated with changes of the sinuses, as revealed by computed tomographic (CT) studies** (3). (See the earlier discussion in the introduction of this chapter.)

**Table 1-5.   Antibiotic options in adults
with acute exacerbations of chronic bronchitis**

Drug	Daily Dosage (for 5 Days)	Comments
Amoxicillin	250 mg po tid	Commonly used
Trimethoprim-sulfamethoxazole	1 DS tab bid	Good sputum levels, commonly used
Erythromycin*	250 mg qid	Not as active against *H. influenzae*
Cefuroxime axetil	250 mg bid	Expensive
Tetracycline hydrochloride	250 mg po qid	On empty stomach
Doxycycline	100 mg bid	Compliance is better

* For patients who cannot tolerate the more cost-effective erythromycin preparations, azithromycin (500 mg on day 1 and then 250 mg once daily on days 2–5) or clarithromycin (250–500 mg bid) can be used.

B. Acute bacterial sinusitis has been reported to follow the common cold in 0.5% to 5% of patients; in other words, **the common cold (i.e., viral rhinosinusitis) is 20 to 200 times more common than acute bacterial sinusitis** (3,39).

C. **The dilemma for the busy clinician is the need to avoid using antibiotics in the patient with just a cold, the viral URI, and yet use antibiotics (usually) in the patient with true bacterial sinusitis.** This problem is compounded by the frequency with which this issue comes up in practice and the ongoing problems with making an accurate diagnosis of acute bacterial sinusitis, usually without x-ray study.

D. Since the paranasal sinuses are not accessible to direct examination and noninvasive sampling for cultures, diagnosis has often been based on clinical evaluations that are insensitive or nonspecific (40). Normally, the paranasal sinuses are sterile (40).

II. **Pathogenesis**

A. **Viral respiratory infection (e.g., rhinovirus).** The exact mechanisms by which virus causes disease in the sinus cavity are not known. Presumably, a viral URI stimulates many inflammatory pathways and the parasympathetic nervous system, resulting in engorgement of the capacitance vessels in the venous erectile tissue of the nasal turbinates, intercellular leakage of plasma into the nose and (presumably) sinuses, discharge of seromucous glands and goblet cells, and stimulation of pain nerve and sneeze and cough reflexes (40). Abnormalities are commonly seen on CT scan. (See Sec. I.A.) Mucus and transudation of plasma into the sinus cavity presumably add to the viscosity of the material accumulating within the sinuses. Sinus disease may result from malfunction of the normal mucociliary clearance process, in part due to the very viscous secretions and partial/total obstruction (because of inflammation) of the usual drainage pathways of the sinuses.

Although some clinicians interpret **mucopurulent rhinitis (thick, opaque, or discolored nasal discharge),** especially in children, as indicating the presence of bacterial sinusitis, this sign should really be recognized as **part of the natural course of a nonspecific, uncomplicated URI.** The nasal discharge in a cold changes from clear to purulent during the first few days of illness. In addition, the color and characteristics of the discharge do not predict whether bacteria will be isolated (39).

B. **Acute bacterial sinusitis. The specific factors that determine whether bacterial invasion of the sinus will occur after a viral URI are unknown.** Sneezing, coughing, and nose blowing may create pressure differentials that cause deposition of bacteria-containing nasal secretions into the sinus. Once bacteria are deposited into the cavity of an obstructed sinus, bacterial growth conditions are favorable; granulocyte phagocytosis may be impaired by the reduced oxygen tension in the obstructed sinus. This process may take weeks to resolve (40).

The seasonal variations of acute bacterial sinusitis reflect the seasonal variations of viral URIs.

C. **Nonviral etiologies of acute bacterial sinusitis.** Allergy, swimming, and nasal obstruction due to polyps, foreign bodies, and tumor can be associated with acute bacterial sinusitis throughout the year. Other, less common risk factors include immune deficiencies such as agammaglobulinemia and AIDS, abnormalities of WBC function, cleft palate, and cystic fibrosis (40). Dental infection can be the source.

III. **Microbiology etiology. Nasopharyngeal cultures do not reflect the bacteriology of the sinuses (39).**

A. The **"gold standard"** is culturing samples obtained by puncture and aspiration of the sinuses, although this is not suitable for routine clinical use (40) and is usually employed only in complex cases.

1. Prior puncture studies have shown that *S. pneumoniae* and *H. influenzae* **account for 50% of cases in adults and children.** *M. catarrhalis* is more common in children (about 20% of isolates) than in adults.

A recent reviewer emphasizes that in children, acute sinusitis is usually caused by the same bacterial pathogens that cause acute otitis media (39). *S. aureus* and streptococcus group A cause less than 5% of cases. Anaerobic infections are infrequent in children. In adults, most anaerobic sinusitis arises from infection of the roots of premolar teeth, thus representing a pure bacterial infection (40). Viruses alone may account for 10% to 15% (39,40).

2. Only about 60% of sinus aspirates in suspected cases of acute sinusitis yield bacteria. The etiology of the cases that are negative on the bacterial culture has not been fully studied, but presumably viruses are important in most. The role of *C. pneumoniae* and *M. pneumoniae* has not been well established (40). Fungi occasionally cause sinusitis and usually present with pressure changes, such as masses, proptosis, and bony erosion (40).

B. **Endoscopic collections,** usually collecting the secretions from the middle meatus and shielding the endoscope to help prevent contamination of the specimen, **may be of limited value, and their utility awaits further study (40).**

IV. **Clinical features.** Unfortunately, **there are no pathognomonic features** of acute bacterial sinusitis.

A. **Nasal versus sinus pathology symptoms are shared** and include sneezing, rhinorrhea, nasal obstruction, facial pressure, and headache.

B. Traditionally, acute bacterial sinusitis has been described (40) as including the preceding sinonasal complaints (Sec. A above) **with the addition of** purulence or color to the nasal discharge, a temperature above 38°C, or erythema over the sinuses; cough is common in children and adults. Hyposomia (decreased smell sensation) is common.

When the sinusitis follows a dental infection, a foul odor of the breath and molar pain are additional characteristics (40).

V. **Diagnosis remains difficult.** Initially, an attempt is made to separate infectious from noninfectious conditions; if it is determined that the condition is infectious, the next step is to discover whether the process is viral, bacterial, or a combination of the two.

A. **An allergic cause** can usually be established by a history of paroxysmal sneezing, itching eyes, allergen exposure, and similar prior episodes. Patients are often accurate in diagnosing this themselves (40).

B. Separating viral versus bacterial versus mixed is difficult, and data suggest impossible, by clinical parameters alone. **CT scans are not recommended for the routine diagnosis** of community-acquired sinusitis because of their lack of specificity, since even patients with a common cold have sinus abnormalities most of the time (3). (See Sec. I.A.) In his excellent review, **Gwaltney emphasized using clinical parameters to define three clinical subgroups (40):**

1. **A "classic"** acute bacterial sinusitis **patient** will have **fever** (>38°C), **and facial pain, marked tenderness** (over the involved sinus), **erythema, or swelling**.

In children with severe URI signs and symptoms, of fever more than 39°C, periorbital swell-

ing, and facial pain or dental pain are suggestive (39).

Also in this group are patients with molar pain
or other evidence of an odontogenic cause of the
infection.

2. **Protracted sinonasal symptoms (>8 to 10
   days)** and the symptoms of colored nasal discharge, nasal obstruction, facial pressure, and
   sometimes cough **that are no better or worse**
   after 8 to 10 days are **clinically suggestive of
   an acute bacterial sinusitis complicating a
   viral URI** that should have resolved or at least
   improved by 10 days. (Sinus aspirate studies of
   patients who initially present with a viral URI
   and then have protracted symptoms after more
   than 1 week are associated with positive bacterial cultures about 60% of the time.)

   In children, prolonged nonspecific URI signs
   and symptoms without improvement for more
   than 10 to 14 days merit therapy, whereas children with symptoms improving by 7 to 10 days of
   onset probably have an uncomplicated viral URI.

3. **Rarely, sinusitis can be complicated by meningitis, brain abscess, or orbital infections**
   that overshadow the underlying sinusitis.

C. **Roentgenographic studies**

1. **For the usual case of acute bacterial sinusitis, no special studies are needed.** (See Sec.
   I.A and I.B.)

2. **Radiographic study is indicated when** (a) episodes of sinusitis are recurrent, (b) complications
   are suspected, (c) the diagnosis is unclear, (d) the
   patient is responding poorly, or (e) sinus surgery
   is contemplated (39).

   a. Normal findings on sinus films make the
      diagnosis of sinusitis highly unlikely (39).

   b. Abnormal findings on plain films, CT scans,
      or magnetic resonance imaging (MRI) in-
      clude air-fluid levels, opacification, or mucosal
      thickening of more than 4 mm (39). **A clas-
      sic air-fluid level on conventional sinus
      roentgenograms usually means an acute
      bacterial sinusitis** (40). Opacification and
      mucosal thickening are often nonspecific
      and may be chronic or due to prolonged URIs.

   c. In young children, the sinuses may not be
      fully developed, making radiographic find-
      ings difficult to interpret. Frontal and sphe-
      noid sinuses begin to appear at about 5 to
      6 years of age but do not develop fully until
      adolescence. Misinterpretation of absent
      sinuses as opacified sinuses in children and
      adolescents can lead to the overdiagnosis
      of sinusitis. In particular, films should be
      read with great caution in children less than
      1 year of age (39).

   D.   **Transillumination** of the sinuses is difficult to perform and standardize.
VI. **Therapy.**
   A.   **Antibiotics.** Randomized, placebo-controlled trials of antibiotics for acute community-acquired bacterial sinusitis with the use of pretreatment and posttreatment sinus aspirate cultures have not been conducted. In several nonrandomized studies, appropriate doses of antibiotics are highly effective in eradicating or substantially reducing bacterial titers in the sinus cavity. When 10-day regimens are used, a bacteriologic cure rate of more than 90% has been achieved (40).

   As with otitis media, acute sinusitis will often resolve even without antimicrobial therapy (39). **Therefore only "classic" cases, or those with protracted symptoms (>8 to 10 days) or complex cases should be treated, as emphasized in Sec. V.B.**
   1.   **Amoxicillin is still successful for initial management of acute uncomplicated sinusitis in most** children (39), and probably most adults, despite beta-lactamase production by most isolates of *M. catarrhalis* and some *H. influenzae* (39). For adolescents and adults, 500 mg po tid and for children 60 to 80 mg/kg/day can be used.
   2.   **For those who do not respond to amoxicillin in 48 to 72 hours, for whom amoxicillin is contraindicated, or who are experiencing recurrent infections,** a beta-lactamase stable agent (e.g., amoxicillin-clavulanate) or a beta-lactamase-stable cephalosporin active against pneumococci (e.g., cefuroxime axetil) is suggested. Some will use these agents as initial therapy (40).
   3.   **See Table 1.6. Antibiotics are usually given for 10 days** (39,40) or for 7 days beyond the point of substantial improvement.
       a.   **One study suggested that selected adult patients with acute maxillary sinusitis** responded as well to a **3-day course of TMP-SMZ** (1 double-strength [DS] tablet bid), as did those with 10 days of therapy. Patients with prolonged symptoms (more than 30 days), prior sinus surgery, antibiotics within the past 1 week, immunocompromised patients, and children were excluded. Also patients who had prominent symptoms of frontal sinusitis (e.g., pronounced frontal headache or tenderness) were excluded; these patients deserve a longer course of antibiotics since the posterior wall of the frontal sinus provides a relatively thin barrier to CNS infection. About 25% of recipients failed the 3-day regimen and these patients need a 10 to 14 day course of antibiotics active against beta-lactamase producing organisms and probably sinus radiographs to confirm the diag-

Table 1-6. Alternative antibiotics for sinusitis

Antibiotics	Oral Dose in Adults	Oral Dose in Children	Comment
Amoxicillin-clavulanate	875 mg bid	*	Some view as an optimal agent of choice for penicillin-resistant *S. pneumoniae* in children (or adults)
TMP-SMZ	1 DS bid	*	May miss some *S. pneumoniae*
Cefuroxime axetil	250 mg bid	*	Expensive[†]
Cefprozil	250 mg bid	*	Expensive[†]
Azithromycin	5-day course (Z pack)	*	See Chapter 26. Macrolide with fewest GI side effects.[†]
Clarithromycin	250 mg bid	*	[†]
Advanced fluoroquinolone (e.g., levofloxacin)	500 mg qd	Avoid	Effective against penicillin-resistant *S. pneumoniae*, useful in adults allergic to penicillin/cephalosporins. Expensive

* For dosages in sinusitis, use same regimens as in Acute otitis media. See Table 1.4 and individual chapter discussions.
† May miss some penicillin-resistant *S. pneumoniae*. See Chapters 2 and 16.

nosis (41). **In general, we have not used this abbreviated course of antibiotics.**

    b. Recently, in a report from the Netherlands, adults with acute maxillary sinusitis and abnormal conventional radiographs (mucosal swelling of more than 5 mm, complete shadowing, or a fluid level) were randomized to receive either amoxicillin 750 mg tid for 7 days or placebo. Amoxicillin did not improve clinical outcomes (42). This preliminary study is difficult to interpret since the critically important duration of sinuslike symptoms was not specified, the number of patients with diagnostic radiographic abnormalities (air-fluid level) was not specified, and it is well known that some patients improve without antibiotics. See Sec. A.

    4. **In severely ill patients** with intracranial or orbital extension, intravenous (IV) therapy with ceftriaxone and vancomycin (to cover high-level penicillin-resistant *S. pneumoniae*) should be started. Infectious disease consultation is advised.

  B. **Ancillary therapy** is directed at drainage of the nasal passages and sinuses and relief of sneezing, coughing, and systemic symptoms (40).

    1. **Decongestants.** Although serial CT scans show that decongestants have little or no effect in promptly draining the sinuses, they are commonly employed. **Oral decongestants are preferred over topical** nasal decongestants, which are often associated with rebound vasodilation and obstruction and pharyngeal irritation. Oral decongestants are safe for patients with stable hypertension who are receiving appropriate antihypertensive treatment (40).

    2. **Topical steroids are useful** if there is evidence of an **allergic component** to the patient's illness. The use of topical (or oral) steroids as decongestants has not been rigorously evaluated. In volunteers with rhinovirus-induced rhinosinusitis, topical steroids had little, if any, beneficial effect on nasal symptoms (40).

    3. **Mucoevacuant drugs** (e.g., guaifenesin) are used on theoretical grounds, but their usefulness has not been **established** (40).

    4. **Nonsteroidal antiinflammatory** drugs are useful in treating systemic symptoms such as fever and malaise, and may be helpful in reducing cough (40). Acetaminophen is also used as an analgesic.

    5. **Cough suppressants** with dextromethorphan or codeine may be needed to control cough.

    6. **Antihistamines.** Although there may be a reluctance to use first-generation antihistamines because of their anticholinergic activity and the possibility of their drying secretions and impair-

ing drainage, testing under randomized, controlled, blinded conditions has shown a reduction of about 50% in sneezing and a reduction of about 30% in rhinorrhea and nasal mucus weights in volunteers with experimental rhinovirus colds. There was no evidence of other symptoms or prolongation of the overall illness, indicating that drying of secretions and impairment of drainage were not problems (40). Therefore **the use of antihistamines (in adults) for symptomatic improvement in the early phase seems reasonable.** Whether antihistamines, by reducing sneezing and nasal secretions, are truly beneficial has not been proven. See related discussion under the common cold, Sec. I.D.

C. **Prevention (40)**
1. Preventing **viral URIs** is impossible but **may be minimized** by avoiding contact with people with colds, and handwashing when contact occurs between infected and noninfected persons. Covering the mouth with disposable nasal tissues when coughing or sneezing is desirable.
2. **Influenza vaccine** is helpful.
3. **Prophylactic antibiotics** to prevent recurrent acute bacterial sinusitis are **not recommended** and will add to the selection of resistant pathogens.

Chronic Sinusitis

Patients with chronic sinusitis need referral to an otolaryngologist for nasal endoscopy, and/or CT study and consideration for drainage procedures. Antibiotics discussed in the section on acute sinusitis are used at times with protracted courses of 3 to 4 weeks. Antibiotics active against ampicillin-resistant *H. influenzae* are preferred (e.g., TMP-SMZ, second-generation cephalosporins, ampicillin-sulbactam, advanced-generation quinolones).

Influenza: More Than the Usual Viral URI

Although influenza may start like a viral URI, it is a **unique** respiratory virus in two ways. First, the epidemiology; **epidemics** are much more obvious and can occur in a community, state, or country. Second, **systemic symptoms** (e.g., fever, myalgias, and malaise) are **more severe** than a usual URI and begin abruptly, often putting the otherwise healthy patient in bed or the older patient in the hospital with a complication. **Influenza is discussed here mostly to emphasize how it differs from the common cold;** it is reviewed in more detail elsewhere (43).

I.   **Epidemiology** (43–44). Influenza A or B viruses typically cause yearly epidemics in the United States, and occasionally there are worldwide pandemics.
   A.   An **epidemic** in a given community lasts about 5 to 6 weeks and may be associated with attack rates as high as 10% to 20% of the population. Although hospitalization rates, as a consequence of influenza, are highest in the elderly, attack rates are highest in children. **Epidemic activity is manifest by increases in school absenteeism, visits to health care facilities, admissions to hospitals for pneumonia, and deaths.**
   B.   **Antigenic variation of the influenza virus.**
      1.   When a **minor** antigenic change occurs due to point mutation (**antigenic drift**), **epidemics** of variable extent result. These antigenic changes occur every 1 to 3 years, which helps explain why there are annual epidemics and why annual vaccinations are needed to protect at-risk patients.
      2.   When a **major** antigenic change occurs (**"antigenic shift"**), worldwide epidemics, called **pandemics**, occur, usually about every 20 years.
II.   **Clinical presentation. The onset is usually abrupt and occurs 1 to 2 days after exposure.**
   A.   **Signs and symptoms.** Although **respiratory symptoms**, particularly sore throat and dry cough, are usually present **at the onset, systemic symptoms predominate** and include (a) **fever** (38° to 41°C),typically for 3 days but possibly for 1 to 5 days; (b) **myalgias**, very frequent and prominent, but not arthralgias; (c) **malaise**, which can be prolonged; (d) **photophobia**; and (e) **headache.**
   B.   **Diagnosis**
      1.   **Epidemiologic data are sufficient to make the diagnosis in most uncomplicated cases.** Therefore when it is documented that influenza virus is prevalent in the community, most people with acute respiratory or acute febrile undifferentiated flulike illness can safely be assumed to have influenza.
      2.   **Laboratory testing** is necessary in establishing initial cases within a community, diagnosing complications of influenza, or helping to determine if patients with respiratory illnesses need droplet, respiratory isolation.
         a.   **Viral cultures** can be performed on respiratory secretions.
         b.   **Influenza A direct antigen assays*** are now available and can be used to test nasopharyngeal secretions (e.g., Directigen Flu A, Becton Dickinson, Cockeysville, MD; or for both influenza A and B, OIA, Optical Immune Assay, Biostar, Boulder, CO). When positive, these are useful, specific tests. When

---

* For summary see Medical Letter. Rapid diagnostic tests for influenza. *Med Lett Drug Ther* 1999;41:121.

compared with cultures, only 60% to 80% of positive cases by culture will be positive by direct antigen test. A negative test should be backed up with an influenza viral culture if a specific diagnosis of influenza is important.

III. **Treatment**
   A. **Symptomatic therapy. Salicylates and salicylate-containing medications should not be given to children with influenza since** the use of salicylates has been associated with Reye's syndrome, especially with influenza B (43). Acetaminophen or ibuprofen have commonly been used as an antipyretic.
   B. **Antiviral agents (43–44, 44A, 44B). There are four anti-influenza agents active against influenza A. Two of these are also active against influenza B.**
      1. **Amantadine and rimantadine are both active against influenza A only.** Each shortens the course of illness and reduces virus titer shedding. Drug resistant viruses are shed by a proportion of treated subjects with either drug; no effect on clinical improvement occurs as a result. Resistant virus has been transmitted to contacts of those receiving either.
         a. **Dose.** 100 mg bid for each: decrease is required for amantadine in the elderly (100 mg qd).
         b. **Side effects** of nervousness/confusion are more prominent with amantadine.
      2. **Zanamivir (Relenza),** which is **inhaled, is active against influenza A and B.** Clinical course and duration of shedding are shortened. Resistance has not been demonstrated.
         a. **Dose.** Two-5 mg puffs bid for 5 days.
         b. **Side effects.** Inhalation may trigger bronchospasm in some patients. Drug-drug interactions do not occur.
      3. **Oseltamivir (Tamiflu)** is an **oral agent active against influenza A and B.** Clinical course and duration of viral shedding are shortened. Resistance has been demonstrated in about 1% of isolates at the end of therapy; no transmission has been demonstrated.
         a. **Dose.** 75 mg bid for 5 days orally.
         b. **Side effects.** Mild nausea occurs. Drug-drug interactions are possible but unlikely.
      4. **Summary.** The advantages of these new agents (activity against influenza A and B and less resistance) favor their use. Cost favors the older agents.*
   C. **Antibiotics should not be used in uncomplicated influenza** since they will not change the natural history of this virus. In addition, antibiotics will alter the bacterial flora of the upper respiratory tract and help select out resistant bacteria.

---

* Approximate wholesale costs for a 5-day course are (44B): $3.50 for amantadine, $8.75 for rimantadine, $44.00 for zanamivir (Relenza), and $53.00 for oseltamivir (Tamiflu).

D. **Hospitalized** patients should be placed on droplet (respiratory) isolation and/or cohorted to help prevent the spread of nosocomial influenza. Patients tend to spread influenza the first 3 to 5 days of their illness.

IV. **Complications**
   A. **Pulmonary**
      1. **Primary influenza viral pneumonia in adults is rare** and occurs predominantly in those with cardiac disease or in pregnant women. Patients rapidly develop bilateral findings on roentgenograms (e.g., diffuse interstitial changes), with severe dyspnea and hypoxemia; they may progress to respiratory failure. **Infectious disease consultation is advised** for these patients. In children, a milder viral pneumonia is fairly common.
      2. **Secondary bacterial pneumonias are common** and can occur early (while the patient is still shedding virus) or occur after initial improvement of a typical influenza illness. The most common pathogens isolated are *S. pneumoniae, H. influenza,* and at times *S. aureus*. Antibiotics are indicated and empiric ceftriaxone, cefotaxime, or ampicillin-sulbactam are often used in this setting. An advanced quinolone (e.g., levofloxacin) can be used in the very ill patient. See Chap. 2.
   B. **Acute sinusitis** often complicates influenza.
   C. **Acute otitis media** can occur (23). (See the related discussion earlier in this chapter.)
   D. **Reye's syndrome** occurs most often after influenza B. Most patients are younger than 16. Lethargy, drowsiness, or abnormal liver function tests are early warning signs.
   E. Myositis with myoglobinuria, Guillain-Barré syndrome, myocarditis, and pericarditis can occur.

V. **Prevention** is discussed in detail elsewhere (44).
   A. **Inactivated influenza vaccines** are aimed at groups at increased risk for influenza or influenza-related complications (e.g., elderly, patients with underlying pulmonary diseases, or other chronic diseases) or groups (e.g., health care workers) that can transmit influenza to high-risk patients. Vaccination is cost-effective in these individuals. It takes 10 to 14 days to develop protective antibody levels after the vaccine is given.
   B. **Live, attenuated, intranasal vaccines** have been tested in healthy children and have been shown to be safe, immunogenic, and effective against influenza A and B (44C). We anticipate these vaccines will be approved for use in the near future.
   C. **Chemoprophylaxis** to prevent influenza A is used in selected settings (44).

External Otitis

I. **External otitis is usually a superficial infection** of the external auditory canal that is typically initiated by moisture and often referred to as "swimmer's ear." It is most commonly caused by *Pseudomonas* spp. Avoiding swimming and/or keeping the ears dry and **using topical treatment usually suffice.** Often the condition responds to careful cleaning of the canal by gentle suction or irrigation. In other instances, antibiotic drops (polymyxin, neomycin, and hydrocortisone [e.g., Cortisporin otic]) or dilute acetic acid or boric acid solutions (to lower the pH) suffice. This topic has been reviewed in detail elsewhere (45).

II. **Malignant external otitis.** This is an important infection caused by *Pseudomonas aeruginosa* and is associated with a high mortality (20%), if untreated. **This disease process begins as an external otitis that may progress into osteomyelitis of the skull base.** Cranial nerve (especially facial), sigmoid sinus thrombosis, and meningitis have resulted in death (46). This disease occurs almost exclusively in elderly diabetics but has been described in nondiabetic patients who have underlying malignancy or are immunocompromised, including AIDS patients.

A. **Diagnosis is often difficult.** One must have **a high index of suspicion. Patients complain of progressively increasing pain and tenderness of the tissues around the ear and mastoid region.** They seldom have fever or systemic symptoms or a peripheral leukocytosis. Cranial nerve abnormalities may develop. **Often there is persistent drainage from the external canal** that yields *P. aeruginosa* on culture. The presence of **granulation tissue at the junction** of the **osseous and cartilaginous portions of the external ear is a highly suggestive finding** (46). Topical therapy is ineffective. **CT scans can help** detect early bone involvement and extent of the disease process. However, technetium phosphate radionucleotide bone scans can identify early bony involvement when there is no destruction on CT scans; Gallium-67 citrate scans are also a sensitive indicator of infection (46).

B. **Therapy.** Most patients require hospitalization and, at least initially, for well-established infection, combination parenteral antibiotics to achieve synergy against *P. aeruginosa.* In this infection, ticarcillin or piperacillin is often combined with tobramycin (or another aminoglycoside to which the pathogen is susceptible). In the penicillin-allergic patient, ceftazidime can be combined with an aminoglycoside. **ENT and infectious disease** consultation are advised. Ciprofloxacin may be useful (46,47) in selected cases (i.e., early disease or for completion of therapy if the organism is susceptible). Serial Gallium scans have been used to monitor response to therapy (46).

Epiglottitis/Supraglottitis

Epiglottitis is an acute and severe inflammation of the epiglottis; some use the term supraglottitis for this condition, indicating inflammation not only of the epiglottis but of the surrounding tissue (48). Before the early 1990s, epiglottitis was primarily an illness of children and due usually to invasive *H. influenzae* b. Since the early 1990s and widespread use of *H. influenzae* b vaccinations in children in the United States, studies have shown a significant change in the epidemiology; **epiglottitis now occurs almost exclusively in adults** (48). Although invasive *H. influenzae* b remains an important etiologic pathogen in adults, *S. pneumoniae* cause a significant number of cases; group A streptococci have also been isolated (49).

I.   **Clinical presentation (48,50).** The onset of epiglottitis **in children** with *H. influenzae* b was classically **abrupt,** with sore throat, fever, and toxicity. The symptoms usually progress rapidly in such a manner that **dysphagia, drooling, and respiratory distress with stridor** become apparent. This diagnosis is still a concern in children who have not been adequately vaccinated against *H. influenzae.*

      In adults, recent series note that symptoms and signs may be more subacute: sore throat, painful or difficulty with swallowing, and muffled voice occur in the majority, and fever or chills, drooling, stridor, sitting erect, dyspnea, cough, and ear pain can occur (48,50).

II. **Diagnosis.** This disease is a **potential medical emergency** and **requires a high index of suspicion** on the basis of the history and clinical findings.

    A.   The diagnosis can be **confirmed by visualization of the epiglottis and supraglottic area. This should only be performed by well-trained personnel; emergency equipment must be available** for maintaining the airway.

    B.   Lateral neck roentgenograms may be useful early, in less toxic patients who are not in respiratory difficulty. The epiglottis appears as an enlarged, rounded shadow resembling a thumb.

    C.   Leukocyte count is usually elevated to more than $15,000/mm^3$, often with a pronounced left shift.

    D.   Blood cultures should be obtained.

III. **Therapy.** Swift and careful management is essential in this disease and directly correlates with the outcome. In the acutely ill patient, valuable time may be unnecessarily wasted obtaining roentgenograms. Ensuring an adequate airway must take priority.

    A.   **Adequate airway.** In young children, nasotracheal intubation and thus emergency consultation (e.g., otolaryngology, anesthesia) is often necessary. In adults, factors predictive of the need for airway intervention were stridor and sitting erect in one study (50).

    B.   **Antibiotics.** Parenteral cephalosporin (second- or third-generation agents; i.e., cefuroxime, ceftriaxone) that is effective against ampicillin-resistant *H. influenzae* or ampicillin-sulbactam or parenteral chloramphenicol in the patient in whom penicillins and cephalosporins are contraindicated, should be initiated immediately. If not contraindicated, **we favor ceftriaxone** or ampicillin-sulbactam, which are also very active against group A streptococcus, mostly *S. pneu-*

moniae, and *S. aureus*. **In a critically ill adult and/or in an area with a high incidence of high-level penicillin-resistant *S. pneumoniae*, we would add IV vancomycin** (along with ceftriaxone) until at least blood culture data are available since more than 20% of adult cases may be due to *S. pneumoniae*. Corticosteroids may be used briefly to help reduce the postintubation edema that develops, but their efficacy has not been proven in this setting (50).

References

1. McCaig LF, Hughes JM. Trends in antimicrobial drug prescribing among office-based physicians in the United States. *JAMA* 1995;273:214.
2. Gonzales R, Steiner JF, Sande MA. Antibiotics prescribing for adults with colds, upper respiratory tract infections, and bronchitis by ambulatory care physicians. *JAMA* 1997;278:901.
   About 50% of the time, antibiotics are given for uncomplicated viral processes in adults. Also see related reference 5 in children.
3. Gwaltney JM Jr, et al. Computed tomographic study of the common cold. *N Engl J Med* 1994;330:25.
   More than 85% of patients had CT abnormalities.
4. Rosenstein N, et al. The common cold—principles of judicious use of antimicrobial agents. *Pediatrics* 1998;101:181 (suppl).
5. Nyquist AC, et al. Antibiotic prescribing for children with colds, upper respiratory tract infections, and bronchitis. *JAMA* 1998; 279:875.
   Written prescriptions given to children were often for viral colds, URIs, or bronchitis in normal children. See related reference 2 in adults.
6. Dowell SF, et al. Principles of judicious use of antimicrobial agents for pediatric upper respiratory tract infections. *Pediatrics* 1998;101:163 (suppl).
   This is an excellent symposium. Series of short papers.
7. Schwartz B, Bell DM, Hughes JM. Preventing the emergence of antimicrobial resistance: a call for action by clinicians, public health officials, and patients. *JAMA* 1997;278:944.
8. Schwartz B, Mainous AG III, Marcy SM. Why do physicians prescribe antibiotics for children with upper respiratory tract infections? *JAMA* 1998;279:881.
   Editorial comment on reference 5.
9. Baucher H, Philipp B. Reducing inappropriate oral antibiotic use: a prescription for change. *Pediatrics* 1998;102:142.
10. Bisno AL, et al. Diagnosis and management of group A streptococcal pharyngitis: a practice guideline. *Clin Infect Dis* 1997;25:574.
    One of the few guidelines for adults. See related reference 16.
11. Sperber SJ, et al. Effects of naproxen on experimental rhinovirus colds: a randomized, double-blind controlled trial. *Ann Intern Med* 1992;117:37.
    Prostaglandins appear to play a role in the pathogenesis of colds. NSAID may minimize some symptoms by blocking these effects. Dose of naproxen used was either a 400-mg load followed by 200 mg tid for 5 days or a 500-mg load, then 500 mg tid for 5 days.

12. Smith MB, Feldman W. Over-the-counter cold medications: a critical review of clinical trials between 1950 and 1991. *JAMA* 1993;269:2258.
13. Turner RB, et al. Effectiveness of clemastine fumarate for treatment of rhinorrhea and sneezing associated with the common cold. *Clin Infect Dis* 1997;25:824.
    This was a study of naturally occurring colds in adults. Similar results were seen with experimentally induced rhinovirus colds published by the same group in Clin Infect Dis 22:656, 1996.
14. Gwaltney JM, Druce HM. Efficacy of brompheniramine maleate for treatment of rhinovirus colds. *Clin Infect Dis* 1997;25:1188.
15. Hayden FG, et al. Effectiveness and safety of intranasal ipratropium bromide in common colds: a randomized, double-blind, placebo-controlled trial. *Ann Intern Med* 1996;125:89.
    Study done in patients 14 to 55 years of age. Treatments were self-administered tid or qid during waking hours for 4 days, two 42-µg sprays per nostril by metered pump spray per dose.
    See a similar report by L Diamond et al (A dose-response study of the efficacy and safety of ipratropium bromide nasal spray in the treatment of the common cold. J Allergy Clin Immunol 1995; 95:1139) in which this nasal spray appeared to be a rational and safe approach to relieving rhinorrhea associated with the common cold in patients 12 to 70 years of age.
15A. Sperber SJ, et al. Pseudoephedrine plus acetaminophen for treatment of "sinus" symptoms in the common cold. Infectious Disease Society of America. 36th Annual Meeting. Denver, CO. November 1998. Abstract 306Sa.
16. Schwartz B, et al. Pharyngitis: principles of judicious use of antimicrobial agents. *Pediatrics* 1998;101:171 (suppl).
17. American Academy of Pediatrics. *1997 Red Book* (24th ed.) Elk Grove, IL: 1997:488–489.
    Useful GAS pharyngitis discussion.
18. Dajani AS, et al. Treatment of acute streptococcal pharyngitis and prevention of rheumatic fever: a statement of health professionals by the Committee on Rheumatic Fever, Endocarditis, and Kawasaki Disease of the Council on Cardiovascular Disease in the Young, the American Heart Association. *Pediatrics* 1995; 96:758.
19. Markowitz M, Gerber, MA, Kaplan EL, Treatment of streptococcal pharyngotonsillitis: reports of penicillin's demise are premature. *J Pediatr* 1993;123:679.
20. Gerber MA. Treatment of failures and carriers: perceptions or problems. *Pediatr Infect Dis J* 1994;13:576.
21. Paradise JL, et al. Otitis media in 2,253 Pittsburgh-area infants: prevalence and risk factors during the first two years of life. *Pediatrics* 1997;99:318.
22. Dowell SF, et al. Otitis media: principles of judicious use of antimicrobial agents. *Pediatrics* 1998;101:165 (suppl).
23. Heikkinen T, Thint M, Chormaitree T. Prevalence of various respiratory viruses in middle ear during acute otitis media. *N Engl J Med* 1999;340:260.
    See editorial comment also.
24. Hirschmann JV. Methods for decreasing antibiotic use in otitis media. *Lancet* 1998;352:672.
    This excellent commentary concludes as follows: "Adoption of all the suggestions discussed—better training in otoscopy, abandonment of

the use of antibiotics for middle ear effusions and for prevention of recurrent acute otitis media, reservation of antimicrobial therapy (given in short courses) for patients who do not improve after brief observation—should substantially reduce antibiotic prescriptions. The result, it is hoped, will be decreased bacterial resistance and the preservation of the efficacy of antimicrobials that unnecessary use has so serious threatened."

For a related discussion see Congeni BL. *Therapy of acute otitis media in an era of antibiotic resistance.* Pediatr Infect Dis J *1999;18:371.*

25. Van Buchem FL, Peeters MF, Van'tHof MA. Acute otitis media: a new treatment strategy. *BMJ* 1985;290:1033.

26. Froom J, et al. Antimicrobials for acute otitis media? A review from the International Primary Care Network. *BMJ* 1997;315:98.

27. Gorbach SL. Reducing antibiotic resistance by less use of antibiotics for otitis media. *Infect Dis Clin Pract* 1999;8:ii.

28. Stool SE, et al. Managing otitis media with effusion in young children: clinical practice guidelines #12. U.S. Department of Health and Human Services. Public Health Service. Agency for Health Care Policy and Research Publications #94-0622, 1994.

29. Poole MD. Implications of drug-resistant *Streptococcus pneumoniae* for otitis media. *Pediatr Infect Dis J* 1998;17:953.
    Part of a symposium on this topic.

30. Berman, S. Otitis media in children. *N Engl J Med* 1995;332:1560.

31. McGracken GH, Jr. Considerations in selecting an antibiotic for treatment of acute otitis media. *Pediatr Infect Dis J* 1994;13:1054.

32. American Academy of Pediatrics. 1997 Red Book. Elk Grove Village, IL: 1997:416.
    Therapy of AOM.

33. Burnett ED. Comparison of ceftriaxone and trimethoprim-sulfamethoxazole for acute otitis media. *Pediatrics* 1997;99:23.
    One dose of IM ceftriaxone is very effective.

34. Kozyrskyj AL, et al. Treatment of acute otitis media with a shortened course of antibiotics: a meta-analysis. *JAMA* 1998;279:1736.

35. Pichichero ME. Changing the treatment paradigm for acute otitis media. *JAMA* 1998;279:1748.
    Editorial comment on reference 34, favoring 5-day therapy in selected patients.

36. O'Brien KL, et al. Cough illness/bronchitis: principles of judicious use of antimicrobial agents. *Pediatrics* 1998;101:178 (suppl).
    Most patients do not need antibiotics.

37. Anthonisen NR, et al. Antibiotic therapy in exacerbations of chronic obstructive pulmonary disease. *Ann Intern Med* 1987; 106:196.
    In this double-blind, crossover trial with antibiotics (TMP-SMZ, or amoxicillin, or doxycycline) or placebo, patients showed a modest improvement, especially those with the most severe exacerbations. Still one of the best studies for this clinical problem.

38. Ball P, Make B. Acute exacerbations of chronic bronchitis: an international comparison. *Chest* 1998;113:199S (suppl).

39. O'Brien KL, et al. Acute sinusitis: principles of judicious use of antimicrobial agents. *Pediatrics* 1998;101:174 (suppl).

40. Gwaltney JM, Jr. Acute community-acquired sinusitis. *Clin Infect Dis* 1996; 23:1209.
    This is a superb review.

41. Williams JW, Jr. Randomized controlled trial of 3 vs. 10 days of trimethoprim-sulfamethoxazole for acute maxillary sinusitis. *JAMA* 1995;273:1015.
Very selected patients may need only short courses.

42. Van Buchem FL, et al. Primary-care-based randomized placebo-controlled trial of antibiotic treatment in acute maxillary sinusitis. *Lancet* 1997;349:683.
Just as with AOM, it has been long recognized some cases of acute sinusitis resolve without antibiotics. See related discussions on p. 1476–1477 of same journal.

43. Treanor JJ, Hall CB. Influenza and infections of the trachea, bronchi, and bronchioles. In: Reese RE, Betts RF, eds. *A practical approach to infectious diseases,* 4th ed. Boston: Little, Brown, 1996:240–257.

44. Centers for Disease Control. Prevention and control of influenza. *MMWR* 1999. 48(RR-4):1–28.
Discusses candidates for influenza vaccine and role of antivirals in preventing infection. Revised annually by the CDC.

44A. Medical Letter. Two neurominidase inhibitors for treatment of influenza. *Med Lett Drug Ther* 1999;41:91.

44B. Long JK, Mossad SB, Goldman MP. Antiviral agents for treating influenza. *Cleveland Clin J Med* 2000;67:92.

44C. Belshe RB, et al. The efficacy of live attenuated, cold adapted, trivalent, intranasal influenza virus vaccine in children. *N Engl J Med* 1998;338:1459.

45. Bojrab DI, Bruderly T, Abdulrazzak, Y. Otitis externa. *Otolaryngol Clin North Am* 1996;29:761.
Discusses also dermatologic problems such as eczematous dermatitis. Also see companion article, CR Shea. Dermatologic disease of the external auditory canal. Otolaryngol Clin North Am *1996;29:783.*

46. Slattery WH, Brackmann DE. Skull base osteomyelitis: malignant external otitis. *Otolaryngol Clin North Am* 1996;29:795.

47. Gehanno P. Ciprofloxacin in the treatment of malignant external otitis. *Chemotherapy* 1994;40(Suppl. 1):35.

48. Mayo-Smith MF, et al. Acute epiglottitis: an 18-year experience in Rhode Island. *Chest* 1995;108:1640.

49. Trollflors B, et al. Aetiology of acute epiglottitis in adults. *Scand J Infect Dis* 1998;30:49.
In 54 patients, blood cultures were positive in 15 (nine H. influenzae, five pneumococci, and one GAS). PCR verified another five cases of H. influenzae and seven cases of pneumococci. Four cases of GAS were verified by serology. Nevertheless, 23/54 (43%) had no identified pathogen.

50. Frantz TD, et al. Acute epiglottitis in adults: analysis of 129 cases. *JAMA* 1994;272:1358.

Pneumonia

Community-Acquired Pneumonia

I. **Introduction. By definition, community-acquired pneumonia (CAP) is** pneumonia in patients who have not been hospitalized or resided in a long-term-care facility at least 14 days before the onset of symptoms. There are about 4 million cases of CAP in the United States per year. Of these, approximately 600,000 patients are hospitalized, with a mortality rate overall of 10% to 15%. Pneumonia is the sixth most common cause of death in the United States (1,2).

   A dilemma for the clinician/caretaker is that a specific pathogen usually cannot be identified; therefore therapy is often empiric. Furthermore, emphasis on outpatient care makes the decision about when to hospitalize the patient more difficult than in the past. This often fosters the desire to use "broad-spectrum coverage"; yet the broader the antibiotic spectrum used, the more likely one will use therapy that is unnecessary and that will lead to excess toxicity, excess cost associated with that toxicity, and increased chance that the patient may become colonized with a resistant organism. What then can the clinician do?

II. **Clinical and epidemiologic features**

   A. **History and physical exam.** The history and chest examination **are not sufficiently sensitive to rule in or rule out the diagnosis of pneumonia.** The sine qua non of pneumonia is a new **infiltrate on chest film.** This topic has recently been reviewed (3). Therefore given the complexities of therapy of CAP, **a chest roentgenogram is essential for an accurate diagnosis.** See Sec. IIIA.

      1. **Cough and sputum production.** In *Streptococcus pneumoniae* pneumonia, sputum production often is minimal unless it is preceded by a viral bronchitis or unless it occurs in someone with chronic bronchitis. For both *Mycoplasma pneumoniae* and *Chlamydia pneumoniae*, sore throat, usually without rhinitis, occurs first followed by protracted cough (usually dry) and lassitude. In gram-negative pneumonias, including *Haemophilus* spp., bronchitis usually precedes the pneumonia and thus cough is very productive. Pleuritic chest pain may occur in any bacterial pneumonia.

      2. **Fever** is usually present unless antipyretics have been used recently; fever may be absent in the elderly.

      3. **Chest findings.** "Crackles" or rales are nonspecific (3). However, in the very ill patient (e.g., with pneumococcal pneumonia) signs of consolidation are often found. Tachypnea may occur

with extensive lobar pneumonia or diffuse interstitial pneumonia.

4. **Other.** In the elderly, a change in eating habits
or alertness may be the first sign of an evolving
pneumonia. Patient "found on the floor" is not an
uncommon presentation in this population. A
single shaking chill is common in patients with
S. pneumoniae.

B. **Epidemiologic factors may provide clues to specific etiologies prior to empiric therapy (1).
Important factors are shown in Table 2.1. Some
points deserve special emphasis.**

1. **Age.** *M. pneumoniae* **and** *C. pneumoniae*
**pneumonia occur more commonly in indi-
viduals less than 45 years old and are
uncommon in those over 65.** *Chlamydia trachomatis* occurs almost exclusively in infants.
Bacteria, especially *S. pneumoniae*, predominate
in older individuals.

2. **Season.** Two infectious agents that are very seasonal are influenza and *Legionella.* Except in patients who acquire infection in the hospital, most
L. pneumophila occurs in the summer and fall.
Influenza occurs in December–March in the
Northern Hemisphere. Once established in a geographic area, any influenza-like illness is probably
influenza. Although primary viral influenza pneumonia is rare in adults, **postinfluenza bacterial
pneumonia** (due to *S. pneumoniae, H. influenzae*,
and to a lessor extent, *S. aureus*) **is very common
in the influenza season.** See Chap. 1. *Legionella*
infection is rare during the influenza season.

3. **Patient setting**
   a. In a patient residing at home, infections are
      likely to be caused by *S. pneumoniae. Haemo-
      philus* spp., *Moraxella* spp., or the organisms
      listed in Sec. 1 above that occur in that set-
      ting as well.
   b. **In the long-term health care facility,**
      S. pneumonia and mixed normal flora pre-
      dominate but gram-negative bacteria, espe-
      cially *Klebsiella* spp. (and rarely *Pseudo-
      monas* spp.) are more common than in
      community-residing individuals.

4. **Host factors**
   a. In all patients, *S. pneumoniae* is common.
   b. In the patient with seizures or in alcoholics,
      mixed aerobic anaerobic (aspiration) pneu-
      monia occurs. Of the patients with *Klebsiella
      pneumoniae* or *Acinetobacter calcoaceticus*
      pneumonia, almost all are alcoholic, although
      even in that group, *S. pneumoniae* is by far
      the most common pathogen.
   c. **AIDS.** If the chest x-ray shows a focal in-
      filtration, bacterial pneumonia, especially

Table 2-1. Epidemiologic and underlying conditions related to specific pathogens in selected patients with community-acquired pneumonia

Common Conditions	Commonly Encountered Pathogens
Alcoholism	*Streptococcus pneumoniae;* anaerobes, gram-negative bacilli
COPD/smoker	*S. pneumoniae, Haemophilus influenzae, Moraxella catarrhalis, Legionella* species
Nursing home residency	*S. pneumoniae,* gram-negative bacilli, *H. influenzae, Staphylococcus aureus,* anaerobes, *Chlamydia pneumoniae*
Poor dental hygiene	Anaerobes
HIV infection (early stage)	*S. pneumoniae, H. influenzae, Mycobacterium tuberculosis*
Influenza active in community	*S. pneumoniae, H. influenzae, S. aureus,* (rarely primary influenza)
Suspected large-volume aspiration	Anaerobes, chemical pneumonitis
Structural disease of the lung (bronchiectasis or cystic fibrosis)	*Pseudomonas aeruginosa, Burkholderia (Pseudomonas) cepacia* or *S. aureus*
Injection drug use	*S. aureus,* anaerobes, *M. tuberculosis*
Airway obstruction	Anaerobes

Less Common Conditions	Pathogens Encountered
Epidemic Legionnaires' disease	*Legionella* species
Travel to the southwestern United States	*Coccidioides immitis*
Exposure to farm animals or parturient cats	*Coxiella burnetii* *
Exposure to bats or soil enriched with bird droppings	*Histoplasma capsulatum*
Exposure to birds	*Chlamydia psittaci*
Exposure to rabbits	*Francisella tularensis*

Source: Modified from Bartlett JC, et al. Community-acquired pneumonia in adults: guidelines for management. *Clin Infect Dis* 1998;26:811.
Abbreviation: COPD, chronic obstructive pulmonary disease.
* Agent of Q fever.

S. pneumoniae and *Haemophilus* spp., is the most likely cause. Some studies suggest that for any given geographic area, penicillin-resistant *S. pneumoniae* may be more common in these patients. *Pseudomonas aeruginosa* can be community-acquired in this patient population. In the patient not on prophylaxis, *Pneumocystis carinii* pneumonia (PCP) is very common. To a much lesser degree *Aspergillus, Cryptococcus,* and *Toxoplasma gondii* can occur. The level of CD4 count affects potential pathogens, see Chap. 12.

III. **Laboratory.** The **common pathogens in CAP are shown in Table 2.2.** As discussed previously and later, in the majority of cases it is not possible to identify an etiologic pathogen.

A. **Chest roentgenogram. A positive chest x-ray is essential to make the diagnosis of pneumonia (3).** The clinician is often tempted to diagnose CAP without a chest radiograph. The recent Infectious Disease Society of America (IDSA) guidelines advises against this emphasizing: "In a time of limited resources, it may be attractive to treat patients for CAP on the basis of presenting manifestations, without radiographic confirmation. However, this approach should be discouraged, given the cost and potential dangers of antimicrobial abuse in terms of side effects and resistance. . . **The Panel recommends that a chest radiograph be obtained for the routine evaluation of patients who are likely to have pneumonia"** (1).

**Table 2-2.   Common pathogens
of community-acquired pneumonia**

S. pneumoniae	15% to 65%
*H. influenzae***	4% to 15%
M. catarrhalis	?%
Atypical	Overall, 10%–45% depending on age and season**
Mycoplasma	
pneumoniae	2% to 30%
Chlamydia spp.	5% to 15%
Legionella spp.	2% to 6%

* Up to 25% to 35% of stains resistant to ampicillin. Although isolated from sputum from patients with pneumonia fairly often, the exact incidence of well-documented lower respiratory tract infections due to this pathogen is unclear. See ref. 4 and text.

** Frequency is difficult to estimate since no reliable diagnostic tests are routinely available. Mycoplasma occurs in those age 5–45.

† In one report, 53% of patients had evidence for mycoplasma, Legionella, or chlamydia. See Lieberman D, et al. Multiple pathogens in adult patients with community-acquired pneumonia: a one-year prospective study of 346 consecutive patients. *Thorax* 1996;51:79.

In another study by Mundy LM, et al., *Chest* 1998;113:1201, in 385 cases of CAP only 29 (7.5%) had an atypical pathogen identified. **Careful studies have shown striking differences in the frequency of atypicals in CAP**.

1. **Bacterial pneumonia** (e.g., *S. pneumoniae, L. pneumophila*):
   a. Usually a single lobe or a single segment is involved, but multiple lobe involvement occurs in about 30% and pleural fluid develops in 10% to 30%.
   b. In very dehydrated patients, the initial x-ray may be negative only to become positive by the next day, after rehydration.
   c. **Upper lobe involvement may occur in any pneumonia, but if there is a non-fluid cavity, this is likely to be tuberculosis. However, in patients infected with human immunodeficiency virus (HIV) with unexplained fever and cough, tuberculosis can occur in the lower lobes or in the face of a normal chest x-ray.**
   d. Aspiration may be accompanied by abscess and air/fluid level; location in the apical segment of the right lower lobe increases the likelihood that an infiltrate in this segment was from aspiration.
2. **Atypical organisms**
   a. **Chlamydia or Mycoplasma.** Pneumonia caused by these organisms usually presents with the same x-ray appearance as bacterial pneumonia. On blinded evaluation of individual films, radiologists cannot differentiate between these etiologies. **The so-called atypical chest x-ray that implies an atypical organism causing the pneumonia is a misconception.**
   b. *Pneumocystis carinii* **pneumonia** (PCP) is usually diffuse and bilateral.
B. **Blood count.** The white cell count in *S. pneumoniae* pneumonia or *L. pneumophila* pneumonia is often between 14,000 and 18,000/mm, sometimes accompanied by an increase in band forms. For the young person with "atypical pneumonia," the white blood cell count is usually less than 10,000/mm without immature forms. In AIDS patients, the white cell count is likely to be below 3,000 on average in PCP infection and often less than 10,000 in bacterial infection.
C. **Sputum gram stain** (when available). A deep-coughed specimen obtained before antibiotics is ideal. Unfortunately, in most series of CAP, only a minority of patients can provide a good sputum sample at admission. It has become policy of many laboratories to reject a sputum as unsatisfactory if, on exam, there are more than 10 squamous epithelial cells or fewer than 25 polymorphonuclear cells per low-power field. These specimens are reasonably "rejected" by the microbiology laboratory for culture or are not worked up extensively. (The exceptions to this rule are spu-

tums for *Mycobacterium* and *Legionella,* which do not have to meet the cytologic criteria to be worked up in the Micro Lab.)

When used thoughtfully, the gram stain can be quite helpful. If a high-powered field where polymorpho-nuclear cells are concentrated is reviewed, the presence of gram-positive cocci of a single morphologic type points strongly to *S. pneumoniae* unless these cocci are large and in clusters that may suggest *S. aureus,* an uncommon cause of pneumonia in adults. Prior studies have shown that the sensitivity of sputum gram stains for patients with pneumococcal pneumonia is 50% to 60% and that the specificity is more than 80% (1). When gram-negative "coccobacillary" forms are seen, *Haemophilus* spp. are likely, whereas if gram-negative diplococci predominate, *Moraxella* spp. are more likely, although *Acinetobacter* spp. in alcoholic patients must be considered. Gram-negative rods suggest *Klebsiella* spp. or members of the Enterobacteriaceae. If polymor-phonuclear cells without organisms are seen, and no antibiotics have been administered, this suggests an organism that does not stain (e.g., *Legionella pneu-mophila, Mycoplasma,* or *Mycobacterium*). Mixed gram negatives and gram positives, both rods and cocci, sug-gest mixed flora, compatible with anaerobic mouth flora aspiration; this pattern occurs in lung abscess.

D. **Sputum culture.** Ideally, **sputum samples should be collected and plated in the laboratory within 2 hours to maximize their yield** (1). Sputum cul-ture often misses the fastidious *S. pneumoniae*, which is detectable in a minority of bacteremic pneumococ-cal pneumonia. By contrast, gram-negative organisms are more easily isolated. **If no gram-negative bac-teria are isolated and blood cultures are nega-tive, gram-negative pneumonia is very unlikely.** If the gram stain yields pure gram-positive cocci and the culture demonstrates a small number of *Klebsiella* spp., it is reasonable to conclude that the etiology is a gram-positive organism.

1. An excellent study of CAP published in 1976 by Davidson et al (4) showed that even when either *Haemophilus* spp. or *E. coli* was isolated along with *S. pneumoniae* in transtracheal aspirates, *S. pneumoniae* was the cause of the pneumonia based on lung aspirate cultures. Furthermore, although *Haemophilus* spp. were often isolated from sputums (in mixed cultures, often with *S. pneumoniae*), the same *Haemophilus* spp. was never isolated from the lung aspirate culture.

    In a more recent study published in 1999 using careful lung aspirates with careful culturing and PCR techniques, Ruiz-Gonzales demonstrated that *S. pneumoniae* remains the leading cause of CAP (4A).

2. **Atypicals.** Most laboratories do not attempt to isolate *M. pneumoniae* or *C. pneumoniae*, and as of early 2000, the technology of PCR is not available for routine use to diagnose these two organisms from sputum. DNA probes continue to undergo investigation (1).

3. Prior antibiotic therapy may suppress the growth of the etiologic pathogen and/or allow the emergence of resistant colonizers that yields a false-positive growth of upper airway organisms (e.g., *S. aureus* or gram-negative bacilli).

4. **If *Legionella* is a special concern** (e.g., in the seriously ill patient without an alternative diagnosis, where epidemiologic data suggest this diagnosis, or in nonresponders to beta-lactam antibiotics), then special laboratory tests are indicated. Negative studies do not exclude the diagnosis, whereas a positive culture or antigen test is usually diagnostic.

   a. **Sputum, even if not a purulent specimen by inspection or by microscopy screening (and/or pleural fluid) for culture, is still suggested. Alert the microbiology lab to culture for *Legionella*.**

   b. **Urinary antigen** (1) is commercially available in kits using radioimmunoassay and enzyme immunoassay (EIA) methods to diagnose serogroup 1 infections rapidly. (Serotype 1 causes about 70% to 80% of cases of Legionnaires' disease in the United States.) This test is about 50% sensitive and presumably 100% specific.

   c. **Acute and convalescent serology** may help with a retrospective diagnosis, but these data are not useful in managing the patient's active infection.

5. ***Mycobacterium* smears and culture** of sputum for selected patients: especially those with a cough that has persisted longer than 1 month, with suggestive radiographic changes, or at especially high risk for *M. tuberculosis* as described in Chap. 13 (see pages 271–272) under *M. tuberculosis* isolation.

E. **Blood cultures** are positive in fewer than 15% of patients with bacterial pneumonia but are definitive if positive. Two sets of blood cultures are advised for patients hospitalized with CAP (1). Coagulase-negative *Staphylococcus* spp. should be ignored as pathogens causing pneumonia.

F. **Arterial blood gases** can help assess the severity of illness and whether hospitalization and/or ICU admission may be necessary.

G. **Acute and convalescent serology** may help in the retrospective diagnosis of such infections as influenza, *C. pneumoniae*, *Legionella* spp., and *Mycoplasma pneu-*

moniae. It is not useful in *S. pneumoniae*. Occasionally, it will be helpful in *C. psittaci* or *Histoplasma capsulatum* infection. **In an unusual case of pneumonia without a clear diagnosis, it may be useful to save a frozen acute serum sample.** A single antibody titer of ≥256 is not specific for *L. pneumophilia*.

H. **HIV serology** may be indicated in any "normal" host from 17 to 55 years of age who is ill enough to be hospitalized with a bacterial pneumonia, since this might be the initial manifestation of underlying HIV infection. This may be especially important for hospitals with more than one newly diagnosed case of HIV per 1,000 discharges (1).

I. **Other laboratory tests** are relatively nonspecific, but bilirubin is often elevated in *S. pneumoniae*, hyponatremia occurs in tuberculosis and *Legionella,* and lactic dehydrogenase (LDH) may be quite high in any pulmonic process, especially PCP.

IV. **When to hospitalize the patient with CAP.** In the managed-care era, guidelines are being developed to determine who should be hospitalized and who can be treated safely as an outpatient.

A. **Investigators from the Pneumonia Patient Outcomes Research Team (PORT)** have recently summarized data on the analysis of more than 14,000 adult patients with CAP and developed and tested a prediction assessment profile (2,5). **They excluded HIV-positive patients and patients hospitalized within the preceding week.** Using their approach, the clinician can assess in the office, clinic, or emergency room whether a patient is **low risk** or **"high risk." This stratification scheme is summarized in Appendix F.**

1. **Low-risk patients can typically be treated as outpatients, or sometimes by an abbreviated hospitalization.** Overall, these patients had a low mortality rate (3%).

2. **High-risk patients need hospitalization.** These patients had mortality rates in the range of 10% to 30%.

B. **Editorial comments on Fine et al (2) risk assessment approach.**

1. In the same issue as the Fine et al paper, in the editorial response, Dr Barry Farr emphasizes that further randomized clinical trials are needed to conclude if these guidelines apply to large numbers of patients safely and that **clinical judgment about admission remains very important (6).**

2. The IDSA Panel on CAP endorses the findings of the PORT studies as valid predictors for mortality from CAP as well as a rational approach for decision making about hospitalization. However, the panel emphasizes that there are many other factors to consider in the decision about the site

of care, including compliance and home support. The panel also notes, "It should be emphasized that the observations of the PORT study were validated as **predictors of mortality** and not as a method of triage" (1).

3. Even the authors of the PORT study emphasize that a prognostic score should not supersede clinical judgment in the decision of when to hospitalize a patient or not.

C. The **American Thoracic Society** (ATS) has also published risk factors associated with poor outcome (7). **When these factors are present, especially multiple factors, hospitalization should be considered. See Table 2.3.**

V. **The dilemmas raised by penicillin-resistant** S. *pneumoniae.* S. *pneumoniae* remains the leading cause of CAP (1,4A), accounting for 15% to 60% of CAP cases, depending on the specific series and probably the majority of cases in those more than 65 years of age, especially those very ill. Therefore **all empiric antibiotic regimens must provide good activity against S.** *pneumoniae* **pneumonia. The antibiotic therapy of S.** *pneumoniae* **pneumonia has become more complex with the advent of the increasing prevalence of penicillin-resistant S.** *pneumoniae.* Therefore this topic is reviewed in some detail so the reader better understands some of the current controversies about therapy of CAP.

A. **The laboratory definition** of and prevalence of *penicillin-resistant S. pneumoniae* is discussed in Chap. 16. Briefly, **against penicillin:**

- **Susceptible** strains have a minimum inhibitory concentration (MIC) <0.1 µg/ml
- **Intermediate** susceptible strains have a MIC 0.1 to 1.0 µg/ml (or sometimes defined as .12 to 1.0 µg/ml)
- **High-level resistant** strains have a MIC ≥2 µg/ml

B. The **prevalence** of *penicillin-resistant S. pneumoniae* from respiratory isolates has increased significantly in the 1990s, as **summarized in Table 2.4. Recent data from the United States suggest 33% to 36% of S.** *pneumoniae* **respiratory isolates are penicillin resistant, the majority of which are intermediately resistant.** There are unexplained regional differences in the United States with higher levels of *penicillin-resistant S. pneumoniae* in the southeast (e.g. 40% of strains) more so than in the northeast (e.g., 20% of strains) (8).

C. **The** *in vitro* **susceptibilities of penicillin-resistant S.** *pneumoniae* **to common antibiotics used for CAP have recently been reviewed and are shown in Table 2.5.**

1. When these data were presented in late 1997, many clinicians were concerned about whether cefuroxime could still be used for initial empiric therapy of CAP, since 47% of intermediate- and

**Table 2-3. Risk factors
for a poor outcome from pneumonia***

Advanced age (≥65 years)

Serious underlying conditions
    Chronic lung, heart, liver, or renal disease
    Diabetes mellitus
    Malnutrition
    Recurrent aspiration
    Alcoholism
    Cystic fibrosis
    Immunodeficiency (including splenectomy)

Hospitalization for pneumonia within 1 year

Physical findings
    Tachypnea >30 breaths/min
    Hypotension
    Fever >38.3°C (101°F)
    Distant sites of infection
    Altered level of consciousness

Laboratory findings
    Leukocytosis >30,000 cells/mm^3
    Leukopenia <4,000 cells/mm^3
    Neutropenia <1,000 cells/mm^3
    Hypoxemia or hypercapnia
    Anemia
    Renal insufficiency

Complications
    Mechanical ventilation required
    Adult respiratory distress syndrome
    Sepsis syndrome

Radiographic findings
    Two or more lobes involved
    Significant pleural effusion
    Cavitation
    Rapid spread

Source: Niderman MS, et al. Guidelines for the initial management of adults
with community-acquired pneumonia: diagnosis, assessment of severity, and
initial antibiotic therapy. *Am Rev Respir Ther* 1993;148:1418.
* These factors have been associated with either death or a complicated course,
particularly if multiple ones are present simultaneously.

        100% of high-level resistance strains were resis-
        tant to cefuroxime *in vitro.*

    2.   However, the *in vivo* observations summarized
        in Sec. D below suggest cefuroxime is still a rea-
        sonable agent to use in mild to moderate CAP.

    3.   In very severe pneumonia, an agent with en-
        hanced *in vitro* activity against *S. pneumoniae* is
        preferred. See related discussion in Sec. VII.A.4.

  D. ***In vivo* observations.** Anecdotal and preliminary
      published data suggest that *in vivo*, many of the anti-
      biotics clinically used for CAP, including the peni-

**Table 2-4. Penicillin susceptibilities
of respiratory isolates S. *pneumoniae* in the 1990s**

Study	% Intermediate Resistance*	% High-Level Resistance[†]	Total % of Penicillin Resistance
Thornsberry et al. *Infect Med* 1993; 93:15; 524 isolates, 7 centers	15.2	2.6	17.8
Barry et al. *Antimicrob Agents Chemother* 1994; 38:2419; 799 isolates, 19 centers	14.9	7.3	22.2
Doern et al. *Antimicrob Agents Chemother* 1996; 40:1208; 1,527 isolates, 30 centers	14.1	9.5	23.6
Thornsberry et al. *Diagn Microbiol Infect Dis* 1997; 29:249;9,139 isolates, 434 centers	19.9	13.6	33.5
Thornsberry et al.[**] ICAAC Abstract E-22 September 1998	22	14[‡]	36

* MIC 0.12–1 µg/ml.
[†] MIC ≥2 µg/ml.
[‡] Approximately 70% of these isolates are resistant to azithromycin, and 93% are resistant to TMP/SMZ in vitro.
[**] Thornsberry C, et al. Sequential surveillance of antimicrobial resistance in the United States: *Streptococcus pneumoniae, Haemophilus influenzae,* and *Moraxella catarrhalis* (1997–1998 vs. 1996–1997). 38th Interscience Conference on Antimicrobial Agents and Chemotherapy. San Diego, California. September 1998. Abstract E-22. Also see related paper by C. Thornsberry et al. *J Antimicrob Chemother* 1999;44:749.

cillins or cephalosporins, are effective, using mortality as the measure of outcome.

1. **Pallares et al** reported from Spain 504 patients with pneumococcal pneumonia; 29% had penicillin-resistant strains (of these 40% were high level). Mortality rates, once controlled for other predictors, were the same (about 28%) for the penicillin-resistant and penicillin-susceptible infected patients, whether penicillin, ampicillin, or ceftriaxone (or cefotaxime) was used. The authors emphasize that their study "was not designed to compare efficacy of various antibiotics and it was not a randomized trial" (9).

Table 2-5. Susceptibilities of respiratory isolates of penicillin-resistant S. pneumoniae (% susceptible)

Strains	Amoxicillin-Clavulanate	Cefuroxime	Ceftriaxone	Clarithromycin	Levofloxacin
Pen-Intermediate	74.5	53.0	91.6	63.5	96.9
Pen-Resistant (High-Level)	6.4	0.0	27.0	38.9	97.1

Source: Modified from Thornsberry C, et al. *Diagn Microbiol Infect Dis* 1997;29:249.

2. **Plouffe et al** reported on 439 cases of pneumococcal bacteremia from 1991 to 1994 with 9%
of strains resistant to penicillin. Mortality rates
were similar for penicillin-resistant and penicillin-
susceptible strains (21% vs. 19%) with little discussion of the specifics of antibiotics used. The
duration of hospital stay was longer (7 vs. 3 days)
in those with penicillin-resistant infections; this
observation was unexplained. The pneumococcal
vaccination status of infected patients was not
studied, but the authors noted that 90% of the bacteremic serotypes identified were in the currently
available vaccine (10).

3. **Dressor et al** reported 92 pneumococcal bacteremic patients (15% due to penicillin-resistant
strains, primarily intermediate) with no difference in clinical outcome whether patients were
treated with penicillin, a cephalosporin, or other
antibiotics (unspecified) (11).

4. **In a neutropenic mouse model** in which serum
levels of amoxicillin or amoxicillin-clavulanate
were similar to those achievable in humans, ex-
perimentally induced penicillin-resistant and
-susceptible pneumococcal infections responded
similarly if the serum level of antibiotic exceeded
the MIC of the pathogen ≥40% to 50% of the dosing interval (12).

5. **Overview.** These data raise the issue of whether
the therapeutic efficacy for beta-lactams correlates best with the duration of time serum levels
exceeding the MIC of the infecting organism,
so-called **time-dependent killing** (see Chapter
14, p. 294). **Possibly this *in vivo* pharmaco-
dynamic observation helps explain why
some beta-lactam antibiotics whose *in vitro*
susceptibility data might predict clinical
failure are nonetheless associated with clinical success.** More clinical correlation and studies are needed in this area of investigation.

VI. **Which bug. . . which drug?**

A. **Try to identify a pathogen.** Since empiric therapy
is commonly used and the optimal antibiotics are
debated, it is important to make sure the diagnosis of
pneumonia is well established (i.e., a positive x-ray
before embarking on therapy). See Sec. III.A.

1. **Sputum. Every effort should be made to
obtain diagnostic specimens before initiating therapy in hospitalized patients.** See Sec.
III.C-D. Identifying a specific pathogen allows the
clinician to pick an optimal antibiotic (or at least
modify the initial antibiotic regimen) and avoid
the direct and indirect costs, potential side effects,
and resistance problems that may be associated
with empiric broad-spectrum antibiotics (1).

2. Unless the patient is severely ill, extra effort should be made to obtain sputum. **In those patients in whom a good sputum is available, the gram stain may suggest an etiologic pathogen** and empiric therapy can be started using these data and **Table 2-6.**

   If a good sputum culture has been obtained before using antibiotics, culture may reveal a predominant pathogen and one can often adjust the initial empiric antibiotics (**Table 2-6**).

   Unfortunately, in many patients a good sputum sample is not available and empiric antibiotics must be used. See Sec. VII.

B. **Epidemiology data** see **Sec. II.B and Table 2-1.**
C. **Common pathogens of CAP** are summarized in **Table 2-2.**
   1. *S. pneumoniae* **remains the most common pathogen in CAP** (1,4A,12A); therefore empiric regimens for CAP should include activity against this pathogen (12A).
   2. *Mycoplasma* and *Chlamydia* account for a significant and variable portion of CAP, especially in young to middle-aged adults, probably in the range of 10% to 45% of cases or more (1,4A,12A). Since these forms of pneumonia are difficult to diagnose, empiric therapy is often directed against these pathogens when appropriate.
   3. *Legionella* spp. likewise account for a variable percentage, which differs dramatically from one geographic area to the next. Empiric therapy aimed at *Legionella* is often necessary if this is an important diagnostic consideration. (See related discussions in Sec. II.B.2, III.C, and III.D.4.)

VII. **Empiric antibiotics for CAP.**
   A. **For patients requiring hospitalization. There is no consensus and the optimal approach is controversial.** Therefore some of the national guidelines will be discussed and then a practical approach will be suggested.
      1. *Medical Letter* (13) suggests cefotaxime or ceftriaxone. A macrolide (e.g., erythromycin, azithromycin, or clarithromycin) can be added to cover for atypical pathogens or an advanced quinolone (e.g., levofloxacin) can be substituted for the beta-lactam. Vancomycin may be required for highly resistant strains of pneumococci and should be added in severely ill patients and those not responding to a beta-lactam. (See Sec. 4.a also.)
      2. **The IDSA Panel Guidelines** (1) support:
         a. **For patients on a general** hospital floor, ceftriaxone (or cefotaxime) or a beta-lactam with beta-lactamase (e.g., ampicillin-sulbactam, Unasyn) with or without a macrolide, *or* an advanced fluoroquinolone (e.g., levofloxacin) as monotherapy.

Alternatives are cefuroxime ± a macrolide or azithromycin alone.

b. **ICU patients** (serious pneumonia) a macrolide or advanced fluoroquinolone (levofloxacin) **plus** ceftriaxone, or cefotaxime, or a beta-lactam/B-lactamase inhibitor.

N.B.: Although *in vitro* an advanced fluoroquinolone (e.g., levofloxacin) is active against most CAP pathogens, some experts are reluctant to use it alone since there are few published data on its clinical efficacy in the very ill patient. However, it is generally agreed that levofloxacin has excellent activity against *L. pneumophilia, Mycoplasma pneumoniae* as well as most pneumococci (13A).

3. **The ATS guidelines** published in 1993 (7). For hospitalized patients, cefuroxime, ceftriaxone, or a beta-lactam/beta-lactamase inhibitor can be used alone or combined with a macrolide. Patients in the ICU were usually treated with a combination, including a macrolide.

4. **A practical approach involves first clinically assessing whether the patient is seriously ill** (i.e., sick enough to be in the ICU because of the pneumonia or at risk for needing intubation because of the pneumonia) **versus moderately ill** (i.e., hospitalized but with easily correctable hemodynamic and/or oxygen parameters).

a. **In the seriously ill** patient, since this is a life-threatening infection, **when no gram stain data are available, broad-spectrum antibiotics seem prudent** until sputum and blood cultures are available. Epidemiologic factors should be considered (Table 2.1). A third-generation cephalosporin (e.g., ceftriaxone or cefotaxime) and a macrolide have commonly been employed. However, since this combination will not uniformly cover high-level penicillin-resistant *S. pneumoniae,* an advanced fluoroquinolone (e.g., levofloxacin, ± ceftriaxone is often used). See Sec. 2b. above.

- If the gram stain shows classic grampositive diplococci and there is a very low likeli-hood of Legionella, antibiotics aimed at *S. pneumoniae*, including high-level resistant forms, are reasonable; e.g., levofloxacin or possibly vancomycin alone.
- For patients with severe structural lung disease, see sec. b.(3) below.
- Once blood cultures and sputum cultures are available, regimens can be tailored appropriately (Table 2.6).
- **Infectious disease consultation is advised** for these very ill patients.

Table 2-6. Treatment of pneumonia according to a specific pathogen

Pathogen	Preferred Antimicrobial	Alternative
S. pneumoniae Mild-moderately ill*	IV penicillin 2 mu q4h or IV ampicillin 1.5–2.0g q6h or IV ceftriaxone 1g q24h or IV cefotaxime	Cefazolin or a macrolide
Very ill**	IV levofloxacin** 500 mg q24h ± ceftriaxone	Vancomycin ± ceftriaxone
H. influenzae (or *M. catarrhalis*) Ampicillin resistant or unknown Ampicillin susceptible	Cefuroxime or Ceftriaxone (cefotaxime) Ampicillin	Ampicillin-sulbactam, fluoroquinolone Cefuroxime, ceftriaxone, or fluoroquinolone
Atypical pathogens— *Legionella* spp.	Macrolides ± rifampin or fluoroquinolone	Doxycycline ± rifampin
Chlamydia spp.	Doxycycline or macrolide, or fluoroquinolone	

Organism		
Mycoplasma pneumoniae	Doxycycline or macrolide, or fluoroquinolone	
Staphylococcus aureus		
Methicillin susceptible	Nafcillin (oxacillin)	Cefazolin, clindamycin, or vancomycin
Methicillin resistant	Vancomycin ± rifampin ± gentamicin	
Pseudomonas aeruginosa	Piperacillin plus aminoglycoside or aztreonam	Ceftazidime plus aminoglycoside; or aztreonam plus aminoglycoside; or ciprofloxacin plus an aminoglycoside (or aztreonam)
Enterobacter spp.	Imipenem or meropenem	Piperacillin plus aminoglycoside
Enterobacteriaceae (e.g., *Klebsiella*, *Proteus* spp., *E. coli*)	Third-generation cephalosporin ± aminoglycoside	Piperacillin and an aminoglycoside (or aztreonam). Beta-lactam plus beta-lactamase inhibitor, or fluoroquinolone
Anaerobes	Clindamycin	Penicillin and metronidazole; or beta-lactam plus beta-lactamase inhibitor (e.g., Unasyn)

Source: Modified from Bartlett et al. *Clin Infect Dis* 1998;26:811, and Medical Letter, *Med Lett Drugs Ther* 1998;40:33 and 1999;41:95.

* Susceptibility data (MIC) may take a couple of days. Once available it may allow you to adjust therapy.

** Once patient is stable, may be able to switch to oral therapy. See Chap. 32.

b. **In the moderately ill patient,** data suggest the clinician has **many options.** The **ideal regimen has not been established.** Therapy needs to be individualized including consideration of epidemiologic factors (Table 2.1) and assessing the risk for gram negatives and atypicals.

(1) **If a sputum is available for gram stain, and shows**

- **Gram-positive diplococci,** IV ampicillin or penicillin are reasonable. Since IV ampicillin is given q6h rather than q4h, overall IV ampicillin is more cost-effective (**Table 2.7**). At the doses of ampicillin and penicillin shown, therapy is adequate for intermediately penicillin-resistant *S. pneumoniae* (13). If the patient is penicillin allergic, a macrolide can be used.

- **Gram-negative organisms** cefotaxime or ceftriaxone, especially for rodlike gram negatives, or ampicillin-sulbactam (for coccobacillary forms) is suggested.
  This is relatively uncommon. Gram-negative pneumonias are usually preceded by a bronchitis and require a high titer of organisms before they become invasive; thus they are visible on the gram stain.

(2) **If no gram stain is available, empiric antibiotics are used, depending on** the patient's age, epidemiologic factors shown in Table 2.1, and miscellaneous issues discussed later. **See options in Table 2.7.**

(3) **Miscellaneous considerations**

- **Ampicillin (or penicillin) alone is still a potential agent for very carefully selected patients (Table 2.7).** Whenever ampicillin (penicillin) can be used, we feel this provides **the moderately ill patient** (who is representative of the vast majority of patients with pneumonia), narrow-spectrum, nontoxic, inexpensive therapy providing the lowest likelihood of colonization with resistant organisms and development of C. difficile or Candida complications. Furthermore, if progression of illness occurs and L. pneumophila or Haemophilus spp. become more likely, experience indicates adjustment of treatment regimen brings rapid resolution.

- If there are epidemiologic or other clinical **data suggesting** *Legionella*, a macrolide (or quinolone) could be used.
- **For oropharyngeal secretion aspiration,** IV penicillin or clindamycin 600 mg q8h or metronidazole plus penicillin is advised.
- **For patients with severe structural lung disease;** i.e., **cystic fibrosis or bronchiectasis**, an antipseudomonal penicillin plus an aminoglycoside ± a macrolide or combination active against *Pseudomonas* spp. ± atypicals is advised.
- **For patients with postinfluenza CAP** (see Chap. 1), antibiotics aimed at *S. pneumoniae, H. influenzae*, and to a lesser extent *S. aureus* are used. Ceftriaxone or cefotaxime or ampicillin-sulbactam are commonly used. An advanced generation quinolone is another option.
- **For patients not responding** to initial antibiotics, **infectious disease consultation is advised.**

B. **For outpatient therapy of CAP.**
   1. *Medical Letter* (13) favors an oral macrolide, or doxycycline, or an advanced fluoroquinolone for adults without significant comorbidity. For older patients and those with underlying diseases, an advanced fluoroquinolone "may be a better choice."
   2. **IDSA** (1) favors macrolides or doxycycline, or an advanced fluoroquinolone. **Modifying factors** include (a) for the young (17 to 40 years of age) doxycycline is preferred since it covers atypicals so well; (b) for suspected penicillin-resistant *S. pneumoniae*, an advanced fluoroquinolone (e.g., levofloxacin) and (c) for aspiration, amoxicillin-clavulanate.
   3. **The 1993 ATS Guidelines** (7) favored a macrolide in young middle-aged adults and older adults with comorbid conditions, amoxicillin-clavulanate or second-generation cephalosporin (e.g., cefuroxime). (N.B.: Advanced fluoroquinolones were not available in 1993.)
   4. **Because ambulatory patients are not as ill as those hospitalized, presumably greater flexibility of choice is available.** Broader-spectrum antibiotics will be necessary if patients fail an outpatient regimen and compliance was not a concern.

Table 2-7. Options for empiric antibiotic therapy of hospitalized community-acquired pneumonia in adults

Agent	Potential Indication	Dose	Comment
Ampicillin	Still potential agent for **carefully selected patients:** • Mild illness, typically >55 yr • No recent antibiotics • No recent hospitalization • Not from nursing home • From area with low % of high-level penicillin-resistant *S. pneumoniae* • If gram stain available it lacks large numbers of gram-negative bacilli or coccobacillary forms, or has gram-positive diplococci Can observe patient	1.5–2 g q6h IV	Will be active against intermediate-resistant *S. pneumoniae* but probably not high-level resistant forms. May miss up to 30% of ampicillin-resistant *H. influenzae.* However, the role of *H. influenzae* in pneumonias may be overemphasized. See text.
Penicillin	**Similar select group as above,** especially when gram-stain reveals characteristic gram-positive diplococci.	2 mu q4h IV	Dose will be active against penicillin intermediately resistant *S. pneumoniae.* In very ill ICU patient, would want to ensure activity against high-level penicillin-resistant *S. pneumoniae,* vancomycin or levofloxacin preferred.

Azithromycin	≤55 yr with no sputum available or non-diagnostic gram stain. No risk factors for gram-negatives (see Table 2-1) Little comorbidity	500 mg IV* × 3 days followed by 250 mg po × 2 days*	Azithromycin is most convenient way to give a macrolide. Active against *H. influenzae* but not against gram-negative bacilli May add to other regimens to cover atypicals
Ceftriaxone	Excellent coverage for most community-acquired gram-negatives, including *H. influenzae* Active against majority of penicillin-resistant *S. pneumoniae*	1–2 g IV q24h	Convenient once-daily regimen **No activity against atypical pathogens** ? role in therapy of known or high risk for high-level penicillin-resistant *S. pneumoniae*. See text; other agents preferred
Cefuroxime	Probably still reasonable to use for mildly to moderately ill patients (admitted to regular floor)	750 mg–1.5 g IV q8h	Not for critically ill ICU patient or patient at risk for or with known high level penicillin-resistant *S. pneumoniae*

continued

Table 2-7. (*Continued*)

Agent	Potential Indication	Dose	Comment
Cefuroxime (continued)	Active against penicillin-susceptible *S. pneumoniae* and may be active in vivo against intermediate strains. See text. Good for *H. influenzae, M. catarrhalis,* and most community-acquired (CAP) gram-negatives.		
Levofloxacin	In vitro, very appealing spectrum of activity against all common CAP pathogens, including most penicillin-resistant *S. pneumoniae* (13A) and atypicals	500 mg IV or po once qd	**Excessive use will select for resistance. Limited clinical experience in critically ill,** therefore, some experts reluctant to use it as monotherapy in critically ill ICU patients though in vitro data suggest monotherapy should work
If patient needs admission but refuses, appealing regimen to provide optimal yet easy oral regimen
Does not cover mouth anaerobes well. Clindamycin can be added to levofloxacin to ensure anaerobic activity. A related agent, trovofloxacin, does and could be considered when anaerobes are a concern (i.e., mixed aerobic-anaerobic). See Chap. 32.

* A 5-day course of azithromycin is providing presumably 10–12 days of adequate tissue levels. A 7-day course provides probably 21 days of tissue levels (e.g., useful in *Legionella* infections).

5. **For a practical approach, age and epidemiologic factors** should be used to select an agent. Usually a sputum gram stain is not available in this setting.

   a. **In the young, otherwise healthy person, less than 50 years of age, azithromycin is a very appealing choice. Alternatives are doxycycline** with a fluoroquinolone a distant third. Azithromycin is selected since it is well tolerated, effective, focused against the likely atypical or most pneumococci and the less likely *Haemophilus* spp., and the once-daily dosing of the 5-day regimen maximizes compliance. If the patient has a history of tolerating erythromycin, that agent qid will be the most cost-effective macrolide.

      The other macrolide, clarithromycin, is another option; it is a bid regimen but must be taken 10 to 14 days.

   b. **In the older patient (over 50–55 years old),** in many ways, this group is approached like the person with an acute exacerbation of chronic bronchitis (Chap. 1). Mycoplasma and chlamydia pneumonia infection is much less common. Usually *S. pneumoniae* or *H. influenzae* will be the offending organism. With the increased frequency of *S. pneumoniae* intermediately-resistant to penicillin and with the observation that high dose amoxicillin-clavulanate is effective in eradicating both *S. pneumoniae* and *H. influenzae* (more so than azithromycin), **amoxicillin-clavulanate is an appealing agent. See Table 2-8.**

Table 2-8.   Oral antibiotic regimens for adults over 55 years old (normal renal function)

Agent	Oral Dose Regimen
Amoxicillin-clavulanate (Augmentin)	500 mg tid or 875 mg bid* for 10–14 days
Azithromycin**	500 mg day 1, then 250 mg days 2–5 (Z pack)
or	
Clarithromycin**	500 mg bid for 10–14 days
or	
Erythromycin**	250–500 mg qid for 10–14 days
Levofloxacin	500 mg once daily for 10–14 days
Cefuroxime axetil	500 mg bid

* The 875 mg bid regimen may cause fewer GI side effects.
** Of the macrolides, azithromycin causes fewest GI side effects, is more active against *H. influenzae*, and is easiest to give. See Chap 26.

If a sputum gram stain is available and is highly suggestive of *S. pneumoniae*, a reasonable approach is full doses of amoxicillin, i.e., at least 500 mg tid for 10 to 14 days.[*]

Hospital-Acquired Pneumonia

I. **Introduction. Hospital-acquired pneumonia (HAP) is** usually **defined as** a pneumonia not incubating at the time of admission and **occurring more than 48 hours after admission.** A comprehensive statement on this topic was published by the American Thoracic Society (ATS) in 1995 (14), and this topic was recently reviewed (15). HAP is the **second most frequent cause of hospital-acquired infections** and remains the **number one cause of nosocomial infection-related mortality;** its presence increases hospital stay by an average of 7 to 9 days per patient and results in additional direct annual hospital costs in the United States of $2 billion (15). Data suggest mortality rates from HAP infection range between 30% and 50%.

As with CAP, **there are many controversies and unanswered questions** in the optional approach to diagnosing and treating HAP. In addition, many patients with fever and stable pulmonary status are treated as if they had pneumonia when they actually do not. This excess treatment may be as great a problem as HAP itself.

II. **Pathogenesis**
  A. **HAP**
    1. **In the absence of an endotracheal tube, microaspiration of oropharyngeal secretions** colonized by pathogenic organisms are the most important factor. Colonization of the oropharynx with *S. aureus* and gram-negative bacilli (GNB) increases with more severe and/or debilitating illness or prolonged hospitalization, especially following administration of antibiotics that eliminate the normal colonizing community flora. Oropharyngeal colonization of GNB in healthy, nonhospitalized patients is less than 10%, whereas 35% of moderately ill and more than 70% of very ill hospitalized patients are colonized with GNB. (See related discussion under Sec. V below.) Once aspirated, pathogenic bacteria overwhelm the lower respiratory defenses and pneumonia results (15).
    2. **Gross aspiration** of large amounts of material occurs less often but can occur with both oropharyngeal and esophageal or gastric contents. Patients with impaired gag reflex, impaired con-

---

[*] Some data suggest that even higher doses of amoxicillin, e.g., 1 g po tid may be useful and effective against many penicillin-resistant *S. pneumoniae*. See report by Piroth L, et al. *Antimicrob Agents Chemother* 1999;43:2484.

sciousness, or with nasogastric (or endotracheal [ET] tubes) are at excess risk.

3. **Following ET intubation,** the ET tube becomes colonized. Since host defense mechanisms have insufficient access to this site, gram-negative bacteria grow to high titer and from there can be inoculated into the lower bronchial tree.

B. **Ventilator-associated pneumonia (VAP).** Not only does the ET tube serve as a barrier to host defenses (e.g., cough, mucociliary clearance), but contaminated secretions pool just above the endotracheal cuff (an area not reached by suctioning) and can drain into the tracheobronchial tree. Also, *Pseudomonas* spp. can colonize the tracheobronchial tree without appearing in the oropharynx at least in part explained by the fact *Pseudomonas* spp. adhere to the tracheal cells better than oropharyngeal cells (15).

Some data suggest up to 25% of ICU patients on ventilators may develop pneumonia, an estimated incidence that is 21 times greater than the non-ICU patient (15)! Although this is probably a high estimate, the incidence of pneumonia is higher among ICU patients than it is among non-ICU patients.

III. **Risk factors for HAP** have been summarized in **Table 2.9.** The most important risk factors are prolonged **ventilator use and** severe and/or debilitating **underlying disease associated with a prolonged period of intubation or length of stay** (LOS). **Prior** use of **antibiotics** also affects which organisms are likely to be isolated.

IV. **Microbiology of HAP.** The organisms causing HAP differ from those of CAP and depend largely on the organisms colonizing the oropharynx, which in large part depends on risk factors (Table 2.9). However, it is noteworthy that 5% to 10% of all cases of HAP are caused by community pathogens.

Several points deserve emphasis.

A. **Enteric GNB are major pathogens** as discussed in Sec. II.A. The longer the LOS, the greater the risk, especially in patients on ventilators. See the discussion on colonization versus infection in Sec. V below.

B. **Hospital-type GNB** (e.g., *Pseudomonas* spp., *Acinetobacter* spp.) are of special concern in patients with **protracted ICU** stay and/or **prolonged ventilator use.** Usually, these patients have had prior courses of antibiotics. Patients with underlying severe **structural lung disease** (e.g., cystic fibrosis or bronchiectasis) are also at risk for these pathogens.

C. *S. aureus* may be a pathogen seen especially in ventilated patients with coma or protracted neurologic problems and patients with prolonged ICU stays, especially if on a ventilator. Intravenous drug abusers and patients with chronic renal failure or diabetes may also be at risk for *S. aureus.*

1. **Methicillin-susceptible *S. aureus*** (MSSR), which is an uncommon cause of pneumonia, is more likely in patients with a short hospital stay

Table 2-9.   **Risk factors for hospital-acquired pneumonia (HAP)**

Patient-Related Factors	Infection Control-Related Factors	Intervention-Related Factors
Elderly age (>70 yr)	Poor hand-washing practices	Prolonged antibiotics[†]
Severity of underlying disease	Improper use of gloves	Repeated courses of antibiotics[†]
Prolonged hospitalization	Contamination of respiratory equipment	Sedatives/analgesics[‡]
Comorbid illness	Contamination of hospital water supply with Legionella spp.[*]	Prolonged ventilator use
Diabetes		Prolonged operations[§]
Renal failure		Nasogastric tube use[″]
Chronic obstructive pulmonary disease (COPD)		Nasal endotracheal (ET) and/or nasal ET tube use[#]
Malnutrition		Transporting intubated patients to/from ICU[**]
Metabolic acidosis		Stress ulcer (bleeding) prophylaxis with antacids or H_2 blockers[††]
Hypotension		Fiberoptic bronchoscopy[‡‡]

Source: Table prepared from data summarized in McEachern R, Campbell Jr GD. Hospital-acquired pneumonia: epidemiology, etiology, and treatment. *Infect Dis Clin North Am* 1998;12:761.

* Up to 20% to 23% of *Legionella pneumonia* cases may be hospital-acquired! Larger hospitals with older, higher-volume hot water tanks may have *Legionella* in the water system. Immunocompromised patients may be especially vulnerable.

[†] Antibiotics can eliminate normal oropharyngeal flora and select for resistant pathogens.

[‡] May increase the risk of aspiration with decreased mental alertness.

[§] Especially **surgery of** thorax, abdomen, or neck **and especially in** the elderly, obese, or patients with underlying COPD.

[″] Nasogastric (NG) tubes may promote gastroesophageal reflux and bacterial migration to the oropharynx.

[#] Nasal tubes may predispose the patient to maxillary sinusitis which may predispose patients to HAP.

[**] The supine position, manipulation of ventilator tubing, and temporary disconnection of suction may predispose to aspiration.

[††] Controversial topic: prophylaxis with these agents raises gastric pH allowing for more GNB colonization (e.g., when compared with sucralfate use).

[‡‡] Bronchoscopy itself may increase risk of aspiration, especially in sedated and/or supine patients.

and in institutions with low rates of methicillin-
(or oxacillin-) resistant *S. aureus* (MRSA or
ORSA). It is relatively infrequent since antibiotics used for other reasons are active against
MSSA and eradicate the colonizing organisms.

2. **MRSA** is more likely in patients with a prolonged
LOS, especially in an ICU and/or in institutions
with high rates of MRSA. MRSA plays a far more
significant role since antibiotics active against
gram negatives eradicate the gram negatives,
paving the way for colonization and replication of
MRSA. See related discussions in Chap. 17.

3. **The sputum gram stain may give a clue** to
this pathogen, demonstrating gram-positive
cocci in clusters.

D. **Common pathogens in CAP** (e.g., *S. pneumoniae*
and *H. influenzae*) can cause HAP and should routinely be covered (see discussion of CAP). If *S. pneumoniae* is seen on gram stain or isolated from a patient
currently or recently receiving a beta-lactam, penicillin resistance is likely. Therefore until susceptibility
data are available, agents active against intermediate-
and high-level penicillin-resistant *S. pneumoniae*
should be used. (See CAP discussion.)

E. **VAP** is **polymicrobial** in up to 50% of cases.

F. *Legionella* spp. occur in hospitals whose water systems are colonized with *Legionella* spp. Patie nts on
steroids or other forms of immunosuppression are
especially at risk.

G. **Miscellaneous.** The role of **viruses** in HAP is **not
well studied.** However, during community epidemics
of influenza and respiratory syncytial virus (RSV) infection, nosocomial viral infections can occur. Likewise,
the role of *Mycoplasma* has not been well studied, but
presumably, an infected health care worker with a
mycoplasmal respiratory infection could infect a hospitalized patient. Occasionally, *Mycobacterium tuberculosis* is spread in the hospital, especially when proper
precautions are not taken with an infectious case; AIDS
patients are especially vulnerable. The disease usually
does not become manifest until after discharge.

V. **Colonization versus infection (superinfection): clinical diagnosis of HAP.**

A. **Colonization** refers to the **presence of organisms**
that are **not causing disease.** Colonizers in the hospital sometimes include community-type organisms,
but hospital gram negatives, such as *Pseudomonas
aeruginosa* and gram positives (e.g., MRSA) are very
common. Therefore **the mere isolation of one of
these organisms from a sputum sample does not
prove they are pathogens** of the lower respiratory
tract; they may just be oropharynx colonizers that "contaminate" the deep cough or suctioned sputum sample.

B. **The determination that "potential pathogens"
isolated from sputum cultures are causing significant pulmonary infection or superinfection**

(i.e., a new pneumonia superimposed on a partially treated pneumonia) **is often difficult.**

1.   **This is usually based on clinical parameters.** See Sec. C.

2.   **Fiberoptic bronchoscopy with quantitative specimens** (with ≥10⁴ bacteria/ml growth implying infection) is sometimes used; but the optimal techniques have not been standardized. The role of diagnostic bronchoscopy varies from institution to institution and must be individualized. When the bronchoscope is passed into the upper airway to obtain a specimen, upper airway colonizers may contaminate the specimen collection unless special techniques are used. A protected (plugged) brush catheter (PBC) has been used to reduce this problem and is best used in conjunction with quantitative sputum cultures. **The exact role of this approach is still undergoing clinical assessment** (16).

C.   **Clinical assessment of colonization versus true infection.**

1.   A formal **"point system"** has been published for patients on a ventilator and summarized in **Table 2.10** (17). Patients with a clinical score of

Table 2-10.   CPIS* used for the diagnosis of VA** pneumonia

1. Temperature °C
    ≥36.5 and ≤38.4 = 0 point
    ≥38.5 and ≤38.9 = 1 point
    ≥39.0 and ≤36.0 = 2 points

2. Blood leukocytes, mm³
    ≥4,000 and ≤11,000 = 0 point
    <4,000 and >11,000 = 1 point + band forms ≥500 = +1 point

3. Tracheal secretions
    <4 + volume of tracheal secretions = 0 point
    ≥4 + volume of tracheal secretions = 1 point + purulent secretion
    = +1 point

4. Oxygenation: PaO_2/FiO_2 mm Hg
    >240 or ARDS = 0 point
    ≤240 and no evidence of ARDS = 2 points

5. Pulmonary radiography
    No infiltrate = 0 point
    Diffused (or patchy) infiltrate = 1 point
    Localized infiltrate = 2 points

6. Culture of tracheal aspirate (semiquantitative: 0-1-2 or 3+)
    Pathogenic bacteria cultured ≤1+ or no growth = 0 point
    Pathogenic bacteria cultured >1+ = 1 point + same pathogenic
    bacteria seen on the gram stain >1+ = +1

Source: Modified from Pugin J, et al. Diagnosis of ventilator-associated pneumonia by bacteriologic analysis of bronchoscopic and nonbronchoscopic "blind" bronchoalveolar fluid. *Am Rev Respir Dis* 1991;143:1121.
* Clinical pulmonary infection score
** Ventilator-associated

more than 6 were felt to have pneumonia, and this clinical impression was supported by bronchoscopy quantitative culture data.

·2. **Besides fever, requisite indicators of new pulmonary infection include leukocytosis, purulence** of sputum, development of **a new infiltrate** on chest x-ray, and **increased oxygenation requirements. We would emphasize the following:**

   a. **Fever** and **leukocytosis** alone can be **nonspecific.** Other infections should be excluded. The elderly may not be able to manifest a fever.

   b. **Purulent sputum.** A good sputum specimen should be obtained by a deep cough or ET suction in ventilated patients. Is it purulent on gross inspection? Does the gram stain suggest a good specimen by cytologic exam?

   In patients with adequate white blood cell response, the absence of sputum production speaks against a gram-negative pneumonia, because most patients produce significant quantities of sputum. Also a nonpurulent sputum (i.e., <25 polys per low-power field) **on gram stain** suggests colonization of bacteria isolated on culture, whereas a **purulent specimen by cytology (>25 polys per low-power field) supports a true infection.**

   In terms of the sputum culture, remember that **gram-negative organisms causing pneumonia usually are isolated from the sputum in large numbers. Therefore if a good sputum on culture reveals no GNB, a pneumonia due to GNB is very unlikely.** Scant growth only of a GNB would also speak against an established GNB pneumonia.

   c. **A new infiltrate on chest x-ray is supportive of the diagnosis of pneumonia, but not pathognomonic, especially in the ICU patient** in whom atelectasis, congestive heart failure (CHF), adult respiratory distress syndrome (ARDS), pulmonary embolism, or pulmonary hemorrhage is an alternate diagnosis. In a recent report of surgical ICU patients, only 30% of pulmonary infiltrates were due to pneumonia (18). **Therefore not all ICU patients with fever and an infiltrate on x-ray have pneumonia!**

   d. **Declining oxygenation on unchanged inspired oxygen** almost always is seen in a true VAP.

D. **Other considerations**

   1. **Blood cultures** should be performed on all febrile patients.

2. **Associated pleural effusions.** If the HAP is associated with a pleural effusion, often a diagnostic thoracentesis is indicated to rule out infected fluid (i.e., empyema) or complex fluid (e.g., pH < 7.2; LDH > 1,000 IU/L; positive gram stain or glucose ≤ 40 mg/dl) which needs drainage. Cultures of pleural fluid may provide a pathogen. However, a febrile ICU patient with **stable** oxygen parameters and an effusion on x-ray probably does not have an underlying pneumonia and the risks of a thoracentesis can be avoided.

3. **Is the patient at high risk for aspiration?** Has the patient had seizures, obtundation, oversedation, a difficult intubation, or very poor oral dentition that may predispose him/her to aspiration?

VI. **Therapy.** Recent studies emphasize that **appropriate, early empiric antibiotics improve mortality rates** (15).

A.   The ATS has published detailed algorithms to address empiric therapy (14).

B.   **We would emphasize the following** points before starting empiric therapy. See **Table 2-11.**

1. **Patients on ventilators in the ICU** are at especially high risk for VAP. Since these patients typically represent complex cases, are debilitated, and have a prolonged LOS, they are **at risk for resistant GNB (including *Pseudomonas* spp., *Enterobacter*, and MRSA** [the latter if a sputum gram stain suggests gram-positive cocci in pairs and clusters]).

   a. If good sputum and gram stains are available, antibiotics may be focused on observed bacteria.

      (1) If large numbers of only gram-positive cocci in clusters, empiric vancomycin is appropriate.

      (2) If only gram-negative bacilli are seen, empiric antibiotics active against the most resistant GNB seen in your ICU is appropriate.

      (3) See Table 2-11. Once culture data are available, the spectrum of antibiotics can be narrowed if susceptibility data allow.

   b. If no good gram stain data are available, combination antibiotics seem prudent; the antibiotics may be able to be revised once culture data are available (**Table 2-11**).

   c. **For very sick patients,** infectious disease consultation is also advised.

2. **In one study, patients admitted to a surgical ICU with trauma** (previously healthy adults) often have early onset of HAP, and in the first week this was due to *H. influenzae* or *S. pneumoniae* (18).

Table 2-11. Empiric therapy of hospital-acquired pneumonia

Setting	Antibiotic Regimen	Alternative
ICU patient on ventilator or prolonged ICU stay or very ill ICU patient	Piperacillin and aminoglycoside* ± vancomycin†	Ceftazidime + aminoglycoside* ± vancomycin or Ciprofloxacin + aminoglycoside* ± vancomycin or Beta-lactam/beta-lactamase‡ + aminoglycoside ± vancomycin
Patient on regular floor, short hospital stay <5 days, mild illness	Cephalosporin§ or beta-lactam/beta-lactamase	
Patient on regular floor Prolonged stay and very sick	Similar to therapy for ICU patient—see above	
Prolonged stay and mildly ill	Ceftriaxone (third generation)	Beta-lactam/beta-lactamase ± aminoglycoside* or Ciprofloxacin ± aminoglycoside

* If an aminoglycoside is contraindicated (Chap. 21) aztreonam can be used.

† Add vancomycin if sputum gram stain shows gram-positive cocci or preliminary cultures suggest *S. aureus.* Vancomycin will also cover *S. pneumoniae* while awaiting cultures.

‡ This combination may be especially useful if a gross aspiration pneumonia is also a concern since, for example, piperacillin-tazobactam would cover oral anaerobes.

§ The choice of a cephalosporin must be individualized. In mild illness, after a short admission on a regular floor, we might elect to use cefazolin, although many may prefer a broader cephalosporin (e.g., cefuroxime or even ceftriaxone).

3. **Patients on a regular floor** for a short stay (<5 days) are less likely to have resistant GNB. If they have a long LOS on a regular floor, they may be at risk for more resistant GNB.

4. **A sputum for gram stain** may help assess if gram-positive cocci are present, raising concerns with *S. aureus* and/or *S. pneumoniae*. See related discussion in Sec. IV.B and IV.D.

5. **If a gross aspiration is witnessed** (e.g., complicated intubation, aspiration during a seizure), and the patient has poor dental hygiene, anaerobes should be covered (e.g., by adding clindamycin [or metronidazole] to agents active against GNB or using a beta-lactam/beta-lactamase combination (e.g., ampicillin-sulbactam or piperacillin-tazobactam, which will also be active against oral anaerobes). Piperacillin is active against many oral anaerobes so piperacillin plus an aminoglycoside is also an option.

6. **For patients who do not initially** respond and/or those at high risk for nosocomial *Legionella* spp. (e.g., in institutions with known *Legionella* in the water supply) empiric use of a quinolone or macrolide may also be indicated in the very ill (e.g., immunocompromised patient).

C. **Duration of therapy.**

1. For GNB the course is usually at least 14 to 21 days, depending on serial clinical assessment, although good clinical data on optimal duration of therapy are not available.

2. For *S. aureus*, a 7- to 14-day course is advised; a longer course for MRSA is sometimes needed.

3. When susceptibility data allow, oral therapy may be able to replace IV therapy once the patient has improved.

D. **In patients not responding,** infectious disease and pulmonary consultations are advised.

References

1. Bartlett JG, et al. Community-acquired pneumonia in adults: guidelines for management. *Clin Infect Dis* 1998;26:811.
   These are consensus guidelines from the Infectious Disease Society of America (IDSA). This is a comprehensive review of CAP with 145 references. Many therapeutic issues remain controversial.

2. Fine MJ, et al. A prediction rule to identify low-risk patients with community-acquired pneumonia. *N Engl J Med* 1997;336:243.
   See reference 5 also. See Appendix F. For a related paper, see Marie TJ, et al. A controlled trial of a critical pathway for treatment of community-acquired pneumonia. JAMA 2000;283:749.

3. Metlay JP, et al. Does this patient have community-acquired pneumonia? Diagnosing pneumonia by history and physical exam. *JAMA* 1997;278:1440.
   To confirm the diagnosis of pneumonia you need a chest x-ray.

4. Davidson M, Tempest B, Palmer DL. Bacteriologic diagnosis of acute pneumonia: comparison of sputum, transtracheal aspirates, and lung aspirates. *JAMA* 1976;235:158.
   Very interesting study but small; 25 acutely ill Native Americans underwent sputum, blood, transtracheal aspirate, and lung aspirate (of infiltrate). S. pneumoniae *was by far the leading pathogen in the lung aspirates. Of interest, no lung aspirates were positive for* Haemophilus *spp., although this was commonly isolated from mixed flora in the sputum cultures.*

4A. Ruiz-Gonzales A, et al. Is *Streptococcus pneumoniae* the leading cause of pneumonia of unknown cause? A microbiologic study of lung aspirates in consecutive patients with community-acquired pneumonia. *Am J Med* 1999;106:385.
   Using conventional (sputum and blood culture, serologic studies) and transthoracic needle aspiration (with culture, antigen detection, and PCR) in 109 adults patients, including 18 patients with AIDS, the most common pathogens were S. pneumoniae *(30%),* Mycoplasma pneumoniae *(22%),* Chlamydia pneumoniae *(13%),* P. carinii *(8%), and* H. influenzae *(7%). An etiologic diagnosis was made in 83% with the lung aspirate providing the sole means in 33%.*
   Nevertheless, lung aspiration studies are not routinely suggested for CAP. See reference 12A for editorial comment on this paper.

5. Auble TE, Yealy DM, Fine MJ. Assessing prognosis and selecting an initial site of care for adults with community-acquired pneumonia. *Infect Dis Clin North Am* 1998;12:741.
   Further discusses approach in reference 2.

6. Farr BM. Prognosis and decisions in pneumonia. *N Engl J Med* 1997;336:288.
   Editorial response to reference 2.

7. Niederman MS, et al. Guidelines for the initial management of adults with community-acquired pneumonia: diagnosis, assessment of severity, and initial antimicrobial therapy. *Am Rev Respir Dis* 1993;148:1418.
   Official statement of the American Thoracic Society (ATS). As of early 2000 these have not been revised. However, see related paper by G.D. Campbell, Jr. Commentary on the 1993 American Thoracic Society guidelines for the treatment of community-acquired pneumonia. Chest *1999;115(suppl.):14S.*

8. Thornsberry C, et al. Surveillance of antimicrobial resistance in *Streptococcus pneumoniae, Haemophilus influenzae,* and *Moraxella catarrhalis* in the United States in the 1996–1997 respiratory season. *Diagn Microbiol Infect Dis* 1997;29:249.
   Related papers summarized in Table 2-4.

9. Pallares R, et al. Resistance to penicillin and cephalosporin and mortality from severe pneumococcal pneumonia in Barcelona, Spain. *N Engl J Med* 1995;333:474.

10. Plouffe JF, et al. Bacteremia with *Streptococcus pneumoniae*: implications for therapy and prevention. *JAMA* 1996;275:194.

11. Dresser LD, McKinnon PS, Rybak MJ. Outcomes of patients with *Streptococcus pneumoniae* bacteremia and pneumonia based on susceptibility and antibiotic regimens from 1996 to 1998. 38th Interscience Conference on Antimicrobial Agents and Chemotherapy. San Diego, CA. September 1997. Abstract L-40.

12. Andes D, Craig WA. *In vivo* activities of amoxicillin and amoxicillin-clavulanate against *Streptococcus pneumoniae:* application to breakpoint determination. *Antimicrob Agents Chemother* 1998; 42:2375.

12A. Dean N. Pneumococcus is number one. *Am J Med* 1999;106:486.
   An editorial comment on reference 4A.

13. *Medical Letter.* The choice of antimicrobial drugs. *Med Lett Drugs Ther* 1999;41:95.
   Includes a discussion of antibiotics for pneumonia.

13A. Chen DK, et al. Decreased susceptibility of *Streptococcus pneumoniae* to fluoroquinolones in Canada. *N Engl J Med* 1999;341: 233.
   The prevalence of pneumococci with reduced susceptibility to fluoroquinolones is increasing in Canada (from 0% in 1993 to 1.7% in 1997), probably as a result of selective pressures from the increased use of fluoroquinolones. See Chap. 32 also.

14. American Thoracic Society. Hospital-acquired pneumonia in adults: diagnosis, assessment of severity, initial antimicrobial therapy, and preventative strategies. A consensus statement. *Am J Respir Crit Care Med* 1995;153:1711.
   Comprehensive review of this topic.

15. McEachern R, Campbell GD Jr. Hospital-acquired pneumonia: epidemiology, etiology, and treatment. *Infect Dis Clin North Am* 1998;12:761.
   Nice recent discussion.

16. Torres A, El-Ebiary M. Invasive diagnostic techniques for pneumonia: protected specimen brush, bronchoalveolar lavage, and lung biopsy methods. *Infect Dis Clin North Am* 1998;12:701.

17. Pugin J, et al. Diagnosis of ventilator-associated pneumonia by bacteriologic analysis of bronchoscopic and nonbronchoscopic "blind" bronchoalveolar lavage fluid. *Am Rev Respir Dis* 1991;143:1121.
   Data from which clinical criteria in Table 2-10 are derived.

18. Singh N, et al. Pulmonary infiltrates in the surgical ICU: prospective assessment of predictors of etiology and mortality. *Chest* 1998;114:1129.
   In this series of 129 patients who developed infiltrates, 30% were due to pneumonia; 29%, to pulmonary edema; 15%, to acute lung injury; and 13%, to atelectasis.

Skin and Soft-Tissue Infections

Cellulitis

Cellulitis is an acute infection of the skin involving the subcutaneous tissues. In adult patients, community-acquired infections are most frequently due to *Staphylococcus aureus* and/or *group A beta-hemolytic streptococci* (GAS). In children, *Haemophilus influenzae* should also be considered. **Erysipelas** is a superficial cellulitis, involving the lymphatics, manifested by warm, shiny, red, edematous, and indurated lesions that begin as small areas of redness and spread peripherally. The majority of cases involve the face or extremities. The etiologic agent is almost always GAS (occasionally group G). The clinical **distinction between streptococcal infections (erysipelas) and cellulitis due to *S. aureus* is difficult and not always reliable. An anatomic approach to cellulitis is clinically more helpful.**

I. **Major anatomic types of cellulitis**
   A. **Cellulitis of the extremities and the trunk** usually causes a warm, erythematous, edematous, and painful spreading inflammation of the skin having poorly defined advancing margins.
      This is usually due to *S. aureus* or GAS.
   B. **Facial cellulitis** may be complicated by extension into the orbit and cavernous sinus.
      1. **Uncomplicated facial cellulitis spares the periorbital area and is usually due to *S. aureus* or GAS.**
      2. Patients with **periorbital cellulitis** may have eyelid erythema, warmth, swelling, and focal pain. **Erythema around or close to the eye is worrisome.** Because periorbital cellulitis is **often due to underlying sinusitis**, sinusitis pathogens (*S. pneumoniae*, *H. influenzae*, and *S. aureus*) should be covered with antibiotic regimens.
         a. **Orbital cellulitis or abscess** is suggested by proptosis and pain with eye movement, decrease in visual acuity, displacement of the globe, limited mobility of the eye, and/or chemosis (edema of the bulbar conjunctiva). An **ophthalmologist should be consulted urgently.** Antibiotics should also be initiated.
         b. **Cavernous sinus thrombophlebitis is a rare** septic phlebitis of the veins draining the orbits that leads to thrombosis of the cavernous sinus. **It should be considered in** severely ill patients and in patients with meningeal signs and/or altered consciousness when there is periorbital cellulitis present.

       c. **Differential diagnosis consideration.**
Rhinocerebral mucormycosis is an uncommon, frequently fatal, necrotizing fungal infection of the paranasal sinuses that may extend into the orbit and the CNS, and is usually seen in poorly controlled diabetics.

       d. **Infectious disease consultation is advised** for severe infections and/or the concern for rare complications.

  C. **Perineal cellulitis.** When the perineal area **(perivulvar, perirectal) or penile and scrotal area** (Fournier's gangrene) is involved with the cellulitis, a **mixed aerobic (usually Enterobacteriaceae, streptococci) and anaerobic** infection is present. Diabetes and obesity are risk factors. **More serious necrotizing soft-tissue infections can occur** (see the following section on Necrotizing Soft-Tissue Infections).

II. **Diagnosis**

  A. The **diagnosis** is typically **made by clinical exam.**

  B. **Cultures**

    1. In the febrile and/or toxic-appearing patient, obtain **blood cultures.**

    2. If there is a cellulitis contiguous with a **draining wound,** gram stains and cultures of the drainage may be useful.

    3. Needle aspirations and/or punch biopsies of an area of cellulitis are not routinely recommended. Typically, their yield is low, except in the severely immunocompromised patient in whom punch biopsy for culture and histopathologic examination may be very useful and in whom occasionally a biopsy is indicated when the patient is not responding to conventional therapy. In addition to bacterial studies, fungal stains, cultures, and histopathologic studies should be done on punch biopsy specimens.

  C. **Invasive streptococcal A disease** has recently been reviewed (1,2).* An early form of this may begin as abrupt onset of **pain** at the soft-tissue infection site with **bullae** formation, **with or without cellulitis and with immature granulocytes** in the peripheral

---

* **Invasive GAS disease** is defined as an infection associated with the isolation of GAS from a normally sterile body site and **includes three overlapping clinical syndromes:** (a) group A **streptococcal toxic shock syndrome** (TSS), with hypotension and multiorgan failure. The case definition for streptococcal TSS has previously been published (*JAMA* 1993;269:390; also see Chap. 7 and Appendix Table E); (b) **necrotizing fasciitis;** and (c) **infections where GAS is isolated from a normally sterile site** in patients not meeting the criteria for TSS or necrotizing fasciitis (e.g., bacteremia without a focus, meningitis, puerperal sepsis, osteomyelitis, septic arthritis, surgical wound infections, etc.). These severe invasive GAS infections rarely occur after an episode of acute GAS pharyngitis.

    The British tabloids coined the term *flesh-eating bacteria* to describe necrotizing infections due to GAS (2).

blood. A magnetic resonance imaging (MRI) scan of the involved area may help clarify the extent of severe soft-tissue infection (1). This **can complicate varicella infection in children** (1,3). Other groups at increased risk are young children, the elderly, and diabetics (1). **Infectious diseases consultation is advised if this diagnosis is suspected.**

    See **related discussions under Necrotizing Soft-Tissue Infections.**

III. **Treatment.** Initial antibiotic therapy should **be based on the clinical impression and anatomical location** of the cellulitis (e.g., extremity vs. perineal, vs. periorbital), as well as the gram stain of the drainage if present. Specific guidelines for **antibiotic therapy** of the various cellulitis are as **shown in Table 3.1.**

    When invasive GAS is highly suspected or known, both IV penicillin and IV clindamycin are advised; see Sec. III.C under Necrotizing Soft-Tissue Infections **(NSTI).**

IV. **Additional measures**
  A. **Surgical consultation** should be obtained for evaluation of any rapidly advancing, fulminant infection and/or if invasive streptococcal A infection is known or highly suspected.
  B. **Intravenous immunoglobulin** (IVIG) (1,2,4,5) may be beneficial **in very severe invasive group A streptococcal infection and/or if hypotension or any features of toxic shock syndrome (TSS) are present.** A dose of 1 to 2 g/kg given once has been suggested (1), but the optimal dose of IVIG in this setting is unknown. **See related discussion under NSTI.**

V. **Follow-up.** Therapy may need to be adjusted in view of blood and wound drainage culture results. **Seven to 10 days of therapy will usually be required.** If there is rapid clinical improvement in severe infections, an initial IV course of therapy may often be completed with oral agents **(Table 3.1).**

Necrotizing Soft-Tissue Infections

Necrotizing soft-tissue infections (NSTI) involve a rapidly progressing inflammation and necrosis of skin, subcutaneous fat and fascia, and sometimes muscle. Therefore they **are deeper and more serious infections than an uncomplicated superficial cellulitis.** When muscle is involved with clostridial infection, it has been referred to as clostridial **myonecrosis. NSTI has been reviewed elsewhere (6,7).**

I. **Clinical setting.** The sine qua non of NSTI is the presence of **fascia necrosis** with widespread undermining of the skin, often coupled with severe **systemic symptoms.** Early in its course, it may be difficult to differentiate NSTI from severe cellulitis. A **high index of suspicion is important.**

Table 3-1.   Empiric therapy of cellulitis in adults

Disease	Primary	Alternative
Facial cellulitis		
Not around the eyes	Nafcillin or oxacillin 1.5 g IV q4h. In mild disease, clindamycin 300–450 mg po q8h	Cefazolin 1 g IV q8h or clindamycin 600 mg IV q8h
Preseptal or periorbital cellulitis	Ceftriaxone 2 g IV q24h or cefuroxime 750–1500 mg IV q8h	Ampicillin-sulbactam or piperacillin-tazobactam
Perineal cellulitis		
Mild	Ciprofloxacin 500 mg po bid and metronidazole 500 mg po q6–8h (or clindamycin 300–450 mg po q6h)	Amoxicillin-clavulanate (Augmentin) the 875 mg/125 mg regimen bid; or TMP-SMX or cefixime and clindamycin
Severe	Ceftriaxone 1–2 g IV q24h and metronidazole 500 mg IV q6h or clindamycin 600 mg IV q8h	Piperacillin/tazobactam or imipenem
Cellulitis of an extremity or trunk		
Mild, outpatient	Cephalexin or cephradine 750–1000 mg po qid	Clindamycin 300–450 mg po q8h or dicloxacillin 500 mg po qid
Severe	Clindamycin 600 mg IV q8h,* plus oxacillin or nafcillin	Oxacillin or nafcillin 1.5 g IV q4h or cefazolin 1 g IV q8h or vancomycin 1 g IV q12h

* Clindamycin is often an agent of choice in this setting because it is active against invasive streptococcus A group. However, in areas with high levels of *S. aureus* resistant to clindamycin, an additional antistaphylococcal agent must be used (e.g., oxacillin or nafcillin). Treatment can be tailored after culture results are available.

A. **Risk factors include** diabetes, peripheral vascular disease, IV drug use, obesity, malnutrition, immune suppression, and chronic renal failure. There usually is a history of trauma or recent surgery.

B. **Clinical clues to early recognition are intense focal pain, swelling of the soft tissue** beyond the area of erythema, skin **vesicles or bullae, crepitus,** and the absence of lymphangitis and lymphadenitis. These infections may spread rapidly along the tissue planes. In postoperative patients, disproportional change in wound appearance, pain, tachycardia out of proportion to fever, and crepitus strongly suggest clostridial myonecrosis (gas gangrene).

II. **Diagnosis** is based on clinical presentation and serial study. Diagnostic aids include the following:

A. **Gram stain** of the tissue exudate.

B. **Blood cultures.**

C. **Aerobic and anaerobic culture of tissue** obtained at surgery or needle aspiration of a soft-tissue abscess.

D. **Serial clinical assessment** may demonstrate rapid progression of this infection within 12 to 24 hours.

E. **Serum creatine phosphokinase (CPK)** levels are useful in detecting the presence of deeper soft-tissue infections. When the level is elevated or rising, there is a good correlation with necrotizing fasciitis or myositis (2).

F. **An MRI** (or computed tomography [CT]) scan of the involved area may demonstrate deep infection, fascia necrosis, and collections that may need drainage. When no deep fascial involvement is revealed on MRI, necrotizing fasciitis can be excluded (8).

III. **Therapy.** Once NSTI is recognized, hospitalization and **prompt and aggressive therapy are essential.**

A. *__Early surgical consultation and debridement__* **are essential.**

B. **Fluid resuscitation is important.**

C. **Antibiotic therapy should be initiated immediately and aimed at streptococci (groups A and B especially),** *S. aureus,* **gram negatives, and anaerobes.** Clindamycin is the most effective drug for experimental streptococcal A infection. Stevens has recently reviewed the multifactorial explanation (2) for this. In a mouse model of GAS myositis, when treatment was started 2 hours after initiation of infection, penicillin was ineffective but clindamycin resulted in a 100% survival rate. However, **in invasive GAS strep infections both IV clindamycin and IV penicillin** should be used because a small portion of strains of GAS are clindamycin resistant (1) (**Table 3.2**).

D. **Supportive therapy** (i.e., nutrition).

E. **In serious invasive streptococcal group A tissue infections with TSS, IVIG may be beneficial** (1,2,4,5). See related discussions under Cellulitis, Sec. II.C and IV.B.

Table 3-2. Antibiotics for necrotizing soft-tissue infections in adults

Clinical Setting	Therapy
Severe infection	
Community-acquired	Ceftriaxone (1–2 g IV q24h) and clindamycin* (600–900 mg IV q8h) and IV aqueous penicillin 2 million units q4h*
Hospital-acquired	Piperacillin 4 g IV q6h and an aminoglycoside and clindamycin 600–900 mg IV q8h
Mild infection	Ceftriaxone and clindamycin or piperacillin-tazobactam
Suspected or known invasive GAS infection	IV penicillin[†] 18 mu/day and IV clindamycin[†] 600–900 mg q8h
Clostridial infection	Penicillin G 18 million units/day or clindamycin

* To ensure maximal activity against group A streptococci, both clindamycin and penicillin are used. See text.
[†] The dose of IV penicillin G in children is 200,000 to 400,000 U/kg per day in divided doses q4 to q6h (1) and for IV clindamycin 30 to 40 mg/kg per day in three divided doses.

Cutaneous Abscesses

I. **Types of cutaneous abscesses (9)**

   A. **Isolated furuncles.** Furuncles (**common boils**) are *S. aureus* infections of obstructed hair follicles or sebaceous glands. Fever and constitutional symptoms are infrequent. Spontaneous or surgical drainage usually affords prompt relief. **Lesions on the lips and nose** can spread via the facial and emissary veins, causing cavernous sinus thrombosis or brain abscess. Therefore lesions of the lips and nose **should not be physically manipulated** in any manner; **surgical drainage of facial lesions is contraindicated.** Warm compresses are often effective therapy. Antibiotic therapy is seldom indicated unless the patient is febrile or has evidence of local extension of the infection or is a high-risk patient with impaired host defenses (e.g., diabetic, immunosuppressed).

   B. **Recurrent furuncles.** Patients with diabetes or on chronic hemodialysis or IV drug users and who are chronic nasal carriers of *S. aureus* are difficult to manage. No treatment regimen has proven to be universally effective. Application of topical mupirocin to the anterior nares with or without long-term oral clindamycin may be an effective regimen to eradicate nasal carriers of *S. aureus*.

Table 3-3. Empiric therapy of cutaneous abscesses in adults

Gram Stain	Route	Primary	Alternative
Gram positive	Oral	Cephalexin (Keflex) or cephradine (Velosef) 750–1000 mg q6h or clindamycin 300–450 mg q8h	Dicloxacillin 250–500 mg q6h
	Parenteral	Oxacillin or nafcillin 1.0–1.5 g q4h	Cefazolin 1 g q8h
Gram negative (perineal abscesses)	Oral	Amoxicillin 875 mg/clavulanate 125 mg bid*	Metronidazole 500 mg po q6h and ciprofloxacin 500 mg bid or TMP-SMX; or clindamycin 300–450 mg q8h and ciprofloxacin or TMP-SMX
	Parenteral	Cefazolin 1 g q8h and metronidazole 500 mg IV/po q6–8h	Piperacillin-tazobactam or ampicillin/sulbactam or cefoxitin

* The 875-mg bid regimen of amoxicillin/clavulanate (Augmentin) may be better tolerated gastrointestinally than the 500-mg tid regimen.

C. **Carbuncles.** Carbuncles are large cutaneous abscesses initiated by *S. aureus* infections of an obstructed hair follicle. Surgical drainage is usually necessary, and systemic antibiotic therapy is required if there are indications as in Sec. A earlier.

D. **Mixed cutaneous abscesses.** Cutaneous abscesses may be caused by a variety of bacterial species other than *S. aureus.* Anaerobes, either in pure culture or mixed with coliforms, are characteristic of abscesses in the perineal region. Nonperineal abscesses are more likely to be secondary to aerobic bacteria, but anaerobic bacteria can be present. **Incision and drainage is the most effective treatment**, and antibiotics are used only in high-risk patients (Sec. A) or when signs of systemic infection are present.

II. **Management of cutaneous abscesses.** The following recommendations are suggested as guidelines for the initial evaluation of cutaneous abscesses:

A. **Clinical evaluation.** Assess degree of illness (i.e., fever, chills, sweats, or constitutional symptoms), risk factors (i.e., diabetes mellitus, valvular heart disease, immunologic disorder, or immunosuppression) and location of abscess (i.e., lips or nose, perineum, or other site).

B. **Incision and drainage (I and D). Surgical drainage of facial lesions is contraindicated.** Antibiotic prophylaxis is suggested for patients with prosthetic joints who undergo incision and drainage of an abscess. (See Chap. 15.)

C. **Gram stains** of drainage or aspirated material should be made.

D. **Culture** drainage or aspirated material for aerobes and anaerobes. If the patient is febrile, **blood cultures** should be obtained.

III. **Antibiotic therapy** will be necessary in certain situations.

A. **High-risk patients with impaired host defenses** (i.e., diabetes mellitus, immunosuppressed patients).

B. **Extension of infection to adjacent tissues** (i.e., cellulitis, osteomyelitis).

C. **Bloodstream invasion** is known or highly suspected.

D. **I and D of an abscess in someone with a prosthetic joint.** (See Chap. 15.)

E. **Initial antibiotic regimens can be chosen based on the gram stain of the abscess drainage or aspirate.** In adults, regimens are shown in **Table 3.3**.

Diabetic Foot Infections

Diabetic patients are 17 times more likely to have gangrene; two-thirds of the major amputations in the United States are performed on patients with diabetes (10,11). Poor host defense, ischemia, and peripheral neuropathy all contribute.

I. **Microbiology.** The organisms isolated are related in part to the severity of the infection.

   A. **Mild non–limb-threatening infections.** Half of these infections are **monomicrobial.** *S. aureus* (>50%) and aerobic streptococci are most commonly isolated.

   B. **Severe limb-threatening infections** are usually associated with severe vascular disease and usually are **polymicrobial** (11A).

      1. **Aerobes.** *S. aureus* and coagulase-negative staphylococci are the most common aerobic isolates. Approximately 20% of isolates are streptococci and enterococci. Enterobacteriaceae account for about 25% of organisms isolated. *Pseudomonas* and *Acinetobacter* spp. are common contaminants in specimens in ulcers or opening draining lesions but are infrequently isolated from deep-tissue cultures. *Corynebacterium* spp. have been isolated from patients with necrotizing infections and should not be considered contaminants in such instances.

      2. **Anaerobes.** The presence of anaerobes is associated with a higher frequency of fever, foul-smelling lesions, and the presence of a foot ulcer. Common anaerobic isolates include anaerobic streptococci (about 15%), *Bacteroides* spp. (10% to 12%), and *Clostridium* spp. (2% to 7%). *Bacteroides* spp. are more frequently found in necrotizing infections and osteomyelitis than in abscesses.

II. **Clinical manifestations.** Most cases of foot or lower leg infection in diabetics begin as chronic perforating ulcers. Patients usually have neglected their ulcers. The severity of the infection may depend on the type of bacteria and host factors. The anatomic location of the infection may affect treatment outcome. Proximal infections (along metatarsals, at the heel, or above the ankle) are associated with lower limb salvage and higher mortality. **Local signs and symptoms predominate and include those related to infection, peripheral vascular insufficiency, and neuropathy.**

   A. **Tenderness is often minimal or absent due to neuropathy.** A **foul odor** may be present due to necrosis or anaerobic infection. It is important to determine the extent of deep-tissue destruction and possible bone and joint involvement by unroofing all encrusted areas and inspecting the wound. Probing the wound is useful. (See Sec. III.D.)

   B. **Systemic signs and symptoms often occur late and indicate severe infection.** Uncontrolled hyperglycemia is a useful sign of uncontrolled infection. **Fever is unusual** except in bacteremic patients.

III. **Diagnosis** is based primarily on clinical findings.

   A. **Leukocytosis** may be minimal or absent, even with severe infection.

   B. The **ESR** is usually elevated during infection but is nonspecific.

C. **Blood cultures** are positive in approximately 10% to 15% of patients. **Though most often positive in febrile patients, they should be collected even if fever is absent** (e.g., two sets 20 to 30 minutes apart).

D. **Probing the base of the ulcer to detect bone is a useful technique to identify osteomyelitis (10).** The ability to reach bone at the base of an ulcer by gently advancing a sterile probe **(prior to any debridement)** has a high specificity and positive prediction value in diagnosing osteomyelitis, but the sensitivity of this test is low. **If bone is detected by probing, treatment for osteomyelitis (not just soft-tissue infection) is recommended.** If bone cannot be detected by probing and the plain radiograph does not suggest osteomyelitis, then some experts suggest treatment can be aimed at a soft-tissue infection only (10).

E. **Wound or tissue cultures.** There is presently **no agreed-on best method for obtaining cultures** in patients with diabetic foot infections. In a deep ulcer, it is useful to clean the superficial area with Betadine, let it dry thoroughly, remove the Betadine with alcohol, and then either insert a needle alongside the ulcer into its base before aspirating or plunge a culture swab into the ulcer, to its base. The deep culture results often parallel those obtained by surgical biopsy. **Deep surgical specimens are very useful to culture.** Specimens should be transported promptly in proper anaerobic transport media to the laboratory and processed **anaerobically and aerobically.**

F. **Gram stains.** Although gram stains usually reveal mixed flora and may not be especially helpful, the lack of an inflammatory response and the presence of gram-positive rods may indicate a clostridial infection, which may be rapidly progressive.

G. **Radiographs.** The differentiation of osteomyelitis from diabetic osteopathy may be difficult; serial radiographic studies may help. The role of radioactive scans to identify osteomyelitis remains somewhat controversial; MRI may be helpful.

V. **Therapy.** Successful therapy requires teamwork among various medical disciplines. **Early surgical and infectious disease consultation is recommended.**

A. **Medical therapy.** Many patients do not need ablative procedures.

1. **Antibiotics** are the mainstay of treatment and are recommended in the presence of surrounding cellulitis, a foul-smelling lesion, fever, and deep-tissue infection. The results of deep-tissue cultures, when available, should be used to direct or modify antibiotic choice. **Empiric therapy** is usually necessary while awaiting cultures (**Table 3.4**). For osteomyelitis, protracted courses of antibiotics (>4 weeks) will be indicated. Optimal **duration of antibiotic therapy** has not been well established

Table 3-4. Antibiotics for diabetic foot infections in adults

Classification	Route	Primary Therapy	Alternative
Non–limb threatening infection (aim at staph/strep)	Oral, mild infection	Clindamycin (300–450 mg tid) or cephalexin or cephradine (500 mg qid)	Dicloxacillin or amoxicillin-clavulanate
	Oral, more severe infection (aimed at staph, strep, gram negatives)	Clindamycin (300–450 mg tid) and ciprofloxacin (500 mg bid)	Amoxicillin-clavulanate or TMP-SMZ and clindamycin
	Parenteral	Cefazolin 1 g IV q8h	Clindamycin or cefoxitin. See options below
Limb-threatening infection	Parenteral	Ampicillin-sulbactam or piperacillin-tazobactam or ceftriaxone and clindamycin	Ticarcillin-clavulanate or cefoxitin or ciprofloxacin and clindamycin
Life-threatening infection	Parenteral	Piperacillin-tazobactam and aminoglycoside (or aztreonam) or imipenem	Vancomycin plus metronidazole plus aztreonam

for soft-tissue infection without osteomyelitis; 10 to 14 days of therapy is often employed.
  2. **Glycemic control** should be reasonably strict.
  3. **Nutritional status** should be monitored and corrected.
  B. **Surgical therapy.** The need for medical stabilization should not delay surgical intervention when needed.
    1. **Nonablative procedures.** Reversal of the septic process may necessitate immediate **surgical debridement of all necrotic tissue** and dependent drainage of all areas with pus. Casts, crutches, or braces may be required to immobilize the inflamed part and allow healing.
    2. **Amputations.** If at all possible, the limb should be preserved. Unfortunately, about one-third of all diabetics having a major amputation of one extremity will have the other extremity amputated within the next few years (11A).

Bite Wounds

The following guidelines can be used for the management of a bite (12–14):

  I. **Cultures** for aerobic and anaerobic bacteria should be obtained from any bite wound drainage. Recent data emphasize that with careful cultures a median of five bacterial species are isolated from dog and cat bite wounds. *Pasteurella* spp. were the most frequent isolates from both dog bites (50%) and cat bites (75%). *P. canis* was the most common isolate from dog bites, whereas *P. multocida* was the most common species in cat bite wounds (12). Other common aerobes included *Streptococci, Staphylococci, Moraxella,* and *Neisseria* spp.; common anaerobes were *Fusobacterium, Bacteroides,* and *Prevetella* spp. Of interest, *S. aureus* and GAS were relatively uncommon (13).
  II. **Copious irrigation and debridement of devitalized tissue and foreign material** are important.
  III. **Rabies and tetanus immunization** need assessment (13).
  IV. **Antibiotic therapy** (12–14).
    A. **Prophylactic antibiotics.** In a recent 1999 editorial comment on this topic, Fleisher emphasized that whether antibiotics prevent infection after bites remains controversial (13). Although early studies reported rates of infection as high as 45% after cat or dog bites, in subsequent studies the incidence was closer to 2% to 3% among patients who were not selected on the basis of the presence of risk factors for infection (13). Therefore Fleisher emphasizes that **currently antibiotics are not given routinely, but they are almost always recommended (prophylactically) for high-risk wounds, such as deep punctures (particularly cat bites), those that require surgical repair, and those involving the hand (13).** Cat

Table 3-5. Antibiotics for bite wounds (adult doses)

Type	Organism	Primary	Alternative*
Dog	*Hemolytic streptococci, P. multocida, S. aureus,* enterococci, *Eikenella corrodens, Capnocytophaga carnimorsus* anaerobes	Amoxicillin-clavulanate 500 mg–125 mg po tid or 875–125 mg po bid[†] or ampicillin-sulbactam (3 g q6h IV)	Ciprofloxacin (500 mg bid) and clindamycin (300 mg tid)
Cat	*P. multocida* more than 50%, otherwise similar to that of a dog	Same	Ciprofloxacin and clindamycin
Human	*S. aureus, E. corrodens, H. influenzae,* beta-lactamase producing oral anaerobes.	Same	Ciprofloxacin and clindamycin[‡]

* In the penicillin-allergic patient, optimal therapy is not well established. Above are the authors suggestions. Other options have been reviewed in detail elsewhere (*Clin Infect Dis* 1992;14:633).

[†] The bid regimen may be better tolerated in terms of GI side effects since less clavulanate is given each day.

[‡] Combination will include activity against anaerobes, *H. influenzae, S. aureus,* and *E. corrodens.*

bites tend to cause deep infections (i.e., septic arthritis or osteomyelitis) due to the cat's sharp, slender teeth that easily penetrate. Therefore **it seems prudent to administer prophylactic antimicrobial treatment for 3 to 5 days after these high-risk dog and cat bite wounds.**

- **Human bites** generally are very serious and more prone to infection and complications than animal bites. Therefore **we tend to use antibiotic prophylaxis for most human bites.**
- Currently, **because of the polymicrobial nature of bite wounds, amoxicillin-clavulanate (Augmentin) remains the favored agent if not contraindicated** (13), including treatment for human bite wounds.

B. **Full therapeutic courses** (e.g., 10 to 14 days) of antibiotics are used for already-infected wounds.

C. **Agents. See Table 3.5.**

Puncture Wounds (of Feet)

Puncture wounds may have complications of tetanus, cellulitis, or deeper local soft-tissue infection, or contiguous osteomyelitis. Initial management of the puncture wound should include the following procedures:

I. **Cleansing of the wound**, including initial soaking in a water-detergent solution to remove debris and residual foreign bodies.

II. **Surgical debridement** of devitalized tissue **is essential**.

III. Proper **tetanus prophylaxis.**

IV. **Antibiotics**

A. **Prophylactic antibiotics** are **not routinely indicated** unless the wound has gone unattended for more than 6 hours or unless adjacent soft-tissue infection has developed, or the wound was contaminated by manure (e.g., nail contaminated by manure) which we view as a dirty wound.

B. **Therapeutic antibiotics** have only partially been studied in this setting. In one report of nail puncture wounds of the foot, 18 of 23 patients had only *P. aeruginosa*, two patients had *S. aureus*, and one patient had both organisms isolated. Ciprofloxacin was effective in all after careful surgical debridement. (15).

1. **Ciprofloxacin** 750 mg po bid for 7 days for cellulitis or deep-tissue abscess and 14 days for adult patients with osteochondritis (on roentgenograms or scans) is suggested (15).

   If the cellulitis is severe, we would add an antistaphylococcal agent (e.g., clindamycin or cephalexin) at least until susceptibility data are available because *S. aureus* may be resistant to ciprofloxacin.

2. Ciprofloxacin and clindamycin can be used for 10 to 14 days in patients with manure-contaminated wounds.
V. **Complications.** Infections developing from the puncture wound, should be managed as outlined in other sections of this chapter; osteomyelitis of the bones of the feet may occur. *P. aeruginosa* **is the most common pathogen in patients wearing sneakers or rubber-soled shoes** and requires proper antibiotic (e.g., ciprofloxacin or piperacillin and aminoglycoside) and, at times, further surgical therapy (15).

References

1. Halsey NA, et al. Severe invasive group A streptococcal infections: a subject review. *Pediatrics* 1998;101:136.
   A nice review sponsored by the Committee on Infectious Diseases, American Academy of Pediatrics.
2. Stevens DL. The flesh-eating bacterium: what's next? *J Infect Dis* 1999;179:S366 (suppl 2).
   This is an update of a prior review of invasive GAS infections by Dr. Stevens published in Clin Infect Dis 1992;14:2.
3. Wilson GJ, et al. Group A streptococcal necrotizing fasciitis following varicella in children: case reports and review. *Clin Infect Dis* 1995;20:1933.
4. Stevens DL. Rationale for use of intravenous gamma globulin in the treatment of streptococcal toxic shock syndrome. *Clin Infect Dis* 1998;26:639.
   Although more data are needed, author favors IVIG in patients with strep TSS. Early initiation may help prevent cytokine-induced shock and organ failure.
5. Perez CM, et al. Adjunctive treatment of streptococcal toxic shock syndrome using intravenous immunoglobulin: case report and review. *Am J Med* 1997;102:111.
6. Lewis RT. Necrotizing soft-tissue infections. *Infect Dis Clin North Am* 1992;6:693.
7. Bosshardt TL, Henderson VJ, Organ CH Jr. Necrotizing soft tissue infections. *Arch Surg* 1996;131:846.
   In this series from an urban community hospital serving an indigent population, 56% of cases were due to parenteral drug abuse.
8. Schmid MR, Kossman T, Duewell S. Differentiation of necrotizing fasciitis using MR imaging. *AJR* 1998;170:615.
9. Magnussen CR. Skin and soft tissue infections. In: Reese RE, Betts RF, eds. *A practical approach to infectious diseases*, 4th ed. Boston: Little, Brown, 1996:Chap. 4.
10. Caputo GM, et al. Assessment and management of foot disease in patients with diabetes. *N Engl J Med* 1994;331:834.
    Also see Gibbons ML, et al. Probing to bone in infected pedal ulcers: a clinical sign of underlying osteomyelitis in diabetic patients. JAMA 1995;273:721.
11. Gibbons GW, Habershaw GM. Diabetic foot infections: anatomy and surgery. *Infect Dis Clin North Am* 1995;9:131.

11A. Nolan RL, Chapman SW. Osteomyelitis and diabetic foot infections. In Reese RE, Betts RF, eds. A practical approach to infectious diseases, 4th ed. Boston: Little, Brown, 1996: Chapter 16.

12. Talan DA, et al. Bacteriologic analysis of infected dog and cat bites. *N Engl J Med* 1999;340:85.
   Review of microbiology of over 100 dog and cat bites. These wounds have complex polymicrobial aerobic and anaerobic flora with many species not isolated in many labs.

13. Fleisher GR. The management of bite wounds. *N Engl J Med* 1999;340:138.
   The editorial comment on reference 12.

14. Goldstein EJC. Bites. In: Mandell GL, Bennett JE, Dolin R, eds. *Principles and practice of infectious diseases*, 5th ed. New York: Churchill Livingstone, 2000;3202–3206.

15. Raz R, Miron D. Oral ciprofloxacin for treatment of infection following nail puncture wounds of the foot. *Clin Infect Dis* 1995;21:194.

4

Urinary Tract Infections (UTIs)

The setting of the UTI is important. Is the UTI in a **male or female?** Is the UTI **"uncomplicated" or "complicated"?** Is the patient elderly? Does the patient have a **catheter** in his or her bladder? These all have a direct impact on the type of therapy one should initiate.

Women are especially prone to UTI via the "ascending route" of infection: Coliform organisms colonize the vaginal introitus first; then urethral organisms can gain access to the bladder easily because of the short urethra in women. Highly specific receptor sites on bladder epithelium contribute.

Hematogenous spread to the kidney or bladder is relatively rare except in the setting of prolonged *Staphylococcus aureus* bacteremia or candidemia.

Although this chapter emphasizes UTIs in adults, **an overview of UTI in children is presented in Sec. VII.**

I. **Clinical presentation** (1–3)
   A. **History.** The classic symptoms of a UTI in older children, teenagers, and adults are urinary **frequency, dysuria** (burning), and **urinary urgency.** Fever may or may not be present. In the elderly patient, fever may be the only manifestation of a UTI. Presentation in the very young child is nonspecific. See Sec. VII.E.
      1. **In women** dysuria and frequency may be seen with cystitis, urethritis alone, or vulvovaginitis. (See Chap. 10.) So-called **external dysuria** is more frequently associated with vulvovaginitis, which may also be suggested by a history of vaginal itching, vaginal discharge, and/or vaginal odor. **Internal dysuria** is more associated with cystitis or urethritis. The sexually active female with multiple partners is at increased risk for urethritis. Gross hematuria is common in acute cystitis but not in urethritis or vaginitis.
      2. **In males,** the classic symptoms of dysuria, frequency, and urgency may be present. However, urethritis should be excluded (Chap. 10) and is suggested by a urethral discharge by history and/or physical examination. Urethritis typically occurs in patients who are sexually active with multiple partners.
      3. **Upper versus lower UTI.** The history may aid in this distinction, which is important clinically since **lower UTI** (e.g., cystitis, urethritis) implies superficial infection, which usually can be eradicated easily. **Upper UTI (acute pyelonephritis)** involves infection of the renal parenchyma (tissue infection) which requires a longer course of antibiotics to eradicate infection.

    a. **Fever** (≥38.4ʏ C) may be the **most reliable clinical finding to differentiate upper from lower** UTI. Patients with lower UTI are usually afebrile or have a very low-grade temperature ("38.2ʏ C).

    b. **Shaking chills or rigors** also suggest upper UTI since this may reflect a bacteremia with underlying tissue infection.

    c. **Upper UTI is also suggested** in a patient who fails to respond to single-dose or 3-day therapy with antibiotics, has prolonged symptoms (>7 days), has a history of complex UTIs, or is in a "high-risk" setting (e.g., diabetes, underlying immunosuppression, transplanted kidney, etc.).

4. **Complicated versus uncomplicated UTI.** This distinction can be determined in part by the patient's history. An **uncomplicated** UTI generally refers to a nonpregnant, young-adult to middle-aged woman with cystitis without known underlying structural abnormality or neurologic dysfunction. This is the single largest group of patients with UTIs. Conventional thinking has been that all UTIs in men are complicated. However, recently a small number of men between 15 and 50 years of age may have developed true uncomplicated UTI (3). (See the related discussion in Sec. III.B.) However, in assessing a male with a UTI, most experts suggest this should initially be considered complicated until proven otherwise (2).

    Complicated UTIs therefore refer to UTIs in other settings: most men, children, elderly patients, patients with obstructive uropathies, catheterized patients, and "high-risk" patients. **Catheter-associated** bacteriuria is the most common source of gram-negative bacteremia in hospitalized patients and has been associated with a threefold increase in mortality, prolonged hospital stay, and increased hospital costs (2).

    Prostatitis is briefly discussed in **Sec. III.C.**

B. **Physical examination** is usually nonspecific.

1. **Fever** is a useful sign and is discussed earlier. UTI should be considered in any febrile (or septic) elderly patient, or child, without an obvious source of fever. However, a significant proportion of the elderly have asymptomatic colonization of the bladder (i.e., asymptomatic bacteriuria). When fever develops for another reason (e.g., influenza or early pneumonia or temporal arteritis), they may have incidental urinary tract colonization to which the fever is inappropriately attributed.

2. **CVA tenderness may be present** in acute pyelonephritis but if absent does not exclude the diagnosis, and it may be a nonspecific finding.

Fever and flank pain are relatively specific indicators of acute renal infection (2).
3. A pelvic examination is indicated in women with a history suggestive of vulvovaginitis.
4. In men with prostatitis, a rectal examination may be useful. If a rectal exam is done, a gentle exam is suggested to check for prostate tenderness. Some experts express concern that a vigorous digital examination may precipitate bacteremia in a patient with acute prostatitis in which the gland can be tender, warm, swollen, and indurated.

C. **Laboratory evaluation**
1. **Pyuria.** Although the patient's state of hydration may affect pyuria, pyuria is still considered a useful indicator of UTI, and **its absence should suggest an alternate diagnosis.** Pyuria in the elderly may be nonspecific, but its absence means that bacteriuria is unlikely. The leukocyte esterase dipstick is an acceptable alternative to a urinalysis to define pyuria.
2. **Gross or microscopic hematuria** occurs in about 40% to 60% of women with acute cystitis but is not present in women with urethritis or vaginitis (2).
3. **Gram stain of the urine. Using one drop of unspun urine,** if you see one bacterium or more in an oil immersion field, this suggests $\geq 10^5$ colony-forming units/ml (CFU/ml) if a culture was done on this sample. **A gram stain of spun urine is useful in urosepsis and acute pyelonephritis,** especially **to help assess for enterococci,** which would appear as gram-positive cocci on gram stain.
4. **Urine cultures** are not routinely advised in young to middle-aged women with uncomplicated UTIs (1–3). However, **cultures are advised** for (a) complicated UTI, including recurrent UTI in women (unless related clearly to sexual activity), and (b) assessment for asymptomatic bacteriuria in pregnancy and after definitive removal of foley or after genitourinary surgical manipulation (4). In some patients, especially in women, in whom antibiotic therapy must be initiated rapidly (e.g., in urosepsis), a single straight catheterization to obtain a urinalysis and culture is reasonable; it poses no risk in the uninfected and eliminates the uncertainty produced by contaminated cultures.
5. **"Clean-catch" urine culture interpretation.** Classically, $\geq 10^5$ CFU/ml has been considered diagnostic of a UTI if the urine was transported and processed properly. Recent data conclude that acutely symptomatic women (with acute dysuria) and pyuria have significant growth if a urine culture has $>10^2$ CFU/ml of a known uropathogen (2,5). In dysuric men, growth of $\geq 10^3$ CFU/ml is presumably significant.

6. **Blood cultures** are advised if bacteremia or sepsis is a clinical concern. (Two sets drawn 20 to 30 minutes apart are suggested.)

II. **Therapy of adult women (not elderly)**

A. **Asymptomatic bacteriuria** (defined as $>10^5$ CFU/ml). **Do not usually treat!** The major **exception is pregnancy,** when it is important to screen (e.g., during the first trimester or at the initial prenatal visit) with a urine culture and treat asymptomatic bacteriuria to reduce episodes of pyelonephritis in the mother and premature labor. Therapy of asymptomatic bacteriuria decreases symptomatic UTI 80% to 90% in pregnant women (6,7). Short courses of antibiotics (3 to 7 days) are preferred over single-dose regimens (6).

Other exceptions may include selected high-risk patients such as those with neutropenia or renal transplant (2).

B. **For uncomplicated UTI.** These infections are most often due to *E. coli*, although *Staphylococcus saprophyticus* is relatively common and a urinary pathogen (2,3). Most experts favor a short **3-day antibiotic regimen** over single-dose therapy or more protracted regimens (2,3). See **Table 4.1** for common regimens.

If patients fail therapy with a 3-day regimen, one should obtain a urine culture and treat the patient with an appropriate antibiotic for 2 weeks (i.e., assume the patient really had subclinical pyelonephritis).

C. **For complicated UTI** (e.g., pyelonephritis) after a urine culture is obtained, empiric antibiotics are started (**Table 4.2**). **If available, a gram stain of the urine can help exclude enterococci** (Sec. I.C), which may help simplify empiric antibiotics. Generally, enterococcus UTI occurs mainly in elderly men. **Therapy is usually given for 2 weeks** and modified by culture susceptibility data.

Table 4-1.   Therapy for uncomplicated cystitis in women

Agent*	Dosage (oral)	Cost
TMP-SMZ (generic)	1 DS bid for 3 days	Under $2
TMP (generic)	100 mg bid for 3 days	Under $2
Ciprofloxacin	250 mg q12h for 3 days	About $16
Ofloxacin	200 mg q12h for 3 days	About $16–$17
Tetracycline	500 mg q6h for 3 days	Under $2
Cephalexin[†] (generic)	250 mg q6h for 7 days	About $16
	500 mg q6h for 7 days	About $30

* Because of the increased resistance of community-acquired *E. coli* to amoxicillin, this agent is no longer recommended for empiric therapy.
[†] Some experts feel cephalosporins should be used for at least 7 days and do not advise 3-day regimens of cephalosporins.

Table 4-2.   Therapy of UTI in adults (normal renal function)

Setting	Antibiotic/Dose	Comment
Pyelonephritis		
Mild	TMP-SMZ 1 DS po bid or Ciprofloxacin 500 mg po bid#	Gram stain of the urine helpful to r/o enterococci
More severe, but first episode	Cefazolin 1 g IV q8h or gentamicin	Gram stain of the urine helpful to r/o enterococci which, if present, is typically treated with ampicillin (or vancomycin) and gentamicin
Recurrent or severe	Gentamicin* or third-generation cephalosporin or ciprofloxacin	
Urosepsis		
No gram stain available	Gentamicin†	Elderly men may be at risk for enterococcal bacteriuria. They seldom get bacteremic. However, in those critically ill, ampicillin 1.5 g q6h (or vancomycin) and gentamicin can be used until culture data are available.
Gram (+) cocci on gram stain	Gentamicin with ampicillin or vancomycin	To cover enterococci
Gram (−) on gram stain	Gentamicin alone if not contraindicated†	If patient has not been recently catheterized, a third-generation cephalosporin (e.g., ceftriaxone 1–2 g qd). If patient catheterized, an aminoglycoside (to ensure *Pseudomonas* spp. activity) until susceptibility data are back. Treat 2 weeks, narrow therapy based on susceptibility data when available.

In areas with relatively high resistant levels of uropathogens to TMP-SMZ and/or diabetics, ciprofloxacin may be preferred. See related discussions in Chapters 24 and 32.

* Although ampicillin and gentamicin have been commonly used in empiric therapy of community-acquired pyelonephritis, because many strains of *E. coli* are now resistant to ampicillin, the attractiveness of using this agent has diminished (2) unless combination therapy for enterococci is desired. See comment. For gram-negative activity, an aminoglycoside or third-generation cephalosporin or quinolone (e.g., ciprofloxacin) is preferred (2).

† If an aminoglycoside is contraindicated, a third-generation cephalosporin, fluoroquinolone, and/or aztreonam can be used, depending on local susceptibility patterns and the risk of resistant pathogens.

1. **Inpatient versus outpatient therapy** must be individualized and requires clinical judgment. Young and healthy patients can often be treated as outpatients unless they are septic, are unable to keep down oral medications, or are noncompliant. Older patients with significant underlying disease, poorly compliant patients, patients with nausea and vomiting, and septic-appearing patients need admission. Intravenous (IV) antibiotics should be used until the patient is able to take fluids by mouth, is symptomatically improved, and has become afebrile (2). The elderly are at increased risk of bacteremia with pyelonephritis.

2. **Urologic workup is indicated if fever and/or lack of clinical response persists for more than 72 hours despite appropriate antibiotic therapy. Renal ultrasonography** is important to exclude an obstructive uropathy or evidence of intrarenal or perinephric abscess. Patients who have symptoms of renal colic or a stone on their admission abdominal x-ray (2) deserve early consideration of a renal ultrasound. Recurrent episodes of pyelonephritis deserve urologic workup once at least.

3. **A follow-up urine culture** 1 to 2 weeks after completion of antibiotics is suggested to make sure the infection has been eradicated.

D. **Recurrent infections in women.** It is important to differentiate **reinfection** (new pathogen causing the UTI) from **relapse** (same pathogen). If symptomatic infection occurs within four weeks of cessation of therapy, it is usually **relapse**. **For relapsing infection,** a longer course (4–6 weeks) of therapy often is successful although a urologic work-up may be required if this does not resolve the issue.

   In young patients with **reinfection** and three or more infections in the preceding 6 to 12 months, **either chronic urinary suppression therapy (Table 4.3) or patient-initiated 3-day treatment courses (our preference),** are options (8). In the patient with recurrent infections clearly related to recent sexual intercourse, a post-coital single dose of antibiotic may be very effective (9,10). Before trying antibiotic prophylaxis, simple measures such as voiding immediately after sexual intercourse, using a form of contraception other than a diaphragm (2), and avoiding prolonged periods of time without urinating (e.g., sometimes an occupational hazard of teachers) may help some women.

E. **Pregnancy.** The therapy of asymptomatic bacteriuria and UTIs in pregnancy has been reviewed in detail elsewhere (6,7).

III. **Therapy of adult men. Prostatitis commonly is associated with UTI in men more than 45 to 50 years of age** (11).

Table 4-3. Chronic suppression regimens in adults

Agent	Dosage*
TMP-SMZ	½ Regular (single-strength) tab at bedtime qo night
TMP	100 mg at bedtime
Nitrofurantoin[†]	50–100 mg at bedtime
Quinolones[‡]	

* There are no clear guidelines as to when to stop prophylaxis, but most often at least 6 months is given initially. Low-dose prophylaxis and postcoital prophylaxis have both been demonstrated to be highly effective, safe, and well tolerated even over periods of 5 years. Emergence of resistant strains while on prophylaxis have been infrequent (2).
[†] **We would avoid nitrofurantoin, and related agents, in the elderly,** who may have increased side effects due to these agents (e.g., interstitial pulmonary infiltrates). (See Chap. 33.)
[‡] We are reluctant to use quinolones for chronic suppression for fear of selecting out more resistant bacteria in the long run. Rather, patient initiated 3-day courses of antibiotic therapy at the first sign of a UTI are preferable in the patient who cannot take TMP-SMZ or TMP. If a quinolone is used, we would favor conventional quinolones (e.g., norfloxacin, ciprofloxacin) rather than the newer, broader quinolones (e.g., levofloxacin, trovofloxacin).
Note: qo, every other.

A. **Asymptomatic bacteriuria** is uncommon in adult males (nonelderly) and **deserves evaluation.**
B. **Uncomplicated UTI. UTIs in otherwise healthy adult men** between the ages of 15 and 50 are **very uncommon.** However, a small number of 15- to 50-year-old men suffer from acute uncomplicated UTI. The exact reasons for such infections are unclear, but risk factors for such men may include homosexuality, intercourse with an infected female partner, and lack of circumcision (2,3). Infecting strains, when tested, are highly urovirulent *E. coli*. Presumably, these strains are more likely to enter the urethra of sexually active men whose partners have vaginal colonization with these *E. coli* or in homosexual men in which insertive anal intercourse may facilitate urethral colonization (3).
   1. **Symptoms** of uncomplicated UTI in men are similar to those in women (i.e., frequency, urgency, suprapubic pain). Urethritis must be ruled out in sexually active men (e.g., with a urethral gram stain [3]). See Chap. 10.
   2. **Microbiology.** *E. coli*, Enterobacteriaceae, and gram-positive organisms are common; *S. saprophyticus* is uncommon. Pre- and posttreatment cultures are advised in men (3). A gram stain of the urine can help exclude enterococci at the time of presentation.
   3. **Therapy.** Agents used for empiric uncomplicated cystitis in women (Table 4.1) can be used. Nitrofurantoin is not suggested. There are no

controlled studies on the duration of therapy, but a minimum of 7 days is advised (3). Early recurrence of the same species suggests a more complicated UTI, a prostatitis or pyelonephritis that warrants a 4- to 6-week course of TMP-SMZ or a ciprofloxacin (3).

C. **Prostatitis.** A detailed review of this common problem is beyond the scope of this handbook; this topic is reviewed elsewhere (11). A few points deserve emphasis.

1. **Acute bacterial prostatitis** is an abrupt febrile illness with signs and symptoms of chills at times, acute perineal pain and discomfort, and symptoms of irritative/obstructive voiding dysfunction: frequency, urgency, dysuria. (See comments on rectal exam in Sec. I.B.4.) Urinalysis usually demonstrates pyuria and bacteriuria.

   a. **Routine urine culture** usually identifies the infecting pathogen because acute cystitis usually is associated with acute prostatitis.

   b. **Prolonged antibiotic therapy** for 2, 3, or 4 weeks, if tolerated, is advised, preferably with agents that penetrate the prostate (e.g., TMP, TMP-SMZ, or a quinolone) and based on susceptibility patterns of the urine culture. An initial episode of UTI (prostatitis) that responds well to therapy does not mandate a urologic workup; in this setting we treat for 3 weeks. In a patient with serial or nonclearing episodes, referral to a urologist is appropriate.

      Antibiotics that do not penetrate the prostate tissue well (e.g., ampicillin, aminoglycosides, cephalosporins) can be used to control acute infections or associated urosepsis. For prolonged therapy, a prostate-penetrating agent is preferred.

2. **Chronic bacterial prostatitis** is a more difficult entity to diagnose and treat. Prostate localization urine cultures may be indicated. The more common entities of **nonbacterial prostatitis and prostadynia** (more of a bladder neck/urethral spasm syndrome) **must be differentiated** (11) **and urologic input is advised for these patients.**

D. **Pyelonephritis.** The same principles of therapy as in women apply, although a male with pyelonephritis probably deserves a urologic workup with the first episode. In addition, drugs that penetrate the prostate are preferred, and in males in whom the prostate is assumed to be involved, a 3- to 4-week duration of therapy is advised.

E. **Recurrent UTI** (>two UTIs in 3 years) merits urologic workup to exclude a structural abnormality and/or chronic prostatitis.

IV. **Therapy of elderly patients** involves special consideration. *E. coli* remain the most common pathogen. Although in
the elderly *S. saprophyticus* causes fewer infections, enterococci are more common, especially in men. Gram negatives
are especially common in patients with a history of UTIs.

    A. **Asymptomatic bacteriuria** is very common in men
and women. **Data do not support therapy** for asymptomatic bacteriuria. It will not progress to renal insufficiency, and therapy of asymptomatic bacteriuria does
not decrease mortality rates but will promote emergence of resistance (12).

    B. **Lower UTI** in women requires 7 to 14 days of therapy
as there are **no data in the elderly for 3-day regimens.** For recurrent infections in postmenopausal
women, a trial of local vaginal **estrogen** or oral estrogen if not contraindicated may be useful as this may
normalize vaginal flora and reduce the incidence of
recurrent UTI. This topic has recently been reviewed
(13). **Cranberry juice** (300 ml daily) may decrease
adherence of uropathogens to uroepithelial cells (14). In
men, conventional 10- to 14-day therapeutic regimens
are advised; longer regimens may be necessary if the
prostate is involved. Chronic suppressive therapy for
recurrent UTI can be used (Sec. II.D), but **prolonged
use of nitrofurantoin should be avoided** as the
elderly may be at increased risk for pulmonary side
effects associated with nitrofurantoin. (See Chap. 33.)

    C. **Upper UTIs** are treated as discussed under Sec. II.C.

V. **Therapy of patients with a chronic foley catheter**
(15). **Routine urine cultures are not indicated** if the
catheter is draining properly. **Asymptomatic bacteriuria should not routinely be treated** (15), unless the
foley is to be removed for a protracted time.

    The overall risk of infection increases with the length of
time the catheter is in place. About 50% of men and women
catheterized for 2 weeks become bacteriuric, and all patients
with permanent indwelling catheters eventually become
infected (2). Provided that the system is not breached, bacteriuria can be prevented in the majority of patients for up
to 10 days with modern sterile closed collecting systems
and catheters (2). The precise role of silver-impregnated
catheters in preventing bacteriuria is undergoing clinical
study.

    A. **The well-appearing patient with low-grade fever.**
Bacteria in the catheterized bladder can release endotoxin, which in turn leads to fever (16). If the catheterized patient has only a low-grade fever and otherwise
is relatively stable, **not every fever needs to be
treated.** Often in this situation, defervescence occurs
without specific therapy and with persistence of the
organism in the bladder. In a way, a bladder that is
infected and drained with a catheter is more like a
drained abscess than an organ that needs to be treated.
If the catheter is left in place, treating the first organism, which is often quite sensitive, will lead to replace-

ment by a resistant bacteria and the cycle will repeat itself. **If, however, the patient is ill, treatment is indicated.**

B. **The ill-appearing patient (symptomatic) with fever and a presumed UTI focus.** Use of systemic antibiotics after blood cultures and a urine culture have been obtained is indicated. The **catheter should be changed** soon after initiation of therapy, to get rid of bacteria that may have "adhered" to the catheter itself (i.e., concretion); biofilms on the internal surface of the catheter often serve as a reservoir for bacteria in which they are protected from antibiotics (2). Ideally, the catheter should be removed whenever possible. Initial empiric therapy needs to include activity against *Pseudomonas.* A gram stain of the urine, when available, is helpful to see if enterococci (gram-positive cocci) are a concern.

1. **Nonbacteremic patients.** The optimal duration of antibiotics in this setting has not been defined (2). Short courses of antibiotics based on susceptibility data are advised to avoid the development of bacterial resistance. Although some advocate 7 to 10 days of therapy, we often use shorter courses in the nonbacteremic patient (i.e., 3 to 5 days of therapy in females and in males the data are less clear, possibly 7 days of therapy).

2. **Bacteremic patients.** These patients need conventional 10 to 14 days of antibiotics based on susceptibility data.

VI. **Candida** in the urine in a catheterized patient usually represents colonization, and true infection is uncommon. **Try to remove the Foley that is usually present in patients with *Candida* spp. in the urine.** Then repeat the culture, as often the candiduria may spontaneously clear with removal of the catheter in about one-third of patients (15).

If no catheter has been used, candiduria may well be a marker of disseminated candidemia.

Poor guidelines are available to diagnose true invasive genitourinary infection. Is the patient at risk for disseminated candidiasis? If yes (i.e., a debilitated patient, often postoperative, often on prolonged antibiotics and/or corticosteroids and/or immunosuppression), **infectious disease consultation is advised to help with the diagnosis and management of this difficult problem** (17,18). Repeated isolation of yeast and/or symptomatic infections need consideration of therapy; this needs to be individualized. Candida cystitis can be confirmed at cystoscopy.

VII. **UTIs in children** pose special considerations. A detailed discussion is beyond the scope of this book; this topic is reviewed in detail elsewhere (19–22). Infection may produce irreversible scarring, an important long-term sequelae of childhood UTIs. To prevent this, there is current emphasis on early and accurate diagnosis, prompt antibiotic treatment, and early evaluation (22). Several points deserve emphasis.

A. **Incidence.** The prevalence of symptomatic and asymptomatic bacteriuria in childhood is influenced by the age and sex of the patient as well as the method of diagnosis. Neonatal bacteriuria is reported in 1.0% to 1.4% of neonates, with boys outnumbering girls. In infancy, symptomatic bacteriuria occurs almost equally in about 1.2% of boys, 1.1% of girls. Symptomatic UTIs in children up to age 7 years may be higher than previously thought, affecting 7.8% of girls and 1.6% of boys (22).

B. **Pathogenesis.** Although hematogenous spread to the kidney is common in neonates, the ascending route of infection is most common in children. The usual organisms originate from fecal flora that colonize the perineum (22).

1. **Obstruction with urinary stasis predisposes to UTI.** Posterior urethral valve, obstruction at the ureteropelvic junction or ureterovesical junction, and ectopic ureterocele are the main causes (19). **Vesicoureteral reflux is the most common abnormality.**

2. **Uncircumcised male infants.** More than 90% of boys with febrile UTIs during the first year of life are uncircumcised. Up to the age of 1 year, data suggest a 10- to 20-fold increase in the incidence of UTIs in uncircumcised male infants compared with female infants and circumcised male infants (22).

3. **Children who also are at increased risk** for bacteriuria or symptomatic UTI **include** premature infants with ICU stays, children with systemic or immunologic disease, children with obstructive uropathies or family history of UTI with anomalies such as reflux, and girls younger than 5 years with a previous history of UTI.

C. **Microbiology.** *E. coli* is the most common pathogen, accounting for about 80% of UTIs (22). Recurrent infections can be associated with Enterobacteriaceae or *Pseudomonas* spp. over time.

D. **Asymptomatic bacteriuria** (ABU). Prior studies suggest ABU occurs in 1.2% to 1.8% of school-aged girls and 0.03% of school-aged boys (19,20,22). Recent reviews tend to treat this condition less.

1. **In infants. Mass screening for bacteriuria in infancy seems to result primarily in the detection of innocent bacteriuric episodes and cannot be recommended.** Instead, in infants and small children with high fever without obvious cause or with uncharacteristic symptoms, such as failure to thrive, urine cultures should be considered and performed as part of the general workup of the child (20). Infants with only ABU tend to become abacteriuric spontaneously over a few months (22).

2. **School girls.** The conclusion from recent studies was not only that ABU can be left untreated,

but that there is also an advantage for the patient to have an asymptomatic growth of low virulent bacteria in the urine. The presence of an established bacterial strain seems to prevent invasion by other bacteria, thus functioning as a kind of biologic prophylaxis (20).

E. **Symptomatic bacteriuria**
  1. **Clinical manifestations. The typical signs and symptoms of UTIs in adults are not present** in young children but are seen in older children (2). Fever may not be present. When fever is present, the diagnosis of UTI should be considered (**Table 4.4**).
  2. **Dysuria, especially without bacteriuria,** when present **may be attributed to** other causes such as vaginitis, local perineal irritation, use of bubble baths, pinworm infections, masturbation, or even sexual molestation (19).
  3. **Diagnosis**
    a. **Pyuria** if present is helpful, but 30% to 50% of children may not have pyuria in a centrifuged urine sample (19).
    b. **Enzymatic dipstick tests.** If the leukocyte esterase and nitrate dipstick tests are negative and the index for suspicion on clinical symptoms is low, it may be reasonable not to do a culture since a UTI is not likely in this setting. If the dipstick findings are positive or the clinical suspicion for a UTI is high, a urine culture should be done (22).
    c. **A urine culture is essential for the diagnosis** and must be obtained properly.

Table 4-4.   Signs and symptoms of urinary tract infections in children at different age groups

Age	Presentation
Neonate and infant	Hypothermia, hyperthermia, failure to thrive, vomiting, diarrhea, sepsis, irritability, lethargy, jaundice, malodorous urine
Toddler	Abdominal pain, vomiting, diarrhea, constipation, abnormal voiding pattern, malodorous urine, fever, poor growth
School-age child	Dysuria, frequency, urgency, abdominal pain, abnormal voiding pattern (including incontinence or secondary enuresis), constipation, malodorous urine, fever
Adolescent	Dysuria, frequency, urgency, abdominal discomfort, malodorous urine, fever

Source: From Sherbotic JR, Cornfeld D. Management of urinary tract infections in children. *Med Clin North Am* 1991;75:328.

(1) **For infants and toddlers.** A "bagged" urine specimen is frequently contaminated, so a positive culture is difficult to interpret; a negative culture helps rule out a UTI (19,22). Contamination is directly related to the length of time the collection device remains applied to the child. If a specimen has not been obtained within 30 minutes of application, reliability begins to decrease. Removing the appliance and plating or refrigerating the urine immediately after the child voids is paramount. Confirmation of all positive urine specimens for culture is advisable before treatment. Consequently, catheterization or suprapubic aspiration (SPA) should be used when the clinical situation dictates immediate treatment (22). The details of SPA are reviewed elsewhere (22).

Although urethral catheterization with growth of more than 1,000 CFU/ml is often said to be significant or any growth by SPA, some authors note that in a true UTI, colony counts from bladder urine are usually more than 50,000 CFU/ml, and colony counts of less than 10,000 CFU/ml may be suspect (22).

(2) **For older and cooperative children,** clean-voided, midstream collection for urinalysis, gram stain, and culture is suggested. Significant colony counts are reviewed in Sec. I.C.5. Gram stain (or unstained examination) of unspun urine, under 40-power microscope lens can be done; if bacteria or leukocytes are seen, UTI is likely (19).

4. **Antimicrobial therapy** is summarized in **Table 4.5**. Children who appear ill or who are at significant risk of becoming seriously ill because of their age (e.g., young infants) or have urinary tract abnormalities should be admitted to the hospital for therapy.

For uncomplicated cystitis, 3 to 5 days of antibiotics are advised; however, in children less than 5 years of age who are awaiting radiographic evaluation, antibiotic prophylaxis should be continued until the radiographic evaluation is complete. For pyelonephritis, a conventional course of antibiotics is 10 to 14 days. Much of this can often be given orally (21,22).

F. **Radiographic evaluation.** The current trend toward early evaluation of young children following their first

Table 4-5.   Suggested antimicrobial therapy for urinary tract infections in children: dosages and alternatives

Parenteral (IV) therapy (suspected upper UTI or sepsis)
    Neonates and infants <4–6 months of age
        Ampicillin, 75–200 mg/kg/day divided into four doses, *plus*
        Gentamicin, 5–7.5 mg/kg/day divided into two or three doses
    Older children
        Ampicillin, 100 mg/kg/day divided into four doses, *plus*
        Gentamicin, 7.5 mg/kg/day divided into three doses, *or* a
        cephalosporin (e.g., cefotaxime 100–200 mg/kg/day divided
        into three or four doses or ceftriaxone)
Oral therapy (acute cystitis, resolving upper UTI)*
    Neonates and infants <4–6 months old
        TMP-SMX[†] 6–12 mg/kg/day TMP with 30–60 mg/kg/day
        SMX, divided into two doses, *or*
        Cephalexin, 50 mg/kg/day divided into three doses
    Older children
        TMP-SMX, 6–12 mg/kg/day TMP with 30–60 mg/kg/day
        SMX, divided into two doses, *or*
    Cephalexin 50 mg/kg/day divided into three doses
Prophylaxis (for recurrent infections)
    TMP-SMX, based on 2 mg/kg/day of TMP as a single nighttime
    po dose, *or*
    Nitrofurantoin, 2 mg/kg/day as a single nighttime po dose

Source: Modified from Sherbotic JR, Cornfeld D. Management of urinary tract infections in children. *Med Clin North Am* 1991;75:335.
Abbreviations: TMP, trimethoprim; SMX, sulfamethoxazole.
* Increasing resistance of *E. coli* to amoxicillin limits the use of this drug (21, 22).
[†] Sulfonamide agents (e.g., TMP-SMX) should not be used in children younger than 6 weeks. Antibiotic dosages should be adjusted for the level of renal function, and serum levels should be followed where appropriate.

documented UTI is based on epidemiologic and clinical data. Significant renal scarring can occur after a single UTI. The yield from the evaluation of children with culture-documented UTIs is high. Radiographic studies of white girls with symptomatic UTIs reveals the presence of vesicoureteral reflux (VUR) in approximately 35% to 50% of cases. Unfortunately, clinical parameters have proven unreliable in distinguishing children with UTIs who also have VUR (22). Imaging studies can detect congenital or acquired abnormalities of the urinary tract, including posterior urethral values, VUR, obstruction, dysplasia, hydronephrosis, renal scarring, and renal stones (21).

    1.   **Indications** include the following (21,22):
        a.   **Any male or female child younger than 5 years with a documented UTI.**
        b.   **Older girls with febrile or recurrent UTIs** should be evaluated (22). A sexually

active adolescent girl with recurrent lower UTI generally does not need a radiographic study.

c. **Any child with pyelonephritis** who has not been previously evaluated.

2. **The choice of radiographic examinations depends on the facilities available, the skills and experience of the radiologist, and clinical findings** (19,21,22). The clinician should review options and plan studies after discussion with the radiologist. These are discussed in detail elsewhere (22).

a. **Renal ultrasonography** is noninvasive and free of ionizing radiation. It can reveal obstruction, renal size and contour, stones, size of the collecting system, and bladder anatomy. Upper tract infection may be associated with increases of renal volume of more than 30%. Therefore ultrasonography **provides anatomic information** and must be combined with a functional study (e.g., special scan). **Children requiring hospitalization for febrile UTI should at least be screened for obstruction with sonography before discharge** (22).

b. **Radionuclide scans** may be used as a screen for VUR, and if abnormal, voiding/cystourethrography can be done. Renal cortical scintigraphy using technetium 99m dimercaptosuccinic acid (DMSA) **can suggest the presence of pyelonephritis,** which can be difficult to diagnose in young children (21) or neonates (22).

c. **Voiding cystourethrography (VCUG)** will detect vesicoureteral reflux, grade the severity of reflux, and provide anatomic as well as functional information of the lower urinary tract. With fluoroscopy VCUG is used to detect the presence of posterior urethral values in boys. The cystogram can be performed whenever the patient is no longer symptomatic and when the urine is sterile (22).

d. **Intravenous urogram** has been the time-honored method to evaluate upper tract abnormalities but exposes the patient to more radiation than other options. In recent years, sonography and radionuclide scintigraphy have provided similar data more safely.

G. **Sequelae** (19,21)

1. As many as 80% of children with uncomplicated UTI will have recurrences.

2. Renal parenchymal infection and scarring are well-established complications of UTI in chil-

dren, especially infants and neonates, and may lead to hypertension and/or renal insufficiency.

3. Children with recurrent infections deserve careful urologic evaluation, and follow up by a pediatric urologist.

4. Bacteremia can occur and is inversely related to age, occurring in 18% of those 1 to 3 months of age and in 6% in those 4 to 8 months, but it is unusual in those more than 1 year of age (21).

References

1. Ward TT, Jones S. Genitourinary tract infections. In: Reese RE, Betts RF, eds. *A practical approach to infectious diseases*, 4th ed. Boston: Little, Brown, 1996:472–518.

2. Stamm, WE Urinary tract infection. In: Waldvogel F, Corey L, Stamm WE, eds. *Clinical infectious diseases: a practical approach.* New York: Oxford University Press, 1999:649–656.
   A concise discussion, emphasizing UTIs in adults, by a recognized expert in the field.

3. Hooton TM, Stamm WE. Diagnosis and treatment of uncomplicated UTI. *Infect Dis Clin North Am* 1997;11:551.

4. Falagas ME, Gorbach SL. Practice guidelines: urinary tract infections. *Infect Dis Clin Pract* 1995;4:241.
   Nice, concise summary of definitions, etiology, epidemiology, natural history, diagnosis, and therapy of UTI.

5. Kunin CM. A reassessment of the importance of "low count" bacteriuria in young women with acute urinary symptoms. *Ann Intern Med* 1993;119:454.

6. Andriole VT, Patterson TF. Epidemiology, natural history, and management of urinary tract infections in pregnancy. *Med Clin North Am* 1991;75:359.

7. Patterson TF, Andriole VT. Detection, significance, and therapy of bacteriuria in pregnancy: update in the managed health care era. *Infect Dis Clin North Am* 1997;11:593.

8. Gupta K, et al. Efficacy of patient self-diagnosis and self-treatment for management of uncomplicated recurrent urinary tract infections in women. *Infect Dis Soc Amer 36th Annual Meeting.* Colorado. Nov. 1998 (abstr 39).
   This approach may decrease antimicrobial use, improve patient convenience, and reduce costs. In this study of 122 college-aged women, 3 days of a quinolone therapy was safe and effective.
   TMP-SMZ for 3 days has also been used in this type of approach.

9. Stapleton A, et al. Post coital antimicrobial prophylaxis for recurrent urinary tract infections: a randomized, double-blind, placebo-controlled trial. *JAMA* 1990;264:703.

10. Stapleton A, Stamm W. Prevention of urinary tract infection. *Infect Dis Clin North Am* 1997;11:719.

11. Pewitt EB, Schaeffer AJ. Urinary tract infections in urology, including acute prostatitis and chronic prostatitis. *Infect Dis Clin North Am* 1997;11:623.

For a concise review of prostatitis, see Meares EM Jr. Prostatitis.
Med Clin North Am *1991;75:405 or* Infect Dis Clin North Am
1987;1:855.
For an update, see Lipsky BA. Prostatitis and urinary tract infec-
tion in men: what's new; what's true? Am J Med *1999;106:327.*

12. Nicolle LE. Asymptomatic bacteriuria in the elderly. *Infect Dis*
    Clin North Am 1997;11:647.

13. Raz R. Role of estriol therapy for women with recurrent urinary
    tract infections: advantages and disadvantages. *Infect Dis Clin*
    Pract 1999;8:64.
    Authors conclude: "In an era of increased antimicrobial resistance
    caused by excessive use of antibiotics, the possibility of avoiding
    UTIs in elderly women by administering estriol therapy must be
    encouraged." More data are needed.
    See related paper by Raz R, et al. Recurrent urinary tract infec-
    tions in postmenopausal women. Clin Infect Dis *2000;30:152.*

14. Avorn J, et al. Reduction of bacteriuria and pyuria after ingestion
    of cranberry juice. *JAMA* 1994;271:751.
    Study was done in 150 elderly women. Findings suggest cranberry
    juice reduces the frequency of bacteriuria and pyuria.

15. Warren JW. Catheter-associated urinary tract infections. *Infect*
    Dis Clin North Am 1997;11:609.

16. Garibaldi RA, et al. Detection of endotoxemia by limulus test in
    patients with indwelling urinary catheters. *J Infect Dis* 1973;
    128:551.

17. Fisher JF, Newman CL, Sobel JD. Yeast in the urine: solutions
    for a budding problem. *Clin Infect Dis* 1995;20:183.
    Detailed discussion of a rational clinical approach to this difficult
    problem.

18. Fan-Havard P, et al. Oral fluconazole versus amphotericin B
    bladder irrigation for treatment of candidal funguria. *Clin Infect*
    Dis 1995;21:960.
    These approaches appeared to be equally efficacious. Fluconazole
    200 mg qd for 7 days was used. Foley catheters were changed at
    the start and after therapy.

19. Zelikovic I, Adelman RD, Nancarrow PA. Urinary tract infections
    in children: an update. *West J Med* 1992;157:554.
    A thoughtful review of the diagnosis and management of UTIs in
    children, including a discussion of appropriate imaging for vesico-
    ureteral reflux.

20. Hansson S, et al. The natural history of bacteriuria in childhood.
    Infect Dis Clin North Am 1997;11:499.

21. Lohr JA, Downs SM, Schlager TA. Urinary tract infections. In:
    Long SS, Pickering LK, Prober CG, eds. *Principles and practice*
    of pediatric infectious diseases. New York: Churchill Livingstone,
    1997:370–377.

22. Rushton HG. Urinary tract infections in children: epidemiology, eval-
    uation, and management. *Pediatr Clin North Am* 1997;44:1133.
    Nice overview.

5

Acute Diarrhea, Gastroenteritis, and Food Poisoning

Acute diarrhea is a common complaint. The annual rate of diarrhea in the United States and western Europe among adults averages about one episode per person per year (1). In developing countries, diarrheal illness is the most common infectious disease and is estimated to cause 3 to 5 billion cases of infectious disease annually with an associated 5 to 10 million deaths per year.

The **mechanisms** of pathogenesis in infectious diarrhea may include one or more of the following: **adherence** to the mucosal surface of the bowel (e.g., important for certain *E. coli*), **invasion** of the mucosal epithelial cells (e.g., *Shigella* spp.), **enterotoxin production** (e.g., *Vibrio cholerae*), and **cytotoxin formation** (e.g., *Shigella* spp.).

I. **Clinical approach to the patient with acute diarrhea** (i.e., diarrhea of recent onset: typically a few days to 2 weeks) and/or gastroenteritis.
   A. **Most cases of diarrhea are managed at home** without need for medical attention. **Medical evaluation should occur for a subset of patients** with more severe illness. Specific **indications for medical evaluation have recently been summarized and include** the following (1):
      1. **Profuse watery diarrhea with dehydration** (suggestive of small bowel secretory diarrhea).
      2. **Dysentery** (i.e., passage of many small-volume stools containing blood and mucus). Patients usually will have prolonged illness without antibiotic therapy.
      3. **Fever** (temp >38.5°C; associated with an invasive pathogen that produces inflammation).
      4. **Passage of more than six unformed stools every 24 hours or a duration of illness lasting more than 48 hours.**
      5. **Diarrhea with severe abdominal pain above 50 years of age** (may have a complicating illness such as ischemic bowel disease).
      6. **Diarrhea in the elderly** (>70 years of age) is more likely to be severe and at times fatal. **The immunocompromised** (patients with AIDS and those who have undergone transplantation or received cancer chemotherapy) often have complicated and difficult-to-manage diarrhea (high morbidity and mortality).
   B. **History.** The clinical and epidemiologic histories are **central to patient evaluation** and management (1).
      1. **Setting.** Patients with a history of recent **travel**, especially camping or international travel, **daycare center exposure, residence in a chronic-**

care facility, family members or **close contacts** of the **index case, male homosexuals,** or **AIDS** patients are at greater risk.

2. **Medications.** Recent **antibiotic** use (preceding 2 months); excessive use of **laxatives, antacids, or alcohol;** or recent **chemotherapy** are important risk factors.

3. **Eating habits.** Ascertain whether the patient recently ate shellfish, seafood, or poultry that may have been improperly handled or prepared. Has the patient been to a picnic or restaurant where others have acquired similar illness?

4. **Less frequent risk factors.** Exposure to turtles and iguanas (e.g., salmonella risk) or sick animals is a risk factor. Is there a setting suggestive of **staphylococcal toxic shock syndrome (TSS),** e.g., menstruation and tampon use, influenza, and persistent sinusitis? See Chap. 7 and Appendix D.

B. **Certain symptoms** may be helpful in making a diagnosis.

1. **When vomiting is the predominant symptom** initially, viral gastroenteritis or food-borne intoxication is suggested. Food poisoning due to a preformed toxin often causes vomiting within 3 to 4 hours of ingesting the food. See **Table 5.1** for a summary of important pathogens and presentations.

2. **Mucus in the stool** when seen in large amounts is consistent with invasive bacterial diarrheas; in small amounts, mucus may raise the question of irritable bowel syndrome.

3. **Blood in the stool** indicates the possibility of inflammatory mucosal disease of the colon (e.g., *Shigella, Campylobacter, Salmonella* spp.). Noninfectious etiologies such as ischemic bowel disease, diverticulitis, ulcerative colitis, and radiation injury are also in the differential diagnosis.

C. **Physical examination** is of **little help** in determining the cause of the diarrhea except in TSS, where hypotension, conjunctivitis, and hand and feet erythema are helpful. **Fever suggests intestinal inflammation** characteristically due to invasive bacteria (*Shigella, Salmonella,* or *Campylobacter* spp.), or a cytotoxic organism resulting in mucosal histologic damage and inflammation (*Clostridium difficile* or *Entamoeba histolytica*) (1). Signs of dehydration should be assessed in severe cases, especially in children. Stool testing for occult blood should be done.

D. **Laboratory.** The **fecal leukocyte exam and testing for occult blood are useful screening tests** in patients with moderate to severe acute diarrhea because they support the use of empiric antibiotics in the febrile patient (Sec. II.C) and when negative may eliminate the need for stool culture in some cases (1).

text continued on page 112

Table 5-1.   Clinical features of agent-specific food

Organism or Agent	Incubation Period	Duration of Illness (Range)	Diarrhea	Fever
Staphylococcus aureus	1–8 h	24 h (8–48 h)	+ (infrequent)	−
Bacillus cereus Emetic illness	1–6 h	9 h (2–10 h)	+	−
Diarrheal illness	6–14 h	20 h (16–48 h)	+++	−
Clostridium perfringens	8–24 h	24 h (8–72 h)	+++	−
Non 0:1 *Vibrio cholerae*	6–72 h	2 days (2–12 days)	++	±
Puffer fish	<2 h	Variable	+	−

borne disease with symptom onset of less than 12 hours

Vomiting	Enterotoxin	Invasion	Foods Most Commonly Implicated	Comments
+++	++	−	Salads, cream-filled pastries, meats (pork, beef, poultry)	High attack rates (80% to 100%) Outbreaks most frequent during summer
+++	++	−	Fried rice	Abdominal cramps often experienced Vomiting occurs more often than diarrhea
+	+	−	Meats, vanilla sauce, cream-baked goods, salads, chicken soup	Diarrhea occurs more often than vomiting Organism may be found in stool of healthy person
±	++	−	Improperly stored beef, fish, or poultry dishes (after preparation); pasta salads, dairy products; Mexican foods	"Pig-bel" or necrotizing enterocolitis is a rare variant Stool has no white blood cells or blood Commercial kit available for detection of toxin in stool
±	+ (a minority produce cholera toxin)	±	Seafood, grated eggs, potatoes	25% can have bloody diarrhea Illness similar to cholera but much less dehydration
+	+ Tetrodotoxin (i.e., a neurotoxin)	−	Fugu (especially prepared Japanese puffer fish), other puffer fish, vividly colored frogs of South America, blue-ringed octopus	Symptoms include paresthesias, ataxia, hypotension, seizures, cardiac arrhythmias, respiratory and skeletal muscle paralysis Mortality 30%–60% Treatment: gastric lavage and cardiorespiratory support Prognosis greatly improves if patient survives first 6 hours

continued

Table 5-1.

Organism or Agent	Incubation Period	Duration of Illness (Range)	Diarrhea	Fever
Paralytic shellfish	1–3 h	3 days (0.5–7 days	–	–
Ciguatera	1–6 h	Variable (can persist for months)	+	–
Scombroid fish	<2 h	Variable (2–10 h)	±	–

Source: From Miranda AG, DuPont HL. Small intestine: infections with common bacterial and viral pathogens. In: Yamada T, ed. *Textbook of gastroenterology.* New York: Lippincott, 1991:1452–1453.
+, present; –, not present; ±, present in some cases.

(Continued)

Vomiting	Enterotoxin	Invasion	Foods most Commonly Implicated	Comments
+	+ (Saxitoxin (i.e., a neurotoxin)	–	Most bivalved mollusks (shellfish) especially from endemic waters experiencing red tide blooms	Symptoms and treatment similar to puffer fish poisoning Mortality 5% to 18% Etiology is concentration of toxic dinoflagellates in mollusks during "red tide" season (spring and fall)
+	+ Ciguatoxin (i.e., a neurotoxin)	–	Barracuda, grouper, snapper, jacks, reef sharks	Most common of fish intoxication in United States Commonly seen in Florida, Hawaii, and the Caribbean Symptoms similar to puffer fish poisoning ELISA available for detection of toxin Treatment suggested with amitriptyline
+	– (preformed histamine causes symptoms; *not* an allergic reaction)	–	"Blood fish" (tuna, albacore, mackerel, skip jacks) under spoiling conditions	Symptoms: flushing, generalized or localized erythema, vertigo, generalized burning sensation Histamine levels can be assayed in implicated fish Treatment with antihistamines very effective Fish with unpleasant odor or clouded eyes should be avoided

1. **Fecal leukocytes or occult blood are found** in inflammatory diarrheal disease.
   a. **The most commonly identified pathogens in patients with a positive test** include *Shigella, Salmonella, Campylobacter, Aeromonas, Yersinia,* noncholera *Vibrios,* and *C. difficile* (1).
   b. Remember that patients with inflammatory bowel disease (ulcerative colitis, Crohn's disease) may have a positive test.
   c. **Fecal leukocytes are not seen in:**
      (1) **Viral gastroenteritis.**
      (2) **Most parasitic infections**, although low numbers of leukocytes are found in patients with intestinal amebiasis.
2. **Stool cultures.** It is **not cost-effective to do stool cultures in all patients with acute diarrhea** (1).
   a. **Cultures should be obtained** in a patient with one of the following (1):

      • **Severe diarrhea**
      • **Fever** > 38.5°C or 101.3°F (oral)
      • **Passage of bloody stools**
      • **Stools with leukocytes or occult blood**
      • **Prolonged diarrhea >2 weeks**

   b. **Special media** are needed to culture from stool many of the bacteria that cause diarrhea. If one suspects a particular special pathogen (e.g., *Yersinia enterocolitica, Vibrio cholerae,* or noncholera *Vibrios*), it is helpful to discuss diagnostic possibilities with the microbiology laboratory so that proper handling of the specimen can be carried out.

      If TSS is a concern, cultures for *S. aureus* (e.g., vagina, cervix, wounds) are indicated. (**Elevated** serum **creatinine** and/or **liver function** tests are usually present in TSS.) See Chap. 7 and Appendix Table D.
3. **Virus detection** is particularly useful in **evaluating children younger than 3 years of age.** For example, a variety of assays are available to detect rotavirus antigen in the stool (2). Viral gastroenteritis is common. See the brief discussion in Sec. III.A.
4. **Ova and parasite** (O and P) stool examinations are not cost-effective in most cases of acute diarrhea. O and P exams are useful in patients not treated with empiric antibiotics with chronic diarrhea, international travelers (especially those traveling to Russia, Nepal, and mountainous regions), homosexual men or patients with AIDS,

contacts at day-care centers with protracted symptoms, those suffering diarrhea as part of a community waterborne outbreak; or those who have bloody diarrhea with few or no leukocytes (possible amebiasis) (1).

Note: ***Entamoeba histolytica is a pathogen that requires therapy*** (3). Nonpathogen amebas include *Entamoeba coli*, *E. nana*, *E. hartmanni*, and *E. polecki* (4).

5. ***C. difficile* toxin assay** may be useful in patients who are on, or who have been on, antibiotics in the preceding 2 months. See Sec. III.B.

E. **Other Studies**
   1. **Proctosigmoidoscopy** may be indicated in the following: homosexual men and in some cases of AIDS related illnesses; in chronic or recurrent diarrhea; in rare potential cases of *C. difficile* diarrhea in which an immediate answer is needed; and in potential cases of *Entamoeba histolytica*.
   2. **Radiographic studies** usually are not indicated.

F. **Miscellaneous**
   1. **Common acute bacterial and viral diarrheal syndromes are summarized in Tables 5.1, 5.2, and 5.3.**
   2. **Noninfectious cause** of the diarrhea **should be considered, especially** for persistent (>14 days) or chronic diarrhea (>1 month) (1). Some of the important diagnoses to consider include irritable bowel syndrome, inflammatory bowel disease, ischemic bowel disease (especially in those older than 50 years of age with other evidence of peripheral vascular disease), partial small bowel obstruction, and pelvic abscess in the area of the retrosigmoid colon. Other less common diagnoses are reviewed elsewhere (1).

II. **Therapy** of acute diarrhea, gastroenteritis, and/or food poisoning. **Most cases** of infectious diarrhea (e.g., viral gastroenteritis, most bacterial etiologies) and gastroenteritis **are treated with supportive care.**
   A. **Fluid replacement**
      1. **Oral fluids** with electrolytes will suffice in most patients. Whereas such treatment is life-saving for young infants in the developing world, in the United States the most important adult groups in which special attention and fluid therapy should be given are the elderly and the immunosuppressed (1) and severely ill children. For these and other patients **with severe diarrhea,** commercially available solutions containing sodium in the range of 45 to 75 mEq/L are recommended (Pedialyte or Rehydrolyte solutions). A homemade version of this oral solution for severe diarrhea is to prepare two separate glasses with sips from each consumed alternately. The first contains

Table 5-2.   Medical importance, clinical and epidemiologic characteristics, and diagnosis of human gastroenteritis viruses*

Virus	Medical Importance Demonstrated	Epidemiologic Characteristics	Clinical Characteristics	Laboratory Diagnostic Tests
Rotavirus Group A	Yes	Major cause of endemic severe diarrhea in infants and young children worldwide (in winter in temperate zone)	Dehydrating diarrhea for 5–7 days; vomiting and fever very common	Immunoassay, electron microscopy, PAGE#
Group B	Partially	Large outbreaks in adults and children in China	Severe watery diarrhea for 3–5 days	Electron microscopy, PAGE
Group C	Partially	Sporadic cases in young children worldwide	Similar to characteristics of group A rotavirus	Electron microscopy, PAGE
Enteric adenovirus	Yes	Endemic diarrhea of infants and young children	Prolonged diarrhea lasting 5–12 days; vomiting and fever	Immunoassay, electron microscopy with PAGE#

Norwalk virus	Yes	Epidemics of vomiting and diarrhea in older children and adults; occurs in families, communities, and nursing homes; often associated with shellfish, other food, or water	Acute vomiting, diarrhea, fever, myalgia, and headache lasting 1–2 days	Immunoassay, immune electron microscopy
Norwalk-like viruses (small, round, structured viruses)	Partially	Similar to characteristics of Norwalk virus	Acute vomiting, diarrhea, fever, myalgia, and headache lasting 1–2 days	Immunoassay, immune electron microscopy
Calicivirus	Partially	Usually pediatric diarrhea; associated with shellfish and other food in adults	Rotaviruslike illness in children; Norwalk-like in adults	Immunoassay, electron microscopy
Astrovirus	Partially	Pediatric diarrhea; reported in nursing homes	Watery diarrhea, often lasting 2–3 days, occasionally longer	Immunoassay, electron microscopy

Source: From Blacklow NR, Greenberg HB. Viral gastroenteritis. *N Engl J Med* 1991;325:252. Copyright 1991, Massachusetts Medical Society.
Abbreviation: PAGE, polyacrylamide-gel electrophoresis and silver staining of viral nucleic acid in stool.
* Laboratory diagnostic tests, other than those for rotavirus Group A, usually are available only in specialized research or diagnostic referral laboratories. Immunoassays are usually ELISAs or radioimmunoassays.

Table 5-3.   Clinical features of agent-specific foodborne

Organism or Agent	Incubation Period	Duration of Illness (Range)	Diarrhea	Fever
Salmonella	8–48 h	3 days (1–14 days)	+++	++
Shigella	24–72 h (up to 7 days)	3 days (1–14 days)	+++	+++
Yersinia	24–72 h (up to 6 days)	7 days (2–30 days)	+++	++
Campylobacter	2–11 days	3 days (2–30 days)	+++	++

disease with symptom onset of greater than 12 hours

Vomiting	Enterotoxin	Invasion	Foods Most Commonly Implicated	Comments
+	+	+ (little mucosal damage)	Eggs, poultry, beef, dairy products	Infection with some serotypes can lead to severe complications in certain patients (those with malignancy, atherosclerosis, and AIDS) Treatment not recommended except in severe or disseminated disease because it prolongs carriage of organism Stool contains white blood cells and may contain blood
±	+	++	Salads (egg, tuna, poultry), milk	Low infective dose (10^2 organisms). Person-to-person transmission common Stools often contain blood, mucus, and pus Systemic symptoms (headache, malaise, lethargy) common
±	+	+	Milk (raw or chocolate), tofu	Abdominal pain is a very prominent feature of illness and may be confused with appendicitis Presence of pharyngitis common in children Rheumatologic postinfectious complications have been reported
±	+	+	Raw milk, poultry, beef, clams, pet animals	Stool contains red and white blood cells

continued

Table 5-3.

Organism or Agent	Incubation Period	Duration of Illness (Range)	Diarrhea	Fever
Escherichia coli (entero-toxigenic)	24–72 h	3 days (1–14 days)	+++	+
Vibrio para-hemolyticus	4–96 h	3 days (2–10 days)	++	±
Clostridium botulinum	12–36 h (may be as long as 8 days)	Weeks to months	±	−
Rotavirus	48-72 h	5 days (3–14 days)	+++	+ (low grade)

(*Continued*)

Vomiting	Enterotoxin	Invasion	Foods Most Commonly Implicated	Comments
				Mostly resistant to trimethoprim-sulfamethoxazole Complications include meningitis and Guillain-Barré syndrome
–	+	–	Salads, peeled fruits, meat dishes, pastries	At least two toxins elaborated: heat-labile (similar to choleratoxin) and heat-stable Most common bacterial agent of travelers' diarrhea
+	+	± (not documented in humans)	Oysters, crabs, shellfish, seawater, contaminated food	Antimicrobials do not shorten illness Fecal white blood cells and blood uncommon
±	++ (neurotoxin)	–	Raw honey (infants), improperly canned products	Neurologic symptoms are results of parasympathetic and neuromuscular blockade Fatality rate 15% Treatment is early administration of antitoxin Infants younger than 1 year should not be fed raw honey
++	–	– (superficial damage to mucosa)	Fresh water, seafood	Primarily an illness of infants and children Endemic in nature Respiratory symptoms common Can cause severe dehydration in children

continued

Table 5-3.

Organism or Agent	Incubation Period	Duration of Illness (Range)	Diarrhea	Fever
Norwalk	24–48 h	1 day (1–3 days)	++	+ (low grade)

Source: Modified from Miranda AG, DuPont HL. Small intestine: infections with common bacterial and viral pathogens. In: Yamada T, ed. *Textbook of gastroenterology.* New York: Lippincott, 1991:1453–1455.
+, present; –, not present; ±, may or may not be present.

8 ounces of orange, apple, or other fruit juice (supplying potassium), ½ teaspoon of honey or corn syrup, and 1 pinch of table salt; the second glass contains 8 ounces of clear water plus ¼ teaspoon of baking soda (1).

For mild diarrhea in most healthy patients, diluted fruit juices, sport drinks, soft drinks, broths, and soups can be used with saline crackers.

2. **Intravenous fluids** (normal saline with potassium chloride or Ringer's lactate) are used in patients who are severely dehydrated or in whom oral rehydration is contraindicated.

B. **Antimotility agent use** in acute diarrhea has recently been reviewed. Several points deserve emphasis (1):

1. **Loperamide** (Imodium) is the preferred agent over diphenoxylate (Lomotil) or opium alkaloids and is viewed as the safer agent. Loperamide works by slowing the intraluminal flow of liquid, thereby facilitating intestinal absorption (1).

2. **Loperamide or related agents should not be used in patients with febrile dysentery** (e.g., shigellosis) in which the disease may be prolonged. In a recent review, the authors note disease prolongation by antimotility agents is not commonly seen, and most clinicians do not need to worry about the use of loperamide in nondysenteric forms of diarrhea, provided antimicrobial therapy is administered (1).

In patients with *E. coli* O157:H7, the hemolytic uremic syndrome may be facilitated by antimotility agents or these agents may worsen neurologic symptoms (1) (Sec. III.C). In *C. difficile* diarrhea, these agents should be avoided (Sec. III.B).

(Continued)

Vomiting	Enterotoxin	Invasion	Foods Most Commonly Implicated	Comments
++	−	− (superficial damage to mucosa)	Shellfish, drinking water	Affects primarily older children and adults Endemic in nature Illness is milder than with rotavirus

3. Given these constraints, except in the therapy of acute travelers' diarrhea (Sec. III.F), we take a **conservative approach using loperamide** and avoid its use in young children.

   We will use loperamide in immunocompromised hosts with persistent/chronic diarrhea. This topic is reviewed elsewhere (1).

C. **Antibiotics. Most patients who present with acute diarrhea do not need antibiotics.** However, there are three settings in which empiric antimicrobial therapy is used (1).

   1. In the patient who is **febrile** (oral temperature >38.5°C) plus has either occult or gross **blood** in the stool or **fecal leukocytes** or patient with acute dysentery, empiric antibiotics are indicated while awaiting cultures. This is especially true for very young or very old or fragile patients with diarrhea in whom dehydration is a significant concern. Antibiotics are essential for patients whose history suggests a bacteremia. Oral ciprofloxacin or IV ceftriaxone are possible options for empiric therapy.

   2. **Travelers' diarrhea** is commonly treated empirically (Sec. III.F).

   3. **Empiric treatment for presumed giardiasis** is sometimes used (Sec. III.D).

   4. **Table 5.4** summarizes antibiotic therapy. **Most patients who present with acute diarrhea do not need antibiotics.** Therapy of common entities have been reviewed in detail elsewhere (1).

D. **Miscellaneous**

   1. **Calories (energy)** should be provided to facilitate electrolyte renewal. Diet follows clinical course. Boiled starches/cereal (potatoes, noodles or rice, wheat, oat) with some salt may be ideal.

Table 5-4.   Therapy of bacterial pathogens

Pathogen	Drug of First Choice*	Alternative	Comments
Salmonella typhi	Fluoroquinolone or ceftriaxone	TMP-SMZ	Duration of therapy of uncomplicated enteric fever is 2 weeks, 4 weeks for metastatic foci.
Salmonella spp.	Fluoroquinolone or ceftriaxone or cefotaxime	TMP-SMZ	Uncomplicated gastroenteritis usually not treated.
Shigella spp.	Fluoroquinolone	Azithromycin or TMP-SMZ	Routinely treated. Optimal duration of therapy unclear (one dose, vs. 3 days vs. 5 days).
Yersinia enterocolitica	TMP-SMZ	Fluoroquinolone or cefotaxime	Intestinal infection is usually self-limited. Therapy is indicated for extraintestinal disease or complications of infection.
Campylobacter jejuni	Erythromycin or azithromycin; or a fluoroquinolone	A tetracycline	Gastroenteritis is self-limited and usually requires no antibiotics. For protracted symptoms, a 1-week course of antibiotics is reasonable.
E. coli 0157:H7			See text III.C. Many experts suggest antibiotics **not be used;** TMP-SMZ may increase the frequency of hemolytic uremic syndrome; antimotility agents and narcotics are **not** advised. **IV isotonic saline is advised to correct dehydration.**
Travelers' diarrhea	Fluoroquinolone	TMP-SMZ, doxycycline	A 3-day course of fluoroquinolones is usually preferred—widespread sulfonamide and tetracycline resistance are now frequent.
Vibrio parahemolyticus			Resolution occurs spontaneously in most cases.

Source: Modified from *Medical Letter.* The choice of antibacterial agents, 1999;41:95.
* If empiric therapy is initiated, susceptibility data should be assessed once available. Dosages discussed in individual chapters on antibiotics.

Crackers, bananas, soup, and boiled vegetables can be used. When stools are formed, diet can be returned to normal as tolerated (1).

2. **Lactose intolerance.** Many authorities would exclude milk products early in the illness but lactose intolerance is not commonly found in cases of acute diarrhea (1). Also see Sec. III.D.

3. **Bismuth subsalicylate** has been used to treat and prevent travelers' diarrhea especially. It has also been used to improve the symptom of vomiting associated with enteric viral infection (1).

4. **Attapulgite (Kaopectate or Diasorb)** is a claylike material that absorbs water and makes stools more formed. Because it is not absorbed, it is quite safe but is not as effective as loperamide (1).

III. **Miscellaneous considerations**

A. **Viral gastroenteritis** is common and may account for 30% to 40% of the cases of infectious diarrhea in the United States. This topic is reviewed in detail elsewhere (2).

1. **Common syndromes** are summarized in **Table 5.2.**

2. **Diagnosis.**

a. **In adults**, the diagnosis of viral gastroenteritis is in part clinical and in part a **diagnosis of exclusion** because techniques are not routinely available to isolate the virus from stool.

(1) **History.** Fever is not prominent. There is no obvious history suggesting a bacterial or parasitic process (e.g., no recent international travel, no recent seafood ingestion or church social). The patient often has been exposed to someone with similar gastrointestinal (GI) symptoms.

(2) **Stool examination.** The **absence of fecal leukocytes** supports, although does not prove, a viral origin. Stools for culture or ova and parasite examination will be negative, and the decision of whether to order these must be individualized.

b. **In children**, similar principles hold, but stools can be examined for rotavirus and, at times, enteric adenovirus.

3. **Therapy** is supportive and fluid replacement is important.

B. *Clostridium difficile* **diarrhea** is a relatively common complication of antibiotic use. This topic has recently been reviewed (5).

1. **Pathophysiology.** Antibiotic therapy alters GI flora, allowing overgrowth of *C. difficile*, which produces a toxin, toxin A, that causes the diarrhea. For unclear reasons, patients older than 50 years of age seem at increased risk.

2. **Clinical manifestations**
   a. **Diarrhea** can occur while the patient is **on antibiotics or 4 to 6 weeks after** a prior course of antibiotics. The diarrhea is usually watery, profuse, and foul-smelling, and bowel movement usually occurs six or more times per day. Bloody diarrhea can occur. Fecal leukocytes are commonly present, but not always. **Crampy abdominal pain** may occur.
   b. **Fever** can be prominent, and temperatures of 39° to 40°C are relatively common and at times may suggest this diagnosis.
   c. **Leukocytosis** is common and high white cell counts (24,000 to 30,000 white cells/mm^3 range) can be seen even in the mildly to moderately ill.
3. **Diagnosis**
   a. **Toxin assay**. Although a tissue cell culture toxin assay is still the most sensitive diagnostic test, most hospital laboratories look for toxin A with a rapid procedure (e.g., enzyme immunoassay [EIA] performed on a stool specimen).
   b. Stool cultures for *C. difficile* are tedious to perform and not pathognomonic if positive; they are not recommended.
   c. **Endoscopy** may be useful if an immediate answer is needed or in patients with relapsing diarrhea in whom another diagnosis may be confirmed with endoscopy. Since routine flexible sigmoidoscopy may miss 10% to 30% of the characteristic lesions, colonoscopy is the most definitive procedure.
   d. **Computerized tomography (CT)** of the abdomen may be helpful, but specific CT features of *C. difficile* are uncommon (6).
4. **Therapy in adults**. The **offending antibiotic should be discontinued whenever possible.** In some mild cases, this alone may be therapeutic. For moderate to severe cases or prolonged symptoms, **oral** antibiotic therapy is required to ensure high stool concentrations of the antibiotic used.
   a. **Oral metronidazole** 250 mg qid for 10 to 14 days **is preferred** (7).
   b. **Oral vancomycin** 125 mg qid for 10 to 14 days is rarely needed. It is no longer recommended for routine use of *C. difficile* since excessive use of oral vancomycin may help select out vancomycin-resistant enterococci (VRE) (Chap. 28). In addition, an oral 10-day course of vancomycin is about 60-fold more expensive than a 10-day course of oral metronidazole! (See Appendix Table C.)
   c. **If oral antibiotics cannot be used**, the best approach is unclear. Intravenous (IV)

metronidazole can be tried. Infectious disease consultation is advised.

d. **Oral cholestyramine resin** (4 g po q6h) may be used alone in adults with mild disease or in relapses. It binds to toxin and helps firm up stool. Since it may bind to oral vancomycin, their simultaneous use should be avoided; staggering oral doses is probably reasonable (i.e., three hours apart).

e. **Opiates and antiperistaltic agents should be avoided.** They may allow for toxin retention in the colon and despite initial improvement symptomatically, more severe colon damage may occur.

f. The role of lactobacilli replacement is unclear.

5. **Therapy in children.** *C. difficile* diarrhea is very uncommon in children. To decrease the emergence of VRE, metronidazole (30 mg/kg/day in four divided doses) is the drug of choice for most patients; oral vancomycin (40 mg/kg/day in four divided doses) is indicated only for seriously ill patients or those who do not respond to metronidazole (8).

6. **Infection control aspects.** *C. difficile* is a common nosocomial pathogen. The hands of care givers are important in nosocomial spread. The use of **gloves** by hospital personnel during routine patient care of positive cases **may help** reduce nosocomial spread.

7. **Relapses after a therapeutic course** of metronidazole or vancomycin are common and seen in 10% to 20% of patients. Some of these cases probably represent new infection, with a new strain of *C. difficile*, rather than true relapse. The best approach in these patients is unclear. A standard 14-day course of oral metronidazole or vancomycin is worth trying again. Infectious disease and/or GI consultation is advisable in refractory cases. Adding oral cholestyramine is also reasonable to try. Since some of these individuals with chronic relapsing illness fail to make antibody to the toxin, IgG has been tried with some success (9,10).

8. **Complications** of unrecognized or severe disease (pseudomembranous colitis) include **toxic megacolon**, colonic perforation, and severe dehydration. Serial abdominal exams are useful in any patient with known or suspected *C. difficile* diarrhea. If toxic megacolon is a concern, abdominal x-rays and surgical evaluation are important.

C. *E. coli* **0157:H7 has emerged as an important cause of both bloody diarrhea and hemolytic uremic syndrome (HUS)**, the most common cause of acute renal failure in children. This topic has been reviewed elsewhere (11).

1. **Pathogenesis.** These *E. coli* produce large amounts of toxins and live in the intestines of healthy cattle and can contaminate meat during slaughter. Outbreaks of human disease have been especially associated with **undercooked hamburger** (12) as well as contaminated lake or municipal water and cider made from fallen apples.

2. **Clinical syndrome** (11,13,14). *E. coli* 057:H7 can cause a **spectrum of illness**, from asymptomatic carriage, nonbloody diarrhea (about 10% to 30% of cases), bloody diarrhea (in majority of diagnosed cases), HUS (in 6% to 10% of children less than 10 years of age), and thrombotic thrombocytopenia purpura (TTP). Watery diarrhea is common; fever is infrequent.

3. **Diagnosis** is made by stool culture on special agar that microbiology laboratories are encouraged to use.

4. **Therapy is supportive.** Recent reviews suggest that **antibiotics not be used** (11). **Antimotility agents and narcotics are not advised** since they may delay the clearance of pathogen and may be a risk factor for HUS. **IV hydration** with isotonic saline **is advised.**

5. **Prevention. Thorough cooking kills** *E. coli* 0157:H7. Therefore ground beef should be cooked thoroughly until the interior is no longer pink and the juices are clear. **Infected patients are highly contagious and should not return to group settings unless hygienic practices can be ensured.** *All confirmed* cases should be reported *immediately* to appropriate public health authorities.

D. **Giardiasis.** *Giardia lamblia* is one of the most frequently isolated intestinal parasites in the United States (15,16).

1. **Transmission.** The most common mode is through **contaminated water** (e.g., surface water contaminated by animals or humans and in which the cysts survive). However, **person-to-person** (e.g., day care centers, male homosexuals, and custodial institutions) and **food-borne** (after fecal contamination) do occur.

   Hypogammaglobulinemic and achlorhydric patients are more susceptible to infection.

2. **Clinical syndrome.** A week or two after ingestion of contaminated water, **acute** explosive **diarrhea** associated with abdominal cramps, flatulence, nausea, vomiting, and low-grade fever may occur. Patients do not pass gross blood, pus, or mucus. **Chronic infections** can occur with milder, intermittent symptoms and malaise. **Lactase deficiency** with or after infection is common.

3. **Diagnosis.** There are two stages in the life cycle of this parasite: the trophozoite, which exists freely in the small bowel, and the cyst, which is passed into the environment (15).
   a. **Fecal leukocytes** are **absent**.
   b. **Stool ova and parasite** exams are still the test of choice, especially if other parasitic infections are possible (e.g., assessing an international traveler). Three liquid stools examined serially over days will maximize results.
   c. *Giardia* **stool antigen**. This test is very useful to rule in, or out, exclusive infection with *Giardia*. A polyclonal or monoclonal antibody against cyst or trophozoite antigens is used with either an immunofluorescent antibody test or capture ELISA. The procedure is highly sensitive and specific for assaying stools (16).
4. **Therapy (15,16). All symptomatic patients deserve treatment**; although some cases resolve spontaneously over 3 to 4 days, most persist until treatment intervenes. **Therapy of asymptomatic infection** (cyst passers) **is controversial**, but therapy is indicated if reinfection is unlikely (e.g., in environments with high levels of sanitation) and in food handlers (15).
   a. **In adults, metronidazole** is commonly used (250 mg tid for 5 days). Quinacrine is currently not available in the United States. **Therapy in pregnancy** remains **unclear.** Ideally, treatment should be avoided in the first trimester. Women with mild disease may delay therapy until after delivery. Paromomycin, a nonabsorbable oral aminoglycoside, is advised in pregnant women, although its efficacy may be in the 60% to 70% range (15–17).
   b. **In children,** some sources suggest metronidazole (15 mg/kg/day in 3 doses for 5 days) (17); other sources (8) suggest that since the safety and effectiveness of metronidazole for children with giardiasis has not been established, furazolidone (6 mg/kg/day divided in four doses for 7 to 10 days) is an option; this drug is available in liquid suspension.
   c. **Other alternative regimens** are reviewed elsewhere (17).
   d. **Lactase deficiency** is common after infection, especially in children. Some experts suggest patients recovering from giardiasis should be counseled to avoid lactose-containing products for approximately 1 month.

e. **Empiric treatment for presumed giardiasis** is sometimes undertaken in patients with persistent diarrhea (2 to 4 weeks), especially if their history suggests some potential for exposure (e.g., use of well water, camping). (See Sec. 1.) Although many clinicians would prefer to evaluate the patient for persistent diarrhea for cause of illness, some elect to treat empirically, with metronidazole, for presumed giardiasis. In a recent review, this approach was considered reasonable in view of the importance of *Giardia* in this syndrome and because half of studied stools of patients with giardiasis may be negative for parasites (1). Workup for those failing empiric therapy for *Giardia* may then be indicated (1).

E. *Cryptosporidium* is an infection due to a coccidian parasite, cryptosporidia, and may cause chronic diarrheal syndromes.

1. **Setting**
   a. **In patients with AIDS**, 10% to 15% of patients in the United States and 30% to 50% of patients in the developing world contract cryptosporidiosis. This topic has recently been reviewed (18).
   b. **Normal hosts** usually manifest self-limiting diarrheal disease. This diagnosis is not uncommon and may occur more frequently in children than in adults (19).
   c. **Outbreaks due to water contamination of municipal water plants** have occurred and affected normal and immunocompromised hosts (20).

2. **Clinical syndrome**. Patients with AIDS have a spectrum of disease ranging from asymptomatic carriage to fulminant, cholera-like diarrhea. Nausea, vomiting, weight loss, and fever can occur. Aggressive antiviral therapy may minimize the risk for developing cryptosporidiosis in AIDS patients (18). In the normal host, the onset of diarrhea may be abrupt, but the illness is usually self-limited and lasts from several days to 2 weeks (19).

3. **Diagnosis** can be made by showing the red-staining organisms on an acid-fast stained stool smear, or the more sensitive **direct immunofluorescence assay** (using a monoclonal antibody directed at the oocyst wall), an **ELISA antigen capture microtiter assay,** and **auramine staining** of formalin-treated concentrated stool specimens.

4. **Therapy**
   a. **In normal hosts**, no therapy is indicated; the disease is self-limited (19).

b. **In AIDS** patients, therapy is often not very effective. Paromomycin (25 to 35 mg/kg/day divided into three to four doses) is suggested (17). Optimal duration of therapy is unclear. High doses of oral azithromycin have been used (21). Consultation with someone experienced in treating AIDS patients is advised in refractory cases. Assuring optimal antiviral therapy may be beneficial in improving the host's overall response.

F. **Travelers' diarrhea** (1,22,23). Travelers' diarrhea affects 4% to 40% of U.S. visitors, depending on where they visit: 4% to low-risk countries (e.g., western Europe), 10% to 15% to intermediate-risk regions (e.g., northern Mediterranean countries, the Middle East, China, and Russia), and 40% to high-risk areas (e.g., most of Latin America, Africa, and southern Asia) (1).

1. **Etiology.** *E. coli* is the most common cause, with *Shigella* or *Salmonella* spp. next and *Campylobacter* and *Vibrio* spp. less commonly isolated when tested. More than 80% of cases are of bacterial origin (1).

2. **Clinical manifestations.** Diarrhea usually occurs in the first week after arrival in another country. Abdominal cramps, nausea, malaise, low-grade temperature, vomiting (in small minority) and at times blood in the stool. The duration of diarrhea, even without therapy, is usually 2 to 4 days.

3. **Prevention.** Careful choice of food and drink and other measures are reviewed elsewhere (22,23). Prophylactic antibiotics are not advised for most healthy travelers (1,22).

4. **Therapy.** Most international travelers to moderate- or high-risk areas usually are advised to carry a course of antibiotics (e.g., in adults, ciprofloxacin 500 mg bid for 3 days) and to take the antibiotic with over-the-counter loperamide when and if mild to moderate diarrhea develops. In children, TMP-SMZ is usually prescribed rather than the quinolone (Table 5.4).

   Patients with high fever or severe bloody diarrhea or persisting diarrhea after the preceding therapy should seek medical attention.

5. **If a returning international traveler has diarrhea** that does not respond to a 3-day empiric course of a quinolone, workup including stool for enteric culture and ova and parasite exam is appropriate.

References

1. DuPont HL, The Practice Parameters Committee of the American College of Gastroenterology. Guidelines on acute infectious diarrhea in adults. *Am J Gastroenterol* 1997;92:1962.

2. Blacklow NR, Greenberg HB. Viral gastroenteritis. *New Engl J Med* 1991;325:252.
   For a recent discussion see Kapikian AZ. Overview of viral gastro-enteritis. Arch Virol *1996;12:7 (suppl).*

3. Aucott JN, Ravdin JI. Amebiasis and "nonpathogenic" intestinal protozoa. *Infect Dis Clin North Am* 1993;7:467.
   For a related summary, see Li E, Stanley SL Jr. Amebiasis. Gastroenterol Clin North Am *1996;25:471.*

4. Healy GR, Garcia LS. Intestinal and urogenital protozoa. In: Murray PR, et al, eds. *Manual of clinical microbiology*, 6th ed. Washington, DC: ASM Press, 1995:Chap. 106.

5. Johnson S, Gerding D. *Clostridium difficile*-associated diarrhea. *Clin Infect Dis* 1998;26:1027.
   One of the "state-of-the-art" series.

6. Boland GW, et al. Antibiotic-induced diarrhea: specificity of abdominal CT for the diagnosis of *Clostridium difficile* disease. *Radiology* 1994;191:103.
   Retrospective review of 64 patients with C. difficile *diarrhea: 39% had normal CT scans; 17% had CT-specific diagnostic features of* C. difficile *disease such as nodular haustral thickening or the "accordion" pattern.*

7. Medical Letter. The choice of antibacterial drugs. *Med Lett Drugs Ther* 1999;41:95.

8. Committee on Infectious Diseases of the American Academy of Pediatrics. Peter G, et al, eds. *1997 Red Book*, 24th ed. Elk Grove, IL, 1997.
   See p. 178 for therapy of C. difficile *and p. 211 for therapy of* Giardia.

9. Leung DVM, et al. Treatment with intravenously administered gamma globulin of chronic relapsing colitis induced by *Clostridium difficile* toxin. *J Pediatr* 1991;118:633.
   Data suggest that a deficiency of IgG anti-toxin A may predispose children to the development of chronic relapsing C. difficile–*induced colitis.*

10. Salcedo J, et al. Intravenous immunoglobulin therapy for severe *Clostridium difficile* colitis. *Gut* 1997;41:366.

11. Tarr PI. *Escherichia coli* 0157:H7: clinical, diagnostic, and epidemiologic aspects of human infection. *Clin Infect Dis* 1995;20:1.
    An excellent summary.

12. Slutsker L, et al. A nationwide case-control study of *Escherichia coli* 0157:H7 infection in the United States. *J Infect Dis* 1998; 177:962.

13. Slutsker L, et al. *Escherichia coli* 0157:H7 diarrhea in the United States: clinical and epidemiologic features. *Ann Intern Med* 1997; 126:505.
    One-third of isolates came from nonbloody specimens. Person-to-person spread is not uncommon. For another review, see Mead PS, Griffin PM. Escherichia coli *0157:H7.* Lancet *1998;352:1207.*

14. Boyce TG, Swerdlow DL, Griffin PM. *Escherichia coli* 0157:H7 and the hemolytic uremic syndrome. *N Engl J Med* 1995;333:364.

15. Hill DR. Giardiasis: issues in diagnosis and management. *Infect Dis Clin North Am* 1993;7:503.
    A nice, concise clinical discussion. For a similar update, see Farthing JJ. Giardiasis. Gastroenterol Clin North Am *1996;25:493.*

16. Orega YR, Adam RD. *Giardia*: overview and update. *Clin Infect Dis* 1997;25:545.
17. Medical Letter. Drugs for parasitic infections. *Med Lett* 1998;40:1. *These tables are serially updated every 2 to 3 years.*
18. Manabe YC, et al. Cryptosporidiosis in patients with AIDS: correlates of disease and survival. *Clin Infect Dis* 1998;27:536.
19. Atkins JT, Caceres E. Cleary TG. Cryptosporidiosis, cyclospora infection, isosporiasis, and microsporidiosis. In: Feigin RD, Cherry JD, eds. *Textbook of pediatric infectious diseases*, 4th ed. Philadelphia: WB Saunders, 1998:Chap. 215.
20. Centers for Disease Control. Assessing the public health threat associated with waterborne cryptosporidiosis. Report of a Workshop. *MMWR* 1995;44(RR-6):1.
21. Dionisio D, et al. Chronic cryptosporidiosis in patients with AIDS: stable remission and possible eradication after long-term, low-dose azithromycin. *J Clin Pathol* 1998;51:138.
    See related report by Hicks P, et al. Azithromycin therapy for Cryptosporidium parvum *infection in four children infected with human immunodeficiency virus.* J Pediatr *1996;129:297.*
22. Centers for Disease Control. *Health Information for International Travel, 1999–2000.* Department of Health and Human Services, Atlanta, 1999.
23. Staat MA. Travelers' diarrhea. *Pediatr Infect Dis J* 1999;18:373.

6

Intraabdominal Infections

Intraabdominal infection should be considered in patients who present with abdominal pain, fever, abdominal tenderness, and leukocytosis. Antibiotic therapy often is started before a specific diagnosis is reached. At times, a lower lobe pneumonia may present with abdominal pain.

This chapter summarizes many areas, including the following:

Principles of antibiotic therapy in intraabdominal infection
Peritonitis
Intraabdominal abscess
Appendicitis
Diverticulitis
Biliary tract infections (cholecystitis, cholangitis) and
Pancreatitis

General Principles

I. **Introduction**
   A. **Initial evaluation** of the patient
      1. **Abdominal percussion tenderness** indicates diffuse or focal peritoneal inflammation.
      2. **A rectal (and pelvic) examination** should be performed on all patients with abdominal pain.
      3. **Signs are difficult to interpret in** patients at the extremes of age and those on corticosteroids.
      4. **Fever** may be modified by antipyretics, corticosteroids, and old age.
      5. **Leukocytosis** and a left shift are commonly but not always present.
      6. **Serial clinical evaluations and surgical evaluation are often important.**
   B. **Cultures**
      1. **Blood cultures** (two sets separated by 20 to 30 minutes) should be performed in febrile patients.
      2. **Peritoneal fluid cultures.** Adequate quantities of infected fluid (and/or tissue if the patient is operated on) should be cultured aerobically and anaerobically. Pus in a syringe is the best transport medium to maintain viability of bacteria. A swab only for culture is inadequate.
II. **Principles of antibiotic therapy of intraabdominal infections**. Empiric antibiotic therapy is often necessary (1,2).
   A. **Microbiologic features.** The infecting microorganisms are the normal microflora of the gastrointestinal (GI) tract.
      1. **Cultures** are polymicrobial, on average, two aerobes, and three anaerobes **(Table 6.1)**.

Table 6-1. Bacteriology of intraabdominal infections

	Frequency of Isolation (%)
Aerobes	
Escherichia coli	65
Proteus spp.	25
Klebsiella spp.	20
Pseudomonas spp.	15
Enterococci	15
Streptococcus spp.	10
(other than groups A or D)	
Anaerobes	
B. fragilis	80
Bacteroides spp. (other spp.)	30
Clostridium spp.	65
Peptostreptococcus spp.*	25
Peptococcus spp.*	15
Fusobacterium spp.	20

Source: From Gorbach SL. Treatment of intra-abdominal infections. *J Antimicrob Chemother* 1993;31:67(suppl. A), with permission.
* Sometimes grouped as anaerobic gram-positive cocci.

2. **Abscesses** are caused primarily by anaerobes in animal models.
3. **Enterococci.** Although enterococci may be isolated from peritoneal fluid cultures, they **usually can be cleared without using antibiotics active against enterococci** (2). **Specific antibiotic regimens aimed at enterococci** are rational in the following settings: (a) initial peritoneal cultures yielding enterococcus in pure culture or a predominance of gram-positive cocci in chains on the gram stain of peritoneal fluid; (b) enterococcus recovered repeatedly from peritoneal flora cultures in the absence of clinical improvement on nonenterococcal treatment; (c) an associated enterococcal bacteremia; (d) life-threatening intraabdominal infection/sepsis while awaiting cultures.
4. *Candida,* guidelines for therapy (2).
    a. When this is the sole isolate or is isolated from both peritoneal (or abscess) fluid and blood, or *Candida* invasion is seen histologically, antifungal therapy is essential.
    b. *Candida* isolated as one of several organisms after perforation of a viscus does not generally require antifungal therapy, especially if adequate drainage was achieved.
B. **Antibiotic therapy is directed at both aerobes and anaerobes.** If the infection has been present more than 48 hours, specific anaerobic antibiotics are indicated **(Table 6.2).**

**Table 6-2. Empiric antibiotics
in intraabdominal infection, including peritonitis**

Severity and Setting	Antibiotic Regimen in Adults (Assumes Normal Renal Function)
Community-acquired	
Mild–moderate	Cefazolin 1 g IV q8h plus metronidazole 500 mg IV q6h*, **or**
	Ampicillin-sulbactam 3 g IV q6h **or** piperacillin-tazobactam or ticarcillin-clavulanate, **or**
	Cefoxitin 2 g IV q6–8h
Severe	Ceftriaxone 1–2 g IV q24h plus metronidazole 500 mg IV q6h, **or**
	Piperacillin-tazobactam ± gentamicin**
Hospital-acquired***	Piperacillin-tazobactam plus an aminoglycoside, **or**
	Piperacillin plus metronidazole plus an aminoglycoside, **or**
	Imipenem plus an aminoglycoside
Oral regimens (after initial IV therapy)	Trimethoprim-sulfamethoxazole (1 DS bid) plus metronidazole 500 mg q6–8h* or clindamycin (300–450 mg tid), **or**
	Ciprofloxacin (500–750 mg bid) plus metronidazole or clindamycin, **or**
	Amoxicillin-clavulanate (Augmentin) 875 mg bid

* Most cost-effective regimen.
** If resistant gram-negatives are a concern, an aminoglycoside can be added.
*** Antibiotics can be adjusted once susceptibility data are available.

1. **For anaerobic activity** of established infection, clindamycin or metronidazole are commonly used options. Since metronidazole is associated with less *Clostridium difficile*–related diarrhea, is more consistently active against *Bacteroides fragilis* and is more cost-effective; **metronidazole** is preferred.
2. **For aerobic activity**
   a. **For community-acquired** infections, a first-generation cephalosporin is not only very effective but cost-effective (e.g., **cefazolin [combined with metronidazole]**) (**Table 6.2**).
   b. **For hospitalized-acquired infections** or seriously ill patients, a third-generation agent (e.g., ceftriaxone or cefotaxime) can be combined with an anaerobic agent. If resistant *Pseudomonas* or *Enterobacter* spp. are a concern, piperacillin and an aminoglycoside combination may be indicated (**Table 6.2**).

c. **Aminoglycoside use**
   (1) **Is not indicated** as initial therapy in **uncomplicated intraabdominal infection.** These agents may not penetrate abscesses well, are inactivated at the low pH within abscesses, and are potentially nephrotoxic (1).
   (2) **Is indicated** when resistant gram-negative bacilli are suspected. These include (a) broad-spectrum antibiotic use in the last 30 days; (b) isolation of cephalosporin-resistant gram-negative bacilli at initial abdominal cultures; (c) reoperation or recurrent infection within the past 4 to 8 weeks; (d) prolonged institutionalization preoperatively (Table 6.2).

3. **Monotherapy** for mild to moderately ill patients (with less well-established infections of less than 48 hours' duration) with community-acquired disease is effective but more expensive than cefazolin/metronidazole combination therapy.
   a. **Ampicillin-sulbactam (Unasyn)** is still commonly used in this setting; however, a significant percentage of community-acquired *Escherichia coli* **may be resistant**. Therefore other choices may be more appropriate (e.g., metronidazole and cefazolin).
   b. **Cefoxitin** alone is a satisfactory treatment, but expensive.
   c. **Piperacillin-tazobactam (Zosyn)** is more active *in vitro* than items a or b immediately preceding, is effective, and can be used as monotherapy.
   d. **Ticarcillin-clavulanate** (Timentin) has been used, especially in gynecologic infections.
   e. **Imipenem** is effective but less active at low pH. In addition, because of its broad spectrum of activity it **should be saved for complex intraabdominal infections** (e.g., nosocomial infections).
   f. **Trovofloxacin** is discussed in detail in Chap. 32. Given its potential side effects and alternative agents, we would favor alternative regimens.

Peritonitis

I. **General principles**. Peritonitis is a localized or general inflammation of the peritoneal cavity. This may be due to microorganisms or irritating chemicals (bile salts, gastric contents, etc). A common classification is shown in **Table 6.3.**

Table 6-3.   Classification of peritonitis

I. **Primary peritonitis**
   A. Spontaneous bacterial peritonitis
   B. Peritonitis in chronic ambulatory peritoneal dialysis (CAPD) patients
   C. Tuberculous peritonitis
II. **Secondary peritonitis**
   A. Acute perforation (with or without necrosis)
   B. Postoperative peritonitis (e.g., anastomotic leak)
   C. Posttraumatic peritonitis (e.g., after blunt or penetrating trauma)
III. **Tertiary peritonitis:** Peritonitis without evidence of a pathogen or due to fungi or low-grade pathogen
IV. **Intraabdominal abscess** with peritonitis
V. **Miscellaneous:** Granulomatous peritonitis, foreign-body peritonitis

Modified from Wittman DH, et al. Peritonitis and intraabdominal infection. In: Schwartz SI, et al, eds. *Principles of surgery,* 6th ed. New York: McGraw-Hill, 1994:1449, with permission.

A. **Clinical presentation**. A detailed history including questions regarding recent surgery, medical history of GI disease, recent travel, or recent accidents is important. Peritonitis typically presents with localized or generalized abdominal pain as the predominant symptom. **Percussion tenderness indicating peritoneal irritation or inflammation is a useful finding on abdominal exam.** Rigidity is commonly seen with early peritonitis but may be absent in peritonitis that progresses slowly or with chemical peritonitis. Associated symptoms might include nausea, vomiting, abdominal distention, intestinal paresis, fever, bacteremia and general toxemia.

B. **Laboratory.** May help, but the clinical history and exam are more important.
   1. **Blood tests.** The leukocyte count is usually elevated but nonspecific. Liver function tests and serum amylase and lipase may be useful in localizing the source of an intraabdominal infection.
   2. **X-rays.** A chest roentgenogram should be obtained to rule out any supradiaphragmatic process. Roentgenographic examination of the abdomen may reveal evidence of a perforation (air under the diaphragm), intestinal obstruction, or lower lobe atelectasis (N.B. Don't attribute a patient's postop fever and upper abdominal pain to pneumonia when, in fact, this is just postop atelectasis.) In general, computed tomography is not required in the initial workup of acute peritonitis unless intraabdominal abscess is a strong consideration.
   3. **Aspiration of peritoneal fluid** is indicated in the setting of ascites or when trauma with hem-

orrhage is a concern. Fluid should be examined for leukocytes (with a differential count), bacterial and fungal organisms, amylase, and so on, and sent for aerobic and anaerobic cultures. Laparoscopy may be considered in certain instances (e.g., trauma).

C. **Therapy.** The cause of the peritonitis should be found and eliminated.

1. **Supportive care** is always necessary (nasogastric suctioning, intravenous fluid).

2. **Surgical consultation is imperative.**

3. **Systemic antibiotics** are chosen to cover coliforms and anaerobes (Table 6.2). The optimal length of therapy is not well defined. In general, nonbacteremic patients are treated for 7 to 10 days with antibiotics, initially intravenously and then orally. Alternatively, one might also treat a patient until all systemic signs and symptoms have resolved, and fever has been absent for 48 to 72 hours. Bacteremic patients should receive a total of 14 days of intravenous and oral therapy to prevent infectious complications at metastatic sites.

II. **Spontaneous bacterial peritonitis** (SBP) (3,4). Patients with SBP do not have evidence of viscous rupture. SBP is most common in adults with cirrhosis or systemic lupus erythematosus. The most frequent organisms isolated are coliforms, with *E. coli* and *Klebsiella* spp. accounting for about 70% of infections.

A. **Clinical presentation**. It may be subtle; a **high index of suspicion** must be maintained.

1. **Clinical features. Ascites is uniformly present** but fever and abdominal pain are seen in only 60% to 80% of patients. **Worsening of hepatic encephalopathy** occurs in about 60% of patients. Clinical deterioration regardless of peritoneal signs should raise the diagnosis of SBP, especially in patients with cirrhosis and ascites.

B. **Laboratory. A peritoneal tap is the most useful diagnostic test. An absolute neutrophil count of greater than 250 cells/mm^3 indicates peritoneal infection.**

1. In approximately one-third of patients organisms will be seen on centrifuged fluid that is subsequently culture positive. If either gram-positive cocci or gram-negative rods are seen as single pathogen types on gram stain, the diagnosis of SBP is supported. (Mixed flora suggests another diagnosis–e.g., perforation.)

2. **Aerobic and anaerobic cultures of peritoneal fluid** should be obtained. To maximize results, 10 ml of fluid should be inoculated at the bedside in blood culture media, but some should be saved for direct plating. Up to one-

third of patients without prior antibiotics may have negative cultures, so-called culture-negative neutrocytic ascites (3).

3. **Blood cultures** are useful. They are positive in about one-third of patients with SBP (3). Urine cultures are also suggested since at times a UTI can be the source of a bacteremia (3).

C. **Therapy.** For definite or highly suspected SBP, intravenous antibiotics are indicated.

1. **Cefotaxime or ceftriaxone** is the drug of choice. In adult patients with normal renal function, 2 g q8h of cefotaxime or 1 to 2 g q24h of ceftriaxone.

2. **Aminoglycosides should be avoided** because their use is associated with excess nephrotoxicity in patients with underlying liver disease. (See Chap. 21.)

3. Other options include piperacillin-tazobactam or cefoxitin but not aztreonam alone (no activity against gram-positive organisms).

4. **A repeat paracentesis 48 hours** after initiation of antibiotic therapy is suggested to confirm decreased cell counts and sterilization of culture-positive cases.

5. **Duration** of antibiotics. Although conventional therapy has been 10 to 14 days intravenously, 5 to 7 days may be effective without relapse.

D. **Prognosis**. The mortality rate for SBP is 30% to 40%. After an initial episode of SBP, the probability of recurrence at 1 year is 70%, and recurrent episodes are associated with high mortality rates. **Prophylaxis** with TMP/SMZ or norfloxacin has been suggested to prevent recurrent episodes (4,5). This topic is reviewed in more detail in Chap. 15.

III. **Peritonitis as a complication of chronic ambulatory peritoneal dialysis (CAPD)**

A. **Clinical presentation.** Turbidity of the dialysate is often the earliest sign of infection and the only finding in one-fourth of cases. Patients may complain of abdominal pain, and have abdominal tenderness (often with rebound). Fever is present in few patients.

B. **Bacteriology**. Gram stains of the effluent generally are negative. Most patients have infection due to coagulase-negative staphylococci or *Staphylococcus aureus*; methicillin-resistant *S. aureus* is common. *Streptococci* spp. are isolated 10% to 15% of the time. Gram-negative bacteria occur in patients with recurrent episodes of infections. **Polymicrobial or anaerobes suggest bowel perforation**.

C. **Diagnosis. When the dialysate fluid contains 100 leukocytes/mm³, peritonitis is present.** Gram stains of the effluent are usually negative. The peritoneal effluent should be cultured. Blood cultures usually are negative.

D. **Therapy** is discussed in detail in a recent comprehensive review (6).
   1. **Intraperitoneal instillation of antibiotics** facilitates outpatient therapy **(Fig. 6.1)**.
   2. **Indications for catheter removal:** persisting peritonitis despite adequate therapy, fungal peritonitis, *Pseudomonas aeruginosa* peritonitis, and severe exit catheter site infection.
   3. **Intravenous antibiotics** that penetrate the peritoneal fluid may be the preferred route of administration by some clinicians or in certain settings. For example, while awaiting cultures, a single intravenous (IV) dose of an aminoglycoside and vancomycin could be used, if the catheter must be removed.

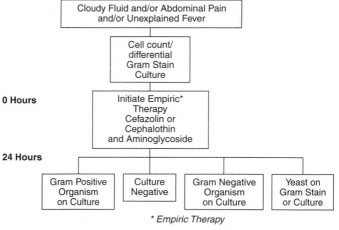

Agent	Continuous Dose	Intermittent Dose (in 1 exchange/day)	
		Residual urine output (mL/day)	
		Anuria (< 500)	Non-anuria (> 500)
cefazolin or cephalothin	500 mg/L load, then 125 mg/L in each exchange	500 mg/L (or 15 mg/kg)	increase dose by 25%
gentamicin netilmicin tobramycin	8 mg/L load, then 4 mg/L in each exchange	0.6 mg/kg body weight	1.5 mg/kg initial loading dose. See footnote for maintenance dose recommendations
amikacin	25 mg/L load, then 12 mg/L in each exchange	2 mg/kg body weight	5 mg/kg initial loading dose. See footnote for maintenance dose recommendations

Figure 6.1. Assessment and therapy. Patients with residual urine output may require 0.6 mg/kg body weight doses with increased dosing frequency based on serum and/or dialysate levels. (Source: Keane WF, et al. Peritoneal dialysis-related peritonitis treatment recommendations: 1996 update. *Perit Dial Int* 1996;16:557.)

Intraabdominal Abscesses

The onset of intraabdominal abscesses may be insidious and should be excluded in any febrile patients without an obvious cause of fever. This is especially true in those who have a potential predisposing cause, such as inflammatory bowel disease, diverticulitis, or history of abdominal surgery or trauma. Mortality with undrained hepatic, pancreatic, and retroperitoneal abscesses is reported to be 45% to 100%.

I. **General principles**
   A. **Etiology.** The GI lesions or events that typically predispose to secondary peritonitis and intraabdominal abscess include organ perforation, extension of preexisting infection, surgical procedures, blunt or penetrating abdominal trauma, or mesenteric ischemia.
   B. **Presentation.** Fever, chills, anorexia, and weight loss may occur. Some patients may have abdominal pain. **Unexplained fever may be the only sign of an intraabdominal abscess.**
   C. **Diagnosis. An abdominal computed tomography (CT) examination is the most efficient means of diagnosing an abscess.**
   D. **Therapy**
      1. **Drainage** is almost always required. Percutaneous needle aspiration and closed-catheter drainage, using CT and ultrasound guidance when technically feasible, is usually preferred to operative drainage (2).
      2. **Empiric antibiotics**
         a. Antibiotics directed at common GI flora **(Table 6.1)** are used primarily to prevent metastatic infection from bacteremia and to treat nondrainable cellulitis around the abscess **(Table 6.2).**
         b. **Duration.** The optimal duration of therapy for a drained abscess is not well defined. Antibiotics active against anaerobes as well as gram-negative aerobes should be continued until all systemic signs of sepsis have resolved and the patient's appetite and sense of well-being have returned. It is not necessary to continue antibiotic therapy simply because drains remain in place. After initial IV antibiotic therapy and clinical improvement, oral therapy can be used to complete a course of therapy of at least 10 days, after drainage, to ensure that contiguous soft-tissue cellulitis has been treated. In bacteremic patients, 14 days of therapy to prevent metastatic infections are suggested.
II. **Hepatic abscess.** Liver abscesses are uncommon and usually develop by local extension or metastatic infection (7). Recent reviews suggest that the **biliary tract disease**

(e.g., obstruction from stones, stricture, or tumors [e.g., pancreatic, cholangiocarcinoma]) **and cryptogenic sources**, with no obvious etiology, are the two most common causes. Bacterial hematogenous seeding (e.g., from another focal site of infection or endocarditis), trauma, or direct extension can occur.

A. **Clinical presentation**. The symptoms of hepatic abscess are **nonspecific** or secondary to the original pyogenic source. Fever, chills, anorexia, nausea, vomiting, and weight loss may be seen. Signs associated specifically with liver abscess may include an enlarged liver, right upper quadrant tenderness, jaundice, and findings in the chest, including pleural effusion.

B. **Diagnosis**
   1. Leukocytosis, **elevated alkaline phosphatase**, and other liver function tests are nonspecific but may be helpful in suggesting the diagnosis. A chest x-ray may suggest hepatic abscess by an elevation or paralysis of the right hemidiaphragm, or a right pleural effusion.
   2. **CT scanning is considered the procedure of choice** for diagnosis. Ultrasonography may be reasonable when gallbladder stones or common bile duct abnormalities are of particular concern.
   3. **Cultures. Blood cultures** are often positive but may not reflect the polymicrobial nature of the abscess. **Specimens obtained using CT or ultrasound guidance should be cultured aerobically and anaerobically.**
   4. **Amebic abscesses should be considered**, especially in young Hispanic men and international travelers. An amebic hemagglutination test on peripheral blood may be helpful. Organisms are not visualized in the aspirated material, which may have a characteristic anchovy color (dark-green).

C. **Therapy**. **Drainage is critical**. Consultation with a surgeon and radiologist is essential. Usually, ultrasound or CT-guided percutaneous catheter drainage is effective, although percutaneous needle aspirations can be done. Preliminary data suggest percutaneous catheter drainage may be preferable to percutaneous needle aspiration, but further study to define the optimal percutaneous drainage techniques is still needed (7). However, occasionally open drainage may be required, usually in the patient who has failed percutaneous drainage. **Antibiotics** are adjunctive. Initial empiric antibiotic therapy involves regimens aimed at mixed aerobic and anaerobic GI-biliary flora (Tables 6.1 and 6.2). Culture and susceptibility results ultimately direct appropriate antibiotic use. Antibiotics are given for **prolonged duration:** 1 to 2 months for a drained solitary abscess and longer therapy for multiple liver abscesses that cannot be drained. **Infectious disease consultation** is advised.

III. **Splenic bacterial abscesses** are rare and are due to metastatic infections associated with bacteremias, contiguous infection, embolic noninfectious events, trauma with subsequent infection of the hematoma, and immunodeficiency (8).

    A. **Clinical presentation** is often subtle. Fever, vague abdominal pain, and pain in the left upper quadrant and/or pleuritic pain may occur. Splenomegaly is seen in slightly more than one-half of patients but is even more common in the immunocompromised patients. Unexplained thrombocytosis in a septic intensive-care-unit (ICU) patient with persistent left pleural effusion is suggestive of splenic abscess.

    B. **Diagnosis.** Leukocytosis is usually seen but is nonspecific. Chest x-ray is surprisingly sensitive and shows abnormalities in 82% of patients. The findings include elevation of the left hemidiaphragm, left pleural effusion, left lower lobe infiltrate and mass effect in the left upper quadrant. Blood cultures may identify a pathogen in patients with bacteremia. **CT scanning is the procedure of choice.** This is superior to ultrasonography and gallium scanning.

    C. **Microbiologic.** Gram-positive aerobes (staphylococci and streptococci) are implicated in 30% of the cases: fungi, usually candida, in up to 25%; gram negatives (with bacteremia); and anaerobes, in about 20% of cases.

    D. **Treatment. Splenectomy is the treatment of choice** for pyogenic abscesses. Antibiotic therapy should be directed against the organisms cultured from the splenic abscess and blood. (N.B. The treatment of hepatosplenic candidiasis involves long-term systemic antifungal therapy.)

IV. **Retroperitoneal abscesses** are uncommon (9), but because of their insidious presentation mortality ranges from 25% to 45%. The most common causes of isolated retroperitoneal space abscess are renal infections and postoperative infections. Other causes include osteomyelitis of the spine with rupture into adjacent tissues, seeding of posttraumatic pelvic hematomas, acute cholecystitis, perforated appendicitis, diverticulitis, perforated colon carcinoma, ischiorectal abscess with penetration to the pelvic retroperitoneum, and a cryptogenic origin (9).

    A. **Clinical presentation.** This is usually **nonspecific** with nonlocalized abdominal pain and variable GI symptoms. The history of chills is seen in 20% of cases; **fever** is documented in nearly 80%. Abdominal tenderness is noted in the majority of cases (9).

    B. **Diagnosis.** Routine laboratory tests are not specific. Blood cultures may be positive in 25% of cases. *E. coli* and *Bacteroides* spp. are the most common isolates. **CT scanning is the most useful imaging test**. Aerobic and anaerobic cultures should be performed on percutaneous or surgical specimens.

    C. **Treatment.** Therapy involves drainage and intravenous antibiotics. Antibiotic coverage is based on clinical setting, blood, and drainage culture results. Aerobic and anaerobic cultures should be performed on percutaneous or surgical specimens. Infectious disease consultation is advised.

V. **Psoas abscesses** were formally synonymous with tuberculous disease of the spine or sacroiliac joint. In recent years most cases are a complication of intestinal disorders. **The psoas muscle is closely associated with and is subject to any uncontrolled infectious process of the ureters, renal pelvis, spine, appendix, and ascending colon**. In the United States the most common cause in adults of psoas abscess is **secondary to** an underlying intestinal disease, especially Crohn's disease, but also diverticulitis, osteomyelitis, and intraabdominal abscess. Primary staphylococcal psoas abscess occurs in less than 10% of adult psoas abscesses, but up to 75% of cases in children are primary staphylococcal abscesses (10). Organisms may enter the retrofascial space directly by extension from an adjacent infection. Primary psoas abscess is due to hematogenous spread of staphylococci with predisposing trauma in at least some patients.

A. **Clinical presentation**
   1. **In adults,** the symptoms often are **nonspecific**. There may be pain in the iliac fossa, groin, or hip and tenderness of the iliac fossa. The patient may complain of a limp and frequently lies with the hip flexed. Weight loss is common. Findings include a positive psoas sign (pain on extension and elevation of the leg). This is common, especially if there is underlying Crohn's disease. Fever and leukocytosis may not be present. Psoas abscess rarely occurs in the elderly.
   2. **In children,** presentation is similar to adults. Often there is a history of trauma. Usually, there is no discomfort on flexion or rotation of the hip.
B. **Diagnosis. CT and ultrasound** are the most accurate test for diagnosis, though neither reliably differentiates abscess from hematoma or neoplasm. Clinical correlation and **ultrasound or CT-guided aspiration with culture is useful diagnostically and therapeutically.**
C. **Treatment. Drainage is necessary**. An open surgical procedure is required if the source is gastrointestinal. A primary psoas abscess responds well to percutaneous drainage. For known or highly suspected primary abscesses, antibiotics aimed at *S. aureus* are used (e.g., nafcillin, first-generation cephalosporin, vancomycin, etc). For a secondary abscess, broad-spectrum antibiotics for the underlying condition can be used until specific culture results are available. Prognosis is generally good for primary psoas abscess; secondary psoas abscesses have been associated with a mortality in the range of 15% to 20% because of delayed or inadequate therapy.
VI. **Pancreatic abscess** is discussed later in this chapter.

Appendicitis

I. **Pathogenesis.** Obstruction is one of the major mechanisms that predisposes the appendiceal wall to bacterial invasion by intraluminal bacteria; fecaliths, enlarged lymphatic follicles, tumors, inspissated barium, and other foreign bodies such as worms all occur. Distention of the appendix leads to impairment of blood supply to the mucosal lining, and bacterial invasion of deeper tissues occurs. Ultimately, tissue infarction can occur, with the potential for perforation at the antimesenteric border (11).

II. **Microbiology. Bacterial cultures** reveal **polymicrobial** involvement. *Bacteroides fragilis* and *E. coli* are almost universally isolated. *Pseudomonas* spp. are commonly isolated, but their significance in this setting is unclear (11).

III. **Clinical presentation** and differential diagnoses are beyond the scope of this handbook. Diagnosis is primarily on clinical grounds, although ultrasonography has been used to complement the clinical evaluation and has helped reduce the rate of unnecessary and delayed operations. CT scanning may be used in special circumstances. Surgical consultation is essential.

IV. **Complications. The major complication of appendicitis is appendiceal rupture and then focal or diffuse peritonitis or abscess formation.** Particularly at risk are the **pediatric** and **geriatric** populations; their presentation may be atypical or difficult to access. In the elderly, fever and leukocytosis may be blunted, and signs and symptoms may be subtle. Therefore diagnosis is delayed, raising the risk for rupture. Consequently, appendicitis is a more serious illness with higher morbidity and mortality rates in these age groups.

V. **Therapy**

    A. **Surgical intervention is routinely indicated.** Antibiotics alone should not be used to delay surgery or substitute for surgery.

    B. **Antibiotics**.

        1. **For acute appendicitis without rupture** (11) a single dose or 1 to 3 doses of antibiotics to prevent wound infection are typically recommended (e.g., in adults, a single dose of cefoxitin [2 g] or three doses IV at q6 to 8h). A more cost-effective regimen would be cefazolin and metronidazole.

        2. **For appendiceal rupture with local peritonitis**, the optimal duration of antibiotic therapy is unclear. It seems prudent to treat the patient until the temperature is normal for 48 to 72 hours and there is clinical improvement. Oral antibiotics can be used to complete the course to avoid prolongation of hospitalization. Antibiotic options would include those discussed under the topics of peritonitis and diverticulitis (**Tables 6.2 and 6.4**).

Table 6-4. Therapy for diverticulitis (normal renal function)

Severity	Preferred Regimen	Alternative
Mild	Oral TMP-SMZ (1 DS bid) and metronidazole (500 mg q6–8h)*	(1) Oral TMP-SMZ and clindamycin 300 mg po tid; **or** (2) Ciprofloxacin 500–750 mg po bid plus metronidazole 500 mg po q6–8h or clindamycin 300 mg po tid; **or** (3) Amoxicillin-clavulanate (Augmentin) 875 mg po bid
Moderate to severe	Cefazolin (1 g q8h IV) and metronidazole 500 mg q6h or 1 g q12h IV	(1) Piperacillin-tazobactam +/– an aminoglycoside**; **or** (2) Ceftriaxone (1 g IV q24h) plus metronidazole (500 mg IV q6h) or clindamycin 600 mg IV q8h; **or** (3) Cefoxitin 2 g*** IV q6–8h; **or** (4) Clindamycin and an aminoglycoside

* Most cost-effective regimen.
** When resistant gram-negative pathogens are a concern.
*** We would not use cefoxitin alone in a very ill patient.
For other options, see Table 6-2.

Diverticulitis

Diverticulosis and diverticular disease usually refer simply to the presence of uninflamed diverticula, herniations of the mucosa through weak portions of the colonic wall. This condition is very common in Western society and affects at least 5% to 10% of the population more than 45 years of age, 60% of those older than 70, and almost 80% of those more than 85 (12,13).

I. **Pathogenesis**. The cause of colonic diverticula is related primarily to two factors: increased luminal pressure and weakening of the bowel wall (13).

A. **Elevated colonic pressure**. Diminished stool bulk, from insufficient dietary fiber, leads to alterations in GI transit time and to elevated colonic pressure. Patients who receive fiber supplementation frequently note relief of pain, nausea, vomiting, and flatulence (13).

B. **Bowel wall weakening.** Hypersegmentation and intracolonic pressure cause herniation of the colonic mucosa at inherent weak spots of the colonic wall (e.g., where branches of the marginal artery penetrate the colonic tunica muscularis) (12,13).

C. **Diverticulitis.** Particles of undigested food may become inspissated within diverticula. Obstruction of the neck of a diverticulum then sets the stage for distention as a result of mucous secretion and overgrowth of normal colonic bacteria (13). Diverticulitis results from a **perforation** in the fundus of the diverticulum, which produces **pericolic inflammation** (12).

II. **Diagnostic considerations**

A. **Signs and symptoms. Left lower quadrant abdominal pain and percussion tenderness** in the setting of **fever** and **leukocytosis** are highly suggestive, especially with a history of prior diverticulitis or known diverticula (12,13).

1. Abdominal complaints may be minimal in the elderly and in those on corticosteroids.

2. **GI bleeding is usually not seen**, though trace blood in the stool may be present (13).

3. Occasionally, a tender mass is present on palpation of the left lower quadrant.

4. Right-sided diverticulitis can occur and is seen more often in Asians (13).

5. The white blood cell and sedimentation rates may be elevated, but not always.

B. **CT scanning** has recently **become the radiographic test of choice, especially if** the clinical diagnosis is not clear; the patient has a palpable abdominal mass; the patient is on corticosteroids, making the physical exam unreliable; a complication is suspected; or the patient is not responding to medical care (12,13).

C. **Plain abdominal films** may be useful to exclude extracolonic air in an abscess or evidence of colonic obstruction or perforation.

D. A water-soluble contrast enema can be a safe and useful adjunct in patients with suspected mild to moderate diverticulitis, but contrast studies have been supplanted by CT (13).

E. Ultrasound is advocated by some but is operator dependent, and abdominal tenderness may preclude the use of the requisite amount of external pressure needed to perform the test (13).

F. **Endoscopy.** Uncomplicated diverticulitis is usually considered a **contraindication** to colonoscopy or flexible sigmoidoscopy because of the risk of perforation with the procedure. However, it may be indicated when the diagnosis remains in doubt (e.g., bleeding, possible ischemic bowel, carcinoma, or Crohn's disease).

III. **Therapy**

A. **The mildest cases** of acute diverticulitis can be handled on an **outpatient basis**. Typically, these involve patients with recurrent mild symptoms.

1. **Clear liquid diets** are suggested until symptoms improve.

2. **Oral antibiotics** are useful (Table 6.4). A 7 to 10 day course is often effective.

3. A high-fiber diet and colonoscopy, to exclude a diagnosis of cancer, is advised once the acute attack has resolved (13).

B. **Moderately to severely ill patients are hospitalized** to provide GI rest (nothing by mouth for 48 to 72 hours) and intravenous fluids. **Nasogastric suctioning** is used if the patient is vomiting or has abdominal distention or obstruction. Severe pain may require meperidine. (Morphine should be avoided.)

1. **Antibiotics** are aimed at mixed aerobic and anaerobic abdominal flora **(Table 6.4).** The optimal duration of intravenous antibiotics must be individualized and is often approximately 5 to 7 days of IV antibiotics with additional oral therapy often to complete a total of 10 to 14 days of antibiotics.

2. **Improvement should occur in 48 to 72 hours. Failure to improve** or worsening in this initial period of maximal medical therapy **is an indication for possible surgical intervention.** To determine whether an abscess is present, a CT scan is suggested for the patient who does not improve.

3. **Indications for surgery** include failure to improve with medical therapy, clinical deterioration despite medical therapy, complications of uncontrolled abscess-related sepsis, fistula, obstruction, and recurrent disease. Frequently, surgery is recommended early for patients younger than 40 years of age with severe disease, although this has recently been debated (13); for immunocompromised patients; and for those with presumed right-sided diverticulitis.

A detailed discussion of surgical considerations has recently been reviewed (13).

Biliary Tract Infections

I. **Introduction**
A. **Anatomic considerations.** The gallbladder lies in a fossa on the undersurface of the liver and in close proximity to the duodenum, pylorus, hepatic flexure, and right kidney. Therefore, diseases of these adjacent organs may clinically mimic some diseases of the gallbladder-biliary system.

B. **Microbiologic features.** The biliary tract of healthy people usually does not harbor bacteria. When obstructed, the biliary tract organisms mimic intestinal flora, except that anaerobic flora are present in far lower concentrations. Although enterococci may be isolated in mixed infections, as with peritonitis, **routine therapy aimed at enterococci in the mild to moderately ill patient is not necessary unless blood cultures reveal enterococci.** In a patient very ill with biliary infection/sepsis, some experts will cover for enterococci at least while awaiting culture data.

II. **Acute cholecystitis (14)**

  A. **Pathogenesis.** Acute cholecystitis **involves** the formation of **calculi** that are associated with inflammation of the gallbladder in 85% to 95% of cases. An impacted stone leads to obstruction of the cystic duct, with an increase in mucosal pressure and subsequent distention of the gallbladder, edema, impairment of venous return, ischemia, and ultimately perforation.

  B. **Clinical presentation.** Acute onset of **right upper quadrant abdominal pain**, nausea, vomiting, and **fever** are the most frequently presenting symptoms. **Right upper abdominal tenderness**, fever, leukocytosis, and **elevated liver function tests (obstructive pattern)** occur when the bile duct is obstructed.

  C. **Diagnosis.** Abdominal **ultrasound** is usually the **preferred initial study**. Cholescintigraphy (HIDA) is reserved for patients with an equivocal ultrasound.

  D. **Therapy**

  1. Initial therapy is conservative, consisting of intravenous fluids, nothing by mouth, parenteral analgesics, and antibiotics aimed primarily at gram-negative bacteria with specific anaerobic coverage only in the critically ill with sepsis or possibly for the elderly. Enterococcal coverage is indicated for the septic or very ill patient. (See Sec. I.B and **Table 6.2.**)

  2. Cholecystectomy remains the treatment of choice for patients with acute cholecystitis. The timing of this and the potential role of laparoscopy cholecystectomy are individualized, and surgical consultation is essential.

III. **Acute acalculous cholecystitis (15).** Acute inflammation of the gallbladder can occur **without stones. Persons at risk include debilitated hospitalized patients**, especially those who are **critically ill** and those who have had **major** nonbiliary **surgery**, trauma, burns, sepsis, or prolonged ICU stay. The etiology is unclear but may involve bile stasis, gallbladder ischemia, or cholecystoparesis.

  A. **Clinical** symptoms and findings are similar to those of calculous cholecystitis but are **often nonspecific** (15).

  B. **Diagnosis** can be difficult and the best imaging procedure is unclear. In a recent report, morphine cholescintigraphy had the highest sensitivity (9 of 10, 90%), followed by CT (8 of 12, 67%), and ultrasound (2 of 7, 29%) (15). Multiple studies in a patient may be necessary to clarify the diagnosis. **Surgical consultation is advised.** To improve morbidity and mortality, a **high index of suspicion** is necessary (15).

  C. **Therapy**

  1. Urgent open cholecystectomy or cholecystostomy is needed.

  2. **Broad-spectrum antibiotics** as per Table 6.2, under hospital-acquired infection.

D. **Prognosis.** High mortality rates are common in these debilitated patients in whom the diagnosis is often delayed. In a recent report, the mortality rate was more than 40% (15).

IV. **Acute cholangitis (acute biliary sepsis)** occurs because of infection of the biliary system. It is a **serious and potentially lethal** disorder requiring prompt recognition and treatment (14,16).

A. **Etiology.** The **most common cause** of acute cholangitis in the United States is **obstruction and infection associated with stones in the common duct.** Malignant obstruction of the bile duct due to pancreatic cancer, cholangiocarcinoma, cancer of the papilla of Vater, or portahepatic metastases occasionally mimics stone disease. Rarely, *Ascaris lumbricoides* infection causes obstruction. The exact site of origin of the bacteria is not well known. Bacteria that are detected may enter the bile duct from the GI tract (blood and lymphatics), especially when obstruction is present.

B. **Clinical presentation.** Right upper quadrant abdominal **pain, fever,** and **jaundice** are common. All three signs (so-called Charcot's triad) occur in only 50% to 60% of patients. **Septic shock** and obtundation are **common**, especially if therapy is delayed.

C. **Diagnosis**
   1. **Leukocytosis** and **elevated liver function tests** are common but not specific.
   2. **Blood cultures** should be drawn.
   3. **CT scanning** may detect stones or define the level of obstruction if secondary to tumor. **Ultrasonography** is useful in differentiating extrahepatic obstruction from intrahepatic cholestasis. The detection rate for choledocholithiasis with ultrasound is poor.

D. **Therapy**
   1. **Supportive care is essential**, including nothing by mouth, intravenous fluids, and evaluation and treatment of sepsis.
   2. **Antibiotics.** See **Table 6.2.**
   3. **Surgical or GI consultation for biliary decompression** is advised. Although approximately 85% to 90% of patients will respond to antibiotics and supportive care alone, endoscopic stone removal reduces complications and shortens the course of illness (14). Those who fail to respond or who deteriorate on medical therapy may require urgent bile duct decompression.

V. **Post–endoscopic retrograde cholangiopancreatography (ERCP) cholangitis** may occur secondary to introduction of bacteria along with contrast media. For patients, especially those already hospitalized, who have had recent ERCP, therapy directed at *P. aeruginosa* and other nosocomial pathogens may be warranted (e.g., piperacillin [or ceftazidime]) and an aminoglycoside.

Pancreatitis

Acute pancreatitis is often a sterile inflammatory process caused by autodigestion of the pancreas. A detailed description of the clinical presentation and criteria of severity are reviewed elsewhere (17–19). **This discussion emphasizes the infectious complications of pancreatitis.** The diagnosis of pancreatitis is reasonably common, especially since the availability of CT scanning. The infectious complications of pancreatitis are serious, yet a concise discussion of them is often not readily available. Therefore we will devote several pages to this important complex topic.

I.   **Etiology. The etiology** of a specific attack is important to help prevent recurrences and possible complications. Etiologies include **alcohol, gallstones, hypertriglyceridemia** (usually >1,000 mg/dl), **abdominal trauma, operations** (upper abdominal, renal, or cardiovascular surgery), **hypercalcemia, pregnancy, pancreatic cancer, tumors of the ampula, post-ERCP, infections** (mumps, rubella, Epstein-Barr virus, cytomegalovirus, coxsackie B, hepatitis (A, B, C), parasites, mycoplasma pneumonia), **drugs**, and systemic **vasculitis**.

II. **Clinical manifestations**

    A.   **Signs and symptoms** include fever, abdominal (e.g., diffuse upper, LUQ, or "boring") and back pain, nausea and vomiting, dyspnea, abdominal tenderness and/or distention, and tachycardia. A sepsislike picture can occur (i.e., a systemic inflammatory response syndrome [SIRS], as described in Chap. 7).

    B.   **Laboratory.** Leukocytosis, elevated serum amylase and/or lipase, abnormal liver function tests, elevated C-reactive protein, pleural effusion on chest x-ray, and small bowel sentinel loop on abdominal flat plate can be seen. **Abdominal CT is the most useful diagnostic test**, for it will help evaluate stones, biliary duct dilation, and the extent of pancreatic inflammation and necrosis (Sec. IV).

III. **Overview of severity.** Approximately **20%** of patients have **severe** pancreatitis with sterile or infected pancreatic or peripancreatic necrosis or pancreatic fluid collections (19). Necrosis of either the duct system or the pancreatic parenchyma is the initiating event in most of the complications of acute pancreatitis and many occur in the absence of bacteria.

    A.   Approximately 10% of the total group have extensive necrosis (greater than 10% to 15% of the gland) and, of these, nearly 50% will become infected (19).

    B.   **The more extensive the necrosis, the higher the risk of infection.** Overall, infections occur in about 5%, but these infections are responsible for 80% of all deaths from pancreatitis. The incidence of infection increases over the first 3 weeks and peaks during the third and fourth week of the illness (19).

IV. **Diagnosis of pancreatic infection.** It may be difficult to determine clinically whether the patient has a superimposed infection, given that leukocytosis and fever are seen with sterile pancreatic necrosis. Also, 50% of patients with infection may not show clinical signs of an active infection. The **CT scan with vascular enhancement is the most useful study for predicting who is at risk for the development of infection.** **Poorly enhanced pancreatic tissue** is shown **by dynamic contrast-enhanced CT and correlates well with** the presence of **pancreatic necrosis.** Between 40% and 70% of those with more than 30% necrosis will become infected (19). **Gas bubbles** seen in the region of the pancreas on CT scan may be **presumed** to result from **infection.**

CT scan–guided aspirations of necrotic pancreatic tissue for gram stains and for aerobic and anaerobic cultures will clarify whether infections actually exist. Commonly isolated organisms include *E. coli, Klebsiella* spp., and other Enterobacteriaceae, anaerobes (in a minority of patients but less well studied), enterococci, and *Pseudomonas* spp. in some patients. The mechanism by which colonic bacteria arrive at the injured pancreatic tissues is unclear and appears to be a secondary phenomenon.

V. **Therapy**
   A. **Prophylactic antibiotics.** The data are **still unclear regarding whether routine early prophylactic antibiotics can prevent later infectious complications.** If prophylactic antibiotics are to be useful in pancreatitis, they should be used at an early stage of tissue damage in the more severe cases before secondary infection has developed. We feel antibiotics are indicated if the precipitating event is stone disease; otherwise, the data are uncertain.
      1. **Pancreatic penetration** of antibiotics (20). Aminoglycosides typically do not penetrate pancreatic tissue. Piperacillin, cefotaxime, ceftizoxime, and the fluoroquinolones penetrate pancreatic tissue well and are active against many gram-negative bacteria but not against anaerobes (except the newer fluoroquinolone, trovofloxacin, which was not available for study by this group). Only piperacillin is active against enterococci. Metronidazole shows good penetration into pancreatic tissue, is active against anaerobes, and is an appealing agent to combine with an antibiotic effective against a gram-negative bacteria.
      2. **Imipenem** penetrates pancreatic tissue well and is active against common aerobic and anaerobic isolates. In a randomized multicenter trial in Italy of antibiotic prophylaxis in severe necrotizing pancreatitis, imipenem prophylaxis was associated with a lower incidence of pancreatic-related sepsis than the placebo group (21). Although this report is exciting, patients with severe necrotizing pancreatitis and infectious complications are prone to have protracted courses and may acquire infections due to resistant bacteria. Therefore, at this point it seems prudent to save a very broad-

spectrum antibiotic such as imipenem for later use in high-risk infected patients.

3. **At this point we suggest a compromise approach:** Use a **third-generation cephalosporin and metronidazole** or an extended penicillin-betalactamase inhibitor (e.g., piperacillin-tazobactam) for prophylaxis **in severe cases** of necrotizing pancreatitis. We do not use prophylactic antibiotics in mild pancreatitis. The duration of therapy is not well defined, but 7 to 10 days seems rational. We save imipenem for future infectious complications. Patients with biliary obstruction–related pancreatitis may provide a particularly good setting in which to use prophylactic antibiotics, but whether these patients benefit more is unclear.

4. We agree with the conclusion of a recent review: A prospective, randomized double-blind multicenter trial of antibiotics, alone or in combination, is really indicated before definitive recommendations can be made about the precise role of prophylactic antibiotics in severe acute pancreatitis (22).

B. **Surgical intervention. When infection occurs, surgical intervention is indicated. Serial surgical evaluation is essential in the management of patients with severe acute pancreatitis, and these patients ideally should be managed on the surgical service.** Aggressive surgical debridement, often requiring serial procedures with open drainage in selected patients with extensive pancreatic and peripancreatic necrosis, is advised (19). Serial CT scanning with vascular enhancement is helpful to assess the progression/status of an individual patient. Large fluid collections, seen on CT, which lack a wall of granulation of fibrous tissue and therefore are not pseudocysts can occur early in the course of acute pancreatitis (days or weeks). Since more than 50% of these collections will disappear spontaneously, aspirating these before 4 to 6 weeks is unnecessary (19). (See the related discussion under Sec. VI.C.)

C. **Fluid resuscitation** is important. Monitoring with a Swan-Ganz catheter often is essential in the care of the severely ill patient (19).

VI. **Infectious complications**

A. **Infected pancreatic necrosis** is discussed earlier. This is a more common problem than true pancreatic abscess or infected pseudocyst.

B. **Pancreatic abscess.** A true pancreatic abscess is a **collection of pus and necrotic pancreatic tissue surrounded by a capsule.** This either occurs within the pancreatic parenchyma or expands into the lesser sac and retroperitoneum. Although the incidence ranges from 2% to 5%, pancreatic abscesses are an important cause of death. Acute necrotizing pancreatitis is the most common antecedent event leading to abscess formation; the more extensive the necrosis, the higher the risk of abscess formation (23).

1. **Clinical presentation** (23). Pancreatic abscess **should be suspected** in acute or resolving pancreatitis with **fever** (>2 weeks) **or recurrent persistent fever**, abdominal pain, and leukocytosis (especially 3 to 4 weeks after onset). Initially, there may be clinical improvement followed by clinical deterioration. Hypocalcemia (<6.0) or worsening renal function (creatinine >3) suggest a worse outcome.

2. **Diagnosis. CT scanning is the best method to demonstrate an abscess.** (See Sec. IV.) Presence of air within fluid collections or within the pancreas itself is strongly suggestive of a pancreatic abscess. Gas is seen in 20% to 90% of abscesses on CT, usually from gas-forming organisms (gram-negative or anaerobic bacteria) (23). Retroperitoneal gas or air within peripancreatic fluid collections may also be seen in uninfected patients who develop a fistulous tract.

   CT-guided percutaneous thin-needle aspiration and culture of the fluid will clarify the diagnosis. Aerobic and anaerobic cultures should be performed. Common isolates include Enterobacteriaceae, streptococci, including enterococci, staphylococci, *Bacteroides* spp.; the majority of cultures are polymicrobial (23). Blood cultures may be positive but are not diagnostic of abscess or its contents.

3. **Therapy**
   a. **Surgical drainage is essential** for true pancreatic abscess. There is a confirmed near 100% death rate if surgical drainage is not performed (23). The optimal surgical approach remains controversial but includes percutaneous catheter drainage and open surgical drainage. The open surgical approach is indicated if the abscess is thick, if rapid improvement does not occur after percutaneous drainage, or if there is CT evidence of considerable surrounding tissue necrosis.
   b. **Nutrition support** with enteral or total parenteral support is favored.
   c. **Antibiotics** are used in conjunction with surgical drainage. The antibiotics should be selected on the basis of susceptibility testing against any organism cultured from blood or abscess cavity at the time of surgery or from prior aspiration. In the absence of culture data, empiric therapy should be instituted as outlined previously. Infectious disease consultation is advised.

C. **Pancreatic pseudocysts.** The term *pancreatic pseudocyst* has been used to refer to all intrapancreatic and peripancreatic fluid collections, usually within a non-epithelialized capsule arising in the setting of acute or chronic pancreatitis (23). Once a fluid collection is diagnosed, it is important to define the functional behavior of the fluid collection, such as a change in size or the development of signs of infection. These characteristics will define appropriate therapy. Presumably, pseudocysts develop as a result of the disruption of the pancreatic ductal system with subsequent leakage of activated pancreatic enzymes leading to necrosis of the gland and surrounding tissue accompanied by the production of larger volumes of exudate (23).

1. **Clinical presentation.** Abdominal pain, nausea or vomiting, weight loss, palpable abdominal mass, jaundice, and abdominal tenderness can be seen. Approximately 50% of cysts are not palpable, and up to 50% of palpable masses in patients with pancreatitis represent inflammation and edema of the pancreas versus pseudocysts. Routine laboratory tests are nondiagnostic.

2. **Diagnosis. CT scanning** is the most accurate imaging technique but does not differentiate between a sterile and an infected fluid collection. Approximately 8% to 43% of pseudocysts undergo spontaneous resolution, usually within 6 weeks after onset. Therefore, **it is suggested that drainage procedures be postponed until the pseudocyst persists for more than 6 weeks or a complication arises** (23). Some suggest prolonged observation in the absence of symptoms.

3. **Complications.** Complications of pancreatic pseudocyst include obstructive jaundice and chemical pancreatitis with acute rupture of the pseudocysts. Pancreatic ascites can occur with a slow leak into the peritoneal cavity, hemorrhage within the cyst or secondary to cyst erosion into a major artery, or perforation into the GI tract. Secondary cyst infection can occur (23).

D. **Infected pancreatic pseudocyst.** Although uncommon (23), secondary infection presumably results from hematogenous seeding, direct transmural passage of bacteria from an adjacent bowel, and possible bacterial seeding after ERCP.

1. **Diagnosis. Persisting fevers**, abdominal pain, and an abdominal mass in a patient with a known pseudocyst may suggest the diagnosis. However, no data exist on the unique features of patients with infected pancreatic pseudocysts. CT scanning will demonstrate whether a pseudocyst exists. **CT-guided or ultrasound-guided percutaneous needle aspiration with aerobic or anaerobic cultures will clarify whether the fluid is infected.** Polymicrobial infection with enteric gram-negative and/or gram-positive organisms is isolated.

2. **Therapy.** It is critically important for therapy to differentiate an infected pseudocyst from a pancreatic abscess. An infected pseudocyst can be effectively treated by drainage alone (e.g., percutaneous catheter drainage), but an abscess requires open drainage and extensive debridement (23). Infectious disease and surgical consultations are essential.

References

1. Gorbach SL. Intra-abdominal infections. *Clin Infect Dis* 1993; 17:961.
   State-of-the-art clinical series and still a nice summary.
2. McClean KI, et al. Intraabdominal infection: a review. *Clin Infect Dis* 1994;19:100.
3. Bhuva M, Ganger D, Jensen, D. Spontaneous bacterial peritonitis: an update on evaluation, management, and prevention. *Am J Med* 1994;97:169.
4. Gilbert JA, Kamath PS. Spontaneous bacterial peritonitis: an update. *Mayo Clin Proc* 1995;70:365.
5. Singh N, et al. Trimethoprim-sulfamethoxazole for the prevention of spontaneous bacterial peritonitis in cirrhosis: a randomized trial. *Ann Intern Med* 1995;122:595.
   Patients were given 1 DS tablet qd, Monday to Friday. For an update see editorial by P Gines and M Navasa. Antibiotic prophylaxis for spontaneous bacterial peritonitis: how and whom? J Hepatol *1998;29:490. This topic is discussed in Chap. 15.*
6. Keane WF, et al. Peritoneal dialysis-related peritonitis treatment recommendations: 1996 update. *Perit Dial Int* 1996;16:557.
   These recommendations are serially updated every 3 to 5 years.
7. Seeto R, Rockey DC. Pyogenic liver abscess: changes in etiology, management, and outcome. *Medicine* 1996;75:99.
   Report of 142 patients from San Francisco Hospital from 1979–1994. For a related report see CJ Huang et al. Pyogenic hepatic abscess: changing trends over 42 years. Ann Surg *1996;223:600.*
8. Allan JD. Splenic abscess: Pathogenesis, clinical features, diagnosis, and treatment. *Curr Clin Top Infect Dis* 1994;14:23.
9. Crepps JT, Welch JP, Orlando R III. Management and outcome of retroperitoneal abscesses. *Ann Surg* 1987;205:276.
   Although a few years old, reviews 50 cases and the importance of their insidious presentation, CT studies, and drainage options.
10. Bresee JS, Edwards MS. Psoas abscess in children. *Pediatr Infect Dis J* 1990;2:201.
11. Schwartz SI. Appendix. In: Schwartz SI, et al, eds. *Principles of surgery*, 6th ed. New York: McGraw-Hill. 1994.
12. Freeman SR, McNally PR. Diverticulitis. *Med Clin North Am* 1993;77:1149.
13. Ferzocs LB, Raptopoulos V, Silen, W. Acute diverticulitis. *N Engl J Med* 1998;338:1521.
    Nice review with concise discussion of current surgical options.
14. Kadaskia SC. Biliary tract emergencies: acute cholecystitis, acute cholangitis, and acute pancreatitis. *Med Clin North Am* 1993; 77:1015.

15. Kalliafas S, et al. Acute acalculous cholecystitis: incidence, risk factors, diagnosis, and outcome. *Am Surg* 1998;64:471.
16. Hanau LH, Steigbigel NH. Cholangitis: pathogenesis, diagnosis, and treatment. *Curr Clin Top Infect Dis* 1995;15:153.
17. Tenner S, Banks PA. Acute pancreatitis: nonsurgical management. *World J Surg* 1997;21:143.
18. Steinberg W, Tenner S. Acute pancreatitis. *N Engl J Med* 1994; 330:1198.
    See recent update Bakon TH, Morgan DE. Acute necrotizing pancreatitis. N Engl J Med *1999;340:1412.*
19. Frey CF. Management of necrotizing pancreatitis. *West J Med* 1993;159:675.
20. Buchler H, et al. Human pancreatic tissue concentration of bactericidal antibiotics. *Gastroenterology* 1992;103:1902.
    Human pancreatic tissue concentrations of 10 different antibiotics were determined in patients undergoing pancreatic surgery.
    See a related paper by Powell JJ, Miles R, Siriwardena AK. Antibiotic prophylaxis in the initial management of severe acute pancreatitis. Br J Surg *1998;85:582, which reviews experimental and clinical literature from 1990 to 1997.*
21. Pederzoli P, et al. A randomized multicenter clinical trial of antibiotic prophylaxis of septic complications in acute necrotizing pancreatitis with imipenem. *Surg Gynecol Obstet* 1993;178:480.
    Interesting report from University of Verona, Italy, from six Italian centers. Data, to our knowledge, have not been confirmed by other investigators.
22. Ho HS, Frey C. The role of antibiotic prophylaxis in acute pancreatitis. *Arch Surg* 1997;132:467.
23. Witt MD, Edwards JE Jr. Pancreatic abscess and infected pancreatic pseudocyst: diagnosis and treatment. *Curr Clin Top Infect Dis* 1992;12:111.

Sepsis

Current estimates indicate there are approximately 500,000 cases of sepsis in the United States every year, with an estimated crude mortality of 35%. The attributable mortality to sepsis is approximately 25%, and 10% of patients die of underlying diseases. Sepsis is the thirteenth leading cause of death in the United States and accounts for an estimated $5 to $10 billion in annual health care expenditure (1,2).

I. **Background**
   A. **Direct effects of bacteria versus bacteria-induced effects**. In a recent review of sepsis and bacteremia (3), the authors emphasize that most systemic symptoms of infections are not due to the proliferation of bacteria themselves but to the inflammatory reactions triggered by the infectious process. Although antibiotics can kill bacteria, they do not inhibit bacterial and host mediators that may induce septic shock and/or multiple organ dysfunction (3).
   B. **Definitions**. In 1992 the American College of Chest Physicians and the Society of Critical Care Medicine had a consensus conference and suggested a series of definitions and criteria for the disease states and physiologic alterations formerly and variously termed *septicemia, sepsis syndrome, septic shock,* and *organ failure* (4). This was done in part to provide some consistency in future clinical studies in prevention and therapy of septic shock. Although there is still some controversy in adopting these definitions, they are now commonly used in the literature and practice.
      1. **See Table 7.1.**
      2. **Systemic inflammatory response syndrome (SIRS). This syndrome is a set of acute physiologic responses to any of various insults, infectious or noninfectious.** SIRS may occur not only from infection but also as the result of burns, trauma, pancreatitis, or other noninfectious severe insults (e.g., postoperative inflammation). (N.B. These noninfectious insults [e.g., early severe pancreatitis] can therefore mimic sepsis.)
      3. **Multiple organ dysfunction syndrome (MODS)** is altered organ function (e.g., manifested by renal failure, respiratory failure often with adult respiratory distress syndrome, cardiovascular failure with shock) requiring intervention. Although MODS may develop as a primary process following, for example, trauma with lung injury or rhabdomyolysis with acute renal failure, with regard to sepsis, **MODS occurs in response to the systemic inflammatory response to infection**. The average

Table 7-1. Definitions of severity of response to infections

Term	Definitions	Comments
Bacteremia	Presence of viable bacteria in the blood.	May be accompanied or not by symptoms but without the signs which define SIRS.
Systemic inflammatory response syndrome (SIRS)	Two or more of the following conditions: • temperature >38°C or <36°C • heart rate >90 per minute • respiratory rate >20 per minute or $PaCO_2$ <32 mmHg • white blood cell count >12,000/cu. mm or <4,000/cu. mm or >10% immature forms	The term SIRS was developed to imply a clinical response arising from a nonspecific insult. The SIRS was included in the original consensus, but has remained controversial in the U.S. and is not accepted by a panel of experts in Europe, because of its lack of specificity.
Sepsis	Same as SIRS, with evidence of a confirmed infectious process.*	Also called sepsis syndrome.
Severe sepsis	Sepsis with hypoperfusion (e.g., lactic acidosis, oliguria, acute alteration in mental status), or organ dysfunction or hypoperfusion not due to another cause. Coagulation abnormalities may occur.	Part of a clinical continuum from mild to severe manifestations of sepsis. Presumably if treated early enough may be able to prevent development of septic shock.

| Septic shock | Severe sepsis with hypotension despite adequate fluid resuscitation (systolic blood pressure <90 mmHg or reduction of >40 mmHg from baseline) | No other cause for hypotension apparent, e.g., no GI bleed, no myocardial infarction. Perfusion abnormalities may persist after a patient has been rendered normotensive by the administration of inotropes or pressor agents. |

Modified from Zanetti G, Baumgartner JD, Glauser MP. Bacteremic sepsis, sepsis, and septic shock. In: Root RK, et al, eds. *Clinical infectious diseases: a practical approach.* New York: Oxford University Press, 1999:471–481; Bone RC, et al. Definitions for sepsis and organ failure and guidelines for the use of innovative therapies in sepsis. *Chest* 1992;101:1644; Rangel-Frausto MS. The epidemiology of bacterial sepsis. *Infect Dis Clin North Am* 1999;13:299.

* **Not all patients with clinical sepsis have positive cultures.** In one study of more than 2,500 patients meeting the criteria SIRS, in those with clinically suspected sepsis, severe sepsis, or septic shock, almost half had negative cultures! **The cause of SIRS in these culture-negative patients is unknown,** but they had morbidity and mortality rates similar to the culture-positive populations. Both culture-negative and culture-positive groups received empiric antibiotics. See Rangel-Frausto MS, et al. The natural history of the systemic inflammatory response syndrome (SIRS): a prospective study. *JAMA* 1995;273:117.

risk of death increases by 15% to 20% with failure
of each additional organ (2).

C. **Miscellaneous** (1,3)

1. SIRS stages represent a hierarchical continuum:
the more severe the inflammatory response syndrome, the higher the possibility that severe sepsis and/or septic shock may develop (1).

2. Sepsis is the most common cause of death in non-
coronary ICUs.

3. About 40% to 60% of gram-negative bacteremias
and 5% to 10% of gram-positive or fungal bloodstream infection patients go on to develop severe
sepsis or septic shock.

4. When sepsis occurs in patients without underlying
disease, virulent organisms (e.g., *Neisseria meningitidis, Streptococcus pyogenes, Staphylococcus
aureus*) are usually involved or sepsis can occur
when a focal infection is inadequately treated (e.g.,
urinary tract infection [UTI], pneumonia). Most
cases of sepsis occur in patients with underlying
disease such as diabetes, cancer, trauma, recent
surgery, splenectomy, or other chronic illnesses.

5. About half of patients with severe sepsis or septic
shock have positive blood cultures (i.e., proven
bacteremia) (Table 7.1).

D. **Pathogenesis** of sepsis and septic shock is only partially understood (1–6).

1. **Endotoxin, lipopolysaccharide (LPs)**, a component of the gram-negative cell wall, appears to
be important in gram-negative sepsis.

2. **Exotoxins** can produce a special form of septic
shock called toxic shock syndrome (**TSS**), which
can be triggered by several exotoxins of *S. aureus*
and *S. pyogenes*, group A streptococci.

3. **Bacterial cell wall components** can activate
the coagulation/fibrinolysis system, complement
system, and kallikrein/bradykinin systems, which
interact in a complex fashion to induce vaso-
dilation, increase vascular permeability and trig-
ger adult respiratory distress syndrome, consume
coagulation factors, and induce disseminated
intravascular coagulation (DIC) and/or hypotension.

   Monocytic cells can produce presumed potent
mediators of inflammation (**cytokines**) such as
tumor necrosis factor and interleukin I, which may
stimulate the inflammatory cascade. However, the
failure of anticytokines to show clinical improvement in sepsis raises doubt as to the importance of
cytokines triggering sepsis.

   Nitrous oxide, from the enzymatic breakdown
of the amino acid L-arginine, may be responsible
for changes in vasomotor tone, decreased vaso-
pressor responsiveness, and decreased myocardial function (6).

4. **Overview. Despite a significant body of information about the probable pathogenesis of septic shock, we still do not understand it well enough to employ specific agents to help reverse the process consistently.**

II. **Clinical approach**

A. **Ruling out a primary site of infection.** The initial history, physical examination, and screening laboratory tests (blood count, urinalysis, chest x-ray, sputum gram stain if available, and gram stains of any exudates) are performed in hopes of establishing a primary site of infection. (See individual chapters on these topics.) **The patient is said to have sepsis of unclear etiology only if the initial evaluation does not yield an obvious focus.**

B. **Further evaluation. Gram-negative, gram-positive, and fungal bloodstream infections may all have a similar clinical presentation.** Nonetheless, certain aspects of the workup may have a bearing on the potential pathogens. A careful approach to sepsis of unclear etiology is important so that the physician can provide appropriate treatment.

1. **History**

a. **Community- versus hospital-acquired infections.** In the hospitalized or recently hospitalized patient (within the past 30 days), the organisms causing sepsis may be more resistant. This affects the choice of antibiotics, particularly aminoglycosides, and possibly vancomycin (e.g., methicillin-resistant *S. aureus* [MRSA]), depending on the resistance patterns of one's local hospital (Sec. III.A).

b. **Prior or current medications.** Recent antibiotics may inhibit positive cultures as well as select out more resistant bacteria. Corticosteroids may minimize the signs and symptoms of infection, especially fever or signs of peritonitis. Antipyretics may suppress or affect the temperature curve.

c. **Recent manipulations or surgery.** Has the patient had recent surgery, cystoscopy, dental extraction, wound manipulation, intravenous or hyperalimentation line placement, or attempted abortion?

d. **Travel history** may be important to alert the physician to unusual diseases that may have a septic presentation such as Rocky Mountain Spotted Fever (RMSF; endemic areas include North Carolina, Virginia, and the middle southeastern states); babesiosis (acquired in Nantucket, Martha's Vineyard, Shelter Island, Long Island); malaria (foreign travel) or infection with *Vibrio* spp. (e.g., exposure to raw oysters or saltwater). Underlying

liver disease markedly increases the risk of the latter.
e. **Underlying conditions.** Certain underlying conditions may predispose the patient to infectious complications (**Table 7.2**).

2. **Physical examination.** The exam as listed needs to be complete. If the initial examination did not reveal an obvious primary focus of infection, repeat examination must be done serially.

a. **Skin. Furuncles** or intravenous **drug abuse marks** should be sought. **Intravenous access sites** should be carefully inspected. A characteristic rash may provide a clue to the underlying bacteremia. A detailed discussion of acute rash and fever in children and adults is reviewed elsewhere (7–9).

(1) **Meningococcemia** can present with a fulminant course. Initially, the rash may be macular or petechial, but it may appear ecchymotic or purpuric. A petechial rash (with tick bite history) may be RMSF.

(2) **Disseminated gonococcal infections** may present with distal extremity (fingers and fingertips), petechial, pustular, papular, or hemorrhagic lesions. These patients may be septic, but severe sepsis or septic shock would be unlikely in this syndrome.

(3) **Pseudomonas bacteremias** occasionally can present with what were previously believed to be characteristic lesions, **ecthyma gangrenosum**. These oval or round lesions have a rim of erythema and induration, and the center may ulcerate.

(4) **Embolic peripheral stigmata of bacterial endocarditis** (e.g., Janeway lesions, Osler nodes) are present only in a minority of patients (fewer than 30%), so their absence in a given patient does not rule out this diagnosis.

(5) A **scarlatiniform rash or diffuse erythroderma** may suggest TSS (especially if with diarrhea). (See Sec. C.2.)

(6) **Macronodular skin lesions of embolic candidemia** are 0.5 to 1.0 cm in diameter, pink or red, usually palpable, single, multiple or generalized.

b. **Head, ears, eyes, nose, and throat examination.** Local infection may provide a source for meningitis (i.e., chronic ear infections or sinus infection), although routine initial physical examination should have raised the possibility of a localized central nervous system (CNS) infection (e.g., lethargy, meningismus).

c. **Heart.** A careful baseline cardiac examination is important for purposes of comparison, in case a murmur develops or changes. The **absence of a murmur** does not exclude the diagnosis of acute bacterial endocarditis, but is strongly against subacute endocarditis.

d. **Lungs.** The lungs initially may sound clear in the elderly, dehydrated patient with an early pneumonia. With hydration and time (12 to 36 hours), rales may become audible and an infiltrate obvious on chest roentgenography. The compromised host may show minimal findings on lung examination but may have an abnormal chest x-ray.

e. **Abdomen, rectal, and pelvic examination.** The **abdominal scar of a splenectomy** should be sought. Localized peritoneal inflammation findings (e.g., **percussion tenderness**) may be subtle in the elderly or in patients on steroids. A rectal abscess may be a primary source of infection in patients with inflammatory bowel disease or in leukopenic patients. Evidence of an attempted abortion or of a pelvic abscess may be found on pelvic examination.

f. **Extremities.** Any potentially septic joints should be aspirated for therapeutic as well as diagnostic purposes, for they may become secondarily infected in the bacteremic patient. Point tenderness over the spine may suggest possible vertebral osteomyelitis or parameningeal focus (e.g., epidural abscess).

g. **CNS.** Obtundation may be seen in the septic patient without CNS infection. In the febrile, toxic patient presenting with a cerebrovascular accident, the possibility of bacterial endocarditis presenting primarily with neurologic findings must be considered. A lumbar puncture should be performed if there is any suspicion of CNS infection. (Also see Chap. 11.)

3. **Special laboratory tests.** Much of the preliminary laboratory work has already been done in searching for a defined focus.

a. **Blood cultures.** Multiple blood cultures should be obtained. Even in critically ill patients, **two and preferably three blood cultures, drawn 15 to 20 minutes apart, can be obtained before any antibiotics are ready to be given. If fungi such as *Histoplasma capsulatum* are a concern (compromised host or hyperalimentation-related sepsis), special blood cul-**

Table 7-2. Empiric regimens in suspected bacteremias or sepsis syndrome in various settings

Setting	Organisms Highly Suspect	Therapy (Adult Doses, Normal Renal Function)
Prosthetic cardiac valve endocarditis	S. epidermidis, streptococci, S. aureus	Vancomycin* and gentamicin.†
Underlying heart disease (congenital, rheumatic) or IV drug abuser, with ? acute endocarditis	S. aureus	See Table 8-3
Splenectomized patient, without an obvious focus	S. pneumoniae, H. influenzae, Neisseria meningitidis	Ceftriaxone (2 g IV q24h) or ampicillin-sulbactam (3 g IV q6h) or piperacillin-tazobactam
Leukopenia without an obvious focal infection (also see Chap. 12)	Enteric gram-negative bacilli, Pseudomonas species	Antipseudomonas penicillin (e.g., piperacillin 3 g q4h or 4 g q6h) or similar agent and an aminoglycoside.‡ See Chap. 12 for other options.
	Gram-positive cocci (if a venous catheter line-related infection is present or highly suspicious)	Vancomycin is also added.*

Possible intraarterial or intravenous or deepline catheter infection (e.g., Hickman or Broviac catheter)	S. aureus, S. epidermidis, nosocomial gram negatives, enterococci, (fungi)	Vancomycin* ± nafcillin, and an aminoglycoside‡ until cultures are available.
Underlying bowel disease (e.g., inflammatory bowel disease, extensive diverticulosis with prior diverticulitis)	Mixture of aerobic and anaerobic flora	Piperacillin-tazobactam ± aminoglycoside‡ or Cefotaxime (ceftriaxone) + metronidazole§

* In patients with normal renal function, the usual starting dose of vancomycin is 1 g IV (slow infusion over 2 h) q12h. **See Chap. 28 for the details of dosing vancomycin,** including in patients with renal failure. See related discussions in Chap. 8.

† In this setting, low-dose gentamicin 1.0 mg/kg/dose is used to help achieve synergy.

‡ Usually tobramycin or gentamicin is used (see Chap. 21 for details). If gentamicin or tobramycin resistance is known or highly likely, amikacin is indicated. Ideally, aminoglycoside serum levels should be monitored. Aztreonam can be substituted if it is desirable to avoid an aminoglycoside. We favor double drugs ± vancomycin in the septic-appearing leukopenic patient rather than monotherapy. See Chap. 12.

§ A third-generation cephalosporin + metronidazole would not be active against enterococci. See related discussion in Chap. 6.

ture media will increase the yield of fungal blood cultures. Candida and similar organisms are isolated equally well in standard blood culture media.

b. **Skin lesion aspirates or biopsy.** Skin lesions can be aspirated, gram-stained, and cultured. Lesions suspicious for disseminated candida should undergo punch biopsy with culture and histopathologic stains for fungi.

c. **Review of recent culture data.** The hospitalized, or recently hospitalized, patient may have recent culture data suggesting a potential pathogen, or antibiotic resistance.

d. **Liver and renal function testing** may affect antibiotic choices and doses.

e. **Arterial blood gases, electrocardiogram,** blood cell count, and stool for blood are indicated.

4. **Hemodynamic studies** using a Swan-Ganz catheter are often used to differentiate septic shock from other causes of shock. The main cardiovascular alterations in septic shock are rather similar whatever the causative organism, have recently been reviewed, and include the following (3):

a. Relative or absolute **hypovolemia** due to both venous and arterial dilation and leakage of plasma in the extravascular space, leading to **low systemic vascular resistance, tachycardia, and normal or increased cardiac output.** (Ventricular function is abnormal with reduction of left and right ventricular ejection fraction, biventricular dilation, and normal stroke volume.)

b. A **decreased oxygen extraction** mainly due to arteriovenous shunting and microvascular alterations. (Given the increased cellular metabolism induced by inflammation, this is particularly harmful for tissue.)

c. A **decreased oxygen transport** resulting from relative myocardial depression, in addition to hypovolemia. These problems may be worsened by a decrease in oxygen saturation of hemoglobin due to respiratory failure.

C. **Differential diagnosis**

1. Remember that noninfectious SIRS conditions may mimic sepsis (e.g., burns, pancreatitis, trauma). However, some of these initially noninfectious etiologies (e.g., pancreatitis) can also be complicated by severe infection, and infectious complications may be hard to sort out. (See Chap. 6 for discussion of pancreatitis.)

2. The **classic criteria for streptococcal** and **staphylococcal TSS** are summarized in **Appendixes D and E**. These diagnoses are raised when there is **fever, hypotension,** and

generalized erythematous or erythrodermal **rash**, and **multisystem involvement**. (See related discussion of streptococcal TSS with soft tissue infections in Chap. 3 and Appendix E.)

3. **Fungemia/candidemia** can present with fever, chills, and a sepsislike picture. Patients at increased risk for disseminated candidiasis include patients with prolonged and severe neutropenia, transplant recipients, postsurgical patients with complex and protracted hospitalizations, burn victims, low-birth-weight neonates, patients with central intravenous lines, those receiving hyperalimentation, and recipients of broad-spectrum antibiotics and corticosteroids (10,11). Macronodular skin lesions may be seen (Sec. B.2.a) and in a significant percentage, suggestive endophthalmitis is present on good ophthalmologic examination. Diagnosis is difficult since blood cultures are typically negative. Infectious disease consultation is advised.

III. **Initial therapy**
   A. **Antibiotics**
   1. **If a focal infection** is defined in the bacteremic or septic patient, therapy is discussed in the chapter devoted to that topic (i.e., UTI, pneumonia).
   2. **Special hosts.** In some hosts, the presumed bacteremic or septic patient may raise special considerations (**Table 7.2**).
   3. **No primary focus** of infection in the patient with sepsis necessitates empiric therapy. Recent studies have shown that the outcome of bacteremic patients is improved and the occurrence of shock is reduced by half when appropriate antibiotic therapy is administered early (3). It is important to separate community-acquired infection from hospital-acquired infection, where more resistant gram-negative, MRSA,* or fungal infections are likely. Therapy can be tapered after cultures return and after serial clinical assessment. The intravenous route should be used to ensure adequate dosage (**Table 7.3**).

   With the availability of new potent antibiotics, the use of an early-generation cephalosporin and an aminoglycoside has been challenged (3), especially in community-acquired infections, in an attempt to avoid the nephrotoxicity of the aminoglycoside. In hospital-acquired infection, an aminoglycoside often is necessary, especially if resistant gram-negative bacteria are common. Also, in hospitalized patients, the incidence of MRSA will affect antibiotic choices.

---

* Recently, MRSA has become more of a concern with community-acquired infection. See Chap. 17.

Table 7-3.   Empiric regimens for sepsis of unknown source

Setting	Organisms Highly Suspected	Therapy (adult doses, normal renal function)	
		First Choice	**Alternative Choice***
Community acquired	Community-acquired gram negatives, S. aureus,** meningococci, streptococci	Ceftriaxone 1–2 g IV q24h (or cefotaxime 2 g IV q8h), **or** Piperacillin-tazobactam	Vancomycin plus an aminoglycoside or aztreonam; **or** Vancomycin and a fluoroquinolone
Hospital acquired	Same as above, plus P. aeruginosa, multiresistant enterobacteriaceae, methicillin-susceptible S. aureus	Piperacillin-tazobactam and an aminoglycoside[†]	Piperacillin, cefazolin and an aminoglycoside,[†] **or** Imipenem plus aminoglycoside,[‡] **or** Vancomycin and an aminoglycoside or aztreonam
	Nosocomial gram-negative and methicillin-resistant S. aureus	Vancomycin,[§] plus aminoglycosides ± piperacillin	Vancomycin plus aztreonam or vancomycin plus quinolone

* Allergy to beta-lactams or special epidemiologic factors raising risk of resistant pathogens such as methicillin-resistant S. aureus.

** Recently, MRSA has become more of a problem with community-acquired S. aureus. In regions with increasing concerns with community-acquired MRSA, vancomycin may need to be added until susceptibility data are available. See Chap. 17 and 28.

[†] The aminoglycoside of choice will depend upon local susceptibility patterns. If an aminoglycoside is contraindicated, aztreonam can be used, although it may not be as active against some strains of Pseudomonas spp.

[‡] Because imipenem monotherapy may not be adequate for severe Pseudomonas infection, we would combine imipenem with an aminoglycoside.

[§] Vancomycin is the antibiotic of choice for known or highly suspected methicillin-resistant S. aureus. See Chap. 28 for dosing.

B. **Supportive care** is critical. Only a few issues are discussed in this handbook. This topic has been reviewed recently (12). Patient monitoring is critical, including vital signs, urinary output, mentation, and often data from Swan-Ganz catheterization (Sec. II.B.4).

1. **Cardiovascular management.** The goals are to reverse tissue hypoxia, restore volume, tissue perfusion, and oxygen delivery (3). Volume replacement is essential. Both crystalloid and colloid solutions have been used; there is no consensus on the optimal fluid. Fluid alone is estimated to restore a normal pulmonary artery wedge pressure in 30% to 40% of cases (3). Often adrenergic agents are necessary (e.g., dopamine, noradrenaline, dobutamine [3,12]), but a detailed discussion of the use of these agents is beyond the scope of this book.

2. **Ventilatory support** is often necessary, especially when adult respiratory distress syndrome develops.

3. **Management of coagulopathy.** The most important component of therapy is directed toward reversal of shock and removal of the septic source (surgery) when indicated. Disseminated intravascular coagulopathy (DIC) may occur in about 10% to 20% of patients with septic shock (3).

4. **Antimediator therapy.** As of early 2000 there are no well-studied agents approved by the Food and Drug Administration that can block the pathogenesis/progression of septic shock. It is hoped that such clinical interventions will be available in the future (6).

References

1. Rangel-Frausto MS. The epidemiology of bacterial sepsis. *Infect Dis Clin North Am* 1999;13:299.

2. Wheeler AP, Bernard GR. Treating patients with severe sepsis. *N Engl J Med* 1999;340:207.

3. Zanetti G, Baumgartner JD, Glauser MP. Bacteremia, sepsis, and septic shock. In: Root RK, et al, eds. *Clinical infectious diseases: a practical approach.* New York: Oxford University Press, 1999:471–481.

4. Bone RC, et al. Definitions for sepsis and organ failure for the use of innovative therapies in sepsis. *Chest* 1992;101:1644.

5. Ognibene FP. Pathogenesis and innovative treatment of septic shock. *Adv Intern Med* 1997;42:313.

6. Opal SM, Cross AS, eds. Bacterial sepsis and septic shock. *Infect Dis Clin North Am* 1999;13:285–509.
   This entire volume is devoted to sepsis. More than 10 articles deal with current hypotheses and data on various factors important in pathogenesis.

7. Katz SL, Gershon AA, Hotez PJ, eds. *Krugman's infectious diseases of children*, 10th ed. St Louis: Mosby, 1998.

8. Levin S, Goodman LJ. An approach to acute fever and rash in the adult. *Curr Clin Top Infect Dis* 1995;15:19.

9. Swartz, M. Infections with rash. In: Root RK, et al, eds. *Clinical infectious diseases: a practical approach*. New York: Oxford University Press, 1999:483–499.
   Nice discussion by a highly respected, seasoned infectious disease expert. Includes series of color photos.

10. Wright WL, Wenzel RP. Nosocomial candida: epidemiology, transmission, and prevention. *Infect Dis Clin North Am* 1997;11:411.

11. Rex JH. Catheters and candidemia. *Clin Infect Dis* 1996;22:467.

12. Dellinger RP. Current therapy of sepsis. *Infect Dis Clin North Am* 1999;13:495.
    Summary written by critical care director.

8

Infective Endocarditis

Infective Endocarditis of the Native Valves

The term *infective endocarditis* includes bacterial, fungal, rickettsial, chlamydial, and possibly viral infection of heart valves or mural endocardium. Bacterial endocarditis (BE) is the most commonly recognized form of the disease and is often characterized as acute (ABE) or subacute (SBE) on the basis of its clinical presentation (1). Fungal endocarditis is seen primarily in narcotic addicts or in patients with prosthetic valves.

I. **Clinical presentation**
   A. **Host factors**
      1. **Underlying heart disease** (1)
         - 25% to 50%—no previously known underlying heart disease
         - 10% to 50%—mitral valve prolapse with a significant murmur
         - Less than 15%—rheumatic valvular damage (used to be common)
         - 10% to 20%—degenerative heart disease
         - 10%—congenital heart disease overall but more common in children with BE (2)

      2. **Age.** The overall median age of patients with BE is more than 50 years. However, BE can occur in children, often with congenital heart disease and prior cardiac surgery, with a median age in one series of 9 years (2).
      3. **Intravenous drug users.** These individuals are at risk even in the absence of valvular heart disease. The tricuspid valve is the most common site, followed by the mitral, aortic, and pulmonic valve.
   B. **SBE versus ABE**
      1. **SBE**. Patients may present either abruptly or insidiously. In the latter instance, fever is almost a constant. Symptoms, weeks or occasionally months in duration, include fatigue or malaise, night sweats, weight loss, arthralgia/myalgia, prominent low back pain, and at times neurologic symptoms including stroke syndromes, and dementia.
      2. **ABE**. Invariably, this disease is abrupt in onset (e.g., over a couple to a few days). Symptoms include fever, chills, myalgia/arthralgia, and back pain, and are more severe than similar symptoms in SBE.
   C. **Signs and symptoms**. The presenting signs and symptoms of BE are variable and are often nonspecific

(1,3). **Always consider BE in the patient with fever and a murmur**.

1. **Fever** is almost always present, although it may be minimal or absent in the very elderly and those with chronic renal failure.
2. **Peripheral stigmata** occur in a minority of patients. Their presence helps make the diagnosis, but their absence does not exclude BE.
   a. **SBE**. Frequency of these findings increases with duration of illness. Conjunctival petechiae are the most common finding; cutaneous petechiae are second, followed by splenomegaly.
   b. **ABE**. Osler nodes, or Janeway lesions, are more common in the ABE than in SBE but are seen only in the minority of patients. Roth spots are uncommon in ABE or SBE.
3. **Cardiac signs**
   a. **SBE**. A murmur is ultimately heard in more than 80% to 85%, although it may be absent in the elderly (1,3). A systolic or diastolic aortic murmur, systolic mitral murmur, or murmur of ventricular septal defect are most commonly heard.
   b. **ABE**. A murmur may not be present initially. A rub may be present with a murmur.
   c. **Heart block** may occur in either.
   d. **Congestive heart failure (CHF)** may develop secondary to valve insufficiency or rupture of the chordae tendineae.
4. **Embolic phenomena**. These are manifested as episodes of vascular occlusion that cause pain in the abdomen (mesenteric or splenic arterial involvement), chest (coronary or pulmonary emboli, embolic pneumonia with *S. aureus*), or extremities. Hematuria may result from emboli to the kidneys, blindness from retinal artery involvement, and acute neurologic symptoms (including embolic stroke, toxic encephalopathy) from cerebrovascular involvement.
5. **Intravenous drug users**. Tricuspid involvement is common (50%), but **a tricuspid murmur is usually difficult to hear**. Peripheral stigmata are rare. Instead, pulmonary emboli and related symptoms are seen. Aortic and mitral valves are involved in 25% to 30% of the time. Pulmonic valve involvement is rare.

II. **Laboratory studies**. With the exception of microbiologic studies and, at times, echocardiographic data, laboratory findings are variable, nonspecific, and often of little definitive value in the diagnosis of endocarditis.

   A. **Nonspecific findings**
      1. **Erythrocyte sedimentation rate** is elevated in almost all patients with SBE who are not in CHF. It is not useful in ABE.

2. **Anemia.** A mild to moderate normocytic/normo-chromic anemia is very common in SBE but usu-ally absent in ABE.

3. **Peripheral leukocyte counts** are usually nor-mal or moderately elevated, although prominent leukocytosis may be seen in ABE.

4. **Thrombocytopenia** may be seen in patients with ABE and in those with splenomegaly accompanying more chronic infections.

5. **Urinalysis**. Microscopic hematuria and protein-uria are common.

B. **Blood cultures and bacteremia. Blood cultures must be obtained whenever the diagnosis of BE is suspected**; they will be positive in 85% to 95% of cases. Blood cultures are the most important test to obtain in the evaluation of a patient with suspected endocarditis (3).

1. **In suspected SBE**. Three separate cultures (more are not helpful) over a 24-hour period are sufficient, or samples can be drawn 1 to 2 hours apart, before any antibiotics. Direct the labora-tory to hold cultures for 2 weeks.

2. **In suspected ABE**. Three cultures from sepa-rate venipuncture sites at 20- to 30-minute inter-vals before treatment are suggested.

3. **Recent/current antibiotic therapy**. Cultures may be negative in SBE unless antibiotics have been discontinued 3 to 5 days.

4. **Culture-negative BE** can occur, but in almost half of the 5% to 15% of cases, antibiotics prior to obtaining blood cultures is the explanation (1,3,4). Culture-negative endocarditis is usually in the setting of underlying valvular heart disease. In-fection can be caused by fastidious organisms or those not recoverable in broth media (3). Infec-tious disease consultation is advised. At times, serologic tests (antibody to *Legionella, Bartonella, Coxiella burnetti, Brucella, Chlamydia* spp.) may be indicated. If patients with culture-negative endocarditis undergo valve replacement surgery, special studies of the resected vegetation should be performed (4).

C. **Echocardiography (Echo)** is not necessary for every case of BE. For example, in the patient with underly-ing valve disease and sustained community-acquired viridans streptococcal bacteremia, an Echo adds lit-tle to the diagnosis itself. A negative Echo cannot ex-clude BE.

1. Recently, the **Duke criteria** for BE have em-ployed an Echo test (**Sec. III**). An Echo may be useful in patients with bacteremia in whom one is trying to determine if BE is present or in patients with negative blood cultures (e.g., after anti-biotics) who are suspected of having BE.

2. In SBE, do not do Echo before culture results are available. In ABE, Echos may help identify myocardial abscess and/or valve dysfunction.
3. Transthoracic testing is less invasive and less sensitive. Transesophageal testing detects 85% to 90% or more of vegetations. (N.B. Previous endocarditis vegetations can persist.)
   a. However, a recent series of more than 130 patients concluded that in **patients without prosthetic valves who have a technically adequate transthoracic Echo, transesophageal Echo is unlikely to be of incremental benefit in diagnosing endocarditis** (5).
   b. The optimal approach is transesophageal echocardiography (TEE) using biplane technology with color flow and continuous as well as pulsed Doppler. **TEE** allows for very small vegetations to be imaged and is the **procedure of choice** for assessing the pulmonic valve, prosthetic valves (especially in the mitral position), and perivalvular areas for abscesses (3).

      TEE is useful to confirm the diagnosis in highly suspect patients and to exclude the diagnosis of endocarditis when the clinical suspicion is not high (3).

III. **Diagnosis**
   A. **Positive blood cultures**, or positive cultures (or histopathologic examination) from the vegetation are required to establish a definitive diagnosis (3). However, obviously not all bacteremic patients have endocarditis, and clinical findings can be variable in BE.
   B. **Duke criteria** for diagnosing BE. Recently, there has been renewed interest in diagnostic criteria to help the clinician (6).
      1. See **Tables 8-1** and **8-2.**
      2. When these criteria are used to assess the entire diagnostic evaluation, they provide a sensitive and specific approach to the diagnosis of endocarditis (3).
         a. Patients who have "definitive" or "possible endocarditis" (Tables 8.1 and 8.2) should be treated for endocarditis.
         b. Vegetations on Echo strengthen the diagnosis, but a negative TEE does not rule out endocarditis. Karchmer notes the false-negative rate for TEE ranges from 6% to 18%. Thus Echo helps exclude the diagnosis of endocarditis only when the index of suspicion is low (3).

IV. **Microbiologic features** (1,3)
   A. **SBE**
      1. **Streptococci** account for approximately 55% to 70% of all cases of native valvular BE in the non-

**Table 8-1. Duke criteria for diagnosis
of infective endocarditis**

Definite infective endocarditis
Pathologic criteria
  Microorganisms: demonstrated by culture or histology in a veg-
    etation, *or* in a vegetation that has embolized, *or* in an intra-
    cardiac abscess, *or*
  Pathologic lesions: vegetation or intracardiac abscess present,
    confirmed by histology showing active endocarditis
Clinical criteria, using specific definitions listed in Table 8.2
  2 major criteria, *or*
  1 major and 3 minor criteria, *or*
  5 minor criteria
Possible infective endocarditis
  Findings consistent with infective endocarditis that fall short of
    "definite," but not "rejected"
Rejected
  Firm alternate diagnosis for manifestations of endocarditis, *or*
  Resolution* of manifestations of endocarditis, with antibiotic
    therapy for 4 days or less, *or*
  No pathologic evidence of infective endocarditis at surgery or
    autopsy, after antibiotic therapy for 4 days or less

Source: Durak DT, et al. New criteria for diagnosis of infective endocarditis:
utilization of specific echocardiographic findings. *Am J Med* 1994;96:200.
* Some experts suggest using the term *sustained resolution* [3].

addict population (**viridans streptococci, 40%
to 60%;** enterococci, 10%; nonhemolytic, microaerophilic, anaerobic, or nonenterococcal group D
streptococci, 10%).

2. **Miscellaneous** (10% of cases). HACEK organisms
    (see Sec. 3) and other fastidious gram-negative
    organisms. Typical gram-negative rods and *Neis-
    seria gonorrhoeae* rarely cause BE in spite of their
    frequency of bacteremia. *Pseudomonas* spp. in the
    drug addict is the exception.

3. **Culture-negative endocarditis.**
    a. The usual cause is prior antibiotic therapy
        (4). See Sec. II.B.4.
    b. HACEK organisms (*Haemophilus* spp., *Ac-
        tinobacillus actinomycetemcomitans, Cardio-
        bacterium hominis, Eikenella corrodens,
        Kingella* spp.) or *Bartonella henselae* or *B.
        quintana* require prolonged incubation.
        (Alert the microbiology laboratory.)
    c. **Legionella** spp. will need special sub-
        cultures.
    d. *Coxiella, Mycoplasma*, or *Chlamydia* spp.
        require special culture methods (1,3).

B. **ABE**
    1. *S. aureus* causes the majority of these cases. In
        the patient with community-acquired *S. aureus*

**Table 8-2. Definitions of terminology
used in the Duke criteria**

Major criteria
1. Positive blood culture for infective endocarditis
   a. Typical microorganism for infective endocarditis from two
      separate blood cultures
      (1) Viridans streptococci,* *Streptococcus bovis,* HACEK group,
          or
      (2) Community-acquired *Staphylococcus aureus* or enterococci,
          in the absence of a primary focus, *or*
   b. Persistently positive blood culture, defined as recovery of a
      microorganism consistent with infective endocarditis from
      (1) Blood cultures drawn more than 12 hours apart, *or*
      (2) All of three or a majority of four or more separate blood
          cultures, with first and last drawn at least 1 hour apart
2. Evidence of endocardial involvement
   a. Positive echocardiogram for infective endocarditis
      (1) Oscillating intracardiac mass, on valve or supporting
          structures, *or* in the path of regurgitant jets, *or* on
          implanted material, in the absence of an alternative
          anatomic explanation, *or*
      (2) Abscess, *or*
      (3) New partial dehiscence of prosthetic valve, *or*
   b. New valvular regurgitation (increase or change in preexisting
      murmur not sufficient)

Minor criteria
1. Predisposition: predisposing heart condition *or* intravenous
   drug use
2. Fever: ≥38.0°C (100.4°F)
3. Vascular phenomena: major arterial emboli, septic pulmonary
   infarcts, mycotic aneurysm, intracranial hemorrhage, conjunctival
   hemorrhages, Janeway lesions
4. Immunologic phenomena: glomerulonephritis, Osler's nodes,
   Roth spots, rheumatoid factor
5. Microbiologic evidence: positive blood culture but not meeting
   major criterion as noted previously[†] *or* serologic evidence of active
   infection with organism consistent with infective endocarditis
6. Echocardiogram: consistent with infective endocarditis but not
   meeting major criterion as noted previously

Source: Durak DT, et al. New criteria for diagnosis of infective endocarditis:
utilization of specific echocardiographic findings. *Am J Med* 1994;96:200.
Abbreviation: HACEK, *Haemophilus* spp., *Actinobacillus actinomycetemcomi-*
tans, Cardiobacterium hominis, Eikenella spp., and *Kingella kingae.*
* Including nutritional variant strains.
[†] Excluding single positive cultures for coagulase-negative staphylococci and
organisms that do not cause endocarditis.

bacteremia with documented prolonged bacteremia, endocarditis is very common and patients need prolonged courses of antibiotics. The hospitalized patient with a removable focus (IV catheter) who responds rapidly to therapy and catheter removal can often be treated for 10 to 14 days (7). Infectious disease consultation is advisable in patients with *S. aureus* bacteremia.

2. **S. pneumoniae** and group B beta-hemolytic streptococci are rare causes of ABE.

V. **Treatment.** Prolonged (4 weeks, sometimes 6 weeks), intravenous, bactericidal agents are used. When appropriate antibiotic therapy is begun, symptomatic improvement, decline in fever, and reversion of blood cultures to negative are usually prompt. With very sensitive organisms, this is likely to occur in 24 to 48 hours, but with more difficult-to-eradicate pathogens such as **S. aureus**, it may take several days to a week before definite improvement is noted. Patients should be serially evaluated for congestive heart failure, which may be a marker of valve dysfunction. Drug fever can occur. (See Chap. 12.)

A. **Empiric therapy** is summarized in **Table 8.3** and reviewed in more detail elsewhere (1,3).

B. **Therapy for a specific organism** is summarized in **Table 8.4** and reviewed in more detail elsewhere (1,3). Infectious disease consultation is advised.

VI. **Role of surgery** is reviewed elsewhere (1,3,8), but a few points deserve emphasis.

A. **Strong indication**

1. Progressive or significant **congestive heart failure** that does not respond to routine medical therapy. Early cardiology consultation is

Table 8-3. Empiric antibiotics for native valve endocarditis (normal renal function)

Acute versus Subacute	Primary	Alternative
ABE*	Nafcillin/oxacillin 1.5g IV q4h and gentamicin 1 mg/kg IV q8h and vancomycin‡ 1g IV q12h	Vancomycin (see Chap. 28) and gentamicin 1 mg/kg IV q8h
SBE†	Aqueous penicillin 3 MU IV q4h and gentamicin 1 mg/kg IV q8h	Vancomycin and gentamicin 1 mg/kg IV q8h

* Therapy aimed at *S. aureus,* streptococci including enterococci.
† Therapy aimed at streptococci, including enterococci.
‡ Vancomycin will be active against enterococci and the possibility of community-acquired MRSA strains. See Chap. 17.
MU, million units.

Table 8-4. Therapy for common organisms causing endocarditis (assumes normal renal function) in adults

Organism	Primary	Alternative
Viridans streptococci Penicillin sensitive (MIC <0.1 ug/ml)	Penicillin 2–3 MU IV q4h × 4 weeks or ceftriaxone 2 g once IV qd × 4 weeks	Cefazolin 1 g IV q6h or 1.5 g q8h × 4 weeks or Vancomycin × 4 weeks
Relatively penicillin-resistant streptococci Penicillin MIC ≥0.2 to ≤0.5 ug/ml	Penicillin 3 MU IV q4h × 4 weeks and gentamicin 1 mg/kg IV q8h × 2–4 weeks	Vancomycin 4 weeks
Enterococci* Ampicillin sensitive	Penicillin 3–4 MU IV q4h × 4–6 weeks and gentamicin 1 mg/kg IV q8h × 4–6 weeks	Vancomycin and gentamicin for 4–6 weeks
VRE†	Request infectious disease consult	
Staphylococci Methicillin sensitive	Oxacillin/nafcillin 1½ g q4h for 4–6 weeks with optional gentamicin 1 mg/kg IV q8h × 3–5 days	Cefazolin 2 g q8h for 4–6 weeks with optional gentamicin 1 mg/kg IV q8h × 3–5 days or Vancomycin × 4–6 weeks
Methicillin resistant	Vancomycin × 4–6 weeks	
HACEK organisms	Ceftriaxone 2 g IV once qd × 4 weeks	Ampicillin 3 g IV q6h and gentamicin 1 mg/kg IV q8h × 4 weeks

Abbreviation: MU, million units.
* For detailed discussion of enterococcal endocarditis, see ref. 3. **All patients with enterococcal endocarditis deserve an infectious disease consultation.**
† VRE = vancomycin resistant. See Chap. 28.

advised to help assess the need for surgical intervention.

   2. **Fungal** endocarditis (most patients).
   3. **Uncontrolled infection: persisting bacteremia** (7 to 10 days) despite appropriate antibiotic therapy.
   B. **Relative indications** (3)
      1. Extension of infection into perivalvular tissue (myocardial abscess)
      2. *S. aureus* infection of aortic or mitral valve
      3. Relapse after maximal antimicrobial therapy
      4. Large (>10 mm) hypermobile vegetations by Echo
      5. Persistent unexplained fever (>10 days) during empiric therapy of culture-negative endocarditis
      6. Endocarditis caused by *C. burnetti* or *Brucella* spp.
VII. **Prevention of bacterial endocarditis** is discussed in Chap. 15.

Endocarditis Associated with Prosthetic Valves

The cumulative incidence of prosthetic valve endocarditis (PVE) (1,3,9) in recent years is approximately 1.4% to 3% at 12 months, 4% to 5.4% at 4 years, and 3.2% to 5.7% at 5 years. The risk of PVE is not uniform over time; it is greatest in the first 6 months after surgery (3).

I. **Time of onset**
   A. **Early PVE**. PVE associated with valve insertion usually occurs within 12 months of surgery but occasionally later.
   B. **Late PVE**. PVE from bacteremia theoretically may occur at any time, but by convention refers to those later than 1 year after valve insertion.
II. **Pathologic features**
   A. **Early PVE** occurs from sewing the organism in with the valve. Ring abscess and valve dehiscence (and associated severe valvular insufficiency) are the hallmarks. Extension to the conduction tissue (especially after aortic valves) and/or obstruction of valve outflow by vegetative material, especially after mitral valves, can occur.
   B. **Late PVE** in bioprosthetic valves is more typically confined to the valve leaflets (9).
III. **Microbiologic features**
   A. **Early PVE**. Staphylococcal species predominate. In the immediate postoperative period, *S. aureus*; at later times it is staphylococcal species coagulase negative (SSCN), which are usually methicillin resistant.

Occasionally, a gram-negative or fungal species will be etiologic.

B. **Late PVE** mimics native valve endocarditis. (See prior discussion.)

C. **Culture-negative endocarditis** occurs occasionally. As with native valve BE, it is usually the result of prior antibiotic therapy, although fastidious organisms can be etiologic (9), as in native valve culture-negative endocarditis. (See prior discussion.)

IV. **Diagnosis.** Signs, symptoms, and diagnostic methods are similar to native valve endocarditis, as discussed in the previous section. When Echo is performed, TEE is preferred (3).

V. **Therapy.** Surgery plays a more prominent role in PVE than in native valve BE.

A. **Antibiotic therapy** follows the same general principles previously outlined for native endocarditis. **See Table 8.5.** One must remember that additive toxicity may result from simultaneous vancomycin and gentamicin. (See Chap. 21.) **Therapy should continue for at least 6 weeks for more sensitive organisms and for 8 weeks for more resistant ones.** In the setting of PVE, every effort should be made to **attain maximum bactericidal blood levels.** Infectious disease consultation is advised.

B. **Surgery. Because of the high mortality associated with early PVE treated with antibiotic therapy alone, some authorities believe that the diagnosis of PVE, with or without evidence of valve dysfunction or failure, may be an indication for valve replacement. Infectious disease, cardiology, and cardiac surgical consultations are advised (Table 8.6).**

Table 8-5.   Antibiotic therapy for PVE (normal renal function)

Clinical Situation	Primary
White awaiting culture results	Vancomycin and gentamicin 1 mg/kg IV q8h and ampicillin 3 g IV q6h[‡]
Staphylococci Methicillin sensitive	Oxacillin/nafcillin* 1½ g q4h and rifampin,* 300 mg PO q8h and gentamicin,[†] 1 mg/kg IV q8h
Methicillin resistant**	Vancomycin* and rifampin,* 300 mg PO q8h and gentamicin[†] 1 mg/kg IV q8h
Other organisms	See Table 8-4.

* For at least 6 weeks duration.
** See Chap. 28 for details of dosing vancomycin.
[†] For 2 weeks duration. See Chap. 21.
[‡] Then antibiotics adjusted based on susceptibility data.

Table 8-6. Indications for cardiac surgery in patients with PVE

1. Moderate to severe heart failure due to prosthesis dysfunction (incompetence or obstruction)
2. Invasive and destructive paravulvular infection
   a. Partial valve dehiscence, unstable hypermobile valve
   b. New or progressive conduction system disturbances
   c. Fever persisting 10 or more days during appropriate antibiotic therapy
   d. Purulent pericarditis
   e. Sinus of Valsalva aneurysm or intracardiac fistula
3. Uncontrolled bacteremic infection during therapy
4. Infection caused by selected organisms
   a. Fungi, *Pseudomonas aeruginosa*
   b. *Staphylococcus aureus**
   c. Coagulase-negative staphylococci*
5. Relapse after appropriate antimicrobial therapy
6. Persistent temperature during therapy for culture-negative PVE in absence of other causes of fever
7. Recurrent arterial emboli[†]
8. Renal failure with severe aortic regurgitation[‡]

Source: Modified from Karchmer AW, Gibbons GW. Infections of prosthetic heart valves and vascular grafts. In: Bisno AL, Waldvogel FA, eds. *Infections associated with indwelling medical devices,* 2nd ed. Washington, DC: American Society for Microbiology, 1994:213–249; Jamieson SW. Surgical therapy for infective endocarditis. *Mayo Clin Proc* 1995;70:598.

* While not a uniformly accepted indication for surgical treatment of PVE, several investigators favor surgical therapy for PVE caused by *S. aureus* or coagulase-negative staphylococci [9]. This may especially apply to patients who do not respond rapidly to antibiotic therapy.

[†] Rather than an indication for surgery, the potential for additional systemic emboli is often viewed as a factor that, in combination with other considerations, might help to justify surgery. Reviews suggest recurrent emboli are rare in patients who are receiving appropriate antibiotics [9].

[‡] The presence of deteriorating renal function in patients with endocarditis associated with severe aortic regurgitation should, in itself, stimulate urgent operation [8].

References

1. Sentochnik DE, Karchmer AW. Cardiac infections. In: Reese RE, Betts RF, eds. *A practical approach to infectious diseases,* 4th ed. Boston: Little, Brown, 1996:350–379.
   Dr. Karchmer is a national expert on IE. See reference 3 also.
2. Martin JM, Neches WH, Wald ER. Infective endocarditis: 35 years of experience at a children's hospital. *Clin Infect Dis* 1997;24:669.
3. Karchmer AW. Infective endocarditis. In: Root RK, et al, eds. *Clinical infectious diseases: a practical approach.* New York: Oxford University Press, 1999:621–635.

See related review by AW Karchmer, Infective endocarditis. In: Braunwald E, ed. Heart disease: a textbook of cardiovascular medicine, *5th ed. Philadelphia: WB Saunders, 1997:Chap. 33.*

4. Hoen B, et al. Infective endocarditis in patients with negative blood cultures: analysis of 88 cases from a one-year nationwide survey in France. *Clin Infect Dis* 1995;20:501.

5. Irani WN, Grayburn PA, Afridi I. A negative transthoracic echocardiogram obviates the need for transesophageal echocardiography in patients with suspected native valve active infective endocarditis. *Am J Cardiol* 1996;78:101.

Series from University of Texas Southwestern Medical Center, Dallas.

6. Durak DT, et al. New criteria for diagnosis of infective endocarditis: utilization of specific echocardiographic findings. *Am J Med* 1994;96:200.

7. Raad II, Bodey GP. Infectious complications of indwelling vascular catheters. *Clin Infect Dis* 1992;15:197.

8. Jamison SW. Surgical therapy for infective endocarditis. *Mayo Clin Proc* 1995;70:598.

9. Karchmer AW, Gibbons GW. Infections in prosthetic heart valves and vascular grafts. In: Bisno AL, Waldvogel FA, eds. *Infections associated with indwelling medical devices*, 2nd ed. Washington, DC: American Society for Microbiology, 1994:213–249.

Acute Joint and Bone Infections

Nonprosthetic Joint Infections

Bacterial arthritis (septic arthritis) most commonly involves a single joint by hematogenous seeding from a distant site (1). *Staphylococcus aureus* is the most common organism in adults. *Gonococcus* is the most common organism in the 15- to 40-year-old group.

I. **Clinical presentation** (1–3). A careful history and physical examination are important in searching for the primary infection site. Risk factors such as rheumatoid arthritis, sickle cell disease, immunosuppression, prior or current sexually transmitted disease (e.g., signs and symptoms of gonococcal disease) or narcotic use are important.
   A. **Clinical features**
      1. **Joint symptoms**. Infectious arthritis typically presents with prominent pain, acute joint swelling, warmth, erythema, and almost complete lack of range of motion of the involved joint. The usual signs of inflammation may be absent in a setting of immunosuppression or rheumatoid arthritis. In patients with rheumatoid arthritis, an inflamed joint that is "out of phase" (i.e., much more painful, swollen) with others is suggestive.
      2. **With bacteremia** multiple joint arthralgias occur, but actual septic arthritis is usually limited to one or two joints. *S. aureus* is the most common organism in this setting.
      3. Tuberculosis and fungal infections of the joint and Lyme arthritis are typically subacute and not discussed in this handbook.
   B. **Physical examination.** Joint inflammation (warmth, possibly erythema, as well as an effusion) is characteristic and should be carefully sought. **In a septic joint, usually the examiner cannot move the joint for more than a few degrees (usually less than 15°) without discomfort.** More than 50% of the time concurrent infections at other sites are found in bacterial arthritis. The characteristic skin rash of disseminated gonococcal (GC) infection (macular, vesicular, or pustular skin lesions most commonly over the distal extremities), may or may not precede the development of arthritis in disseminated GC infection. Previous evidence of a skin lesion(s) due to *S. aureus* should be sought.
II. **Laboratory**
   A. The **mainstay of diagnosis is joint fluid examination**, gram stain, and culture (4).
      1. **Inflammatory versus noninflammatory**. Total white blood cell (WBC) and differential counts should be performed on all synovial fluids (4).

a. **Traditionally, fluids with a WBC count of less than 2000/mm³ are considered noninflammatory.** For example, in uncomplicated osteoarthritis the usual WBC count is less than 1,000/mm³, and fewer than 30% of these are neutrophils (4).

b. **Fluids with a cell count of more than 100,000/mm³ should be assumed to be "septic" (infected) until proven otherwise (4).**

c. Fluids between 50,000 and 100,000/mm³ are problematic: Some early infections are in this range, and fluids from patients with crystal-induced or idiopathic inflammatory arthritis (e.g., rheumatoid arthritis, Reiter's syndrome) may be in this range (4). Fluids between 2,000 and 50,000/mm³ are inflammatory, but usually not infected.

d. A noninflammatory fluid generally has less than 50% neutrophils, whereas **infected fluids generally have more than 95% neutrophils**, but many crystal-induced effusions have elevated neutrophils (4).

2. **Joint fluid culture** is discussed in Sec. B.

3. **Fluid should be examined for crystals** under polarized light, since crystal-induced effusions can mimic septic joints. Therefore it is especially important to rule out gout and pseudogout.

B. **Culture** and gram stains

1. Two separated **blood cultures** and, if present, **cultures of other infected sites** should be obtained. Open and/or draining skin lesions should be cultured.

2. **In the proper setting** and age group, joint fluid can be directly plated on chocolate agar media to culture **gonococci**. Pharyngeal, rectal, cervical, or urethral surfaces can be cultured for *Neisseria gonorrhoeae* in patients at risk (e.g., sexually active patients 15 to 40 years of age especially). (See Chapter 10.)

3. **Joint fluid cultures** for aerobic bacteria should be plated as quickly as possible. In subacute cases special cultures for tuberculosis and fungi may be indicated.

C. **Radiography** may be helpful in deep-seated infections, such as the hip; in patients with underlying joint disease, such as rheumatoid arthritis; or in a prosthetic joint to assess loosening of the prosthesis.

D. **Synovial tissue biopsy** is indicated in ill-defined, chronic processes.

III. **Therapy** (1–3)

A. **Joint aspiration.** At the outset, the joint should be tapped dry. If fluid reaccumulates, frequent aspiration is an important adjunct to therapy. An infected joint is like an abscess and needs to be serially drained if fluid reaccumulates. **A septic hip joint usually requires surgical drainage and immediate orthopedic consultation.**

B. **Antibiotic therapy** is based on the initial gram stain in adults and children (**Tables 9.1 and 9.2**). In neonates cefotaxime or cefotaxime and an aminoglycoside can be used. See Appendix Table A.

Prosthetic Joint Infections

With the increasing use of prosthetic joint devices, the primary care provider may be initially involved in the diagnosis of those infections whose definitive management involves orthopedic and infectious disease involvement early on.

I. **Background**
   A. **Risk factors** associated with the development of infection in prosthetic joints include advanced age, rheumatoid arthritis, diabetes mellitus, use of corticosteroids,

Table 9-1. Empiric antibiotic therapy for septic arthritis based on the initial gram stain in adults (normal renal function)

Gram Stain	First Line of Therapy	Alternative
Gram (+) cocci	Nafcillin/oxacillin 1.5 g IV q4h or vancomycin 1 g IV q12h (in areas of MRSA)[a]	First-generation cephalosporin (cefazolin) *or* clindamycin
Gram (−) cocci	Ceftriaxone 1 g IV qd	Cefotaxime *or* spectinomycin
Gram (−) bacilli	Piperacillin-tazobactam (see Chap. 18) ± an aminoglycoside[b]	Piperacillin and an aminoglycoside; *or* gentamicin plus third-generation cephalosporin *or* ceftriaxone alone if gentamicin contraindicated
No organism seen	Ceftriaxone 1 g IV qd or cefotaxime 2 g IV q8h	Cefoxitin

Abbreviation: MRSA, methicillin-resistant *Staphylococcus aureus*.
[a] For details of vancomycin dosing, see Chap. 28.
[b] For the patient at risk for *Pseudomonas aeruginosa* or nosocomial gram-negative pathogens, an aminoglycoside can be added until susceptibility data are available.

Table 9-2. Empiric therapy for septic arthritis based on gram stain in children

Gram Stain	Drug of Choice	Alternative
Gram (+) cocci	Nafcillin or oxacillin 100–200 mg/kg/day in divided doses q4h	Cefazolin **or** clindamycin **or** vancomycin*
Gram (−) cocci	Ceftriaxone (50 mg/kg/day, max 1 g) IV once daily	Cefotaxime
Gram (−) bacilli	Third-generation cephalosporin ± gentamicin[†]	Gentamicin (see Chap. 21) and piperacillin or ticarcillin (see Chap. 18)
No organism seen	Ceftriaxone (as above)	Cefuroxime with or without nafcillin

* Preferred in known or high-risk methicillin-resistant *Staphylococcus aureus*.
[†] If local resistance patterns dictate, tobramycin or amikacin can be used.
An aminoglycoside can be added if the patient is at risk for *Pseudomonas aeruginosa* or other resistant gram-negatives.

malnutrition, infection at another site, prior surgery of the affected joint, type of implant (knees at greater risk than hip prostheses), and prior postoperative wound infection at the site of surgery (2).

B. **Initiation of infection**. Bacterial contamination of the joint may be initiated either during or after implantation. Series suggest that 80% to 90% of prosthetic joint infections evident in the first 2 years after surgery originate in the operating room and account for the high frequency of staphylococcal infections. Later infections may be due to hematogenous spread from a distant focal infection (2).

C. **Microbiologic features** (5). The majority of infections are due to coagulase-negative staphylococci or *S. aureus*. Gram-negative bacilli account for less than 15%.

II. **Clinical aspects** (2,5)

A. **Presentation.** Prosthetic joint infections are generally indolent and the degree of pain and systemic symptoms often considerably less pronounced than in septic arthritis of a native joint. (See Sec. 3.)

1. **Pain** of the involved joint nevertheless **is a prominent** feature, usually is constant, is worsened by weightbearing, and increases over time.

2. Fever or localized erythema is common but occurs in a minority of patients.

3. A chronic indolent course is suggestive of coagulase-negative staphylococci, whereas an acute or fulminant presentation is more common with virulent pathogens (e.g., *S. aureus* or group A streptococci).

4. In prosthetic joint infection, passive range of motion may persist but active movement is limited (by pain).

B. **Diagnosis**

1. Although radiographic studies and/or scans may be suggestive, careful **aspiration of joint fluid with culture** remains the test of choice for definitive diagnosis. (A meticulous skin prep should be done to avoid contaminating the aspirated fluid with skin flora, the same organisms that are often true pathogens.)

   Loosening of the prosthesis on x-ray may suggest infection, but it is often difficult to distinguish mechanical from infectious loosening.

2. **Blood cultures** should be obtained.

3. Subsequent **histologic and microbiologic examination** of tissue samples obtained at surgery are also definitive and may be especially useful in patients on prior antibiotics, which may suppress bacterial growth of aspirated joint fluid.

C. **Therapy.** The **optimal approach** to treatment of the infected arthroplasty remains **unclear.** Because of the "foreign-body" nature of these prostheses, infection is typically difficult to eradicate without removal of the device, which may not be feasible. We suggest close cooperation with the orthopedic surgeon and infectious disease specialist.

   After obtaining a joint fluid for study, empiric therapy with vancomycin (± an aminoglycoside) is reasonable while awaiting culture data.

III. **Preventive antibiotics**. The role of antibiotics, if any, to prevent prosthetic joint infection is discussed in Chap. 15.

Osteomyelitis

Osteomyelitis is an inflammatory process in bone and bone marrow. It is caused most often by pyogenic bacteria but may be caused by other microorganisms, including mycobacteria and fungi. It is helpful to think about osteomyelitis in terms of mechanism of onset (i.e., hematogenous osteomyelitis versus contiguous focus osteomyelitis versus peripheral vascular disease-related osteomyelitis). This topic has recently been reviewed (6–8), but several points deserve emphasis.

I. **Clinical presentation**

A. **Hematogenous osteomyelitis** results from a bacteremia seeding bone.

1. **Long-bone** involvement is more common in children. *S. aureus* is common, although in sickle cell

disease *Salmonella* spp. may occur, especially in developing countries (7).

2. **Vertebrae. In adults the vertebrae** are the most common sites of localization. *S. aureus* is the most common organism. IV drug users (*Pseudomonas*) and hemodialysis patients (gram-negative organisms) are especially at risk.

3. **Localized signs and symptoms** such as pain (e.g., focal back pain in involvement of the vertebrae); soft-tissue swelling, erythema, and warmth over the involved long bone; and systemic symptoms such as fever, chills, night sweats, and weight loss are common. The presentation may be acute or subacute.

B. **Contiguous focus osteomyelitis** is secondary to an adjacent area of infection.

1. **Associated with diabetic foot ulcer.** The area of soft-tissue infection associated with a foot ulcer in a diabetic with peripheral neuropathy often leads to osteomyelitis. *S. aureus* is a common cause in early infections with mixed gram-negative bacteria and *S. aureus* in more subacute infections. Anaerobes may be found in conjunction with gram negatives in advanced vascular disease of diabetes with more chronic infections. See Chap. 3.

2. **Other clinical situations**. Postoperative infections, open fractures, prosthetic joint infections, direct inoculation from trauma, or contiguous wounds may be predisposing conditions.

3. **Symptoms.** Especially in the diabetic foot infections, patients may be without systemic symptoms. See related discussions in Chap. 3. Infection with *S. aureus* or group A streptococcus is more likely to produce symptoms. Following prosthetic joints, infection with coagulase-negative *Staphylococci* spp. is likely to cause only focal joint pain.

C. **Peripheral vascular disease–associated osteomyelitis** usually occurs in diabetic patients with or without large-vessel insufficiency or patients with severe vascular insufficiency. These infections are commonly due to mixed pathogens and involve the feet. They are a variant of contiguous focus osteomyelitis. (See diabetic foot infection in Chap. 3.)

II. **Diagnosis. Vigorous attempts at isolating the etiologic agent are warranted** to optimize therapy and to minimize potential antibiotic toxicity. **The gold standard for diagnosing osteomyelitis is histopathologic and microbiologic examination of the bone** (7). Other adjunctive approaches include the following:

A. **Blood cultures**. Approximately 50% of patients with acute hematogenous osteomyelitis will have positive blood cultures. In contiguous osteomyelitis, blood cultures are usually negative. Two blood cultures drawn 30 to 60 minutes apart are advised.

B. **Wound culture** drainage. The technique of culturing diabetic foot wounds and "probing" the wound to bone is discussed in Chap. 3.

C. **Needle aspirations** of soft-tissue collections, subperiosteal abscesses, and intraosseous lesions to obtain culture material are often diagnostic.

D. **Open biopsy** should be considered in those patients in whom the response to therapy is unusually slow or incomplete, or in situations in which tuberculosis, fungi, metastatic tumor, or Ewing's tumor (which may clinically and radiographically mimic osteomyelitis) are being considered. Biopsy material should be submitted for histopathologic examination as well as special stains for bacteria, acid-fast bacilli, and fungi. Aerobic, anaerobic, mycobacterial, and fungal cultures should be performed.

E. **Leukocyte count** may be normal or minimally elevated.

F. **Erythrocyte sedimentation rate** (ESR) may be normal early but will usually rise as the duration of illness increases. However, a normal ESR does not exclude the diagnosis. When the ESR is elevated, it provides an excellent parameter to monitor appropriate therapy.

G. **C-reactive protein**, like the ESR, is an acute-phase reactant but is relatively insensitive and nonspecific (7). (See Chap. 13A.)

H. **Simple plain-film evaluation** is very helpful when positive. Cortical destruction with periosteal new bone formation strongly suggests the diagnosis, and when the clinical suspicion is high, further studies add little information (7). However, in hematogenous osteomyelitis the radiologic changes often lag days to a week or two behind the clinical presentations. In contiguous osteomyelitis, x-ray changes may be difficult to discern but usually develop over time.

I. **Radionuclide scanning** is most helpful early in the course of acute disease, prior to the development of roentgenographic changes. Positive scans may be seen as early as 24 hours after the onset of symptoms. For nuclear imaging, technetium scanning is still often preferred. This and other scanning options have recently been reviewed (7,8). **Magnetic resonance imaging (MRI) is particularly helpful in vertebral osteomyelitis** and superior to computed tomography (CT) in differentiating bone and soft-tissue involvement. Because of the many radiographic approaches available, when routine x-rays are not diagnostic, we suggest the role of radionuclide scanning versus CT versus MRI be reviewed with your radiologist to help pick the best test, or tests, depending on the individual case, resources available, and experience of your radiologists.

Table 9-3.   Empiric antibiotic therapy of acute osteomyelitis for adults

Clinical Presentations	Treatment
Hematogenous osteomyelitis	
Acute	Nafcillin/oxacillin*
Subacute	Nafcillin/oxacillin **or** third-generation cephalosporin
Contiguous focus osteomyelitis	Piperacillin-tazobactam ± an aminoglycoside[†] **or** third-generation cephalosporin[†]
PVD associated osteomyelitis	See diabetic foot infections, Chap. 3.

* If gram-negatives are a concern (e.g., in patients with a history of urosepsis or nosocomial infection), a third-generation cephalosporin or an aminoglycoside can be added until cultures are available.

[†] Therapy may be modified by culture data of contiguous wound. An aminoglycoside may be added initially if there is concern with *P. aeruginosa* or a resistant nosocomial gram-negative.

V.   **Therapy** involves prolonged antibiotics (4 to 6 weeks), and **infectious disease consultation is advised.** For empiric therapy, see **Tables 9.3** and **9.4.**
   A.   **Hematogenous osteomyelitis.** In children and neonates, osteomyelitis may have a rapid course. In acute osteomyelitis, it is important to treat the patient optimally to achieve a cure rather than risk the chance of

Table 9-4.   Empiric therapy of acute osteomyelitis for children

Clinical Presentation	Treatment
Hematogenous osteomyelitis	
Without hemoglobinopathy	Nafcillin/oxacillin if more than 6 years of age
	If under 6 years, ceftriaxone (or cefotaxime) ± oxacillin or nafcillin
With hemoglobinopathy	Ceftriaxone (cefotaxime) ± oxacillin or nafcillin
Contiguous focus	Third-generation cephalosporin **or** nafcillin/oxacillin and aminoglycoside*

* Therapy may be modified by culture data of contiguous wound.

Note: Ceftriaxone should be avoided in neonates in whom cefotaxime is preferred. See Chap. 19.

partial or inadequate regimens that will fail and be associated with a relapse or chronic osteomyelitis.

B. **Contiguous osteomyelitis**. Especially in adults, isolating the specific organism should be the initial goal of the physician before starting antibiotics, unless the patient is very ill, which is uncommon. After obtaining cultures, suggested therapy is shown in **Table 9.3 and 9.4.**

C. **In neonates,** *S. aureus*, enteric gram-negative bacilli and streptococci must be considered. Oxacillin and an aminoglycoside can be used if no organisms are seen. If gram-negative bacteria are seen, ampicillin and an aminoglycoside can be used. See Appendix Table C for dosages.

D. **Diabetic foot infections** are discussed in Chap. 3.

References

1. Smith JW, Piercy EA. Infectious arthritis. *Clin Infect Dis* 1995; 20:225.
   "State of the art" series.
2. Roberts NJ Jr, Mock DJ. Joint infections. In: Reese RE, Betts RF, eds. *A practical approach to infectious diseases,* 4th ed. Boston: Little, Brown, 1996:Chap. 15.
3. Espinoza LR, ed. Infectious arthritis. *Rheum Dis Clin North Am* 1998;24:211.
   This symposium has a series of articles dealing with orthopedic management of septic arthritis, septic arthritis in children, gonococcal arthritis, and postinfectious arthritis.
4. Hasselbacher P. Arthrocentesis, synovial fluid analysis, and synovial biopsy. In: Klippel JH, ed. *Primer on the rheumatic diseases*, 11th ed. Atlanta: Arthritis Foundation, 1997:98.
5. Steckelberg JM, Osman DR. Prosthetic joint infections. In: Bisno AL, Waldvogel FA, eds. *Infections associated with indwelling medical devices*, 2nd ed. Washington, DC: American Society of Microbiology, 1994:Chap. 11.
   This is an excellent discussion.
6. Nolan RL, Chapman SW. Osteomyelitis and diabetic foot infections. In: Reese RE, Betts RF, eds. *A practical approach to infectious diseases,* 4th ed. Boston: Little, Brown, 1996:Chap. 16.
7. Haas DW, McAndrew MP. Bacterial osteomyelitis in adults: evolving considerations in diagnosis and treatment. *Am J Med* 1996; 101:550.
8. Lew DP, Waldvogel FA. Osteomyelitis. *N Engl J Med* 1997;336:999.

Sexually Transmitted Diseases and Pelvic Inflammatory Disease

This chapter presents a very brief overview of the common sexually transmitted diseases (STDs) for the practitioner who only occasionally or rarely sees a patient with a STD. For the practitioner who frequently sees such patients or wants more detailed information for the occasional patient, other, more comprehensive resources are advised (1–3).

General principles in seeing a patient with a STD include the following (1):

- **Patients with one STD often have another.**
- **All patients with STDs should have serologic studies for syphilis and HIV.**
- **Partners of patients with STDs should be evaluated and treated when indicated.**
- **All STD patients should be counseled for safer sex practices.**
- **Screening should be performed on asymptomatic patients that are at risk.**

Urethritis in Men

Urethritis, or inflammation of the urethra, is caused by an infection characterized by the **discharge** of mucopurulent or purulent material and by **burning** during urination (2). Initial evaluation **requires differentiating gonococcal urethritis (GCU) from nongonococcal (NGU) infection.** Causes for NGU include *Chlamydia trachomatis, Ureaplasma urealyticum, Trichomonas vaginalis,* and Herpes simplex virus.

I. **Epidemiologic features** (1). NGU, which appears disproportionately in higher socioeconomic groups, is now twice as common as GCU in the United States. GCU is relatively more common among homosexual than among heterosexual men.

II. **Clinical features in men** (1). There are similarities and differences between GCU and NGU. Clinicians must ask about oral sex and pharyngeal symptoms for possible gonococcal pharyngitis and get appropriate throat cultures.

A. **Incubation period.** Seventy-five percent of men with GCU develop symptoms.

   1. **GCU:** 75% develop symptoms within 4 days, 80% to 90% within 2 weeks.
   2. **NGU:** 50% develop symptoms within 4 days but the range is 2 to 25 days.

B. **Onset** is abrupt in GCU and less acute in NGU.

C. **Urethral discharge** is described by 75% of men with GCU.

1. **GCU:** 75% with **profuse, purulent** discharge present at the meatus without stripping and usually stains the underwear.
2. **NGU:** 10% to 30% and often clear.

D. **Dysuria** is common in both GCU and NGU.

E. **Urethritis is documented by** the presence of any of the following signs (2):
   1. Mucopurulent discharge or purulent discharge, or
   2. Gram stain of urethral secretions demonstrating ≥5 white blood cells (WBCs) per oil immersion field, or
   3. Positive leukocyte esterase test on a first-void urine or microscopic examination of first-void urine demonstrating ≥10 WBCs per high-power field.

F. **Note: Pharyngeal gonococcal infection** is often asymptomatic. History of orogenital contact should be carefully obtained in laymen terms since pharyngeal infection has certain treatment implications, which are summarized in Table 10-1.

III. **Diagnosis and differential diagnosis in men** (1). All patients who have urethritis should be evaluated for the presence of GC and chlamydial infection.

A. **Examination of the patient.** Men should stand before the seated examiner, and the entire genital area should be examined preferably at least 2 hours after micturition for adequate recovery of discharge. If discharge is not spontaneously present, the urethra should be gently milked. The mucosa is often friable and bleeds easily in GCU.

B. **Examination of the urethral specimen.** If no discharge is expressed, urethral material should be obtained by inserting a small swab. Calcium alginate or rayon swab on a metal shaft is inserted approximately 2 to 4 cm into the urethra and then removed while rotating the swab. Even small numbers of PMNs on a urethral smear provide objective evidence of urethritis. If characteristic **gram-negative, intracellular diplococci are seen, the diagnosis of gonorrhea is established. If PMNs are present but organisms are not observed, the patient has NGU.** This test is more than 95% accurate in men with symptomatic acute urethritis (4). One cannot diagnose coincident NGU by gram staining in the presence of gonorrhea.

C. Testing for chlamydia in patients with NGU is strongly recommended because a specific diagnosis might improve compliance and partner notification (2).

D. **Pharyngeal cultures** should be obtained in patients with history of orogenital contact.

IV. **Treatment**

A. **All sexual partners exposed within 60 days should be evaluated (2) and treated even if asymptomatic.** If the patient's last sexual intercourse was more than 60 days before onset of symptoms or diagnosis, the patient's most recent sex partner should be treated.

B. Because coincident infections with chlamydia are very common in GCU, one should assume the patients with gonorrhea are coinfected. Hence **all GCU patients should also receive NGU therapy as well.**

C. **Suggested regimens** are shown in **Table 10.1.** Treatment should be initiated as soon as possible after diagnosis. Single-dose regimens have the important advantage of improved compliance and of directly observed therapy. If multiple-dose regimens are used, the medication should be provided in the office or clinic (2) to help improve compliance.

For patients with recurrent or persistent symptoms, alternate approaches are described (2).

V. **Follow-up.** Patients who have uncomplicated GC and/or NGU and who are treated with any recommended regimen need not return for a test of cure (2) but should be evaluated if symptoms persist or recur after therapy. Patients should be instructed to abstain from sexual intercourse until therapy is completed (7 days after single-dose regimen or after completion of a 7-day regimen). If patients with GC have persisting or recurring symptoms after treatment, reevaluation is indicated with cultures for *N. gonorrhoeae* and any GC isolated should be tested for antibiotic susceptibilities.

Table 10-1. Therapy of urethritis*

Type of Urethritis	Primary	Alternative
GCU		
Oral	Ciprofloxacin,[†, ‡] 500 mg po once plus regimen for NGU[‡]; or cefixime 400 mg po once plus regimen for NGU	Ofloxacin*,[‡] 400 mg po once plus regimen for NGU[‡]
Parenteral	Ceftriaxone 125 mg IM[‡] plus regimen for NGU[‡]	Spectinomycin (see Chap. 31) plus regimen for NGU
NGU	Azithromycin 1 g po once or doxycycline 100 mg po bid for 7 days	Erythromycin base 500 mg po qid × 7 days or Ofloxacin 300 mg bid for 7 days

Abbreviations: GCU, gonococcal urethritis; NGU, nongonococcal urethritis.
* For other options for therapy, see reference 2.
† Ciprofloxacin and other quinolones are contraindicated in pregnant women and children younger than 15. See Chap. 32.
‡ **Therapy which can also be used for gonococcal pharyngitis.** Although chlamydial coinfection of the pharynx is unusual, coinfection at the genital sites sometimes occurs. Therefore, treatment for both gonorrhea and chlamydia (with azithromycin or doxycycline) is suggested for gonococcal pharyngitis.

VI. **Complications**. Epididymitis and prostatitis are possible complications; Reiter's syndrome is a possible complication of chlamydial disease (1,2).

Mucopurulent Cervicitis

Mucopurulent cervicitis (MPC) is characterized by a purulent or mucopurulent endocervical exudate visible in the endocervical canal or on an endocervical swab specimen (2).

I. **Etiology. Similar to that of urethritis in men.** *Chlamydia trachomatis* and *N. gonorrhoeae* are the two most common infectious causes. Cervicitis and pelvic inflammatory disease (PID) are a continuum. Clinicians should have a low threshold to consider PID in their differential diagnoses.

II. **Diagnosis**
   A. The diagnosis of mucopurulent cervicitis is based on the presence of one of the two following criteria:
      1. Yellow **mucopurulent discharge** on a cotton swab that has been inserted into the endocervix.
      2. Ten or more **polymorphonuclear leukocytes** per oil-immersion field on a gram-stained endocervical smear suggests the diagnosis of MPC, though other experts feel this test is not standardized enough in women (2). **The cervical gram stain has very limited utility in the management of MPC (1).**
   B. Microbiologic studies for gonorrheal and chlamydial infection should be performed as discussed under urethritis.

III. **Treatment**. Empiric treatment should be initiated for all symptomatic and asymptomatic women. Because of poor sensitivity of the gram stain in women for *N. gonorrhoeae*, therapy should cover both *N. gonorrhoeae* and *C. trachomatis*, since 30% to 60% of women with GC cervicitis also have chlamydial infection (1,2). **All male sexual partners should be treated as well. Treatment regimen is the same as that for urethritis (Table 10.1).**
   A. **Follow-up.** See Sec. V under "Urethritis in Men."
   B. **Management of sex partners.** Partners should be notified, examined, and treated for the STD identified or suspected in the index case (2). See Sec. IV under "Urethritis in Men."

IV. **Complications**. Cervical gonorrheal and chlamydial infection can ascend to cause PID.

Ulcerative Lesions

The following discussion is a brief overview of genital ulcer disease.

I. **Genital herpes simplex infection (HSV)** (1,2)
   A. **Epidemiology.** Approximately 70% to 95% are due to HSV type 2. Type 1 genital infections may result

from orogenital sexual contact. Patients developing initial HSV-2 infection who have antibody to HSV-1 have milder initial episodes than do patients with no antibody. Many patients (perhaps up to 60%) have asymptomatic initial episodes and/or recurrence, perhaps explaining the onset of herpetic lesions in a long-term, stable, monogamous sexual relationship. Initial episodes are classified as primary if the patient has no prior exposure to HSV.

B. **Clinical features. The diagnosis can often be made on clinical grounds alone.**

1. **Lesions** that appear **2 to 20 days after exposure** are initially **vesicular**, are often grouped, and surmount an **erythematous base**. Particularly in women, the vesicles quickly erupt to form equal-sized, shallow, markedly nonindurated, **painful ulcers**. Lesions are usually located on the penis or on the labia, vulva, or cervix, and often spare the vagina. Lesions heal by crusting over. Primary disease often **lasts 3 weeks**; occasionally, primary disease can be severe and may require hospitalization (2).

2. **Regional lymphadenopathy,** usually tender, develops generally toward the end of the first week of illness and is common.

3. **Extragenital manifestations.** Fever, malaise, and anorexia are common in primary infection.

4. **Recurrence.** Within the first year after infection, lesions occur in approximately 90% of patients with HSV-2, but in only 25% to 50% of those infected with HSV-1 patients (5). Therefore identification of the type of infecting strain has prognostic importance and may be useful for counseling purposes (2). Recurrence, which is triggered by stress, fever, or trauma, may be preceded by a prodrome of itching, tingling, or burning 6 to 24 hours before lesions appear. Recurrences generally last 7 to 10 days and proceed through the same stages as primary disease; systemic manifestations are far less common.

C. **Diagnosis can be made clinically.**

1. **The Tzanck smear** has only limited utility because vesicles are diagnostic.

2. **Direct immunofluorescent techniques** are becoming available.

3. **Culture** carried out in the first 24 to 48 hours is positive in nearly 100% of cases and becomes positive within 24 hours of inoculation. It is the only method useful for diagnosis of asymptomatic shedding. Virus yield diminishes for lesions that are just a few days old.

4. **Syphilis and HIV serologic studies are indicated** in these patients.

D. **Treatment.** Genital HSV is a recurrent, incurable disease. Systemic antiviral drugs can suppress signs and symptoms of initial and recurrent episodes, but available agents neither eradicate latent virus nor affect the risk, frequency, or severity of recurrences after the drug is discontinued (2). The lesions should be kept clean and dry.

1. **Topical acyclovir** is relatively ineffective.
2. **Intravenous acyclovir** is rarely indicated except for severe disease requiring hospitalization.
3. **Oral treatment** is used in three situations:
   a. **Initial infection** is treated **for 7 to 10 days** or until clinical resolution occurs.
   b. **Recurrent disease** may be **treated for 5 days,** but its impact is minimal.
   c. **Frequently recurring disease** (i.e., six episodes or more per year) can be controlled with **long-term suppressive therapy.** (See Sec. 5.)
4. **Therapeutic agents** (2)
   a. **Acyclovir. For initial** infection, 200 mg five times a day or 400 mg tid; **for recurrence**, 200 mg five times a day, or 400 mg tid, or 800 mg bid.
   b. **Famciclovir**. 250 mg tid for initial treatment; for recurrence, 125 mg bid.
   c. **Valacyclovir.** One gram bid for initial treatment; for recurrence, 500 mg bid.
5. **Suppressive therapy** (2). Daily suppressive therapy reduces the frequency of genital recurrences by 75% or more among patients with frequent recurrences, but it does not completely prevent viral shedding. The extent to which suppressive therapy may prevent HSV transmission is unknown. Safety and efficacy of acyclovir for suppression has been shown for as long as 6 years; for valacyclovir and famciclovir, 1 year. **Regimens** for chronic suppression **include** acyclovir 400 mg bid, famciclovir 250 mg bid, and valacyclovir 250 mg bid or 500 or 1,000 mg once a day (2).

   After 1 year of continuous suppressive therapy, discontinuation of therapy should be discussed and reassessed on an individual basis (2).

E. **AIDS patients** may have more severe and/or prolonged episodes of genital or perianal HSV infections. The optimal dosage of antiviral drugs for these patients is controversial, but they may benefit from higher doses until clinical resolution (e.g., acyclovir 400 mg po three to five times daily). Famciclovir 500 mg bid has been useful in decreasing recurrences (2). **High doses of valacyclovir** (8 g/day) have been associated with a syndrome resembling either hemolytic uremic syndrome or thrombotic thrombocytopenic purpura; these high-dose regimens **should be avoided** (2). We tend to avoid using valacyclovir in AIDS patients.

For severe cases, acyclovir 5 mg/kg intravenously (IV) q8h may be necessary (2).

F. **Pregnancy**
   1. **The safety of systemic acyclovir** and valacyclovir therapy in pregnant women has not been established, and a registry of recipients is maintained (2). Current registry findings do not indicate an increased risk for major birth defects after acyclovir treatment (2).

      Although the first clinical episode of genital herpes during pregnancy may be treated with oral acyclovir, routine administration of acyclovir to pregnant women who have a history of recurrent genital herpes is not advised at this time (2). Infectious disease consultation is advised if acyclovir use is being considered.

   2. **Perinatal infection.** Most mothers of infants who acquire neonatal herpes lack histories of clinically evident genital herpes. The risk for transmission to the neonate from an infected mother is high among women who acquire genital herpes near the time of delivery (30% to 50%) and is low among women who have a history of recurrent herpes at term and women who acquire genital HSV during the first half of pregnancy (3%). **Therefore prevention of neonatal herpes should emphasize prevention of acquisition of genital HSV infection late in pregnancy (2).**

      At the onset of labor, all women should be examined and carefully questioned regarding whether they have symptoms of genital herpes. Infants of women who do not have symptoms or signs of genital herpes infection or its prodrome may be delivered vaginally (2). Cesarean section does not completely eliminate the risk for HSV infection in the neonate (2).

      This topic is reviewed elsewhere in more detail (2,6).

G. **Management of sex partners.** The sex partners of patients with genital herpes are likely to benefit from evaluation and counseling. Symptomatic sex partners should be evaluated and treated in the same manner as patients who have genital lesions (2).

II. **Syphilis**. A complete review of this topic is beyond the scope of this handbook. Several issues deserve emphasis.

A. **Epidemiologic features** (1,2)
   1. **Incidence**. The incidence among male homosexuals has declined considerably as a result of behavior modification in response to AIDS. At the same time, the rate among heterosexuals has increased as a result of sex-for-drugs prostitution.
   2. **Transmission**. Transplacental transmission is the second major route of acquisition. Transfusion syphilis is no longer a problem.

B. **Clinical manifestations** (1,2)
   1. **The incubation period** averages 3 weeks but ranges from 10 to 90 days. During this interval,

infected patients have neither clinical nor serologic evidence of disease.

2. **Primary syphilis.** One or sometimes multiple, **ulcerated, painless** lesions, called **chancres**, appear at the site of initial infection and multiplication of the spirochetes. Chancres are usually **minimally painful or nontender** and are usually clean ulcerations with distinctly indurated edges. Several discrete, nontender inguinal nodes are seen within the first week. Untreated, primary syphilis usually resolves in 3 to 6 weeks. **Nontreponemal serologic tests for syphilis are positive in approximately 50% of patients when the chancre first appears.**

3. **Secondary syphilis.** *Treponema pallidum* disseminates even before the appearance of the chancre; often after its resolution, a nonspecific, constitutional illness that commonly includes a sore throat and myalgia ushers in a **generalized maculopapular**, symmetric, and nonpruritic **rash, often involving the palms and soles**. It almost always involves the oral mucous membranes and the genitalia. The dry lesions do not pose a contagion risk, for they contain very few organisms, whereas the painless, shallow ulcers of the mucous membranes are highly contagious. **Patchy alopecia** is frequent. **Condylomata lata**, hypertrophic lesions resembling flat warts, occur in moist areas (e.g., around the anus) and are highly contagious. **Serologic tests are almost always reactive in secondary syphilis,** usually in high titer. These manifestations resolve without treatment. Approximately 25% of untreated patients will again develop the manifestations of secondary syphilis, termed **mucocutaneous relapse,** during the subsequent 1 to 2 years. Such patients are contagious to sexual partners. This phase is known as the **early latent period**.

4. **Latent syphilis** is clinically silent, and diagnosis can be made only on the basis of serologic tests.

5. **Late (tertiary) syphilis** eventually develops in nearly one-third of infected, untreated patients. Briefly, syphilis should be suspected in the following clinical settings. (See references 2 and 3 for details.)

   a. **Lymphocytic meningitis** may be a manifestation of secondary syphilis or appear somewhat later as meningovascular syphilis.

   b. **Destructive lesions of skin and bones** may represent so-called late benign syphilis.

   c. **Dementia** may be due to general paresis.

   d. **Posterior column** disease (i.e., tabes dorsalis).

   e. **Disease of the aorta or incompetence of the aortic valve.**

C. **Serologic diagnosis. Potential pitfalls in sero-diagnosis must be recognized.** There is a lack of sensitivity of the nontreponemal tests in late syphilis. **The treponemal test is the best serologic test.**

   1. **Nontreponemal tests.** Screening tests for syphilis exploit the observation that patients with syphilis develop antibodies reactive with a variety of poorly defined lipids. Nontreponemal tests include the **VDRL** (Venereal Disease Research Laboratory), **RPR** (rapid plasma reagin), and **ART** (automated reagin test) tests.

      a. **Nontreponemal tests are nonspecific.** False-positive reactions occur in a variety of acute and chronic conditions such as acute viral illnesses, collagen vascular disease, pregnancy, and intravenous drug use. A nontreponemal test is considered diagnostic in the setting of a highly suggestive clinical syndrome (e.g., chancre) but cannot be used to diagnose latent syphilis without confirmation by a treponemal test.

      b. **Quantification.** The tests are often quantitated and reported as the highest twofold dilution of serum eliciting a positive reaction. Titers of 1:8 or higher are unusual among false-positive cases. The highest titers are seen in secondary syphilis; 1:256 or higher is not unusual.

      c. **Sensitivity.** Nontreponemal tests are insensitive in primary and late syphilis. In suspected late syphilis one should obtain a treponemal test even when the nontreponemal test is nonreactive. In suspected primary disease, repeat serologic study (nontreponemal and treponemal) in 3 months is advised.

      d. **Response to therapy.** If therapy is adequate, titers should undergo a fourfold decline within 3 months in treatment of early syphilis and within 6 months in late syphilis.

      e. **Posttreatment.** Serial serologic studies are important. Nontreponemal tests must be used. They convert to nonreactive within 2 years in approximately 90% of primary syphilis and in nearly 75% of secondary syphilis. Reappearance or fourfold risk in titer indicates relapse or reinfection. The same nontreponemal tests should be used in follow-up serologic studies.

   2. **Treponemal tests.** The fluorescent treponemal antibody absorption (**FTA-ABS**) test is the most sensitive (90%) but requires a fluorescence microscope. More easily performed is the microhemagglutination test for antibody to *T. pallidum* (**MHA-Tp**) (80% sensitive), which requires no special equipment. The treponemal tests are more

specific and more sensitive than the nontreponemal tests and are particularly useful in very early primary and late syphilis.

   a. Treponemal tests confirm the diagnosis in patients with reactive nontreponemal tests or where suspicion is high and the nontreponemal test is negative. The treponemal tests are **not used for screening** because of their cost and because they are most effective when used in the high-prevalence population already defined by a reactive nontreponemal test.

   b. The treponemal tests are not quantitated but are reported as nonreactive or weakly to strongly reactive.

   c. The **treponemal tests remain positive for extended periods, for life (even after adequate treatment of syphilis).**

   d. **False positives** can occur in other treponemal diseases (e.g., yaws, pinta, bejel) and in some other spirochetal diseases (e.g., Lyme disease).

3. **Interpretation.** Serologic evaluation of syphilis is an imperfect science, and the clinician is well advised to take all clinical and epidemiologic information into account before making decisions regarding treatment. **It is useful to seek input from someone experienced with serologic interpretation when one sees only occasional cases of syphilis.** Patterns of seroreactivity are summarized in **Table 10.2**.

D. **Treatment**. The discussion below is to provide an overview only. **Before initiating/completing therapy for a patient with syphilis, an infectious disease consultant or someone experienced in treating syphilis ideally should be consulted.**

1. **Penicillin remains the drug of choice for all stages of syphilis** unless the patient is hypersensitive. See **Table 10.3.**

2. **All patients being treated for syphilis should be strongly advised to undergo testing for HIV antibody.**

3. **Follow-up.** All patients treated for syphilis should have follow-up serologic studies every 3 months for early syphilis and every 6 months for latent syphilis for at least 2 years after treatment. Pregnant women should have monthly serologic studies.

4. **In penicillin-allergic pregnant women**, erythromycin is no longer recommended. Patients should be skin tested; if they are positive, patients should be desensitized in consultation with an expert (2).

5. The **Jarisch-Herxheimer reaction**, which is self-limited and usually requires only antipyretics,

Table 10-2. Serology for syphilis

Nontreponemal Test (e.g., RPR, VDRL)	Treponemal Test (e.g., FTA-ABS, MHA-Tp)	Interpretation
Nonreactive	Nonreactive	Past or present treponemal infection highly unlikely; very early primary syphilis still possible
Reactive	Nonreactive	Biologic false-positive reaction; treponemal infection extremely unlikely
Nonreactive	Reactive	Early primary syphilis; secondary syphilis with prozone; late syphilis; adequately treated syphilis or false positive, another treponemal disease (e.g., yaws) or spirochetal disease (Lyme disease)
Reactive	Reactive	Syphilis, any stage; adequately treated latent or late syphilis; other treponemal disease; reinfection with syphilis; inadequately treated syphilis
Reactive with rising titer	Reactive	Relapse of or reinfection with syphilis; adequately treated syphilis with superimposed condition generating a false-positive NT

Abbreviation: NT, nontreponema test.

manifests as fever, increased rash, adenopathy, and sometimes hypotension 1 to 6 hours after beginning treatment. It is seen in approximately 50% of patients with primary syphilis and in almost all patients with secondary syphilis. It probably results from the release of treponemal antigens upon lysis of the organisms.

E. **Therapy of HIV-infected patients** involves **special considerations**, which are reviewed elsewhere (2). HIV-infected patients who have either late latent

Table 10-3. Therapy for syphilis (adults) without HIV infections

	Primary	Alternative[†]
Contact (within 90 days)* or early syphilis	Benzathine penicillin G, 2.4 MU IM × 1 dose	Tetracycline 500 mg po qid for 2 weeks or doxycycline 100 mg po bid × 2 weeks
Latent syphilis (with normal CSF exam if performed)	Benzathine penicillin G 2.4 MU IM qw × 3 weeks	Doxycycline 100 mg po bid × 4 weeks or tetracycline 500 mg qid for 4 weeks
Neurosyphilis[†]	Aqueous crystalline penicillin G 18–24 million units a day, administered as 3–4 million units q4h for 10–14 days**	Procaine penicillin 2.4 million units IM a day plus probenecid 500 mg po qid; both for 10–14 days.** Compliance must be ensured

Abbreviation: CSF, cerebrospinal fluid; MU, million units; qw, weekly.
* Patients whose exposure was more than 90 days previously may be evaluated serologically to determine whether they need treatment. Those exposed <90 days preceding the diagnosis of primary, secondary, or early latent, might be infected even if seronegative; therefore such patients should be treated presumptively.
[†] **Pregnant patients, HIV-infected patients, or patients with neurosyphilis should be desensitized, if necessary, and treated with penicillin.**
[‡] See text for comments on therapy of HIV-infected patients.
** After completion of these neurosyphilis regimens, some experts also administer benzathine penicillin 2.4 MU IM (2).

syphilis or syphilis of unknown duration should have a CSF examination before treatment (2). Penicillin regimens should be used in the therapy of all stages of syphilis; skin testing and desensitization may be needed in penicillin-allergic patients. Careful follow-up serologic studies have been detailed elsewhere (2).

III. **Chancroid**. This infection is caused by the gram-negative rod *Hemophilus ducreyi*. Small epidemics have occurred in the United States, usually associated with prostitutes. Chancroid is a major public health problem in the developing world, and its significance is compounded by its striking association with HIV infection (i.e., chancroid is a cofactor for HIV transmission) (2).

   A. **Clinical manifestations** (1,2). The incubation period is 4 to 7 days. **Painful**, ragged, necrotic-appearing, nonindurated **ulcers** occur on the genitalia. The ulcers are often dirty and may vary in size. "Kissing lesions" of the thighs may occur by autoinoculation. Painful inguinal nodes that may become fluctuant and rupture occur in more than 50% of patients. Occasionally, super-infection with mixed anaerobic occurs.

B. **Diagnosis.** Differential diagnoses include herpes simplex and syphilis. Differentiation between these is often not possible clinically. Gram staining of the lesion, which is insensitive and nonspecific, is not recommended. Culture of the organism is definitive but difficult to perform and usually not available.

Therefore a probable diagnosis, for both clinical and surveillance purposes, may be made if the following criteria are met: (a) the patient has one or more painful genital ulcers; (b) the patient has no evidence of *T. pallidum* infection by darkfield examination of ulcer exudate or by a serologic test for syphilis performed at least 7 days after onset of ulcers; and (c) the clinical presentation, appearance of genital ulcers, and regional lymphadenopathy, if present, are typical for chancroid and a test for HSV is negative. The combination of a painful ulcer and tender inguinal adenopathy, which occurs among one-third of patients, suggests a diagnosis of chancroid; when accompanied by suppurative inguinal adenopathy, these signs are almost pathognomonic. Polymerase chain reaction (PCR) testing for *H. ducreyi* might become available soon (2).

C. **Treatment.** Development of resistance to traditional agents occurs. Uniformly effective in all geographic areas are the following (2):
1. Azithromycin 1 g po once, or
2. Ceftriaxone, 250 mg intramuscularly (IM) as a single dose, or
3. Ciprofloxacin 500 mg po bid for 3 days (contraindicated in pregnancy), or lactating women, or persons less than 18 years of age, or
4. Erythromycin base, 500 mg po qid for 7 days.

D. **Miscellaneous** (2)
1. **Patients should be tested for HIV** infection at the time chancroid is diagnosed.
2. Patients should be retested 3 months after the diagnosis of chancroid if the initial tests for syphilis and HIV were negative.
3. **Patients should be reexamined** in 3 to 7 days after initiation of therapy. If treatment is successful, ulcers improve symptomatically within 3 days and objectively within 7 days after therapy (2). Approaches to nonresponders are discussed elsewhere (2). HIV patients need to be monitored carefully and many need longer courses (2).
4. **Sex partners** of patients with chancroid should be examined and treated regardless of whether symptoms of the disease are present, if they had sexual contact with the patient during the 10 days preceding onset of symptoms in the patient (2).
5. No adverse effects of chancroid on **pregnancy** outcome or on the fetus have been reported (2).

Ceftriaxone or erythromycin therapy are options for the pregnant woman needing therapy.

Venereal Warts

Warts (condylomata acuminata) are caused by human papillomaviruses (HPV). HPV is discussed in more detail elsewhere (1–3) and only a brief discussion follows here. More than 20 types of HPV can infect the genital tract.

I. **Clinical features** (1,2). Most HPV infections are asymptomatic, subclinical, or unrecognized. Visible genital warts are usually caused by HPV types 6 or 11 and form soft papules with irregular, verrucous surfaces that appear 4 to 6 weeks after exposure. Lesions are usually located around the external genitalia and inside the urethra, inside the vagina, and on the cervix. Perianal warts in women may result from spread from a primary genital focus, but perianal warts in men strongly suggest receptive anal intercourse, and such patients should be evaluated for other anal infections such as gonorrhea, chlamydia, or HIV.

II. **Diagnosis** is usually made clinically. Subclinical involvement is detected by swabbing suspect epithelium (i.e., the vagina, cervix, or the penis) with 3% to 5% acetic acid, which turns infected areas white. Subsequent colposcopic examination in women reveals smaller lesions.

III. **Treatment**. The goal is elimination of overt warts and relief of signs and symptoms. The relapse rate approaches 75%. Regimens are discussed in detail elsewhere (1–3).

None of the available treatments are superior to other treatments, and no single treatment is ideal for all patients or all warts (2). Therapy must be individualized and, therefore, ideally supervised by someone experienced in treatment of venereal warts.

A. **Provider-administered** therapy includes the following (2):

1. **Cryotherapy** with liquid nitrogen or cryoprobe, destroys warts by thermal-induced cytolysis. Its major drawback is that proper use requires substantial training, without which warts are frequently overtreated or undertreated, resulting in poor efficacy or increased complication (2).

2. **Podophyllin resin 10% to 25%** in compound of benzoin must be applied carefully and allowed to air-dry to avoid spread of the compound to adjacent areas with focal irritation. The **safety** of this agent in **pregnancy has not been established**.

3. **Trichloroacetic acid (TCA) or bichloracetic acid (BCA)** 80% to 90% can be applied weekly; these are caustic agents that destroy warts by chemical coagulation of the proteins. Spread to adjacent normal tissue should be avoided.

B. **Patient-applied therapy** (2)

1. **Podofilox 0.5% solution or gel** is applied cyclically by the patient after proper education on its

application (2). The safety of this agent in pregnancy has not been established.

2. **Imiquimod 5% cream** is applied three times a week qhs for as long as 16 weeks. The safety of this agent during pregnancy has not been established.

C. **Other techniques** include **laser surgery** and **intralesional interferon**, which are discussed elsewhere (2).

D. Because of the shortcomings of available treatments, some clinics employ combination therapy (i.e., simultaneous use of two or more modalities on the same wart at the same time). Most experts believe that combining modalities does not increase efficacy but may increase complications (2).

IV. **Miscellaneous**

A. **Sequelae**. It is important to remember that some types of HPV are a **risk factor for cervical dysplasia. Female patients and female partners of infected male patients should be advised to have yearly PAP smears.**

B. **Follow-up**. After visible warts have cleared, a follow-up evaluation is not mandatory. Patients should be counseled to watch for recurrences, which occur most frequently within the first 3 months.

C. **Sex partners**. Examination of sex partners is not necessary for the management of genital warts because the role of reinfection is probably minimal and, in the absence of curative therapy, treatment to reduce transmission is not realistic. However, examination of partners may be beneficial to exclude other STDs and early genital warts.

Vulvovaginitis

Vulvovaginitis is a common problem for women. **Vulvovaginal candidiasis, trichomoniasis, and bacterial vaginosis** are the three most common vaginal infections, which are summarized in **Table 10.4** briefly. For further data, see basic references (1–3,7).

Bacterial vaginosis (BV) has been associated with adverse pregnancy outcomes (e.g., premature rupture of membranes, preterm labor, and preterm birth). The screening and treating of high-risk pregnant patients are reviewed elsewhere (2).

Pelvic Inflammatory Disease

Pelvic inflammatory disease (PID) comprises a spectrum of inflammatory disorders of the upper female genital tract, including any combination of endometritis, salpingitis, pelvic peritonitis, and early tuboovarian abscess (2). In the United States, PID is most often a polymicrobial infection. The major causative organisms include *N. gonorrhoeae* (25% to 50%), *C. trachomatis* (10% to 40%), and mixed aerobic/anaerobic bacteria (25% to 60%).

I. **Risk factors**
   A. Teenage girls
   B. Multiple sexual partners
   C. Exposure to STD
   D. Use of IUD
   E. Prior PID
   F. Failure to use barrier contraceptives
II. **Clinical characteristics** (1–3). **The diagnosis of acute PID on clinical grounds alone is notoriously inaccurate** in that fewer than two-thirds of suspected cases are confirmed at laparoscopy. No one sign or symptom is pathognomic. **The most common signs are lower abdominal pain, increased vaginal discharge, and adnexal tenderness.** Fever, irregular menstrual bleeding, and/or urinary tract symptoms are found in less than a third of the patients. Asymptomatic infection is frequent among adolescents. **Experts recommend maintaining a low threshold of suspicion.**
III. **Laboratory.** WBC, ESR (erythrocyte sedimentation rate), and pregnancy test may help. Cervical cultures for gonorrhea and chlamydial infection and serologic tests for syphilis should be performed.
IV. **Centers for Disease Control (CDC) criteria for clinical diagnosis of PID**. Although the diagnosis of PID is based on clinical findings, the clinical diagnosis of acute PID is imprecise. Consequently, many episodes go unrecognized (2).
   A. **Minimal criteria**. Empiric therapy should be instituted in sexually active young women and other women at risk for STDs if all three of the minimal criteria present and no other cause for the illness is identified (2).
      1. **Lower abdominal tenderness**
      2. **Adnexal tenderness**
      3. **Cervical motion tenderness**
   B. **Additional criteria.** These additional criteria will further increase the specificity of the diagnosis.
      1. **Additional criteria** that support the diagnosis of PID include the following:
         a. Oral temperature >38.3°C (>101°F)
         b. Abnormal cervical or vaginal discharge
         c. Elevated ESR
         d. Elevated C-reactive protein, and
         e. Laboratory evidence of cervical infection with *N. gonorrhoeae* or *C. trachomatis*.
      2. The **definitive criteria** for diagnosing PID in select cases include (a) histopathologic evidence of endometritis on endometrial biopsy, (b) transvaginal sonography or other imaging techniques showing thickened fluid-filled tubes with or without free pelvic fluid or tuboovarian complex, and (c) laparoscopic abnormalities consistent with PID (2).
V. **Principles of management**. A practical approach to this problem taking into account the CDC criteria, difficulties in making the diagnosis, and need to not undertreat this problem, has been proposed by MacDonald and Samson (8).

Table 10-4.   Summary of vulvovaginitis

	Candidiasis	Trichomoniasis	Bacterial Vaginosis
Predisposing factors	Pregnancy Diabetes mellitus Oral contraceptive use Broad-spectrum antibiotics use Corticosteroid therapy Tight or nylon undergarments	Multiple sexual partners Menstruation Pregnancy	Often sexually transmitted but not always
Symptoms	Premenstrual onset Pruritus External dysuria Vaginal discharge is not malodorous	Yellow vaginal discharge Dysuria Vulvar itching	Mild-to-moderate discharge or vaginal odor Unrelated to the menstrual cycle Pruritus may be present Patient may be asymptomatic
Examination	Vulvar erythema Thick, white, cheesy discharge	Copious, purulent, frothy discharge, with foul odor (50%) Erythematous vagina and cervix	Discharge is **thin**, at times frothy, gray, and **adherent** to the vaginal walls Vaginal pH >4.5 Erythema or tenderness of vulva and vagina is usually absent
Microscopy	10% KOH wet prep is used to identify **pseudohyphae**	Saline wet mount is used to identify **motile, flagellated organisms** surrounded by a polymorphonuclear infiltrates	Positive **whiff test** (fishy, amine odor with KOH). On saline wet mount **clue cells** (epithelial cells studded with coccobacilli, different from the vaginal flora), few polymorphonuclear cells seen

Treatment*		
Clotrimazole; e.g., Gynelotrimin 3-day combination pack (200-mg vaginal insert tablets for 3 nights and vaginal cream 1% locally bid 3–7 days)** **or** Clotrimazole 1% cream or 100 mg tablets intra-vaginally for 7 days[†] **or** Fluconazole 150 mg oral dose once only Sexual partners usually do not need treatment except possibly in women with recurrent disease	Metronidazole 2 g PO × 1 dose[‡] **or** metronidazole 500 mg PO bid × 7 days. **All sexual partners should be treated**	**For nonpregnant women:** metronidazole gel 0.75% intravaginally bid × 5 days **or** metronidazole 500 mg po bid × 7 days **or** clindamycin cream 2%, 1 applicator qhs × 7 days **or** clindamycin 300 mg po bid for 7 days **or** metronidazole 2 g po once. **Male sexual partners should be treated in recurrent cases.** **In pregnancy,** metronidazole 250 mg po tid for 7 days, or metronidazole 2 g po once or clindamycin 300 mg po bid for 7 days has been suggested (2)

* Many other regimens are available (2).

[†] **Regimen preferred in pregnancy;** 7 days suggested for topical therapy.

[‡] This regimen can be used in pregnancy (2).

** OTC, over the counter (available without a prescription).

A. Exclude acute appendicitis, ectopic pregnancy.
B. Use CDC minimal criteria to guide the diagnosis.
C. Err on the side of the overdiagnosis.
D. Treat early with broad-spectrum antibiotics (**Table 10.5**).
E. **Consider hospitalization for patients:**
   - Who are unlikely to adhere to or be able to tolerate oral therapy (e.g., because of nausea and vomiting)
   - Who fail to respond to outpatient therapy in 48 to 72 hours
   - Who have tuboovarian abscess
   - Who are pregnant
   - Who are immunocompromised, including HIV infection with a low CD4 count
   - Who may have a surgical emergency (e.g., appendicitis)

F. Reassess patient 48 to 72 hours after initiating therapy.
G. Identify, evaluate, and treat sexual partners for *C. trachomatis* and GC.
H. **Screen for and treat lower genital tract infections, obtain serologic studies for syphilis and HIV from all patients.**

VI. **Sequelae.** One-fourth of all women who have had acute salpingitis will experience one or more long-term sequelae.

Table 10-5.   Therapy for PID*

Setting	Primary	Alternative
Outpatient	Ofloxacin 400 mg po bid and metronidazole 500 mg po bid both for 14 days	Ceftriaxone 250 mg IM × 1 dose and doxycycline 100 mg po bid × 14 days
Inpatient†	Cefoxitin 2 g IV q6h (or cefotetan 2 g IV q12h) and doxycycline 100 mg IV or po q12h	Clindamycin 900 mg IV q8h plus gentamicin 2 mg/kg load then 1.5 mg/kg IV or IM q8h maintenance‡

* Common regimens described. For more options see reference 2. Ofloxacin and doxycycline are contraindicated in pregnancy.
† When possible, doxycycline should be administered orally even when the patient is hospitalized because of the pain associated with its IV infusion. See Chap. 27. Parenteral therapy of antibiotics may be discontinued 24 h after the patient improves clinically (2).
   Doxycycline (100 mg po bid) in the primary regimen and clindamycin (450 mg po qid) in the alternative regimen should be continued on an outpatient basis to complete 10–14 total days of therapy. Doxycycline is contraindicated in pregnancy.
‡ Single daily doses of gentamicin may be substituted (2). See Chap. 21. **This is the regimen preferred in pregnancy.** IV therapy can be discontinued 24 h after the patient improves clinically. Oral therapy should be continued with doxycycline 100 mg bid or clindamycin 450 mg qid to complete a total of 14 days of therapy. Clindamycin is preferred in the pregnant patient once doxycycline is contraindicated in pregnancy.

These include tuboovarian abscess, infertility, ectopic pregnancy, chronic pelvic pain, and recurrent episodes of salpingitis.

VII. **Therapy**
    A. Early initiation of **empiric antibiotic therapy** is important for optimal efficacy. See **Table 10.5**.
    B. For **tuboovarian abscess** cases, surgical intervention should be undertaken if there is no response to therapy within 48 to 72 hours or if there is clear-cut worsening at any point during therapy. Most patients will respond to IV antibiotics, which often can be given at home after improvement has been ensured with a short hospitalization. Oral therapy may be reasonable in selected patients, and clindamycin is preferred over doxycycline (2). Infectious disease consultation is suggested.

References

1. Jernigan JA, Rein MF. Sexually transmitted diseases. In: Reese RE, Betts RF, eds. *A practical approach to infectious diseases*, 4th ed. Boston: Little, Brown, 1996:519–558.
   This is an excellent clinical summary of STDs.
2. Centers for Disease Control and Prevention. 1998 Guidelines for Treatment of Sexually Transmitted Diseases. *MMWR* 1998;47 (RR-1):1–116.
   These recommendations are serially updated about every 4 to 5 years. A very useful resource for the practitioner. Every clinician who sees patients with STDs should get a copy.
   For further information on syphilis, see Augenbraun MH, Rolfs R. Treatment of syphilis, 1998: nonpregnant adults. Clin Infect Dis *1999;28:S21 (suppl 1).*
3. Holmes KK, et al, eds. *Sexually transmitted diseases,* 3rd ed. New York: McGraw-Hill, 1999.
   A comprehensive text edited by national experts in the field. Excellent resource.
4. Goodhart ME, et al. Factors affecting the performance of smear and culture tests for the detection of *Neisseria gonorrhoeae. Sex Transm Dis* 1982;9:63.
   For a related paper, also see Kleris GS, Arnold AJ. Differential diagnosis of urethritis: predictive value and therapeutic implications of the urethral smear. Sex Transm Dis *1981;8:110.*
5. Benedetti J, Corey L, Ashley R. Recurrence rates in genital herpes after symptomatic first-episode infections. *Ann Intern Med* 1994; 121:847.
6. Peter G, et al, eds. *1997 Red Book: Report of the Committee on Infectious Diseases*, 24th ed. Elk Grove Village, IL: American Academy of Pediatrics, 1997:266–278.
7. Sobel J. Vaginitis. *N Engl J Med* 1997;337:1896.
8. MacDonald NE, Samson LM. Pelvic inflammatory disease. In: Long SS, Pickering LK, Prober CG, eds. *Principles and practice of pediatric infectious diseases.* New York: Churchill Livingstone, 1997:397–402.
   For a recent discussion of the role of anaerobes in PID see Walker CK, et al. Clin Infect Dis *1999;28:S29 (suppl 1).*

Fever and Apparent Acute CNS Infection

Meningitis

The **diagnosis** of meningitis ultimately is based on the findings in the cerebrospinal fluid (CSF), with blood culture data providing corroborative data at times. **Since examination of the CSF is essential in the diagnosis of meningitis, whenever this diagnosis is seriously considered, a lumbar puncture (LP) is necessary unless contraindicated.**

I. **Clinical presentation** (1,2). Meningitis should be considered in any patient with fever and headache (typically severe, bilateral, associated with photophobia), lethargy, confusion, vomiting, and/or stiff neck (meningismus). However, presenting signs and symptoms can be nonspecific, especially in infants, young children, and the elderly. Neonates may present with poor feeding, listlessness, and altered respiratory patterns. Elderly patients may present with lethargy or obtundation with minimal or no fever and variable signs of meningeal inflammation (2).

   A. **Prodrome**
       1. **Bacterial. Onset** can be rapid (over several hours to 24 hours; e.g., with meningococcal meningitis) or slowly evolving (from a couple to a few days) typically after an upper respiratory tract infection (URI).
       2. **Nonbacterial.** In viral meningitis, the prodrome is usually over days and patients appear less ill, although the onset of fever can be abrupt. Headache is common and can be severe; photophobia is common. Diarrhea, cough, pharyngitis, pleurodynia, and myalgias may occur.

           Fungal and mycobacterial meningitides typically evolve over 1 to 3 or more weeks. (Since these are subacute processes, we will not really address them).

   B. **Physical exam (1)**
       1. **In bacterial meningitis**
           a. **Meningismus** may be subtle or marked.
               (1) **Kernig's sign** is elicited with the patient in the supine position; the thigh and knee are flexed into the patient's abdomen followed by passive leg extension. In the presence of meningeal irritation, the patient will resist leg extension, which constitutes a positive sign.
               (2) **Brudzinski's sign**, a positive sign, is elicited when passive flexion of the

neck results in flexion of the hips and knees.

    b. **Cranial nerve palsies** and **seizures** occur in a minority of patients.

    c. **Signs of increased intracranial pressure** (coma, hypertension, bradycardia, and cranial third nerve palsy) may occur with disease progression. Papilledema in early infection is seen in fewer than 1% and should suggest an alternative diagnosis.

    d. **Rash in meningococcemia** (with or without meningitis). About 50% to 60% of patients with meningococcemia will present with a rash on their extremities. This is typically erythematous and macular early on but quickly evolves into a petechial phase and at times, purpuric phase.

    e. **CSF rhinorrhea or otorrhea** may occur in patients who have had a basilar skull fracture; in these patients, meningitis may be recurrent and is usually caused by *Streptococcus pneumoniae*.

    f. **In patients with head trauma**, signs and symptoms of bacterial meningitis may be masked by the underlying injury. Mental status changes in these subgroups and/or unexplained fever mandates CSF examination to exclude underlying meningitis.

2. **In viral meningitis**

    a. **Rashes** (exanthems) can occur as well as myopericarditis and conjunctivitis.

    b. **Salivary gland enlargement** may be present in about 50% of patients with **mumps**.

    c. **Neurologic complications**—including urinary retention, dysesthesias, paresthesias, neuralgias, motor weakness, paraparesis, and impaired hearing—have occurred in herpes simplex 2 infections. Neurologic findings usually subside within 6 months.

    d. **In neonates** less than 2 weeks of age, fever is accompanied by vomiting, anorexia, rash, or URI signs. Nuchal rigidity and a bulging fontanelle may be seen, but infants under 1 year of age are less likely to demonstrate meningeal signs. Focal neurologic signs are uncommon.

II. **Pathogens** (1,2)

  A. **Bacterial** pathogens are summarized in **Table 11.1.** A few points deserve emphasis.

    1. **In adults,** *S. pneumoniae* and *Neisseria meningitidis* are the most common pathogens, although *Listeria monocytogenes* is also a concern in the elderly or those on immunosuppression.

    2. **In children** who have been vaccinated with the conjugated *Haemophilus influenzae* vaccine, this

Table 11-1. Bacterial meningitis

Organism	Setting	Predisposing Conditions	Estimated Mortality Rates Despite Therapy	Special Issues
Neisseria meningitidis	Children and young adults especially	Deficiencies in the terminal complement components (C5-9)	10–13%	Can be fulminant
Streptococcus pneumoniae	All ages	CSF leak; may have recurrent meningitis. Patients often with contiguous or distant foci of pneumococcal infection; e.g., pneumonia, otitis media, mastoiditis, sinusitis, bacteremia/endocarditis. Increased risk of bacteremia/serious infection in asplenic states, multiple myeloma, hypogammaglobulinemia, alcoholism, malnutrition, chronic liver/renal disease, malignancy, diabetes.	20–25%	Rise of penicillin-resistant, cephalosporin-resistant *S. pneumoniae* has complicated empiric therapy and therapy of resistant pneumococci. **All CSF isolates need to undergo careful susceptibility studies,** with MIC determination to penicillin.

continued

Haemophilus influenzae (usually encapsulated strains)	Infants, children especially <6 years of age	No prior history of *H. influenzae* B vaccination. Older children/adults at increased risk with underlying: sinusitis, otitis media, epiglottitis, pneumonia, splenectomy, head trauma, hypogammaglobulinemia, diabetes.	3–6%
Listeria monocytogenes	Neonates,* elderly	Immunosuppression; e.g., chronic steroids. Underlying chronic disease: hepatic, renal, diabetes, malignancy, collagen vascular, conditions with iron overload, and alcoholism.	22–29%
Streptococcus agalactiae (group B streptococcus)	Usually neonates, occasionally adults: incidence may be increasing	Neonates usually acquire from asymptomatic colonization (vaginal, rectum) of mother. Adult risk factors: age >60, diabetes, parturient women, cardiac disease, collagen vascular disease, hepatic or renal failure, corticosteroid use, but no underlying disease in about 40%.[†]	

Table 11-1. (*Continued*)

Organism	Setting	Predisposing Conditions	Estimated Mortality Rates Despite Therapy	Special Issues
Aerobic gram-negative bacilli (Klebsiella spp., *E. coli, Serratia marcescens, Pseudomonas aeruginosa, Salmonella* spp.)	S/P head trauma S/P neurosurgery Neonates	Elderly, immunosuppressed, patients with gram (−) septicemia.		
S. aureus	S/P neurosurgery S/P head trauma *S. aureus* endocarditis	CSF shunts Diabetes, chronic renal failure, IVDA, underlying malignancy Underlying sinusitis, osteomyelitis, pneumonia	15–75%	MRSA may be a concern (Chap. 17)
S. epidermidis	CSF shunt in place			Foreign body (e.g., CSF shunt) makes therapy difficult.
Nocardia		Immunosuppression, malignancy, head trauma, CNS procedures, sarcoidosis, chronic granulomatous disease		Request infectious disease consultation.

CNS, cental nervous system; CSF, cerebrospinal fluid; IVDA, intravenous drug abuser; MIC, minimum inhibitory concentration; MRSA, methicillin-resistant *S. aureus*. * **Listeria in the neonate may be transmitted from the maternal genital tract and rectum.** † See review in *Medicine* 1993;72:1.

pathogen seldom causes invasive disease. Therefore *S. pneumoniae* and *N. meningitidis* remain major pathogens.

3. **In neonates**, *Escherichia coli* and group B streptococci cause the great majority of cases, but *L. monocytogenes* may occur.

B. **Viruses** cause an acute aseptic meningitis with an early polymorphonuclear pleocytosis and then more prolonged lymphocytic pleocytosis.

1. **Enteroviruses** account for **most cases** in which a pathogen is identified. **Echovirus** and **Coxsackie virus** are the most common enteroviruses. They are worldwide in distribution and spread by the fecal/oral route. Infants and young children are most susceptible because there is absence of previous exposure and immunity.

2. **Lymphocytic choriomeningitis virus** is transmitted to humans by contact with rodents (e.g., hamsters, rats, mice) or their excreta; the greatest risk of infection is to pet owners, persons living in nonhygienic situations, and laboratory workers. This is an uncommon cause.

3. **Human immunodeficiency virus** (HIV). Acute HIV infection can be associated with an aseptic meningitis. Other patients may have a more chronic aseptic meningitis with cranial neuropathies or long track findings.

4. **Herpes virus,** including herpes simplex virus (HSV), varicella zoster virus (VZV), Epstein-Barr virus (EBV), and cytomegalovirus (CMV), can cause an aseptic meningitis. The neurologic complications associated with HSV are the most important; an aseptic meningitis is associated with genital herpes, HSV type 2. (HSV encephalitis is discussed later, separately.)

5. **Arboviruses** (e.g., St. Louis encephalitis, California encephalitis group of viruses) can cause an aseptic meningitis in addition to an encephalitis (see the section on encephalitis).

C. **Nonbacterial, nonviral etiologies** include fungal, spirochetal (*Borrelia burgdorferi, Treponema pallidum*), and mycobacterial (*M. tuberculosis*). Since these are **subacute processes,** we will not discuss them here. They are discussed elsewhere (1). Also see special later comments on the HIV-infected patient.

III. **CSF examination is the most important investigation in the diagnosis of meningitis** and should be performed with the utmost urgency, care, and attention to detail.

A. The **contraindications to** a carefully done **LP** are few. When present, empiric therapy is initiated after blood cultures.

1. If a **mass lesion or increased intracranial pressure** is clinically suspected because of **focal or asymmetric neurologic findings or papilledema or** the Cushing response (**bradycar-**

dia and hypertension) or ophthalmoparesis is present, immediate neurologic evaluation with **a computed tomography (CT) scan or magnetic resonance imaging (MRI) is indicated**, before the LP (**Fig. 11.1**).

If raised intracranial pressure appears likely or is known, a neurosurgeon's help can be enlisted in whether CSF can be safely obtained.

2. A **significant coagulopathy** (e.g., anticoagulation, thrombocytopenia with platelet counts below 40,000 to 50,000, or a prolonged prothrombin time) preclude the LP unless the coagulopathy can be carefully corrected under supervision of a specialist. (Empiric therapy is usually advised in these patients, without an LP.)

3. **Severe scoliosis and a contaminated or infected lumbar area** may preclude doing the LP.

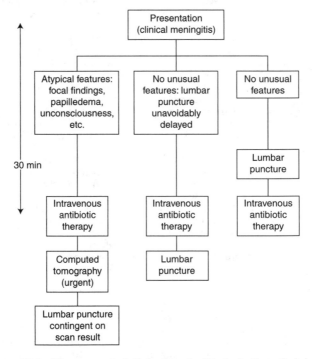

Figure 11-1.   Management of clinical meningitis, including administration of antibiotics within 30 minutes after presentation, in addition to intensive monitoring of vital signs, neurologic status, and urine output, with prompt and aggressive treatment when required. (Source: Archer BD. Computed tomography before lumbar puncture in acute meningitis: a review of the risks and benefits. *Can Med Assoc J* 1993;148:961.)

B. **CSF findings** in meningitis are shown in **Table 11.2.**
   Several points deserve emphasis (1,2).
   1. **In bacterial meningitis** there is usually a **neu-
      trophilic pleocytosis,** although in 10% a lym-
      phocytic predominance (in neonatal meningitis,
      some cases of *L. monocytogenes* and possibly in
      patients with early bacterial meningitis) is seen
      (1,2). Up to 4% of cases may have no CSF pleocy-
      tosis, especially in premature infants and neo-
      nates (3). The CSF white blood cell (WBC) count is
      typically more than 1,000/µl with a neutrophilic
      predominance but many patients will have <1,000
      WBC/µl (2). A gram stain and culture should be
      done routinely.
      a. **Gram staining** of the CSF permits an accu-
         rate diagnosis of an etiologic organism in 60%
         to 90%; the specificity is 90% to 100% in an
         experienced lab (1,2), but in practice the gram
         stain sensitivity is more in the range of 40%
         to 60%. Prior antibiotic therapy diminishes
         the usefulness of gram stains and cultures.
         In infants and children 90% to 100% of CSF
         cultures become sterile with 24 to 36 hours of
         appropriate antibiotic therapy (3).
      b. **CSF cultures** are positive in 75% to 85% of
         cases but in less than 50% of patients receiv-
         ing prior antibiotics (2). See Sec. a also.
      c. A **decreased CSF glucose** concentration
         (<40 mg/dl) is found in 60% of patients; a
         CSF/serum glucose ratio of <0.31 is seen in
         70% of patients (1,2).
            The protein level is nonspecifically ele-
         vated.
      d. **Several rapid diagnostic tests** have been
         developed (1) to aid in the diagnosis of bac-
         terial meningitis. Currently available **latex
         agglutination** techniques detect the anti-
         gens of *H. influenzae* type B, *S. pneumoniae*,
         N. meningitidis, *E. coli* K1, and group B strep-
         tococci. These newer tests are more rapid and
         sensitive than the older counterimmunoelec-
         trophoresis tests. Many of the test kits do not
         include a detection method for group B menin-
         gococcus. Rapid diagnostic tests should ide-
         ally be performed on all CSF specimens from
         patients with presumed bacterial meningitis,
         especially if the CSF gram stain is negative.
         They may also be useful if CSF cultures are
         anticipated to be negative due to prior anti-
         biotic therapy. It must be emphasized that a
         negative latex agglutination test does not rule
         out an infection.
      e. **Polymerase chain reaction (PCR)** has
         been utilized in cases of *N. meningitidis* and

Table 11-2.   "Typical" cerebrospinal fluid findings in meningitis

	Normal	Bacterial	Viral	Fungal/TB	Parameningeal Focus/Abscess
Leukocyte count (WBC/µl)	0–5	>1,000	100–1,000	100–500	10–1000
% PMNs	0–15	90	<50	<50	<50
Glucose (mg/dl)	45–65	<40	45–65	30–45	45–65
Protein (mg/dl)	20–45	>150	50–100	100–500	50 to >150

Source: Modified from Segretti J, Harris AA. Acute bacterial meningitis. *Infect Dis Clin North Am* 1996;10:797.
Abbreviations: WBC, white blood count; PMNs, polymorphonuclear neutrophils; CSF, cerebrospinal fluid.

L. monocytogenes, and its role continues to undergo evaluation (1).

f. **Radiography** (1). Cranial CT and MRI do not aid in the diagnosis of acute bacterial meningitis. (See Sec. A and B.) They should be considered in patients who have prolonged fever, clinical evidence of increased intracranial pressure, focal neurologic findings and seizures, enlarging head circumference (neonates), persistent neurologic dysfunction, or persistently abnormal CSF parameters or cultures. CT may be particularly useful in the subset of patients with meningitis as a result of basal skull fracture with a CSF leak. High-resolution CT scanning with water-soluble contrast enhancement of the CSF (metrizamide cisternography) is the best available test for defining the site of CSF leakage.

2. **In viral meningitis** (1). **See Table 11.2.**

a. **Enteroviruses**. The cell count is usually 100 to 500 WBC/µl, occasionally up to 1,000; although neutrophils may be predominant in the CSF early, this quickly gives way to lymphocytic predominance (6 to 48 hours). If present, a decrease in glucose is minimal (1). PCR technology will facilitate the diagnosis of enteroviral infection when it becomes more available (4). Isolation of enterovirus from the throat or rectum (stool) in a patient with aseptic meningitis is suggestive of an etiologic diagnosis, but since viral shedding may persist up to several weeks, previous coincidental infection cannot be ruled out.

b. **Mumps**. There is typically a lymphocytic pleocytosis. The glucose is usually normal but may be decreased in up to 25% of cases. Serologic tests, both complement fixation and hemagglutination inhibition, are reliable for diagnosis. Testing of paired acute and convalescent sera should demonstrate a diagnostic fourfold rise in mumps antibody titer (1).

c. **Lymphocytic choriomeningitis**. The CSF will show a lymphocytic pleocytosis; hypoglycorrhachia is seen in up to 25%. The virus may be cultured from CSF and blood early and later in urine. Diagnosis can be made by demonstrating a fourfold rise in antibody titer from acute to convalescent serum.

d. **Herpes viruses**. In patients with HSV 2 meningitis, there is a lymphocytic pleocytosis with normal glucose. Although the virus may be cultured in some cases, PCR is promising also.

e. **HIV**. The CSF typically shows a mild lymphocytic pleocytosis (20 to 300/mm³), mildly elevated protein, and normal or slightly decreased glucose. HIV can be isolated from the CSF (1).

C. **Blood cultures** should be drawn before therapy even if an LP is contraindicated.

IV. **Therapy** should be expedited since it is generally agreed that early effective antibiotic therapy improves survival and decreases neurologic sequelae (2). Some experts have suggested that antimicrobial treatment should be begun within 30 minutes of presentation for medical evaluation (1,2).

A. **Therefore in the patient with suspected meningitis and without focal neurologic findings on physical examination, one should carry out a lumbar puncture as quickly as possible** without antecedent CT and then initiate therapy before the results of gram stain or culture are available.

Others have suggested first obtaining a CT and, in the interim, providing antibiotics. Since most such patients do not have meningitis, the administration of antibiotics before LP leads to confusion, since the cultures return negative (and would have been negative had the LP preceded the antibiotics) but the negative cultures after antibiotics are uninterpretable. Furthermore, there are many studies indicating that LP is extremely safe in meningitis (and even safe in the face of mass lesions). **However, if there is clinical evidence of mass lesion or if the patient is HIV positive, CT should be carried out. If a mass lesion is demonstrated, LP is highly unlikely to be useful, and with the even minute risk that it entails, probably should not be carried out.**

If for any reason the LP will be delayed beyond 30 to 60 minutes in the very ill patient, empiric antibiotics would be in the patient's best interest.

1. **Blood cultures should be obtained before therapy.**
2. See **Table 11.3 for empiric therapy.**

B. **In patients who present with focal neurologic findings or who have papilledema, a CT scan of the head should be performed prior to lumbar puncture** to rule out the presence of an intracranial mass or lesion. This is because of the potential risk of herniation, which is estimated to be lower than 1.2% in patients with papilledema and about 12% in patients without papilledema but with elevated intracranial pressure. The time involved in waiting for a CT scan significantly delays therapy with an increase in morbidity and mortality. **Therefore emergent empiric antimicrobial therapy should be initiated before sending the patient to the CT scanner. Blood cultures should be obtained before therapy** (1).

C. **For patients with a subacute presentation** (over days) **and/or those in whom the diagnosis of meningitis is not clear,** if not contraindicated, the LP should be expedited before empiric therapy is started.

Table 11-3. Empiric antibiotics
for presumed bacterial meningitis

Setting	Antibiotics
Adults	
<55 yo	Ceftriaxone (2 g IV q12h) and vancomycin* (± rifampin)
>55 yo and/or at risk for Listeria (immunocompromised)	Ceftriaxone, vancomycin, and ampicillin
Children over 3 months	Cefotaxime or ceftriaxone and vancomycin*
Children[†] 1–3 months	Ampicillin plus cefotaxime or ceftriaxone and vancomycin
Neonates[‡] 0–4 weeks	Ampicillin plus cefotaxime or ampicillin plus aminoglycoside (if hospital-acquired)

* Because S. pneumoniae may be penicillin or cephalosporin resistant, empiric vancomycin is used until culture data are back. See Chap. 16.
[†] Organisms of concern include S. agalactiae, E. coli, L. monocytogenes, H. influenzae, S. pneumoniae, and N. meningitidis.
[‡] Organisms of concern include S. agalactiae, E. coli, L. monocytogenes, K. pneumoniae, Enterococcus spp., and Salmonella spp.

    1. If purulent CSF is obtained, empiric antibiotics should be started before CSF gram stain data, become available.
    2. If the CSF is clear, whether to await laboratory results on the CSF or initiate therapy empirically must be individualized.

  D. **Empiric antibiotics** are summarized in **Table 11.3.**
    1. Because of increasing concerns with penicillin-resistant S. pneumoniae, especially high-level resistance, vancomycin is now part of regimens for possible or known S. pneumoniae meningitis until actual minimum inhibitory concentration (MIC) data are available. (See Chaps. 16 and 28.)
    2. For L. monocytogenes, ampicillin is the agent of choice. TMP-SMZ can be used in the penicillin-allergic patient.

  E. For **specific pathogens** that are isolated, antibiotics can be tailored, depending on the organism and susceptibility data. Infectious disease input is advised. (For a detailed discussion of penicillin-resistant S. pneumoniae issues, see Chap. 16.) **All pneumococcal isolates need careful MIC testing.** Infectious disease consultation is advised for cases of penicillin-resistant S. pneumoniae meningitis.

  F. **Viral meningitis.** There is no specific antiviral chemotherapy for the enteroviruses. Antiviral treatment in the form of intravenous acyclovir may be indicated for

HSV type 2 meningitis. This is generally indicated in severe primary genital herpes infection. Infectious disease consultation is advised. Specific antiretroviral therapy is not indicated for the aseptic meningitis of acute HIV infection.

Herpes simplex **encephalitis** is treated with intravenous (IV) acyclovir. See later discussion.

G. **Steroid adjunctive therapy**. Hearing loss after bacterial meningitis in infants and children may occur in 5% to 30% of patients. This is in part due to CNS inflammation, which may in part be modified by dexamethasone.

1. **In adults, the role of dexamethasone is not clear, and dexamethasone is not recommended.**

2. **The role of dexamethasone in children and infants has recently been reviewed (5).** The 1997 *Red Book* recommendations are as follows:

- Dexamethasone therapy should be considered when bacterial meningitis in infants and children 6 weeks and older is diagnosed or strongly suspected on the basis of the CSF tests, including gram-stained smears, after the physician has weighed the benefits and possible risks and before the etiology has been established.

- Dexamethasone **is recommended for treatment of infants and children with *H. influenzae* type B meningitis.***

- Dexamethasone should be considered for the treatment of infants and children with pneumococcal or meningococcal meningitis. However, its efficacy for these infections is unproven, and some experts do not recommend its use.

- The recommended dexamethasone regimen is 0.6 mg/kg/day in four divided doses, given intravenously, for the first 2 days of antibiotic treatment. A regimen of 0.8 mg/kg/day in two divided doses also is appropriate.

- If dexamethasone is given, it should be administered as early as possible, preferably at the time of, or shortly before, the first dose of antibacterial therapy. Dexamethasone when initiated 4 or more hours after administration of parenteral antimicrobial therapy is unlikely to be effective. Some experts consider that an interval of more than 1 or 2 hours precludes possible effectiveness.

- If dexamethasone is given to patients with pneumococcal meningitis, a repeat lumbar puncture should be considered after 24 to 48 hours to assess the response to therapy.

- Dexamethasone should not be used for suspected or proven nonbacterial meningitis. If

---

* Invasive *H. influenzae* b disease, including meningitis, has decreased significantly in recipients of the conjugated *H. influenzae* b vaccines.

dexamethasone has been started before the diagnosis of nonbacterial meningitis was made, it should be discontinued.
- "Partially treated" meningitis with negative cultures is not an indication for continued dexamethasone therapy.
- The decision to give dexamethasone in patients with presumed bacterial meningitis should not be based on severity of the presenting illness.
- No data are currently available on which to base a recommendation concerning the use of dexamethasone for treatment of bacterial meningitis in infants younger than 6 weeks, or of meningitis in those with congenital or acquired abnormalities of the central nervous system, with or without a prosthetic device.

V. **Indications for prophylaxis** after exposure to an index case of bacterial meningitis are discussed in Chap. 15.
VI. **Special considerations in HIV-positive patients.** *Cryptococcus neoformans* is the most common cause of meningitis in these patients, although bacterial causes such as *S. pneumoniae* must be excluded.
   A. Cryptococcal infection is usually an **indolent presentation** with onset of headache, fever, and malaise **over weeks.** However, sometimes patients present with only minimal cognitive changes.
   B. **Diagnosis**
      1. **Serum latex** agglutination test for cryptococcal polysaccharide antigen is positive in most patients (>90%).
      2. Patients with a positive serum cryptococcal antigen should undergo a spinal tap (usually after a head CT), and CSF antigen studies and routine and fungal cultures should be performed.
   C. Often these patients have elevated intracranial pressure that can lead to nerve damage if unattended. This may be caused by accumulation of the capsular material of the *Cryptococcus*. Therefore if opening pressure is elevated, then either repeated serial taps, lumbar shunt, or CSF peritoneal shunt should be carried out to prevent blindness and deafness.

Encephalitis

The syndrome of acute encephalitis shares many features with acute meningitis, with the likelihood of **mental status changes** occurring early in disease. Clinically, **seizures** are more likely to occur with encephalitis and systemic illness is more prominent. **Encephalitis caused by herpes simplex virus (HSV) represents the most common treatable form of encephalitis**. HSV infections of the CNS are among the most severe of all human viral infections of the brain and are associated with significant morbidity and mortality. Varicella zoster virus can cause CNS involvement during active varicella infection. A direct correlation exists between cutaneous dissemination and visceral involvement.

I.   **Clinical presentation** (1)

    A. **Herpes simplex virus (HSV)**. Most patients with herpes simplex encephalitis (HSE) present with the **focal encephalopathic process** characterized by altered mentation, and decreasing levels of consciousness with focal neurologic findings. **Fever and personality changes** are uniformly present. Two-thirds of patients develop either focal or generalized **seizures**. The clinical progression of HSV encephalitis may be slow or rapid. Severe obtundation and coma can occur. The differential diagnosis includes abscess, subdural empyema, tuberculosis, cryptococcosis, toxoplasmosis, CMV, tumor, and subdural hematoma.

    B. **Varicella zoster virus**. The most common neurologic abnormality seen is **cerebellar ataxia**. Meningoencephalitis and cerebritis may be severe complications. Headache, fever, and vomiting often are accompanied by an altered sensorium with associated seizures. Cranial nerve dysfunction, aphasia, and hemiplegia have also been described. Encephalitis associated with herpes zoster is seen **most commonly in** people of **advanced age**, following **immunosuppression,** and in those with **disseminated cutaneous zoster**.

II.   **Diagnosis** (1)

    A. **HSV**. The CSF white count is often elevated (mean of 100 cells/mm^3) with a lymphocytic predominance. However, the CSF white count can be normal initially or even throughout the course. The presence of red blood cells in the CSF suggests the diagnosis in the appropriate clinical setting but is not diagnostic. CSF protein is elevated (approximately 100 mg/dl). The CSF can be normal in 3% to 4% of patients.

        1. **PCR for HSV in CSF** is the **optimal way to diagnose HSE** (6).

        2. **MRI** is more sensitive than CT and is considered the optimal imaging technique. **A negative MRI is therefore against the diagnosis of HSE** (7).

        3. Brain biopsy is seldom indicated now with the availability of PCR. HSV isolation from CSF is difficult and successful only in a small minority of patients even when attempted.

    B. **Varicella zoster virus**. CSF shows a lymphocytic pleocytosis and elevated protein. However, this is also seen in uncomplicated zoster. The electroencephalogram typically shows diffuse slowing but may also reveal focal abnormalities. The virus has been cultured from brain tissue and CSF. Zoster ophthalmicus with associated contralateral hemiplegia one to two months later implies unilateral arteritis or thrombosis of vessels leading from the carotid siphon.

III. **Antiviral therapy**. At this point, only encephalitis caused by herpes viruses is treatable.

A. **HSV.** Acyclovir should be given intravenously at 10 mg/kg q8h (if renal function is normal) for 14 to 21 days. Infectious disease consultation is advised. Since PCR data may take a couple to a few days to get back, empiric IV acyclovir is necessary in the suspicious case with a suggestive MRI. (If the MRI is normal, empiric IV acyclovir is not suggested.)

B. **Varicella zoster virus.** IV acyclovir is the drug of choice for VZV-associated CNS infection for those who are at high risk for progressive disease. Despite the lack of clinical trials, acyclovir has been used for herpes zoster–associated encephalitis. Infectious disease consultation is advised.

IV. **Arboviral infections** (e.g., eastern or western equine encephalitis, St. Louis encephalitis) are uncommon and therapy is supportive. Typical infections occur in the latter part of summer, and clinical disease is more common in the very young and very old.

Brain Abscess

I. **Pathogenesis.** The majority of patients with a brain abscess (1,8,9) have a predisposing condition or source, such as paranasal sinusitis, otogenic or mastoid infections, recent trauma (injury or surgery), and at times metastatic spread (e.g., bacteremia with multiple brain abscesses, especially if with congenital heart disease with a right-to-left shunt; the high hematocrit that is present, which leads to vascular stasis, probably contributes to the susceptibility).

II. **Pathogens**

A. **Common bacteria** include the following:

1. **Streptococci** (aerobic, anaerobic, and microaerophilic) are seen in 60% to 70% of cases. *S. milleri* (also called *S. intermedius*, part of the viridans streptococci group) are common abscess formers.

2. **Gram-negative bacilli** (e.g., *E. coli*, *Klebsiella* spp., *Pseudomonas* spp.) are isolates in 20% to 30% of cases.

3. **Anaerobes**, especially *Bacteroides* spp., are common and isolated in 20% to 40% of cases.

4. ***Staphylococcus aureus*** may occur in 10% to 15% of cases, especially after cranial trauma or staphylococcal bacteremia.

B. **Nocardia** may be isolated in patients on immunosuppression, including transplant recipients and those on chronic corticosteroids, and patients with AIDS.

C. **Fungal** infections can occur, especially in the immunocompromised.

1. **Candida** focal lesions can occur.

2. ***Aspergillus* species** may disseminate to the brain from the lungs or by direct extension from an adjacent site. **Most patients with *Aspergillus* brain abscess are neutropenic and have an**

underlying hematologic malignancy. Other risk factors include Cushing's syndrome, diabetes mellitus, hepatic disease, chronic granulomatous disease, and IV drug use. Postcraniotomy patients, organ transplant recipients, HIV infected patients, and those receiving chronic corticosteroid therapy are also at risk.

3. **Mucormycosis** is usually seen in those with predisposing conditions such as diabetes mellitus (often with acidosis); acidemia from systemic illness; hematologic neoplasia; renal transplantation; IV drug use; use of Deferoxamine. CNS infection may occur by direct extension (rhinocerebral form) or by dissemination.

4. *Pseudallescheria boydii.* This organism may enter the CNS by direct trauma, by hematogenous dissemination, from an IV catheter site, or by direct extension from the sinuses in both normal and immunocompromised hosts. *P. boydii* may be found in contaminated water and manure, and thus **infection may follow near drowning**.

III. **Clinical presentation** (1)

A. **Bacterial brain abscess**. The presentation of bacterial brain abscess is usually indolent but occasionally fulminant.

1. The **clinical manifestations occur secondary to the presence of a space-occupying lesion** rather than the systemic signs of infection and include **headache** (70%), which may be moderate to severe, hemicranial or generalized; **nausea and vomiting** (50%); **seizures** (25% to 30%), which are usually generalized; **nuchal rigidity and papilledema** (25%); focal neurologic deficits (50%); and the majority of patients will have **mental status changes** ranging from lethargy to coma. Nuchal rigidity implies rupture of the abscess into the CSF.

2. **Fever** is observed in only 40% to 50% of cases.

3. Approximately half of patients with bacterial brain abscess present with headache, fever, and focal neurologic signs.

B. **Fungal brain abscess**. The clinical presentation of fungal brain abscess is also dependent on its intracranial location and the growth pattern of the organism. Certain fungal pathogens may, however, present with specific symptoms and signs.

1. *Aspergillus* **spp.** Patients most commonly present with signs of **stroke** referable to the involved area of the brain. Headache, encephalopathy, and **seizures** may be seen. Fever is not a constant finding, and meningeal irritation is rare.

2. **Mucormycosis.** Symptoms of rhinocerebral mucormycosis are referable to the eyes or sinuses and include headache, facial pain, diplopia, lacrimation, and nasal stuffiness or discharge. Fever and

lethargy have been described. Signs include **nasal ulceration,** facial swelling, nasal discharge, proptosis, and external ophthalmoplegia. **Cranial nerve abnormalities are common.** Blood vessel invasion and secondary thrombosis occurs commonly.

3. *Pseudallescheria boydii.* **CNS infection usually becomes manifest 15 to 30 days after an episode of near drowning**. Clinical presentation depends on localization in the CNS and includes seizures, altered consciousness, headache, meningeal irritation, focal neurologic deficits, abnormal behavior, and aphasia.

IV. **Diagnosis**

A. **Bacterial brain abscess. CT scanning** is an **excellent** imaging technique to examine the brain parenchyma, paranasal sinuses, mastoids, and middle ear. Characteristically, the CT will show a hypodense lesion with a peripheral uniform ring enhancement following injection of contrast. There may also be a surrounding hypodense area of edema. **MRI may be superior to CT** in the diagnosis of brain abscess, including early detection of cerebritis.

B. **Fungal brain abscess.** Noninvasive studies (e.g., **CT, MRI**) are usually **nonspecific**, but some exceptions exist. For example, the finding of a cerebral infarct in a patient at risk for invasive aspergillosis suggests that diagnosis. In patients with rhinocerebral mucormycosis, CT and MRI typically show sinus opacification, erosion of bone, and obliteration of deep facial planes. Cavernous sinus involvement may also be seen by MRI. **Definitive diagnosis requires biopsy with appropriate stains and culture for fungal organisms.**

IV. **Approach to the patient with brain abscess**

A. **Microbiologic diagnosis.** A presumptive diagnosis of brain abscess by radiologic studies should be followed by microbiologic analysis. Aspiration can often be performed stereotactically with the use of CT scanning. **Neurosurgical consultation is essential.** Specimens should be sent for gram stain, Ziehl-Neelsen stain for mycobacteria, modified acid-fast stain for *Nocardia,* and silver stains for fungi. Cultures for *Mycobacteria, Nocardia,* and fungi should also be performed.

B. **Empiric antibiotic therapy for bacterial process.** Once a diagnosis is made either presumptively or by aspiration, antimicrobial therapy should be initiated. If an aspiration cannot be performed or if the gram stain is unrevealing, empiric therapy should be started. **Infectious disease consultation is advised.**

1. **Empiric therapy** needs to be active against common pathogens. (See Sec. II.) Meningeal doses of penicillin, a third-generation cephalosporin, and metronidazole (triple therapy) are commonly used.

If *S. aureus* is a concern, nafcillin (or vancomycin in the allergic patient) can be substituted for penicillin. If penicillin-resistant *S.
pneumoniae* or methicillin-resistant *S. aureaus*
is a major concern, vancomycin will be an important agent.

2. **Therapy can be adjusted on the basis of culture results.** For *Nocardia,* TMP-SMZ is the
   agent of choice.

3. **Duration of therapy**. High-dose IV antimicrobial therapy should be continued for 4 to 6 weeks
   and often is followed by oral antibiotics if appropriate agents are available. In patients who have
   undergone surgical excision, 3 to 4 weeks of therapy may be appropriate.

   Nocardial brain abscess should be treated for
   3 to 12 months following surgical drainage.

C. **Surgical therapy** (1). Most patients with bacterial
   brain abscess require surgical excision for optimal
   therapy. Aspiration by stereotactic CT guidance is
   rapid, accurate, and safe, and allows for swift relief
   of intracranial pressure. Multiloculated lesions may
   be incompletely evacuated and may require crani-
   otomy.

   Certain subsets of patients may require only medical therapy. These include patients with medial conditions that increase surgical risk, multiple abscesses,
   abscesses in deep or dominant location, concomitant
   meningitis or ependymitis, early abscess reduction
   with clinical improvement following antimicrobials,
   and an abscess measuring less than 3 cm.

D. **Fungal brain abscesses**. A combined medical and
   surgical approach is necessary.

   1. Surgical drainage is the cornerstone of therapy.
   2. Infectious disease consultation is advised for anti-
      fungal therapy.

Spinal Epidural Abscess

Spinal epidural abscess, a rare entity, will be reviewed only
briefly.

I. **Pathogenesis**. Spinal epidural abscess follows hematogenous dissemination from a focus elsewhere to the epidural
   space (25% to 50% of cases) or by direct extension from vertebral osteomyelitis. Blunt spinal trauma may also provide
   a devitalized site that is susceptible to infection from a
   transient bacteremia. Other predisposing conditions
   include penetrating injuries, extension of decubitus ulcers,
   or paraspinal abscesses, back surgery, lumbar puncture,
   or epidural anesthesia (8).

II. **Microbiology**. Staphylococci (*S. aureus*) account for about
    65%; streptococci, about 8%; and aerobic gram negatives,
    about 17% (8).

III.   **Clinical manifestations** include **focal vertebral pain**, followed by root pain; defects of motor, sensory, or sphincter function; and finally paralysis. **Focal tenderness** of the spine is present in more than 90% of cases. **Fever** is present in most cases (8).

IV.   **Diagnosis.** MRI imaging is preferred over CT since MRI can visualize the spinal cord and epidural space well (7). Osteomyelitis may also be present.

V.   **Therapy** (8)

   A.   **Antimicrobial therapy.** Empiric therapy must include antistaphylococcal therapy (either nafcillin or vancomycin). Coverage for gram-negative bacilli (e.g., ceftazidime) is added for a patient with a history of spinal procedure or injection drug use. Infectious disease consultation is advised.

   B.   **Surgical therapy** is often essential and neurosurgical consultation is necessary.

References

1.   Tunkel AR, Scheld WM. Central nervous system infections. In: Reese RE, Betts RF, eds. *A practical approach to infectious diseases,* 4th ed. Boston: Little, Brown, 1996:Chap. 5.

2.   Segretti J, Harris AA. Acute bacterial meningitis. *Infect Dis Clin North Am* 1996;10:797.

3.   Bonadio WA. The cerebrospinal fluid: physiologic aspects and alterations associated with bacterial meningitis. *Pediatr Infect Dis J* 1992;11:423.

4.   Rothart HA. Enteroviral infections of the central nervous system. *Clin Infect Dis* 1995;30:971.

5.   Peter G, et al, eds. *1997 Red Book: Report of the Committee on Infectious Diseases,* 24th ed. Elk Grove Village, IL: American Academy of Pediatrics, 1997:620–621.

6.   Lakeman FD, et al. Diagnosis of Herpes simplex encephalitis: application of polymerase chain reaction to cerebrospinal fluid from brain-biopsied patients and correlation with disease. *J Infect Dis* 1995;171:857.
     See related discussion by Tebas P, et al. Use of the polymerase chain reaction in the diagnosis of herpes simplex encephalitis: a decision analysis model. Am J Med *1998;105:287.*

7.   Bleck TP. Imaging for central nervous sytem infections. In: Mandell GL, Bennett JE Dolin R, eds. *Principles and practices of infectious diseases: update.* 1995;4(1):1–13.

8.   Tunkel AR, Scheld WM. Focal central nervous system infections. In: Root RK, et al, eds. *Clinical infectious diseases: a practical approach.* New York. Oxford University Press, 1999:Chap. 76.
     Concise discussions of brain abscess, subdural empyema, and epidural abscess.

9.   Mathisen GE, Johnson JP. Brain abscess. *Clin Infect Dis* 1997; 25:763.

Approach to the Febrile Patient Without an Obvious Source

I. **Introduction.** Although infection is the most common cause of fever, many other processes are associated with fever. Usually, infections will manifest with obvious organ involvement. (See Chapters 1 to 11.) Noninfectious causes of fever are briefly summarized in Sec. V below.

This chapter will address some of the initial clinical considerations raised, especially in adults, by

- Recent onset (<72 hours) of unexplained fever
- Subacute fever (several days)
- Fever in the patient in intensive care unit (ICU)
- Fever in the HIV-positive patient
- Fever in the leukopenic patient

Extensive discussions of these topics are beyond the scope of this handbook.

This is in contrast to the patient with a more "classic" fever of unknown origin (FUO) lasting for more than the preceding 2 or 3 weeks without obvious explanation. Because of the expense of hospitalization and the frequent ability to investigate an apparent FUO as an outpatient (e.g., with blood and urine cultures, computed tomography [CT] scans, erythrocyte sedimentation rate [ESR], temporal artery biopsies when indicated in the elderly), only a minority of persisting unexplained fevers of unknown origin are due to infection. These complex FUO patients may need hospitalization and infectious disease consultation for careful evaluation and are discussed in detail elsewhere (1–4).

II. **Clinical diagnostic approach to fever**
   A. **Normal host: Fever present for 72 hours or less**
      1. **The bacteremic or septic-appearing febrile patient** is discussed separately in **Chap. 7**.
      2. **Epidemiologic factors**
         a. **Age.**
            (1) **Viral infection explains many fevers occurring in infants and small children** but far fewer in older individuals. Influenza commonly is associated with fever, but typically, respiratory symptoms are prominently present in adults, and, during epidemics, influenza is recognized in the community.
            (2) **Occult bacteremia.** *Streptococcus pneumoniae* or *Haemophilus influenzae* bacteremia **occurring in the infant or child** may present as nonlocalizing fever. Risk factors include a toxic or unhappy, irritable child, children under the age of 24 months, high fever (<40°C),

leukocytosis (>15,000/mm^3) often with toxic granulations or vacuolation of polymorphonuclear leukocytes, and underlying disease (5). The use of the *H. influenzae* type b conjugated vaccine has dramatically reduced bacteremia with this organism. *Staphylococcus aureus* bacteremia, often without an obvious source, has to be considered in any adult with abrupt onset of unexplained fever and true rigors.

  (3) **In the elderly** patient, quite often bacterial infection presents without localizing symptoms. Fever may be minimal.

  b. **Season.** Outside of the influenza season (December through March), a fever of more than 100.5°F in an adult usually is clinically significant and may suggest infection.

  c. **Travel history.** If the patient has recently returned from international travel with potential exposure to malaria, typhoid fever, or amebiasis, then special studies will need to be done (e.g., malaria blood smears, stool cultures, and stool exam for trophozoites or cysts). Long flights with inactivity may predispose to prostatic abscess and to phlebothrombosis.

B. **Fever present for less than 72 hours, in abnormal host.**

  1. **The bacteremic or septic patient is discussed in Chap. 7.**

  2. **Malignancy**

    a. **With leukopenia (white blood cell [WBC] count <500/mm^3), fever is assumed to be due to an infection.** See separate discussion (Sec. III under "Fever in Special Host Settings") later in this chapter.

    b. With normal WBC count, a variety of other possibilities are raised besides infection (e.g., drug fever, tumor fever, and infections seen in normal patients).

  3. **AIDS.** Fever in these patients is discussed later in Sec. II under "Fever in Special Host Settings." Bacterial infection usually presents in a manner similar to that in the normal host.

  4. **Intravenous drug user**. The substances injected, either the filler or the active moiety, can produce short-term and usually low-level fever. However, if the temperature exceeds 100.5°F, a bloodstream infection, possibly endocarditis, is a concern.

C. **Fever lasting 72 hours or more** may begin slowly or with shaking chills and fever.

  1. **Normal host**

    a. **Infection**. Most aggressive bacterial infections will localize by 72 to 96 hours; see separate chapter discussions. Certain infectious syndromes are less aggressive.

(1) **Subacute bacterial endocarditis** must be considered in anyone with unexplained fever, especially if he/she has a murmur and/or prosthetic valve. (See Chap. 8.)

(2) **Intraabdominal abscess.** Patients may have fever, often without focal gastrointestinal complaints, for several days. Abdominal CT is essential in making this diagnosis. (See Chap. 6.) (N.B. Don't forget the pelvic/rectal exam!)

(3) **Infectious mononucleosis and related syndromes** typically take days to weeks to present. Approximately 20% of young adults with infectious mononucleosis will present with fever and malaise without pharyngitis. Primary **cytomegalovirus** (CMV) typically presents without pharyngitis or adenopathy and can be overlooked for many days. The patient may feel well between fever and usually does not have weight loss. Remember that **acute HIV** disease may present like mono. A minority of patients with acute HIV disease will have a truncal maculopapular rash. The incubation period is between 1 and 12 weeks, most commonly 2 to 4 weeks, so risk factors should be elicited in the proper setting. The duration of acute HIV disease is 3 to 14 days typically (6).

(4) **Miscellaneous considerations**

(a) **Miliary tuberculosis** may not initially be obvious on chest x-ray and may be very difficult to diagnose. (Liver and bone marrow biopsy, cultures, and histopathology are needed.) **Pulmonary tuberculosis** must be considered in patients with a suggestive chest x-ray, especially if they are in a high-risk setting (homeless, prior history of tuberculosis, exposure history, etc., see related discussion in Chap. 13, Part B, I.B. under "Airborne Isolation").

(b) **Dental or sinus** abscess can sometimes present with fever without focal signs.

b. **Noninfectious** considerations. See Sec. V.

2. **Abnormal host**

a. **Malignancy**

(1) **Normal WBC.** Fever is usually due to the tumor, to medications, or to an

infection. Most infections will have localizing symptoms. Consider central line infection if applicable. If the tumor initially presented with fever, at recurrence, fever will also often recur.

(2) **WBC count of less than 500/mm³; fever is usually due to infection**. See Sec. III under "Fever in Special Host Settings."

b. **AIDS.** Opportunistic infection is the most common cause, but lymphoma and drug fever are also important considerations. (See Sec. II under "Fever in Special Host Settings.")

c. **Noninfectious   considerations.** (See Sec. V.)

III. **Clues from the physical examination in the normal host.** In the febrile patient, a careful physical examination is essential to exclude an obvious focal infection. Furthermore, **in the persistently febrile patient it is imperative that the physical examination be repeated at intervals** since signs may evolve. **Special considerations** of examination include the following:

A. **Head and neck.** After a routine ear and oropharyngeal exam, do not forget to see if the thyroid gland is tender, which would suggest thyroiditis. Are the areas over the sinuses tender? The conjunctivae should be examined carefully for petechiae seen in endocarditis.

B. **Careful cardiac exam.** A murmur may be the only clue to bacterial endocarditis (BE). A soft, flow murmur is less suggestive of BE. The patient should be examined both in the sitting and leaning forward positions to help assess for an aortic insufficiency murmur or a rub. In acute *S. aureus* endocarditis, there may be no murmur.

C. **The spleen.** A palpable spleen may be found in malignancy, in chronic infection, and in collagen vascular disease. (To feel for the spleen, remember also to roll the patient onto his/her right side facing the examiner.)

D. **Soft-tissue infection.** Streptococcal disease as well as *S. aureus* can present with fever before the soft-tissue signs are manifest. Serial exams may be helpful. (See Chap. 3.)

E. **Genital-rectal.** Prostatic abscess is not always tender, but bogginess may be present. Tenderness along the epididymis suggests either epididymal infection or noninfectious inflammation of the artery, as is seen in polyarteritis. If initially pelvic and/or rectal exams were not performed, then they should be.

F. **Extremities.** Careful palpation along the course of major veins in the leg and the plantar surface of the foot can uncover tender veins.

G. **Lymph nodes** should be carefully examined.

IV. **Clues from the laboratory**

A. **WBC and differential.** The WBC count, by itself, is often not helpful since WBC count between 10,000 and

20,000 cells/mm^3 can occur from a variety of insults, including the stress from being ill from a viral infection. Corticosteroids may increase the WBC count, but typically to less than 20,000 cells/mm^3. If the total count WBC count exceeds 20,000 cells/mm^3 and the differential does not suggest a hematologic malignancy, bacterial infection is frequently the cause. In the hospitalized patient currently or recently on antibiotics, disseminated candidiasis or *C. difficile* colitis must also be considered as sources for this degree of leukocytosis.

1. **Band forms** ("shift to the left"). If, however, there are a substantial number of band forms (e.g., >10% to 15%), even when the WBC count is in the low or low normal range, bacterial infection is very likely. **The many clinical noninfectious problems that produce leukocytosis are far less likely to produce band forms.**

2. **Eosinophilia.** A reaction to a drug can cause eosinophilia with and without fever. Malignancy invading bone marrow or other tissue, some collagen vascular syndromes (e.g., polyarteritis nodosa), and infrequently invasive parasitic disease (e.g., *Strongyloides*) can cause eosinophilia. If the suspect medication is discontinued, the eosinophilia resolves rather promptly (e.g., 2 to 4 days) if the medication was the offending agent.

B. **Liver function tests**
   1. **Bilirubin.** Elevated bilirubin and/or lactic dehydrogenase (LDH) elevation suggests possible hemolysis, possible lymphoma, or collagen vascular disease. Bacteremias can be associated with hyperbilirubinemia.
   2. If alkaline phosphatase, gamma glutyl transferase (GGT), and bilirubin are elevated, often with normal or mildly elevated liver enzymes (AST/ALT), common duct obstruction with stones must be considered, even in the absence of localizing signs. If the bilirubin is normal, with an elevated alkaline phosphatase and GGT, granulomatous or drug-induced intrahepatic cholestasis is a consideration; granulomas such as miliary tuberculosis may present in this way.

C. **Sedimentation rate (ESR).** If the sedimentation rate is elevated above 50 to 60 mm/hour Westergren, a more serious underlying process must be considered. If the ESR is more than 100 mm/hour, possible causes are arteritis/collagen vascular disease, a malignancy, or infection such as miliary tuberculosis, bacterial endocarditis, or silent intraabdominal abscess. False ESR evaluations can occur in myeloma; C-reactive protein often helps sort this out.

D. **C-reactive protein** is discussed in Chap. 13, Part A.

E. **Monospot test.** This is a very useful test if infectious mononucleosis (EBV) is suspect. An initial test can be false negative early in mono, and repeat tests in 7 to 10 days are useful in suspicious cases. The monospot test typically remains positive only for 3 to 4 months, so a positive test does not reflect illness from years ago.

F. **Miscellaneous.** In a monolike illness in which acute CMV is a concern, serology is a practical way to clarify the diagnosis. In acute CMV "mono," by the time the patient is symptomatic, both IgG and IgM CMV antibodies are positive. Therefore if the CMV IgG antibody is negative, acute CMV is unlikely. If the CMV IgG is positive, the CMV IgM antibody should be performed. If it is negative, the positive IgG antibody is consistent with prior (old) CMV infection; if positive, acute CMV causing a monolike syndrome is likely. (Unfortunately, some rheumatologic conditions, such as rheumatoid arthritis, may cause a false-positive CMV IgM antibody.) To diagnose early, **acute HIV disease**, a quantitative plasma HIV RNA viral load test is suggested since it is more sensitive early in disease than HIV antibody titers (6A).

V. **Noninfectious causes** of fever can be low grade or spiking and hectic.

A. **Drug fever** usually develops within 2 weeks of initiation of therapy but may develop at any time, including months after initiation of a specific drug. **The patient typically looks and feels well**. Rigors and spiking fever can occur. A rash and/or eosinophilia is suggestive but often not present. When the offending agent is stopped, the fever will resolve in 48 to 96 hours. Commonly implicated agents are antibiotics (especially penicillin and sulfonamides), diphenylhydantoin, amphotericin B, allopurinol, and procainamide. This topic has recently been reviewed (7).

B. **Malignancy.** Lymphoma is the classic example, both Hodgkin's and non-Hodgkin's. Any solid tumor, especially renal cell carcinoma even before its "physical presence" is obvious can present with fever. Acute leukemia is usually obvious on blood smear.

C. **Collagen vascular disease.** Most of the arthritides and vasculitis syndromes present with a finding to suggest the diagnosis. Polymyalgia presents with muscle pain without weakness and polymyositis with weakness without pain. **A rash with palpable purpura suggests vasculitis.** Childhood/adult juvenile rheumatoid arthritis may present only with fever. Giant cell (temporal) arteritis may present in the elderly without focal findings or complaints of headaches, even without tender temporal arteries (1). A normal ESR helps exclude many of these entities.

D. **Other considerations include** sarcoidosis, Crohn's disease (sometimes even before bowel manifestations become obvious), atrial myxoma, phlebothrombosis, and/or pulmonary embolism, factitious fever, surreptitious injection of pyrogen, thyroiditis, and adrenal insufficiency.

VI. **To treat or not to treat fever?**

A. **Antipyretics.** Fever in and of itself does not require therapy. Antipyretics **are indicated to** avoid the potential harmful secondary effects of hypermetabolism in the elderly patient or those with underlying pulmonary and/or cardiovascular disease or to avoid high fever in the child with a history of febrile convulsions. Antipyretics are often used for improving the patient's comfort (1).

Remember that aspirin (salicylates) should be avoided to treat fever in children with viral illnesses, especially chickenpox and influenza-like illnesses, because salicylate use has been associated with Reye's syndrome.

B. **Antibiotics**
1. **In the patient with subacute fever** (>72 hours) with no localizing findings and stable clinical condition, often one can hold antibiotics pending cultures and serial assessments. This in the long run may cause less confusion in the patient's work-up.
2. **In the patient with recent onset of fever**
   a. Antibiotics are indicated in the moderately to severely ill and/or toxic-appearing patient. (See Chap. 7 for choices in the septic patient and individual chapters for presumed organ-related infections.)
   b. In children with possible occult bacteremia, intramuscular ceftriaxone or oral amoxicillin-clavulanate tid are often employed.
   c. In the stable adult, often antibiotics are not needed empirically.

Fever in Special Host Settings

I. **Fever in the adult patient in the ICU**. Fever is a common and complex problem in these patients, who are often very ill with multiple possible sites of infection (e.g., central lines, endotracheal tubes, indwelling bladder catheters, etc.). This topic has been reviewed (8,9,9A).
   A. **Fever** can be difficult even to measure in the ICU. Oral temperatures are not accurate in intubated patients. Axillary temperatures are not reliable. Tympanic membrane probes are not ideal and must be maintained very well to be reliable. The "gold standard" is probably the **pulmonary artery catheter temperature** when available. Second best is the **rectal temperature** in the nonleukopenic patient (9). **A fever above 38.3°C deserves evaluation**.
   B. **History** may be difficult since patients are often intubated or heavily sedated. Focal symptoms should be elicited when possible. The nursing staff may have useful observations.
   C. The **physical exam** is often difficult to perform and nonspecific. Considerations are shown in **Table 12.1**.
   D. **Cost-effective laboratory work-up** is undergoing evaluation. In the postoperative patient, a physical

Table 12-1. Physical exam of the febrile ICU patient

SKIN	*ABDOMEN*
Drug rashes	Percussion tenderness
Wounds	Abdominal distension
IV catheter sites	Wounds
Deep line exit/tunnel sites	*PERINEUM*
Vasculitis rash	Genital inspection for cellulitis
Tissue necrosis with peripheral vascular disease	Rectal exam (prostatitis)
Nodular lesions of disseminated candidemia	Pelvic exam if indicated
HEENT	*EXTREMITIES*
Parotitis	IV phlebitis/cellulitis
Wounds	Phlebitis
Sinus tenderness or erythema	Ischemia
CHEST	*NEUROLOGICAL*
Often nonspecific or difficult to interpret findings	Confusion
Dullness/changes of pleural effusion	Meningismus

Source: Modified from Masur H, Malangoni M. Evaluation of fever in the ICU. Symposium. Infectious Disease Society of America (IDSA). 35th Annual Meeting. San Francisco. Sept. 1997.

examination, chest physical therapy, and careful wound exam is appropriate for the evaluation of a 24- to 48-hour postoperative fever, since fever is so common on the first or second postop day. **For fever occurring 3 or more days after surgery, a more vigorous laboratory work-up is usually necessary,** as it is in the toxic, possibly septic patient or the medical ICU patient (9).

1. **Blood cultures.** For temperatures of 38.3°C or more, two sets of blood cultures separated in time by 15–20 minutes from a peripheral vein are preferred (9).

   a. If access is a problem, one blood culture peripherally and one via a "deep line" is a reasonable compromise (9).

   b. Quantitative blood cultures are not usually necessary unless an institution has a particular interest in these. (See the following discussion.)

2. **Sputum culture**, with gram stain, is advised when purulent sputum is available. The sputum culture should be plated in the microbiology laboratory within 2 hours of being collected.

3. **Chest x-ray.** A portable exam, preferably taken in the sitting position, is suggested.

4. **If diarrhea is present**, enteral feeding and drug side effects (especially antibiotic) are the most common explanation.

a. *Clostridium difficile* toxin assay is indicated in the patient who has recently received or is receiving antibiotics. (See Chap. 5.)

b. Stool for enteric culture and ova and parasite exam is indicated only for community-acquired diarrhea, diarrhea within 3 days of admission, or especially for the patient who has recently been involved in international travel and/or the HIV patient with no recent stool work-up.

5. **Urine culture** is indicated in those patients with a Foley catheter and/or those after urologic manipulation and/or with obstructed uropathy.

6. **Wound cultures** and gram stains are indicated for draining wounds.

7. **Any IV or vascular catheter exit site purulence** should be cultured and gram-stained (and the catheter removed) (9,9A).

   If there is evidence of a deep-line tunnel infection, embolic phenomenon, or sepsis, the catheter should be removed and cultured.

a. If the catheter tip culture is positive ($\geq$15 colony forming units) and the blood cultures are positive, catheter-related sepsis is likely (9).

b. If only the catheter tip is positive, the significance is unclear. See detailed discussion of catheter-related infection elsewhere (9,9A).

E. **Consider noninfectious etiologies** of fever. **Fever in the ICU may not be infectious in origin (Table 12.2).** The frequency of these entities is not well known.

F. **Miscellaneous issues**

1. Colonization of an indwelling bladder catheter or endotracheal tube by bacteria that release endotoxin may cause fever without these bacteria producing invasive disease at that site (10). How often this occurs clinically is not clear. See Chap. 4.

2. Although deep-line infection is often blamed for fever, if the blood culture drawn through the deep line is negative, this "explanation" is probably not correct.

3. By definition, ventilator-associated pneumonia has focal findings (i.e., a new infiltrate on chest x-ray). (See Chap. 2.)

4. Disseminated candidemia can cause fever with negative blood cultures.

5. Very early *C. difficile* colitis may cause fever and leukocytosis even before diarrhea develops.

6. Consider drug fever.

7. In patients with a nasotracheal or nasogastric tube **nosocomial sinusitis** can occur and cause fever. Since technically it is difficult to perform plain radiographs, a CT scan is the best radi-

Table 12-2.   Noninfectious etiologies of fever in ICU patients

Drug reactions (with or without rash)	Adrenal insufficiency
Resolving hematomas	Acute gout
Pancreatitis	Ischemic colitis
DVT (deep vein thromboses)	Thyrotoxicosis
Pulmonary hemorrhage	Underlying tumor
Seizures	With obstruction
CNS bleed	With perforation
Myocardial infarction/ischemia*	Peripheral vascular disease with tissue necrosis
Pericarditis	Aspiration (gastric) pneumonia (chemical pneumonitis)
Pulmonary emboli	Unusual syndromes
Alcohol withdrawal	Malignant hyperthermia[†]
	Neuroleptic malignant syndrome[‡]

Modified from Masur H, Malangoni M. Evaluation of fever in the ICU. Symposium. Infectious Disease Society of America (IDSA). 35th Annual Meeting. San Francisco, September 1997.

* Low-grade temperatures (38°C) are common; temperatures above 38.5°C due to myocardial infarction are uncommon. (*Am Heart J* 1978;96:153.).

[†] **Malignant hyperthermia** can occur 24 hours after anesthesia (especially after halothane, succinyl choline use) with temperatures ≥41°C. Sodium dantrolene is considered the treatment of choice (*Semin Neurol* 1991;11:220. *Med Clin North Am* 1993;77:477. *Pediatr Clin North Am* 1994;41:221. *Crit Care Clin* 1997;13:785.).

[‡] **Neuroleptic malignant syndrome** (NMS) is precipitated by neuroleptic drugs (e.g., phenothiazines, antidepressants, butyrophenones, loxapine, antiemetics, and thioxanthenes). Hyperthermia (≥41°C), hypertonicity of skeletal muscle, fluctuating consciousness, and autonomic nervous system lability (diaphoresis, tachycardia, blood pressure instability, and/or cardiac arrhythmias) are present. Elevated serum CPK levels can be seen (secondary to myonecrosis). Sodium dantrolene is the therapy of choice along with discontinuation of the drug (*Med Clin North Am* 1993;77:477. *Crit Care Clin* 1997;13:785.).

ographic test. If findings of sinusitis are present on CT, puncture and aspiration of the involved sinuses for aerobic and anaerobic culture and gram stain, by an ENT consultant, is advised (9). Gram-negative bacilli are commonly isolated.

8. **The role of a lumbar puncture (LP) must be individualized** (9,10A). In patients who have undergone recent neurosurgical procedures, with or without intracranial devices, unexplained fever necessitates an LP, unless contraindicated, to exclude nosocomial meningitis. (See Chap. 11.) In patients who have not undergone a neurosurgical procedure and do not have headache, the yield of a LP in hospitalized patients was very low in one study (10A).

G. **Empiric antibiotics.** It is often reasonable to withhold antibiotics in the stable patient. If antibiotics are
deemed clinically indicated, then **use local susceptibility patterns and focal findings to select antibiotics.** See **Table 12.3** for an overview of antibiotic
considerations in adults. Once culture data are available, antibiotics can be modified. **A few points
deserve special emphasis.**

1. **If intravenous catheter-related infection** is
   a concern, vancomycin is indicated to ensure
   activity against gram-positive bacteria, including
   methicillin-resistant *S. aureus* (MRSA). Also consider gram negatives if the patient is receiving
   anti–gram-positive therapy.

2. **For nosocomial pneumonia**, gram-negative
   pathogens are often a concern. (**See Chap. 2.**) A
   gram stain of the sputum will help identify gram-
   positive cocci suggestive of *S. aureus*, including
   MRSA or *S. pneumoniae*. Penicillin-resistant
   S. pneumoniae is becoming more of a concern,
   especially with nosocomial acquisition. (See Chap.
   16.) The role of bronchoscopy to obtain cultures
   must be individualized.

3. **Occult candidemia.** In patients receiving broad-
   spectrum antibiotics, or immunosuppression
   (including corticosteroids) or with recent abdomi-
   nal/bowel surgery, empiric antifungal therapy
   may be a consideration if routine causes of fever
   have been excluded. Infectious disease consultation is advised.

4. **See Table 12.3.**

Table 12-3.   ICU fever and empiric antibiotics

Setting	Possible regimens
Pneumonia (see Chap. 2 for details)	
Gram negative	Aminoglycoside* plus piperacillin or piperacillin-tazobactam
Gram positive	Vancomycin
No gram stain data	Triple therapy (e.g., vancomycin, piperacillin, and an aminoglycoside) pending cultures
Fever alone	None or above triple therapy, depending upon severity of illness
Possible candidemia	Amphotericin B or fluconazole
Bacteremia	Vancomycin plus aminogly-coside* and piperacillin

* The aminoglycoside used will depend on local susceptibility data. If an aminoglycoside is contraindicated, aztreonam is often substituted.

II. **Fever in HIV-positive patients** (11,12)
   A. **Causes.** The level of CD4 count influences common considerations. **If the CD4 count is more than 200 to 300, the patient can be evaluated as a "normal host,"** although *Mycobacterium tuberculosis*, candidal infection, disseminated varicella zoster infections occur at this level.
      1. **Community-acquired bacterial infection may occur at any CD4 count.**
         a. *S. pneumoniae* or *Haemophilus* spp. pneumonia are common. *Pseudomonas aeruginosa* can be seen in community-acquired pneumonia (especially in patients with advanced disease). Patients with HIV may be at increased risk for infections due to penicillin-resistant *S. pneumoniae*. (See Chaps. 2 and 16.)
         b. *S. aureus* from intravenous drug use is common. The latter can be complicated by bacterial pyomyositis.
         c. Bacterial sinusitis may be accompanied by fever. (See Chap. 1.)
         d. Salmonella can be a persistent and recurrent problem when it develops.
      2. **Opportunistic infections are common as the CD4 count progressively decreases (Table 12.4).**
         a. **When the CD4 count is below 200/mm³**
            (1) *Pneumocystis carinii* **pneumonia (PCP)** can present with fever and minimal respiratory complaints (e.g., mild shortness of breath).
            (2) **Fungi infections** with *Cryptococcus neoformans*, *Histoplasma capsulatum*, and *Coccidioides immitis* can be seen.
            (3) *Toxoplasma gondii* may present with fever and possible focal neurologic complaints.
         b. **When the CD4 count is below 50/mm³** disseminated cytomegalovirus (CMV) and/or *Mycobacterium avium* complex disease are more likely.
      3. **Noninfectious fevers**
         a. Lymphoma (CD4 counts often <500/mm³), or phlebothrombosis secondary to hypercoagulable state.
         b. Drug fever, especially due to TMP-SMZ or diphenylhydantoin, may be present.
      4. **Fever without explanation is common.** A frequency of 15% to 30% is reported in the literature. This may be the fever of unrestricted HIV replication if most common causes of fever have been excluded; CD4 counts are usually less than 100/mm³.
   B. **Evaluation** has been reviewed in detail elsewhere. A few points deserve emphasis (12).

Table 12-4.   Fever in HIV-positive patients and correlation of complications with CD4 cell counts

CD4+ cell count	Complications
>500/mm³	Acute retroviral syndrome*
	Candida vaginitis
	Persistent generalized lymphadenopathy
200–500/mm³†	Pneumococcal and other bacterial pneumonia*
	Tuberculosis (pulmonary)*
	Herpes zoster*
	Thrush
	Candida esophagitis
	Cryptosporidiosis (self-limited)
	B-cell lymphoma†
<200/mm³†	*Pneumocystis carinii* pneumonia*
	Disseminated/chronic herpes simplex*
	Toxoplasmosis*
	Cryptococcosis*
	Disseminated histoplasmosis and coccidioidomycosis*
	Cryptosporidiosis (chronic)
	Microsporidiosis
	Tuberculosis (miliary/extrapulmonary)*
<50/mm³	Disseminated CMV*
	Disseminated *Mycobacterium avium* complex*

Source: Sullivan M, Feinberg J, Bartlett JG. *Infect Dis Clin North Am* 1996; 10:149.
* Associated with fever.
† Most complications occur with increased frequency at lower CD4+ counts.

1. **The CD4 count influences the type of evaluation.**
   a. **If the CD4 count is above 200**, the evaluation should focus on community-acquired infection including pneumonia, *M. tuberculosis,* and lymphoma.
   b. **If CD4 count is 50 to 200/mm³**, pneumocystis, fungi, and *T. gondii* are of concern, as well as the processes listed in Sec. a.
   c. **If CD4 count is less than 50/mm³**, *M. avium* and cytomegalovirus infections as well as the preceding considerations in section a. and b. need assessment.
2. **Specimens to identify infectious agents**
   a. **Blood cultures**. Except for mycobacterium, the dimorphic fungi (e.g., *H. capsulatum*), and viruses, BACTEC system (Becton Dickinson Diagnostic Instrument Systems, Sparks, MD) cultures are comparable to lysis centrifugation isolator cultures.
   b. **Sputum**. Gram stain, silver or special stains for *P. carinii*, "concentrated" myco-

8. Cunha BA, Shea KW. Fever in the intensive care unit. *Infect Dis Clin North Am* 1996;10:185.

9. Masur H, Malangoni M. Evaluation of fever in the ICU. Symposium. *Infect Dis Society of America* (IDSA). 35th Annual Meeting. San Francisco. Sept. 1997.

9A. O'Grady NP, et al. Practice guidelines for evaluating new fever in critically ill adult patients. *Clin Infect Dis* 1998;26:1042.

10. Garibaldi RA, et al. Detection of endotoxemia by limulus test in patients with indwelling urinary catheters. *J Infect Dis* 1973; 128:551.

10A. Metersky ML, Williams A, Rafanan AL. Retrospective analysis: are fever and altered mental status indications for lumbar puncture in a hospitalized patient who has not undergone neurosurgery? *Clin Infect Dis* 1997;25:285.
See editorial comment in this same issue.

11. Sullivan M, Feinberg J, Bartlett JG. Fever in patients with HIV infection. *Infect Dis Clin North Am* 1996;10:149.

12. Mirales P, et al. Fever of unknown origin in patients infected with the human immunodeficiency virus. *Clin Infect Dis* 1995;20:872.
Study points out that visceral leishmaniasis has been an important cause of FUO where such infection is prevalent. See related discussion by Berenguer J, et al. Visceral leishmaniasis in patients infected with HIV. Ann Intern Med *1989;111:129.*

13. Hughes WT, et al. 1997 Guidelines for the use of antimicrobial agents in neutropenic patients with unexplained fever. *Clin Infect Dis* 1997;25:551.
Guidelines from Infectious Disease Society of America.

14. Silva IC, High KP. Outpatient treatment for febrile neutropenic patients. *Infect Dis Clin Pract* 1998;7:307.
See also related paper Freifield AG, Pizzo PA. The outpatient management of febrile neutropenia in cancer patients. Oncology *1996; 10:599.*

15. Freifeld A, et al. A double-blind comparison of empirical oral and intravenous antibiotic therapy for low-risk febrile patients with neutropenia during cancer chemotherapy. *N Engl J Med* 1999; 341:305.
Low-risk patients were randomly assigned to receive either oral ciprofloxacin (30 mg/kg/day in three divided doses with maximal dose 750 mg q8h) plus oral amoxicillin-clavulanate (40 mg/kg/day of amoxicillin component in three divided doses with maximum dose 500 mg q8h) versus IV ceftazidime (maximum dose 2g q8h).

16. Kern WV, et al. Oral versus intravenous empirical antimicrobial therapy for fever in patients with granulocytopenia who are receiving cancer chemotherapy. *N Engl J Med* 1999;341:312.
In low-risk patients, oral ciprofloxacin plus amoxicillin-clavulanate was compared with IV ceftriaxone and amikacin.

17. Finberg RW, Talcott JA. Fever and neutropenia—how to use a new treatment strategy. *N Engl J Med* 1999;341:362.
Thoughtful and conservative editorial on references 15 and 16 . . . further studies are needed before outpatient oral antibiotics can be routinely used safely in the low-risk febrile neutropenic patient.

Miscellaneous

Part A: Microbiology Lab Pointers

Because of time constraints, state and/or federal regulations, and relative inaccessibility of most hospital microbiology laboratories, most primary-care providers have little interaction with their micro labs. However, **a few special areas deserve emphasis**. More detailed discussions are provided elsewhere (1–3).

I. **Conventional susceptibility testing.** Guidelines for the preparation of media, incubation factors, and interpretation of results for commonly used techniques are provided by the National Committee for Clinical Laboratory Standards (NCCLS) (2).
    A. **Disk diffusion test, agar diffusion test (Kirby-Bauer).** Worldwide, this remains the most widely used method for testing the activity of antimicrobials against rapidly growing bacteria. It **remains popular because of its ease of performance, reproducibility, and proven value** (3).
        1. **Method.** Paper disks impregnated with a standardized quantity of an antimicrobial agent are applied to the surface of an agar plate that has been inoculated with a suspension of organisms to be tested. The antimicrobial agent diffuses from the paper disk through the agar in a continuously decreasing gradient. After 16 to 20 hours of incubation, a concentric zone of growth inhibition around the paper disk can be measured. Standards for interpretation of the zones of inhibition are available.
        2. **Interpretation** (3)
            a. *Susceptible* **(sensitive)** implies that an infection due to the tested strain should respond to an appropriate dose of the active antibiotic.
            b. *Resistant* indicates that the strain is not completely inhibited by antimicrobial concentrations within the therapeutic range, and it strongly predicts failure when that particular antibiotic is used alone.
            c. *Intermediate* indicates that a clinical response may occur if unusually high concentrations of relatively nontoxic antibiotics can be achieved at the site of the infection. **For most situations, however, a strain classified as intermediate should be considered resistant until proven otherwise. Some laboratories will routinely report all intermediate zones of inhibition as resistant.**

3. **Limitations** include the following: (a) Some organisms grow too slowly for this method to be used; (b) only bacteriostatic (inhibition of growth) information is provided; and (c) interpretation standards are based on achievable serum concentrations, and this must be considered for urinary tract isolates since some antibiotics achieve much higher urine concentrations than serum.

B. **Dilution susceptibility tests** are used commonly to determine the **minimum inhibitory concentration** (MIC) of an antibiotic for an infecting organism. The **MIC of the drug is defined as the lowest concentration that prevents visible growth of the test organism** under a standardized set of conditions. Dilution susceptibility testing can be done by a broth dilution or agar dilution method, usually broth dilution. In clinical labs, this is done with **semiautomated/automated microdilution techniques** employing serial twofold dilutions of antimicrobials in **commercially available microtiter trays.** These trays are inoculated with a standard number of organisms, incubated for 6 to 9 hours with "rapid" or 15 to 24 hours with "conventional" techniques. The organism (i.e., concentration at which visible growth is inhibited) can be determined and recorded (3).

The Vitek System (bioMerieux Vitek, Hazelwood, MS) and the Baxter Microscan (Baxter Diagnostics, Inc., West Sacramento, CA) are two examples of automated microtiter techniques commonly used in North America (2).

C. **Gradient diffusion (Epsilometer testing)**. This is commercially available as the **E test** (AB Biodisk NA, Piscataway, NJ).

1. This *in vitro* technique was created to overcome several of the disadvantages of the disk diffusion and dilution techniques and to retain the principle of the agar dilution method by **producing an accurate, reproducible, quantitative MIC result** (2–4).

2. **Procedure** (2–4)
   a. An inert thin plastic carrier strip with a predefined continuous concentration gradient of dried and stabilized antibiotic on one side and a continuous MIC interpretive scale corresponding to a range of 15 $\log_2$ dilutions on the other side is used.
   b. After an agar plate is inoculated with a broth suspension of the test organism, four to six E strips can be placed on the plate, which is incubated.

3. **MIC result.** After incubation, 18 to 48 hours, an ellipse of inhibition is formed around the strip, and the MIC is visually read at the point where the ellipse intersects the strip edge (**Fig. 13.1**). Studies evaluating E-test performance compared

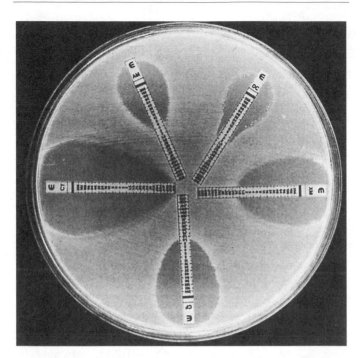

Figure 13.1.   E tests with a beta-lactamase-producing *Haemophilus influenzae* strain performed with HTM agar. Antibiotic abbreviations on the E-test strips and minimum inhibitory concentration interpretations (indexed to base 1) are as follows: AM, ampicillin, 8 µg/ml; DC, doxycycline, 4 µg/ml; XM, cefuroxime, 1 µg/ml; CF, cefaclor, 2 µg/ml; CT, cefotaxime, 0.015 µg/ml. (From Jorgensen JH, et al. Quantitative antimicrobial susceptibility testing of *Haemophilus influenzae* and *Stretococcus pneumoniae* by using the E test. *J Clin Microbiol* 1991;29:109.)

with routine susceptibility testing methods have demonstrated excellent agreement.

4. **Uses. The E test is commonly used to determine the MIC against penicillin for *S. pneumoniae*,** allowing the micro lab to clarify if an isolate has "intermediate" or "high-level" resistance (4). (See Chap. 16.) It also is useful in determining MICs for fastidious organisms (e.g., *H. influenzae,* anaerobes, and enterococci).

D. **Susceptibility testing of anaerobic bacteria and fungi is not routinely available in most hospitals.** In special circumstances, susceptibility data may be desired, and consultation with someone in infectious diseases and the microbiology laboratory is advised.

E. **Mycobacterium susceptibility testing** is routinely advised for clinical isolates of *Mycobacterium tuberculosis.* Large laboratories may be able to do this testing on site; often the isolate must be sent to a reference lab when isolated in smaller laboratories. Whether susceptibility data are performed on other mycobacteria must be individualized; infectious disease consultation is advised.

F. **Genotypic susceptibility tests** are reviewed elsewhere (2).

II. **Cultures**

A. **Blood cultures.** Blood cultures are indicated whenever there is reason to suspect clinically significant bacteremia or fungemia. In severely ill patients, blood cultures might be the only source demonstrating the causative agent. **Attention to strict aseptic technique** when drawing blood cultures **is imperative to minimize the risk of contaminating blood cultures with resident skin flora** (e.g., coagulase-negative staphylococci, diphtheroids, and *Propionibacterium acnes*) since contaminated cultures are often misleading. Furthermore, some organisms, which are usually skin contaminants can, under certain circumstances (e.g., catheter-related sepsis, prosthetic valve endocarditis), be true bloodborne pathogens. Therefore adequate preparation of the skin is an important aspect of this procedure (3). (See related discussions in Chap. 7.)

1. **Blood culture methods** (3). Most laboratories use an **aerobic and anaerobic** broth medium into which the blood is inoculated. Growth of microorganisms can be detected by visual examination of the bottles for turbidity, by blind subculture to solid media, or by a variety of automated systems that detect microbial metabolism. With older instruments, cultures are read at intervals (one to three times) during the day. However, reading is essentially continuous with newer systems.

a. **Volume of sample.** The ideal volume of blood to be collected for broth culture is unknown. Because of the low density of most bacteremias, 10- to 20-ml samples (e.g., **5 to 10 ml per bottle, depending on the manufacturer's recommendation**) **for adults** and 1- to 5-ml samples for children commonly are recommended.

b. **Timing and number of blood cultures. Two to three blood cultures, drawn at intervals of at least 20 minutes, are recommended** to help exclude contaminants and assess the duration of the bacteremia. Venous blood can be drawn from the same anatomic site.

c. **Blood lysis tubes** are available in two forms—one designed for centrifugation and concentration of organisms and the other, a smaller pediatric tube, from which the contents can be plated directly onto solid media.

Blood lysis permits quantitation of organisms in blood, results in increased recovery and decreased detection time for certain microorganisms (e.g., *Histoplasma capsulatum,* mycobacterium such as *Mycobacterium avium* complex [MAC]) and certain fastidious organisms. (See Sec. 2.) The major disadvantages of the blood lysis technique identified thus far are a high contamination rate and poor recovery of anaerobic organisms.

2. **Fastidious organisms require special techniques.** Blood cultures for brucellosis, tularemia, leptospirosis, systemic fungal infections, *Bartonella henselae* (formerly, *Rochalimaea henselae*, the organism believed to be responsible for cat-scratch disease), and *Mycobacterium avium* complex require special media and incubation for optimal isolation. **Your own microbiology laboratory should be consulted about these diagnostic concerns for specific recommendations regarding optimal collection and processing of the specimens at your laboratory**.

B. **Anaerobic cultures** (3) of abscesses, body fluids, etc.
1. **Sites for anaerobic culture.** Because many body sites are colonized with anaerobes, only certain sites are appropriate for anaerobic cultures: (a) **normal sterile bodily fluids** (e.g., blood, bile, pleural, peritoneal, etc), (b) **abscess contents**, (c) surgical biopsy specimens, (d) culdocentesis fluid, (e) suprapubic bladder aspirates, and (f) deep-wound aspirates (e.g., diabetic foot infection; see Chap. 3).

Inappropriate sites include sputum, fecal specimens, vaginal, bronchoscopy washings, etc.

2. **Special anaerobic containers are recommended** and provided by your micro lab for collection and transport of specimens that should be expedited. **Aspirated fluid specimens, or tissue, are preferred over swabs** from surgical specimens. If a culture swab must be used, it should be placed in an oxygen-free transport system.

C. **Mycobacterial cultures.** The major obstacle in culturing specimens for mycobacteria is the presence of large numbers of contaminating organisms. Prompt processing of individually collected fresh specimens is preferable to pooled samples, in which overgrowth of other microorganisms can occur.
1. **Take appropriate specimens (Table 13-1).**
2. If delays in processing are anticipated, specimens should be refrigerated at 4°C. **If gastric specimens cannot be processed promptly, they should be adjusted to pH 7** with sodium bicarbonate so that the gastric acidity will not affect the viability of the organisms.

Table 13-1. Specimens for culture of mycobacteria

Source	Recommended Number	Volume	Comments
Respiratory tract sputum	3	5–10 ml	Saliva inappropriate
Bronchoscopy washing (e.g., bronchoalveolar lavage [BAL])	1		Useful especially when spontaneous or induced sputums fail to provide diagnostic specimens.
Gastric washing	2–3	30–50 ml	Useful if respiratory secretions are not available; early-morning fasting specimens required (before eating or activity); small volume of sterile water can be used in the tube placement (20–30 ml); requires rapid delivery (within 30–60 min) to microbiology laboratory to prevent inactivation of organisms; stains may at times be helpful (saprophytes may cause false-positive smears).
Urine	2–3	Maximum volume of single specimen	Use first-voided midstream collection; avoid 24-h collection (too much bacterial overgrowth); stains may at times be helpful (saprophytes may cause false-positive smears).
Cerebrospinal fluid		Maximum volume available	
Other; joint, pleural, and peritoneal fluid		Maximum volume available	
Blood	1–2	10 ml	Useful for the recovery of *Mycobacterium avium* from patients with AIDS.

Source: Modified from Graham PS, Menegus MA. Microbiology laboratory tests. In: Reese RE, Betts RF, eds. *A practical approach to infectious diseases*, 4th ed. Boston: Little Brown & Co., 1996, Chap. 25.

3. Because mycobacteria may be present in the sample in low numbers, multiple specimens of relatively large volumes should be cultured when possible (e.g., sputum, fluid [cerebrospinal fluid in particular]). Sterile, wide-mouth containers with fitted caps should be used. Mycobacteria sometimes adhere to wax-coated surfaces; therefore **waxed containers should be avoided.**

4. During specimen collection and handling, care should be taken to avoid the production of infectious aerosols, and **specimens should be labeled clearly to indicate a possible biologic hazard.**

5. **Mycobacterium sputum smears** are discussed under Sec. IV.D.

III. **Interpretation of culture results**

A. **Contamination, colonization, and true pathogens causing infection.** Growth of microorganisms in culture does not necessarily represent infection (3).

1. **Contamination** refers to the introduction of extraneous organisms into the culture during specimen collection or processing. Contaminating organisms may originate from the skin of the patient, the clinician, or the laboratory technician, or from laboratory materials and the inanimate environment.

2. **Colonization** of body site refers to the **presence of organisms,** including potential pathogens, that are **not causing infection** (i.e., without evidence of illness, tissue invasion, or inflammation). Colonizing bacteria, for example, normally inhabit the oropharynx, skin, colon, vagina, and surfaces of wounds.

3. **To determine the clinical significance of culture data, the clinician must interpret all culture results in the context of (a) the clinical condition of the patient, (b) the site cultured, (c) the method of specimen collection, and (d) the identity and quantity of organisms recovered.**

   For example, *S. aureus* is a common wound pathogen, especially when the wound is warm, erythematous, tender, and draining purulent material. However, if the wound is benign on physical exam and has scant drainage that is clear but yielded *S. aureus* on culture, in this case *S. aureus* is just a colonizer and no treatment is necessary. Therefore **clinical correlation is necessary in interpreting cultures**.

B. **Failure to culture or detect a suspected pathogen** can be caused by a number of factors (3).

1. **Incorrect diagnosis** can occur. Infection may not be present or may be caused by organisms that are not cultured routinely (e.g., viruses).

2. **Misinterpretations of gram-stained smears** can occur; artifacts might be interpreted as organisms.

3. **Inadequate specimens** that are not representative of material at the true site of infection may be examined.

4. **Improper technique or delayed transport of specimens** may cause overgrowth by indigenous flora or loss of anaerobes or fastidious organisms.

5. **Antimicrobial therapy prior to specimen collection** may kill or inhibit the growth of organisms.

6. **Improper culture methods** may be employed. Special isolation techniques are necessary for anaerobes, mycobacteria, viruses, and certain fungi and bacteria. The physician must inform the microbiology laboratory of clinically suspected pathogens so that appropriate cultures can be performed.

C. **Preliminary identification of bacteria**, though not definitive, may assist the clinician in early diagnosis and choice of empiric antibiotic therapy. Clinical microbiology personnel can provide guidance in the interpretation of preliminary results. In addition to the gram stain, results of several tests often are available before an organism is finally identified (1,3). A few points deserve special emphasis.

1. **Gram-positive cocci**

   a. **Nomenclature of gram-positive cocci** is a frequent source of confusion.

      (1) **Group A** beta-hemolytic streptococci are *Streptococcus pyogenes*.

      (2) **Group B** beta-hemolytic streptococci are *S. agalactiae*.

      (3) **Group D** streptococci include the following:

      • *Enterococcal* **spp.** The majority of clinical isolates of enterococci will be *Enterococcus faecalis* (80% to 90%) and *E. faecium* (5% to 10%). Infrequently, *E. avium, E. raffinosus*, and *E. gallinarum* will be found.

      • **Nonenterococcal species** (*S. bovis*).

      (4) **Viridans group streptococci**, often referred to as *strep viridans,* is **not a single species** but encompasses many species of alpha-hemolytic streptococci, including the *S. milleri* group (*S. anginosus, S. constellatus, S. intermedius*), *S. mitis, S. sanguis, S. mutans,* and *S. salivarius*. Viridans strep are reviewed in detail elsewhere (1).

   b. **Blood agar hemolysis.** Colonies of streptococci may produce various patterns of hemolysis on blood agar plates (3).

      (1) **Beta-hemolysis is a clear, colorless zone** in the agar surrounding colonies of group A streptococci (*S. pyogenes*),

group B streptococci (*S. agalactiae*), and other, less common streptococcal pathogens.

(2) **Alpha-hemolysis,** or **partial hemolysis**, refers to a **greenish zone** surrounding colonies of *S. pneumoniae* and many species of viridans streptococci.

(3) **Gamma-hemolysis** actually denotes **nonhemolysis** and is observed typically with group D streptococci, including enterococcal and nonenterococcal species.

N.B. The **Lancefield serogrouping** of streptococci (groups A, B, C, D, etc.) is based on antigenic differences in cell wall carbohydrates and is an independent classification system that **should not be confused with the hemolysis patterns** of streptococci.

c. **Catalase test.** The gram stain often will help to distinguish between streptococci (chains or pairs) and staphylococci (clusters). If the distinction remains uncertain, a simple catalase test can be helpful. Hydrogen peroxide will bubble on exposure to catalase-positive organisms on a culture plate. Streptococci are catalase negative, and **staphylococci are catalase positive.**

d. **Coagulase test.** Coagulase-positive staphylococci produce an enzyme that coagulates rabbit plasma. A coagulase **slide test can be performed in minutes** but is less sensitive than an overnight coagulase **tube test.** Negative results of a coagulase slide test should be confirmed with a coagulase tube test. *S. aureus* **is coagulase positive;** *S. epidermidis, S. saprophyticus,* and other staphylococcal species **are coagulase negative.** Many laboratories have adopted latex agglutination tests instead of the traditional coagulase test for differentiation between *S. aureus* and other staphylococcal species.

2. **Gram-negative bacilli** (3).

a. **Lactose fermentation.** MacConkey agar plates are used to promote selective growth of gram-negative bacilli. Colonies of **lactose fermenters** (*E. coli* and species of *Klebsiella, Enterobacter,* and *Citrobacter*) appear red on MacConkey plates within 24 hours. **Non-lactose fermenters** (species of *Proteus, Serratia, Salmonella, Shigella, Pseudomonas,* and others) appear colorless or white. **Caution:** Although certain species are typically lactose fermenters (e.g., *E. coli*) some strains of these species are occasionally non-lactose fermenters.

b. **Oxidase test.** When oxidase reagent is applied to colonies on a culture plate, oxidase-positive colonies appear purple. ***Pseudomonas* spp. are oxidase positive** and Enterobacteriaceae are oxidase negative.

3. **Gram-positive bacilli** are often nonpathogens and viewed as contaminants. At times, they may be true pathogens. These organisms can be spore-forming or non–spore-forming. The most commonly isolated non–spore-forming bacilli are "diphtheroids"–corynebacteria that normally inhabit the skin. However, when repeatedly isolated from normally sterile fluids or sites, they may be pathogenic (e.g., in prosthetic device infections). **When isolated from blood or CSF, it is important to distinguish corynebacteria from another non–spore-forming bacilli, *Listeria monocytogenes,*** which is motile at room temperature and may cause meningitis in newborn infants, immunocompromised hosts, and the elderly.

The clinical significance of gram-positive bacilli and *Bacillus* spp. is reviewed in detail elsewhere (1,5,6). (Anaerobic gram-positive bacilli often may be important *Clostridia* spp.)

IV. **Miscellaneous** (3)

A. **Immunodiagnostic tests detecting microbial antigens in clinical specimens.**

1. **"Rapid strep tests."** More than 20 different immunodiagnostic kits are available for the detection of **group A beta-hemolytic streptococci** in pharyngeal specimens. (See detailed discussion of these tests in Chap. 1.)

2. **Respiratory syncytial virus** immunodiagnostic tests are now widely available. Most have very good performance characteristics, with sensitivities and specificities in excess of 90% and 95%, respectively. The good performance of such tests is in part due to intrinsic deficiencies of the gold standard (growth in cell culture) against which they are measured (3).

3. **Legionella urinary antigen** (7). Commercially available kits using radioimmunoassay or enzyme immunoassay (EIA) (Binax, Portland, ME) can detect *Legionella pneumophila* serogroup 1 in the urine. Although the urinary assay detects only *L. pneumophila* serogroup 1, this serogroup causes about 80% of cases of Legionnaires' disease; the test could also be positive from a prior and no longer active infection.

4. **Influenza direct antigen test.** For example, the Directigen Flu A antigen detection test (Becton Dickinson, Cockeysville, MD) employs an enzyme immunomembrane filter assay to detect influenza

A antigen extracted from suitable patient specimens. Nasopharyngeal washes or aspirates are preferred, as they have more viral particles than do nasal and/or pharyngeal swabs. In patients in whom wash or aspirate techniques are contraindicated, swabs can be used. **When positive, this rapid test** (which takes less than 1 hour to perform in the laboratory) **is very useful in making a rapid diagnosis.** The manufacturer reports a specificity of 95%. The sensitivity of the test in multiple laboratories awaits further experience. **A negative antigen test therefore should be processed for influenza A viral cultures before the diagnosis of influenza A is excluded.** By using a direct antigen test as an adjunct to culture isolation in nursing homes, influenza A often can be identified rapidly so that proper antiviral therapy and infection control measures can be initiated. A positive test also helps plan isolation and/or therapy in the acute-care setting (3). **(See related discussions in Chap. 1.)**

B. **Nucleic acid techniques for the direct detection and characterization of microbial pathogens in clinical specimens.**

1. The **polymerase chain reaction** (PCR) is a nucleic acid amplification method. Within hours, as many as 1 billion copies of DNA can be made from a single target segment of DNA or RNA. The technique **has been applied to amplify target microbial nucleic acid in many types of clinical specimens.** The amplified product can be detected by any one of a number of methods. The specific advantage of the PCR is its enormous potential for increasing the sensitivity of probe and other nucleic acid–based detection methods (1,3). For a recent review of this topic, see reference 1.

   a. **Potential limitations. PCR technology is evolving and at present many of the tests available through commercial, hospital, and research laboratories cannot be considered standardized.** Significant variation in both sensitivity and specificity of such tests has been observed in blinded, interlaboratory comparisons. Until PCR tests are better standardized, the results of such testing for clinical diagnostic purposes must be interpreted with great caution. Experts emphasize that this **methodology requires extreme care to prevent false-positive reactions due to contamination.**

   b. **Current clinical applications** for PCR include early clinical diagnosis of (a) **human immunodeficiency virus (HIV) infection**, (b) **herpes simplex encephalitis** when careful PCR is done on CSF, (c) viral hepatitis C infection, (d) cytomegalovirus (CMV) infection (e.g., of CSF). These and other applications are summarized in detail elsewhere (1).

2. **Nucleic acid probe assays** are based on the combination of labeled, single-stranded DNA or RNA molecules (probes) with single-stranded target nucleic acid. Several techniques—including filter, liquid, Southern blot, Northern blot, and *in situ* hybridization—are in common use, and each exploits the technology in a slightly different way (1,3). Nucleic acid probes are pieces of DNA or RNA labeled with chemoluminescent (light-emitting), affinity (antibody-based), or radioactive reporter molecules that are able to bind to complementary sequences of either DNA or RNA in the target organism. **Probe technology exploits the presence of nucleotide sequences that are unique to a given organism or species** as a molecular fingerprint for identification (8).

   a. Nucleic acid probes have been used to detect directly a wide variety of **microorganisms in clinical specimens**. Very successful commercial probe systems include those used for the direct detection of *N. gonorrhoeae* and *C. trachomatis* in cervical samples (1,8). Probes to detect *M. tuberculosis* and group A streptococci in clinical specimens are also available (1).

   b. Nucleic acid probe–based tests have also been developed to identify rapidly grown organisms *in vitro*, to detect virulence determinants (e.g., toxins), and to localize antibiotic resistance determinants (1,8).

      (1) *Mycobacterium* **spp.** The probes that have made the greatest impact on the diagnosis of respiratory disease are the culture confirmation assays designed to identify organisms growing on solid medium or in a liquid medium, such as BACTEC (Becton Dickinson Diagnostic Instrument Systems, Sparks, MD). Probes are available for *M. tuberculosis, M. avium* complex (MAC), *M. kansasii, M. gordonae,* and *M. intercellulare* (1). When a combination of the BACTEC and DNA probe is used, *M. tuberculosis* frequently can be identified in less than 2 weeks from the time of specimen collection. Mixed infections (e.g., *M. tuberculosis* and MAC) can likewise be identified.

      (2) *N. gonorrhoeae* culture confirmation probes are available and do not require viable organisms.

(3) **Other probes** are available (1) for *S. pneumoniae, S. aureus,* group A and B streptococci, enterococci, *Haemophilus influenzae, Campylobacter* spp., *Listeria monocytogenes, Coccidioides immitis, Blastomyces dermatidis, Histoplasma capsulatum,,* and human papillomavirus.

C. **C-reactive protein (CRP)** is a nonspecific acute-phase reactant to inflammation and tissue necrosis. CRP synthesis is by hepatocytes beginning 4 to 6 hours after the onset of inflammation and peaking at 36 to 50 hours. CRP will rise and fall (with appropriate therapy) faster and earlier in the clinical course than the erythrocyte sedimentation rate (9).

1. **Normal serum level** in children and adults is 10 mg/L or less.

2. In general, CRP elevations **in invasive bacterial infections tend to be in the range of 150 to 350 mg/L. In contrast, most acute viral infections tend to be much lower,** less than 20 to 40 mg/L, but this distinction is not absolute since levels of more than 100 mg/L can occur in uncomplicated influenza, CMV, and other viral infections (9).

   CRP will be elevated in rheumatoid arthritis, other inflammatory joint conditions, and congestive heart failure (9).

3. **Uses**. The clinical role of CRP has recently been reviewed (9). Based on current data, serial CRP measurements are most useful for **monitoring patient response** to therapy after the primary diagnosis of invasive infection or inflammatory process has been made. **CRP is not really useful or recommended for differential diagnosis of bacterial versus viral diseases** (including meningitis, acute otitis media, and lower respiratory tract infection) or diagnosing acute appendicitis or distinguishing upper from lower urinary tract infections because of the inconsistencies among studies in which CRP has been used (9).

D. **Sputum smears for mycobacterium** (i.e., acid-fast bacteria [AFB]). Culture for mycobacterium is discussed in Sec. II.C. Since mycobacterium cultures may take 2 to 6 weeks to grow and allow a preliminary identification, **sputum smears are essential to expedite the diagnosis of active pulmonary tuberculosis.**

1. **Sputum specimens should be concentrated** for microscopic exam as well as culture. To enhance microscopic identification and recovery of AFB, a mucolytic agent is used to digest/liquefy the sputum sample, and sodium hydroxide is used to decontaminate (remove competing organisms) the specimen, which is centrifuged (to concentrate AFB); the sediment is then stained and cultured (1,3).

2. **Direct sputum smears** can also be prepared
   (i.e., the sputum specimen is directly applied to
   the slide without the processing mentioned in
   Sec. 1 above), but their yield on microscopic identification and culture is much lower than the concentrated method, unless there is overwhelming
   infection.
3. **Staining techniques** (3)
   a. The **Kinyoun** or **Zichl-Neelsen** basic fuch-
      sin stain combined with conventional light
      microscopy has usually been replaced by
      fluorochrome stains.
   b. **Fluorochrome stains** offer the advantages
      of speed and ease of observation. The most
      well-established technique, Truant stain,
      employs auramine/rhodamine fluorescent
      dyes. Smears are examined under low power
      using a fluorescent microscope. Large areas
      can be easily examined in a short time, mak-
      ing fluorochrome stains more sensitive than
      conventional basic fuchsin stains (1,3).
   c. **The number of tubercle bacilli in respi-
      ratory secretions is directly related to
      the risk of transmission. Consequently,
      results of smears are used to help
      determine the role of "airborne isola-
      tion"** in potentially infected patients. (See
      related discussion in Part B, Sec. I.B.)
   d. One cannot, on the basis of smear results, dif-
      ferentiate *M. tuberculosis* from other myco-
      bacterium. Special DNA probes and culture
      with identification tests will allow this.

Part B: Infection Control Issues

The following discussion is not intended to be an in-depth review
of infection control and isolation issues, which are well covered in
basic infection control textbooks (10,11). However, **the rationale
and principles of isolation procedures and special concerns generated by certain nosocomial resistant pathogens**
are summarized.

The resistant organisms of increasing concern include the
following:

MRSA: Methicillin-resistant *Staphylococcus aureus*, sometimes
   called oxacillin-resistant *S. aureus* (ORSA)
VRE: Vancomycin-resistant enterococci
VISA: Vancomycin intermediately susceptible *S. aureus*
MDR tuberculosis: Multidrug-resistant tuberculosis
MDR gram-negative bacilli

I. **Isolation practices.** The Centers for Disease Control and
   Prevention (CDC) revised its recommendations for isolating
   patients in 1996 (12). A historical review of prior isolation
   procedures (e.g., categories [strict, respiratory, enteric,
   wound, blood] and universal precautions [UP] or body sub-

stance isolation [BSI]) is provided elsewhere (12). In the **current recommendations** (12):

A. **Standard precautions** (12) **apply to all hospitalized patients** and are designed to reduce the risk of transmission of bloodborne and other pathogens in the hospital. Thus UP and BSI precautions are really covered by this designation. Major aspects include the following:

  1. **Hand washing** with a nonantimicrobial soap is essential after patient contact, even if gloves are used.

  2. **Gloves** are used when touching blood, body fluids, secretions, excretions, and contaminated items.

  3. **Gowns** are worn to protect skin and prevent soiling of clothing during procedures and patient-care activities that are likely to generate splashes or sprays of blood, body fluids, secretions, or excretions.

  4. **Eye and facial (mask)** protection is advised for any procedures or contact that may produce splashes or sprays of blood or body secretions/excretions.

  5. Precautions to reduce needle/sharp injuries should be routinely followed.

B. **Transmission-based precautions involve the preceding standard isolations plus additional precautions** to interrupt transmission in hospitals (12).

  1. **Airborne precautions.** Airborne transmission occurs by dissemination of small-particle residue of evaporated droplets that may remain suspended in the air for long times or in dust particles containing the infectious agents.

      Diseases of concern include the following:

      • **Tuberculosis** (pulmonary)
      • **Measles**
      • **Varicella (chickenpox or disseminated herpes zoster)**

    a. **Private room with negative airflow** ensuring six to 12 air exchanges/hour is essential.

    b. **For pulmonary tuberculosis all health care workers (HCWs) need to wear an approved, fit-tested, respiratory mask.** (For bearded HCWs, special hoods are available to provide a negative airflow.)

    c. **For measles or varicella** (chickenpox or disseminated zoster):

      (1) **Immune HCW** need not wear respiratory protection.

      (2) Ideally, **nonimmune HCWs** should not enter these rooms; if they must, respiratory protection should be used (12).

  2. **Droplet precautions.** Droplet transmission involves the infected patient coughing, sneezing, or talking or undergoing oral/airway suctioning or

bronchoscopy. The transmission of large-particle droplets requires close contact of the infected patient and HCW (i.e., usually less than 3 feet). **Because these droplets do not remain suspended in the air, special ventilation and negative airflow rooms are not required** (as in airborne precautions) (12).

Diseases of concern include the following:

- Invasive *Haemophilus influenzae b,* including meningitis, epiglottitis, pneumonia, and sepsis
- Invasive *Neisseria meningitidis* meningitis, pneumonia, sepsis
- **Viruses** such as **influenza, rubella, mumps, parvovirus** B19, and known **adenovirus**
- Certain bacterial respiratory infections, including *Mycoplasma pneumoniae*; **pertussis; streptococcal pharyngitis**, pneumonia, or scarlet fever in children and infants; pneumonic **plague**

   a. **Private room is advised.**
   b. **Masks** (standard type, not what is used for airborne isolation) when entering the room, especially when within 3 feet of the infected patient.

3. **Contact precautions** are used to reduce the spread of important microorganisms from direct contact (e.g., skin-to-skin contact) of patients and HCWs or patients and patients, or, indirect contact, with contact of a susceptible host with a contaminated intermediate object, usually inanimate (12). **Diseases of concern are shown in Table 13.2.**
   a. **Private room** is advised.
   b. **Gloves.** In addition to wearing gloves as in standard precautions (Sec. A.2. above), gloves are **worn routinely when entering** the room. When leaving the room, wash hands after glove removal.
   c. **Gowns.** In addition to wearing a gown as in standard precautions (Sec. A.3.), gowns are worn when entering the room if you anticipate your clothing will have contact with the patient or environmental surfaces or items in the room.

C. **Empiric use of airborne, droplet, and contact isolation.** In many instances, the risk of nosocomial transmission may be highest before a definitive diagnosis can be made and before precautions based on that diagnosis can be implemented. Certain clinical syndromes and conditions carry a sufficiently high risk to warrant empiric precautions while a definitive diagnosis is being pursued. **See Table 13.3.**

Table 13-2.   Indications for contact precautions

Skin infections that are potentially contagious
  Decubiti (noncontained)
  Draining abscesses
  Staphylococcal wounds
  Viral infections such as herpes simplex or varicella zoster
  Certain dermatologic problems: impetigo, pediculosis, scabies
Clostridium difficile **diarrhea**
Certain viral infections
  Respiratory syncytial virus
  Parainfluenza virus
  Enteroviruses in infants and young children
  Conjunctivitis
Multidrug-resistant bacteria infections or colonization

Modified from Centers for Disease Control and Prevention. Guideline for isolation precautions in hospitals. *Infect Control Hosp Epidemiol* 1996;17:53.

II.   **Infection control principles and isolation procedures are critical to prevent the spread of certain pathogens** to other patients or HCWs. Certain problem organisms are reviewed in the next section.

Problematic Pathogens

I.   **MRSA** is an important nosocomial pathogen (13) that can cause serious nosocomial outbreaks. The incidence of MRSA at a particular hospital may vary from 5% to 40% or more, depending on the size, complexity of care provided, compliance with infection control practices, and geographic location.
  A.   **Pathogenesis and transmission** (14). Colonization with MRSA often precedes infection. The most common mechanism by which MRSA is introduced into an institution is the admission of a colonized or infected patient. Health care workers may disseminate MRSA. Patients from chronic-care facilities and dialysis units are often colonized and/or infected.
    1.   The **principal mode of transmission** within an institution is from patient to patient via the **transient colonized hands of hospital personnel**.
    2.   **Airborne transmission** may be important for patients **with tracheostomies** who are unable to handle their secretions and/or patients with MRSA **pneumonia** who may undergo suctioning.
    3.   Transmission via the **inanimate environment** may be important for special populations (e.g., **burns, major open wound infections**).
    4.   Although classically viewed almost exclusively as a nosocomial pathogen, **"community-acquired" MRSA can occur** among patients

Table 13-3. Clinical syndromes or conditions warranting additional empiric precautions to prevent transmission of epidemiologically important pathogens pending confirmation of diagnosis*

Clinical Syndrome or Conditions[†]	Potential Pathogens[‡]	Empiric Precautions
Diarrhea		
Acute diarrhea with a likely infectious cause in an incontinent or diapered patient	Enteric pathogens[§]	Contact
Diarrhea in an adult with a history of recent antibiotic use	*Clostridium difficile*	Contact
Meningitis	*Neisseria meningitidis*	Droplet
Rash or exanthems, generalized, etiology unknown		
Petechial/ecchymotic with fever	*Neisseria meningitidis*	Droplet
Vesicular	Varicella	Airborne and contact
Maculopapular with coryza and fever	Rubeola (measles)	Airborne
Respiratory infections		
Cough/fever/upper lobe pulmonary infiltrate in an HIV-negative patient or a patient at low risk for HIV infection	*Mycobacterium tuberculosis*	Airborne
Cough/fever/pulmonary infiltrate in any lung location in an HIV-infected patient or a patient at high risk for HIV infection**	*Mycobacterium tuberculosis*	Airborne
Paroxysmal or severe persistent cough during periods of pertussis activity	*Bordetella pertussis*	Droplet
Respiratory infections, particularly bronchiolitis and croup, in infants and young children	Respiratory syncytial or parainfluenza virus	Contact

continued

Table 13-3.   *Continued*

Clinical Syndrome or Conditions[†]	Potential Pathogens[‡]	Empiric Precautions
Risk of multidrug-resistant microorganisms		
History of infection or colonization with multidrug-resistant organisms[|]	Resistant bacteria	Contact
Skin, wound, or urinary tract infection in a patient with a recent hospital or nursing home stay in a facility where multidrug-resistant organisms are prevalent	Resistant bacteria	Contact
Skin or wound infection		
Abscess or draining wound that cannot be covered	*Staphylococcus aureus*, Group A streptococcus	Contact

Source: Centers for Disease Control and Prevention. Guideline for isolation precautions in hospitals. *Infect Control Hosp Epidemiol* 1996;17:53.
* Infection control professionals are encouraged to modify or adapt this table according to local conditions. To ensure that appropriate empiric precautions are implemented always, hospitals must have systems in place to evaluate patients routinely according to these criteria as part of their preadmission and admission care.
† Patients with the syndromes or conditions listed below may present with atypical signs or symptoms (e.g., pertussis in neonates and adults may not have paroxysmal or severe cough). The clinician's index of suspicion should be guided by the prevalence of specific conditions in the community, as well as clinical judgment.
‡ The organisms listed under the column "Potential Pathogens" are not intended to represent the complete, or even most likely, diagnoses, but rather possible etiologic agents that require additional precautions beyond Standard Precautions until they can be ruled out.
§ These pathogens include enterohemorrhagic *Escherichia coli* 0157:H7, *Shigella*, hepatitis A, and rotavirus.
|Resistant bacteria judged by the infection control program, based on current state, regional, or national recommendations, to be of special clinical or epidemiological significance.
** See text discussion.

with direct or indirect contact with hospitalized patients; **more recently, true community-acquired MRSA, without obvious contact exposure, appears to be on the rise (15,15A).**

B. **Infection control.** In response to the increase in prevalence of MRSA, some have recommended that isolation procedures be abandoned, arguing that the expenditure of time and money for these measures cannot be justified. However, a **recent report favors isolation procedures for those patients colonized or infected with MRSA,** emphasizing that MRSA is a virulent pathogen (30% of colonized patients become infected) and that many MRSA infections are preventable. Furthermore, the author recommends that routine screening of patients transferred from nursing homes and hospitals be done to identify patients who are colonized and/or infected with MRSA (so they can be appropriately isolated). This appears to be a **cost-effective measure** (16). **Contact isolation is** commonly recommended for patients colonized or infected with MRSA. For patients with colonization and/or infection with burns, a major draining wound, extensive skin involvement, or a lower respiratory tract infection, contact and droplet isolation (i.e., a private room; gowns, gloves, and masks for all entering the patient's room) may be reasonable in an attempt to limit nosocomial spread.

Very careful hand washing is mandatory after caring for patients colonized or infected with MRSA.

C. **Therapy.** The drug of choice for MRSA is **vancomycin** and in some clinic settings (e.g., prosthetic valve endocarditis), vancomycin ± gentamicin ± rifampin can be used (17). Also **see Chap. 16.**

II. **Vancomycin-resistant enterococci (VRE)**

A. **Incidence**. After VRE was initially reported in 1988, the CDC reported a 20-fold increase in strains being isolated from 1989 to 1993 (18). Now up to 14% or more of ICU- or other hospital-acquired enterococci are VRE (especially strains of *E. faecium*), an alarming increase for such a short time, especially since enterococci have become the third or fourth leading pathogen causing nosocomial infections. **Excessive use of oral and IV vancomycin may have contributed to the selection of VRE, prompting the CDC to urge clinicians to use vancomycin only when indicated.** (See Chap. 28.)

B. **Significance of VRE** (19)

1. Fortunately, colonization with VRE is more frequent than infection with VRE. **Colonization or infection** with VRE is **more likely** to occur **in hospitalized patients with the following:** prolonged length of stay (LOS), debilitation, prior broad-spectrum antibiotic therapy, complex medical problems, and prior residence in nursing homes.

    2. **Infections** with VRE do occur, including bacteremias (with 60% to 70% mortality rates), catheter-related UTI, wound, and intraabdominal infections.

  C. **Therapy** has recently been discussed (17,19A). Agents normally used to treat enterococci are not active against VRE (17–19).

    1. **Only two currently available antibiotics are effective against many strains of VRE,** quinupristin/dalfopristin (Synercid) and linezolid (Zyvox), which are discussed in detail in Chap. 28.

    2. Chloramphenicol may be active *in vitro* against up to 25% of strains but often fails *in vivo*.

    3. **Investigational agents.** As of March 2000 ramoplanin (for bowel decontamination) is being studied.

    4. **Infectious disease consultation is advised** for therapy of VRE.

  D. **Infection control** measures **are very important to prevent nosocomial spread** of VRE, especially since active antibiotics against VRE are limited. Isolation has been recommended by the CDC (18,19) and recently reviewed (19A), and although the best approach remains unclear, for patients colonized or infected with VRE we recommend the following:

    1. **Private room** (or cohorting the patient with another patient with VRE)

    2. **Masks** when entering the room

    3. **Gowns** when there is contact with the patient

    4. On leaving the patient's room, **careful hand washing with an antimicrobial soap**

    5. **N.B.** The **duration of these isolation procedures is unclear** at this point, possibly indefinitely (i.e., isolate with future admissions). You should confer with your infection control coordinator before discontinuing VRE isolation.

III. **VISA** (vancomycin intermediately susceptible [or **reduced susceptibility to vancomycin**] *S. aureus*) has only rarely been reported from clinical isolates in the United States but is very worrisome since routine antibiotics are not active against it. This topic has recently been reviewed (20,21).

  A. **Implications. If your lab reports a possible or definite VISA, you should follow the isolation procedures below and notify the infection control coordinator. Regional public health officials should also be notified** since this is a very unusual and worrisome pathogen that needs careful epidemiologic investigation. Patients at special risk may include those with prior MRSA infections and prolonged vancomycin use (e.g., dialysis patients with repeat MRSA infections) (21).

  B. **Isolation.** The patient should be placed as soon as possible in a **private room with precautions** that include a gown, mask, and gloves for anyone having contact with the patient. The number of persons with access to colonized/infected patients should be minimized. An antibacterial soap should be used for hand washing. A detailed discussion is available (22). Special efforts to ensure compliance are advised (22).

C. **Infectious disease consultation** is advised for patients with colonization or infection with VISA.

IV. *M. tuberculosis,* including multidrug-resistant **(MDR) tuberculosis.** Transmission of *M. tuberculosis* is a recognized risk to patients and HCWs in health care facilities. **Transmission is most likely to occur from patients who** have unrecognized or laryngeal tuberculosis, are not on effective antituberculous therapy, and/or are noncompliant, and have not been placed in respiratory isolation. Patients who have MDR tuberculosis can remain infectious for prolonged periods, which increases the risk for nosocomial and/or occupational transmission of *M. tuberculosis,* especially to HIV-infected patients or HCWs (23). See Sec. B.

A. **Guidelines for preventing the transmission of *M. tuberculosis* in health care facilities** have been reviewed and discussed in detail elsewhere (23).

B. **Patients at risk for mycobacterium infection should be placed on "airborne" (AFB-respiratory) isolation and be in a negative-pressure-airflow room, with caretakers using properly fitted and approved respiratory masks** (12) (Sec. I.B.1 under "Infection Control Issues") until the diagnosis of *M. tuberculosis* has been excluded (e.g., three negative concentrated sputum smears for acid-fast bacilli or one negative bronchoalveolar lavage sputum for acid-fast bacilli smear if routine sputum is not available). (See the earlier discussion on p. 262, bottom.)

Our "rules of thumb" for placing patients on AFB-respiratory isolation at the time of admission include the following:

1. **All patients who are clinically suspected to have *M. tuberculosis* until that diagnosis has been ruled out.** This includes (a) those with a chest x-ray with pulmonary cavitation or unexplained hilar adenopathy and cough; (b) those with known significant (+) PPD (Purified Protein Derivative) or history of *M. tuberculosis* and now with a cough and/or fever and/or abnormal chest x-ray; (c) those with cough/fever and/or abnormal chest x-ray and a history of exposure to an active case of tuberculosis.

2. **All patients who have been diagnosed as having *M. tuberculosis* and are undergoing therapy for this diagnosis.** These patients should be isolated until their infectivity and susceptibility status have been formally evaluated by an infectious disease or pulmonary consultant.

3. **All known HIV-positive patients or those at high risk for HIV with unexplained abnormal chest x-ray** (i.e., any focal infiltrate, diffuse infiltrates, CHF (congestive heart failure) versus diffuse pulmonary infiltrates, pleural effusion). Even if the patient has a known pulmonary

process (e.g., *Pneumocystis carinii* pneumonia), until *M. tuberculosis* has been excluded, airborne isolation is important, since these two infections can coexist.

4. **All HIV-positive patients or those at high risk for HIV infection who have unexplained fever and cough**, even if their chest x-rays are "normal"—since these patients with *M. tuberculosis* can have normal chest x-rays.

5. **Patients who may have been exposed to MDR tuberculosis** (e.g., **prisoners, prison guards, those living in crowded or poor sanitary conditions from major metropolitan areas**, such as New York City and Miami) and have an abnormal chest x-ray or unexplained fever or cough.

6. **Patients with hemoptysis** and an unexplained pulmonary process (e.g., infiltrate). (If the patient has known underlying lung cancer with no other risk factors for tuberculosis, isolation is unnecessary. This must be assessed on a case-by-case basis.)

7. Patients with unexplained chronic fever, with or without weight loss, night sweats, etc., and x-ray abnormalities—even if not pathognomonic of tuberculosis.

References

1. Murray PR, et al., eds. *Manual of clinical microbiology*, 7th ed. Washington, DC: American Society for Microbiology, 1999.
   This encyclopedic text is the premier reference source for the micro lab.
2. Cockerill FR. Conventional and genetic laboratory tests used to guide antimicrobial therapy. *Mayo Clin Proc* 1999;73:1007.
   Nice discussion of genetic susceptibility test methods.
3. Graham PS, Menegus MA. Microbiology laboratory tests. In: Reese RE, Betts RF, eds. *A practical approach to infectious diseases*, 4th ed. Boston: Little, Brown, 1996:Chap. 25.
4. Jorgensen JH, et al. Quantitative antimicrobial susceptibility testing of *Haemophilus influenzae* and *Streptococcus pneumoniae* by using the E test. *J Clin Microbiol* 1991;29:109.
   For a related paper, see Kiska DL, et al. Comparison of antimicrobial susceptibility methods for detection of penicillin-resistant Streptococcus pneumoniae. J Clin Microbiol *1995;33:229.*
5. Sliman R, et al. Serious infection caused by *Bacillus* species. *Medicine* (Baltimore) 1987;66:218.
6. Berkowitz FE. The gram-positive bacilli: a review of the microbiology, clinical aspects, and antimicrobial susceptibilities of a heterogeneous group of bacteria. *Pediatr Infect Dis J* 1994;13:1126.
7. Plouffe JF, et al. Reevaluation of the definition of Legionnaire's disease: use of the urinary antigen assay. *Clin Infect Dis* 1995; 20:1286.
8. Tenover FC. DNA hybridization techniques and their application to the diagnosis of infectious diseases. *Infect Dis Clin North Am* 1993;7:171.

9. Jaye DL, Waites KB. Clinical applications of C-reactive protein in pediatrics. *Pediatr Infect Dis J* 1997;16:735.
   This is a nice review and applicable to adults and children.
10. Wenzel RP, ed. *Prevention and control of hospital infections*, 3rd ed. Philadelphia: Lippincott Williams & Wilkins, 1997.
11. Bennett JV, Brachman PS. *Hospital infections*, 4th ed. Philadelphia: Lippincott Williams & Wilkins, 1997.
12. Centers for Disease Control and Prevention. Guideline for isolation precautions in hospitals. *Infect Control Hosp Epidemiol* 1996;17:53.
13. Martin MA. Methicillin-resistant *Staphylococcus aureus.* The persistent, resistant nosocomial pathogen. *Curr Clin Top Infect Dis* 1994;14:170.
14. Mulligan ME, et al. Methicillin-resistant *Staphylococcus aureus*: a consensus review of the microbiology, pathogenesis, and epidemiology with implications for prevention and management. *Am J Med* 1993;94:313.
15. Herold BC, et al. Community-acquired methicillin-resistant *Staphylococcus aureus* in children with no identified predisposing risk. *JAMA* 1998;279:593.
   A disturbing trend noted in Chicago. See editorial comment in same issue which favors still using beta-lactam antibiotics for empiric therapy of suspected community-acquired S. aureus infections. See related paper by Frank AL, et al. Community-acquired and clindamycin-susceptible methicillin-resistant Staphylococcus aureus in children. Pediatr Infect Dis J 1999;18:993.
15A. Kak V, Levine DP. Community-acquired methicillin-resistant Staphylococcus aureus infections. Where do we go from here? *Clin Infect Dis* 1999;29:801.
   Editorial comment on this emerging problem. See two related papers in same journal and related CDC report in JAMA 1999; 282:1123.
16. Jerrigan JA, et al. Control of methicillin-resistant *Staphylococcus aureus* at a university hospital: one decade later. *Infect Control Hosp Epidemiol* 1995;16:686.
17. The Medical Letter. The choice of antibacterial drugs. *Med Lett Drugs Ther* 1999;41:95.
18. Centers for Disease Control. Nosocomial enterococci resistant to vancomycin—United States 1988–1993. *MMWR* 1993;30:597.
   Also see MMWR 1995;44(RR12):1–13 for isolation procedures.
19. Murray BE. What can we do about vancomycin-resistant enterococci. *Clin Infect Dis* 1995;20:1134.
19A. Murray BE. Vancomycin-resistant enterococcal infections. *N Engl J Med* 2000;342:710.
20. Centers for Disease Control. *Staphylococcus aureus* with reduced susceptibility to vancomycin—United States, 1997. *MMWR* 1997; 46:765.
21. Waldvogel FA. New resistance in *Staphylococcus aureus. N. Engl J Med* 1999;340:556.
22. Wenzel RP, Edmond MD. Vancomycin-resistant *Staphylococcus aureus*: infection control considerations. *Clin Infect Dis* 1998; 27:245.
23. Centers for Disease Control. Guidelines for preventing the transmission of *Mycobacterium* tuberculosis in health care facilities. *MMWR* 1994;49(RR-13):1–32.

PART II

Antibiotic Use

14

Introduction to Antibiotic Use

Part A: Principles of Antibiotic Use

I. **Introduction**
   A. **Background.** The benefit to society of antibiotics is one of the most important advances in medicine this century (1).

   - Preventive/prophylactic antibiotics given at the time of surgical procedures that may lead to wound infection have been proven to reduce the incidence of wound infection and its consequences. Guidelines for use of prophylaxis are discussed in Chap. 15.
   - Early appropriate therapy for individuals with a specific acute infectious process provides symptomatic relief and a better outcome than delayed therapy or inappropriate therapy. This has been especially true in the leukopenic patient with gram-negative bacteremia (see Chap. 12) but is also true in many other infections.
   - As a consequence, clinicians have been quick to use antibiotics for any clinical problem that might be a bacterial infection (e.g., the febrile patient), even when it is mild and often even when they think that it is likely caused by virus. In controlled studies of such viral syndromes, antibiotics have shown no benefit (e.g., upper respiratory tract infections, Chap. 1) **This "standard" approach has led to a striking overuse of antibiotics, which in turn has led to evolution of bacteria (e.g., *S. pneumoniae* or *S. aureus*) that cause common serious infections that have become resistant to antibiotics that had been successfully used to control them.**
   - A summary of bacterial resistance issues is provided in Part B of this chapter.
   - The many advantages of effective antibiotics are in jeopardy and **appropriate use of antibiotics is of paramount importance.**

   B. **A different approach.** Clinicians are being forced to consider new and/or different approaches to deal with the practical considerations of treating a given patient and yet minimize excess antibiotic use. This approach must virtually always provide effective antibiotics for those who are most ill and at the same time withhold antibiotics when they are not indicated. **Two components of this approach are especially important.**
      1. **First, of those who are seriously ill, potentially resistant pathogens need to be covered, often necessitating broader antibiotics than in the past.** For example, in severe community-

acquired pneumonia (CAP), agents active against penicillin-resistant *S. pneumoniae* are needed. For bacterial meningitis in which *S. pneumoniae* is suspected or known, again an agent active against resistant strains is necessary (Chap. 11).

As a corollary to this, in some settings (e.g., CAP) it is useful to separate seriously ill patients from mildly ill patients. (See Chap. 2.)

2. **Second, we must minimize the use of antibiotics for clinical situations in which the patient will not benefit from receipt of an antibiotic** (e.g., avoid antibiotics in viral upper respiratory tract infections). (See Chap. 1.)

3. If we can do this successfully, we should be able both to benefit our patients and, at the same time, to prolong the useful life of the new classes of antibiotics we have been forced to use. **If we are unsuccessful,** we may find that the pharmaceutical industry has not had sufficient time to provide new safe and effective agents with which to treat our patients before our new approach to common serious infecting agents is no longer effective.

II. **Ten important questions to ask before selecting an antibiotic.** To provide a framework for a logical, stepwise approach to select an antibiotic for a given patient, we suggest the 10 questions **summarized in Table 14.1** be answered. This topic has been reviewed in more detail elsewhere and will only be summarized below (2).

A. **Question 1. Is an antibiotic indicated on the basis of clinical findings?**

1. **For urgent/serious infections, antibiotics are indicated.** For example, patients with suspected

Table 14-1. **Important questions to answer routinely before selecting an antibiotic**

1. Is an antibiotic **indicated?**
2. Have appropriate **specimens** been obtained, examined, and cultured?
3. **What organisms** are most likely?
4. If several antibiotics are available, **which is best?** (This question involves such factors as drugs of choice, pharmacokinetics, toxicology, cost, narrowness of spectrum, and bactericidal compared with bacteriostatic agents.)
5. Is an antibiotic **combination** appropriate?
6. What are the important **host factors?**
7. What is the best **route of administration?**
8. What is the appropriate **dose?**
9. Will initial therapy require **modification** after culture data are returned?
10. What is the optimal **duration** of treatment, **and** is development of **resistance** during prolonged therapy likely to occur?

or known bacterial meningitis or endocarditis, or patients who are febrile and neutropenic are at risk for life-threatening infections and deserve empiric antibiotics.

2. **For localized infections** (pneumonia, urinary tract infection [UTI], wound infection, cellulitis), **antibiotics are indicated.** See individual chapter discussions.

3. **Antibiotics are not indicated** in uncomplicated viral upper respiratory infections (URIs) or uncomplicated influenza, yet antibiotics are commonly prescribed in 50% or more of URIs, as discussed in Chap. 1.

4. Often antibiotics can be withheld in the mildly ill patient until cultures are available.

B. **Question 2. Before antibiotics are initiated, have appropriate clinical specimens been obtained, examined, and cultured?**

1. **Gram stains** of wound drainage or sterile body fluids may help identify whether the pathogens are gram-positive cocci or gram-negative bacilli.

2. **Routine cultures** (urine, blood, wound drainage) **should be obtained before antibiotics are started.**

C. **Question 3. What organisms are most likely to be causing the infection?** Often the clinician must start antibiotics empirically. Based on clinical information and gram stains, an educated guess about the likely pathogens is useful to help select empiric antibiotics with good activity against the most likely pathogen(s).

1. **Focal findings** (i.e., genitourinary, pulmonary, skin, or biliary) will strongly influence the decision about whether coverage will be directed against gram-positive, gram-negative, or anaerobic organisms.

   For example, if a patient presents with urosepsis and the gram stain of the patient's urine shows only gram-positive cocci, enterococci must be covered. If a patient with community-acquired pneumonia has a sputum gram stain loaded with gram-positive diplococci, therapy must be aimed at *Streptococcus pneumoniae*.

2. **The age** of the patient may provide clues to likely organisms. For example, in meningitis, certain pathogens are common in different age groups. (See Chap. 11.)

   In the elderly, infections may present atypically with inadequate histories, blunted signs on exam, and lack of fever; yet **morbidity rates are higher** in the elderly with infections. Pneumonias are more apt to be associated with bacteremia and slow resolution. UTI is commonly associated with bacteremia. Intraabdominal infection is more commonly associated with perforation, bacteremia, or abscess formation than in younger patients.

Therefore **in the elderly, early empiric antibiotics, broad-spectrum antibiotics, careful dosing, and assessment of drug/drug interactions are especially important** (3).

3. **Hospital-acquired** infections are more likely to be due to gram-negative bacilli with antibiotic resistance or methicillin-resistant *S. aureus* (MRSA) or at times vancomycin-resistant enterococci (VRE). (See Chap. 13, Part B.) Severe nosocomial infections may be due to *Pseudomonas* spp., often necessitating the use of an aminoglycoside until culture data are back.

4. **Severity of illness** dictates not only whether antibiotic therapy should be initiated but also, at times, whether multiple agents or very broad-spectrum agents should be used. (**See related discussion under Sec. I.B.1.**)

5. **Prior culture data** often provide helpful clues. For example, in a patient with repeated UTIs, if the last urine culture revealed a resistant gram-negative bacillus, one should assume this UTI may be due to similar or, especially, resistant bacteria while awaiting culture data.

D. **Question 4. If several antibiotics are available to treat the likely or known pathogen, which agent is best for a particular patient?** This question involves many variables.

1. Is there an obvious **drug of choice** (4)? (**Table 14.2**). If so, can this agent be used?

2. **Are there antibiotic allergies?** For example, if a patient is allergic to a penicillin, the patient must be presumed to be allergic to all the penicillin derivatives unless appropriate skin tests can be done to test specifically for cross-reactivity. It is important to **consider both trade and generic names of antibiotics** when evaluating a patient's allergic history. (**See the discussion of penicillin allergies in Chap. 16.**)

3. **Will the antibiotic** under consideration **penetrate** the infected area? This is especially important in meningitis, osteomyelitis, and prostatitis.

4. **Because of potential side effects,** some agents may be contraindicated in certain settings. Examples include the following:

   a. Chloramphenicol use is tempered by the rare occurrence of aplasia (probably 1/25,000 to 1/50,000 courses of therapy).

   b. The dental effects of tetracycline limit its use in children younger than 8 years and during pregnancy.

   c. The fluoroquinolones may affect cartilage formation and therefore are not currently recommended for use in prepubertal children and pregnant women. (See Chap. 32.)

Table 14-2. Antibiotics of choice for common pathogens

Pathogen	Antibiotic of First Choice*	Alternative Agents*
Gram-positive cocci		
Staphylococcus aureus or *S. epidermidis*[†]		
Non-penicillinase-producing	Penicillin	A first-generation cephalosporin preferred, vancomycin, imipenem, or clindamycin; a fluoroquinolone[‡]
Penicillinase-producing	Penicillinase-resistant penicillin (e.g., oxacillin or nafcillin)	A first-generation cephalosporin, vancomycin, clindamycin, imipenem, amoxicillin–clavulanic acid, ticarcillin–clavulanic acid, ampicillin–sulbactam, piperacillin–tazobactam; a fluoroquinolone[‡]
Methicillin-resistant	Vancomycin with or without gentamicin with or without rifampin	TMP-SMX, minocycline; a fluoroquinolone[†]
Streptococci		
Group A, C, G	Penicillin	Clindamycin, a cephalosporin,* vancomycin, erythromycin; clarithromycin; azithromycin
Group B	Penicillin (or ampicillin)	A cephalosporin,* vancomycin, or erythromycin
Enterococcus[†]		
Endocarditis or other serious infection	Penicillin (or ampicillin) with gentamicin	Vancomycin with gentamicin; quinupristin/dalfopristin; linezolid (see Chap. 28)
Uncomplicated urinary tract infection	Ampicillin or amoxicillin	A fluoroquinolone, nitrofurantoin, fosfomycin

continued

Table 14-2. (*Continued*)

Pathogen	Antibiotic of First Choice*	Alternative Agents*
Viridans group[†]	Penicillin G (with or without gentamicin)	A cephalosporin,* vancomycin
S. bovis	Penicillin G	A cephalosporin,* vancomycin
S. pneumoniae[†]	See text (Chap. 2, 11, 16)	
Gram-negative cocci		
Neisseria gonorrhoeae[†]	Ceftriaxone or cefixime or ciprofloxacin or ofloxacin, see text (Chap. 10)	Cefotaxime, spectinomycin, cefoxitin (see Chap. 10)
N. meningitidis	Penicillin G	Third-generation cephalosporin, chloramphenicol
Moraxella (Branhamella) catarrhalis	TMP-SMX	Amoxicillin–clavulanic acid; an erythromycin; clarithromycin, azithromycin, defuroxime, cefixime, third-generation cephalosporin, tetracycline
Gram-positive bacilli		
Clostridium perfringens (and Clostridium spp.)	Penicillin G	Metronidazole, clindamycin, imipenem, meropenem, chloramphenicol
Listeria monocytogenes	Ampicillin with or without gentamicin	TMP-SMX
Gram-negative bacilli		
Acinetobacter[†]	Imipenem or meropenem	Tobramycin, gentamicin, or amikacin, usually with ticarcillin or piperacillin (or similar agent); TMP-SMX, a ciprofloxacin

Aeromonas hydrophila	TMP-SMX	Gentamicin, tobramycin; imipenem; a fluoroquinolone
Bacteroides[†]		
Bacteroides spp. (oropharyngeal)	Penicillin G or clindamycin	Cefoxitin, metronidazole, cefotetan, ampicillin-sulbactam, piperacillin-tazobactam, chloramphenicol
B. fragilis strains (gastrointestinal strains)	Metronidazole	Clindamycin; imipenem or meropenem; ampicillin-sulbactam; piperacillin-tazobactam; ticarcillin-clavulanic acid; cefoxitin[§]; cefotetan[§]; piperacillin[§]; chloramphenicol
Campylobacter fetus[†]	Imipenem or meropenem	Gentamicin
Campylobacter jejuni[†]	Erythromycin or azithromycin; a fluoroquinolone	A tetracycline, gentamicin
Enterobacter spp.[†]	Imipenem or meropenem	An aminoglycoside and piperacillin or ticarcillin or mezlocillin; a third-generation cephalosporin[‡‡]; TMP-SMX; aztreonam; ciprofloxacin
Escherichia coli[†]		
Uncomplicated urinary tract infection	TMP-SMX[†] or ciprofloxacin (see Chaps. 24 and 32)	A cephalosporin or a fluoroquinolone
Recurrent or systemic infection	A cephalosporin[#]	Ampicillin with or without an aminoglycoside, TMP-SMX, oral fluoroquinolones useful in recurrent infections, ampicillin-sulbactam, ticarcillin-clavulanic acid, piperacillin-tazobactam, aztreonam

continued

Table 14-2. (Continued)

Pathogen	Antibiotic of First Choice*	Alternative Agents*
Haemophilus influenzae (coccobacillary)[†] Life-threatening infections	Cefotaxime or ceftriaxone	Chloramphenicol; cefuroxime (for pneumonia but not meningitis), meropenem
Upper respiratory infections and bronchitis	TMP-SMX	Cefuroxime; cefuroxime-axetil; third-generation cephalosporin, amoxicillin–clavulanic acid, cefaclor, tetracycline; ampicillin or amoxicillin; clarithromycin; azithromycin; cefixime, a fluoroquinolone
Klebsiella pneumoniae[†]	A cephalosporin[#]	An aminoglycoside, imipenem or meropenem, TMP-SMX, ticarcillin–clavulanic acid, ampicillin-sulbactam piperacillin-tazobactam; aztreonam; a fluoroquinolone; amoxicillin–clavulanic acid
Legionella spp.	Azithromycin or a fluoroquinolone or erythromycin with or without rifampin	Doxycycline ± rifampin; TMP-SMX
Pasteurella multocida	Penicillin G	Tetracycline, cefuroxime, cefuroxime-axetil; amoxicillin–clavulanic acid, ampicillin-sulbactam, piperacillin-tazobactam
Proteus spp., indole-positive[†]	Cefotaxime, ceftizoxime, ceftriaxone or cefepime**	An aminoglycoside; ticarcillin or piperacillin or mezlocillin; TMP-SMX; amoxicillin–clavulanic acid; ticarcillin–clavulanic acid, ampicillin-sulbactam, piperacillin-tazobactam; a fluoroquinolone; aztreonam; imipenem

Providencia stuartii[†]	Cefotaxime, ceftizoxime, ceftriaxone or cefepime**	Imipenem or meropenem; an aminoglycoside often combined with ticarcillin or piperacillin or similar agent; ticarcillin–clavulanic acid; piperacillin-tazobactam; TMP-SMX; a fluoroquinolone; aztreonam
Pseudomonas aeruginosa[†] Non-urinary tract infection	Gentamicin or tobramycin or amikacin (combined with ticarcillin, piperacillin, etc., for serious infections)	An aminoglycoside and ceftazidime; imipenem or meropenem, or aztreonam plus an aminoglycoside; cefepime plus an aminoglycoside; ciprofloxacin; trovofloxacin
Urinary tract infections	Ciprofloxacin	Carbenicillin; ticarcillin, piperacillin, or mezlocillin; ceftazidime; imipenem or meropenem; aztreonam, an aminoglycoside; cefepime
Pseudomonas (Burkholderia) cepacia[†]	TMP-SMX	Ceftazidime, chloramphenicol
Salmonella typhi[†]	Ceftriaxone or a fluoroquinolone	TMP-SMX, chloramphenicol; ampicillin, amoxicillin
Other species	Cefotaxime or ceftriaxone or a fluoroquinolone	TMP-SMX, chloramphenicol; ampicillin or amoxicillin
Serratia[†]	Cefotaxime, ceftizoxime, or ceftriaxone**	Gentamicin or amikacin; imipenem; TMP-SMX; ticarcillin, piperacillin, or mezlocillin, which can be combined with an aminoglycoside; aztreonam; a fluoroquinolone

continued

Table 14-2. (*Continued*)

Pathogen	Antibiotic of First Choice*	Alternative Agents*
Shigella†	A fluoroquinolone	TMP-SMX; ceftriaxone; ampicillin, azithromycin
Stenotrophomonas maltophilia††	TMP-SMX	Minocycline, ceftazidime; a fluoroquinolone
Vibrio cholerae (cholera)	A tetracycline	TMP-SMX; a fluoroquinolone
Vibrio vulnificus	A tetracycline	Cefotaxime
Yersinia enterocolitica†	TMP-SMX	A fluoroquinolone; an aminoglycoside; cefotaxime or ceftizoxime
Yersinia pestis (plague)	Streptomycin ± a tetracycline	Chloramphenicol; gentamicin, TMP-SMX

Source: Modified from Medical Letter. The choice of antibacterial drugs. *Med Lett Drugs Ther* 1999;41:95.

Abbreviation: TMP-SMX, trimethoprim-sulfamethoxazole.

* **See later individual discussions of agents for details of agent use and contraindications of use.** Choice presumes susceptibility studies indicate that the pathogen is susceptible to the agent.

† Resistance may be a problem; susceptibility tests should be performed.

‡ The experience with fluoroquinolone use in staphylococcal infections is relatively limited. Resistance during therapy may occur. See Chap. 19.

§ Up to 15–20% of strains may be resistant.

‡‡ *Enterobacter* spp. may develop resistance to the cephalosporins. See discussion in Chap. 19.

Specific choice will depend on susceptibility studies. Third-generation cephalosporins and cefepime may be exquisitely active against many gram-negative bacilli (e.g., *E. coli, Klebsiella* spp.). In some geographic areas, 20–25% of community-acquired *E. coli* infections may be resistant to ampicillin (amoxicillin).

** In severely ill patients, this often is combined with an aminoglycoside while awaiting susceptibility data.

†† Formerly called *Pseudomonas maltophilia*.

Note: The fluoroquinolones should be used only in adults. See Chap. 32.

5. **Bactericidal agents.** In minor infections of the healthy host, bacteriostatic or bactericidal agents are probably of equal efficacy. However, **in severe, life-threatening infections (particularly bacteremias in leukopenic patients or patients with endocarditis or meningitis), bactericidal agents, which depend less on host factors, are necessary.**

   Bactericidal agents include the penicillins, cephalosporins, aminoglycosides, vancomycin, aztreonam, fluoroquinolones, metronidazole, and imipenem.

6. **Cost of antibiotics.** From the 1950s through the 1970s, the cost of an antibiotic and its administration seemed to have had little impact on the prescribing habits of house officers and many physicians. Now, with the spiraling costs of these agents and, in particular, the expense of hospitalization, the cost of administering antibiotics is an important consideration. **This is a complex issue,** and only a brief summary follows. A hospital's pharmacy and therapeutic committee (or formulary committee) will consider all factors when evaluating new versus old agents (2).

   a. **The cost of the antibiotic itself** is the easiest component to sort out. See Tables B and C in the Appendix. **Generic preparations** should be ordered whenever possible, e.g., generic oral trimethoprim-sulfamethoxazole (TMP-SMX). It is **essential that the clinician recognize that the cost per day of the antibiotic itself is only one component of the cost of antibiotic administration in hospitalized patients.** Other factors are discussed later.

   b. **Frequency of administration** per day. The more frequently the antibiotic is given (q4h versus q8h versus q24h), the more expensive it is to administer in terms of personnel time, intravenous materials used, and so on. In one study, the estimated average nonantibiotic cost associated with the mixing and administration of a single intravenous antibiotic dose was $3.35 (5). Agents with longer half-lives may be more cost-effective since they are given less often.

   c. **Number of antibiotics.** Multiple antibiotics may be more expensive than monotherapy. However, in some settings, two antibiotics may be cheaper than one (e.g., the use of cefazolin plus metronidazole is less expensive than ampicillin-sulbactam for intraabdominal infection). (See Chap. 6.)

   d. **Intravenous (IV) versus oral therapy.** Since it is easier to give oral therapy than IV antibiotics (drug costs and nursing time), oral therapy, when appropriate, is very cost-effective.

e. **Monitoring of serum levels and toxicity.** The potential for toxicity with certain agents (e.g., aminoglycosides, chloramphenicol) is real, and the toxicity, if it occurs, may prolong the patient's hospitalization, increase the level of care of the patient (e.g., dialysis), or be associated with increased morbidity and even mortality. Monitoring for potential toxicities is expensive. Therefore if an alternative choice of a "safer" agent is available, it often is wise and cost-effective to use the alternative. See individual agent discussions.

f. **Narrow versus broad spectrum of activity.** For empiric therapy, antibiotics with a broad spectrum of activity are used initially. Once susceptibility data are known, it is preferable to use an agent with as narrow a spectrum as possible.

E. **Question 5. Is an antibiotic combination indicated?** In a few situations, antibiotic combinations are appropriate.

1. **Synergism.** When one antibiotic greatly enhances the activity of another, with more than an additive effect, this interaction is called **synergy.** Synergy can be measured in the laboratory by timed killing curves and checkerboarded methods, but these tests are time-consuming, can be difficult to interpret, and are not routinely performed. Examples of mechanisms of synergy include the following:

   a. **Serial inhibition of microbial growth.** Fixed combinations of trimethoprim (80 mg) and sulfamethoxazole (400 g) will block successive steps in the synthesis of folic acid. (See Chap. 24.)

   b. **One antibiotic enhances the penetration of another.** The synergistic interaction between **penicillin** (or ampicillin) **and aminoglycosides against enterococci** may be mediated by this mechanism. It is believed that enterococci are impermeable to aminoglycosides. The penicillin alters the cell wall, allowing the aminoglycoside to penetrate the bacteria and thereby act effectively at the ribosomal level.

   c. **An extended-spectrum penicillin (e.g., piperacillin) and an aminoglycoside are often synergistic against _Pseudomonas aeruginosa_ and other Enterobacteriaceae.**

2. **In the febrile, bacteremic, leukopenic patient**, use of a synergistic combination may be

associated with improved outcome over a single agent (6).

3. **In infections in which multiple organisms are likely or proved** (e.g., intraabdominal sepsis or pelvic abscess), more than one antibiotic may be required for adequate treatment.

4. **Limiting or preventing the emergence of resistance.** This principle applies primarily to the treatment of tuberculosis. More than one agent is used routinely in an attempt to prevent the replication of preexisting resistant organisms. Whether or not two agents minimize the occurrence of resistance with gram-negative bacilli is unclear (6), but available data suggest they do not.

5. **Beta-lactam/beta-lactamase combinations** (e.g., ampicillin-sulbactam, Unasyn) are used to enhance the activity of the beta-lactam antibiotic. (See Chap. 18.)

6. **Unique drug combination. Imipenem/cilastatin** is another type of combination. The enzyme inhibitor (cilastatin) prevents metabolic breakdown of imipenem by the kidney. (See Chap. 20 for a detailed discussion.)

7. **Disadvantages of multiple antibiotics**
   a. **An increased risk of drug sensitivities or toxicity** is more likely when more agents are used.
   b. **An increased risk of colonization with a resistant bacterial organism** may occur. If superinfection develops, such resistant organisms are more difficult to treat.
   c. **Possibility of antagonism**. Antagonism is present when the combined effect of two drugs is less than the effect of either drug alone; one of the drugs appears to interfere with the action of the second. How often this occurs clinically is unknown (6). Prior data suggest that the combination of tetracycline and penicillin for treatment of meningitis resulted in a poorer outcome than when penicillin was used alone, presumably due to the inhibition of growth by tetracycline, which interferes with the bactericidal action of penicillin.
   d. **Higher costs.** Combination antibiotics often are more expensive than single agents.
   e. **False sense of security.** Although appealing at times, the use of multiple agents to treat all possible organisms often is not possible, practical, or necessary and may be associated with an increase in side effects.

F. **Question 6. Are there important host factors?** There may be special characteristics of the host that must be considered in choosing an antibiotic for use in individual patients. Some examples are given here.

1. **Genetic factors.** Patients with glucose-6-phosphate dehydrogenase (G-6-PD) deficiency may develop hemolysis from sulfonamides, nitrofurantoin, and chloramphenicol (6).
2. **Pregnancy and lactation.** Certain drugs may pose special problems (e.g., the tetracyclines, which may cause hepatotoxicity in the mother and dentition problems in the infant). Because of the physiologic changes that occur in the mother during pregnancy, overall serum drug levels of antibiotics are lower during gestation. Therefore in critical infections, serum levels of antibiotics may need to be monitored and compensatory dosage adjustments may be necessary (7).
   a. **Placental transfer of antibiotics.** Whenever possible, pregnant women should avoid all drugs because of the risk of fetal toxicity. This topic has been reviewed elsewhere (7,8) and is summarized as follows:
      (1) **Antibiotics considered safe in pregnancy** include the penicillins (with the possible exception of ticarcillin) (6), the cephalosporins, erythromycin base, and probably aztreonam.
      (2) **Antibiotics to be used with caution** include the aminoglycosides, vancomycin, clindamycin, imipenem-cilastatin, trimethoprim, and nitrofurantoin.
      (3) **Antibiotics contraindicated in pregnancy** include chloramphenicol, erythromycin estolate, tetracycline, fluoroquinolones, and TMP-SMX (Bactrim, Septra). Although controversial, we would try to avoid using metronidazole because of its carcinogenic potential. (See Chap. 29.) Sulfonamides should be avoided in the last trimester of pregnancy. Some experts suggest avoiding ticarcillin, as it has been shown to be teratogenic in rodents (6). (See Chap. 18.)
   b. **Antibiotics in breast milk**. Data regarding the adverse effects in nursing neonates from antibiotics administered to their mothers are limited. If possible, nursing mothers should avoid all drugs. As in pregnancy, chloramphenicol, tetracycline, sulfonamides, fluoroquinolones, and probably metronidazole should be avoided. See discussions of individual agents.
   c. **The US Food and Drug Administration's (FDA's) use-in-pregnancy drug-rating system is shown in Table 14.3.** These pregnancy categories are based on the degree to which available information has ruled out

Table 14-3. FDA Use-in-Pregnancy Ratings

The U.S. Food and Drug Administration's use-in-pregnancy rating system weighs the degree to which available information has ruled out risk to the fetus against the drug's potential benefit to the patient. The ratings, and their interpretation, are as follows:

Category	Interpretation
A	**Controlled studies show no risk.** Adequate, well-controlled studies in pregnant women have failed to demonstrate a risk to the fetus in any trimester of pregnancy.
B	**No evidence of risk in humans.** Adequate, well-controlled studies in pregnant women have not shown increased risk of fetal abnormalities despite adverse findings in animals, or, in the absence of adequate human studies, animal studies show no fetal risk. The chance of fetal harm is remote, but remains a possibility.
C	**Risk cannot be ruled out.** Adequate, well-controlled human studies are lacking, and animal studies have shown a risk to the fetus or are lacking as well. There is a chance of fetal harm if the drug is administered during pregnancy; but the potential benefits may outweigh the potential risk.
D	**Positive evidence of risk.** Studies in humans, or investigational or post-marketing data, have demonstrated fetal risk. Nevertheless, potential benefits from the use of the drug may outweigh the potential risk. For example, the drug may be acceptable if needed in a life-threatening situation or serious disease for which safer drugs cannot be used or are ineffective.
X	**Contraindicated in pregnancy.** Studies in animals or humans, or investigational or post-marketing reports, have demonstrated positive evidence of fetal abnormalities or risk which clearly outweighs any possible benefit to the patient.

Source: *Physicians' desk reference,* 53rd ed. Montvale, NJ: Medical Economics, 1999:347.

risk to the fetus balanced against the drug's potential benefits to the patient. This topic has recently been reviewed (7).

The human embryo is most vulnerable to teratogenic insult during the first trimester (days 1 to 70 of gestation). During the second trimester (days 70 to 154 of gestation), the fetal organs have been developed and growth continues; agents with antimetabolic activity, such as the folate antagonists, have the most theoretical potential for adverse effects. The third trimester (day 154 to delivery) is characterized by an impaired fetal ability to metabolize toxic agents and competition of the drugs with endogenous substances (e.g., bilirubin) for plasma protein-binding sites (7).

3. **Renal function**. Renal failure may affect not only the choice of antibiotic but also its dosages (9). (See discussions of individual agents.) Consequently, **renal function should be monitored in patients treated with antibiotics that are potentially nephrotoxic** and primarily excreted by the kidney. **These are summarized in Table 14.4.** Serum antibiotic levels, especially when aminoglycosides are used, should be monitored, as should serum creatinine, every 2 to 4 days.

a. **Dosages of antibiotics excreted by the kidney are modified based on the patient's creatinine clearance.**

b. **The serum creatinine may not accurately reflect the patient's renal function, especially in the elderly,** who may have decreased creatinine production. The **creatinine clearance is a better measure** of renal function. By modifying the equation of Cockcroft and Gault (10), it is possible to estimate the patient's creatinine clearance from the patient's age, gender, body weight (in kilograms), and serum creatinine (10) as follows:

Table 14-4.   Major pathways of antibiotic excretion

Antibiotics Primarily Excreted by the Liver*	Antibiotics Primarily Excreted by the Kidneys
Cefoperazone	Aminoglycosides
Chloramphenicol	Aztreonam
Clindamycin	Cephalosporins (other than cefoperazone)
Doxycycline	Imipenem
Erythromycin	Fluoroquinolones[†]
Metronidazole	Penicillin and penicillin derivatives
Nafcillin	Trimethoprim
Rifampin	Tetracycline
Sulfamethoxazole	Vancomycin

* In renal failure, dosages usually do not need modifications. See individual chapter discussions.
† The fluoroquinolones are excreted by the kidneys to a variable degree depending on the specific agent (see Chap. 32).

(1) **Male estimated creatinine clearance =**

$$\frac{(140 - \text{age}) \times (\text{weight})}{(72 \times \text{serum creatinine})}$$

   (a) **Female estimated creatinine clearance = 85% of male value**

   (b) **Some prefer to use ideal body weight (IBW),** which can be calculated as:

Male = 50 kg + 2.3 kg per each inch over 5 feet (in height)

Female = 45.5 kg + 2.3 kg per each inch over 5 feet

   (c) **In the obese patient,** we use IBW to estimate the creatinine clearance.

(2) **In patients with severe hepatic insufficiency,** this formula may overestimate the creatinine clearance. (See Sec. 4.d later.)

4. **Liver function.** Our understanding of modifying dosages in hepatic insufficiency is not as sophisticated as it is for renal insufficiency (11). However, **four issues deserve special emphasis** in patients with hepatic insufficiency.

   a. **Aminoglycoside use in patients with cirrhosis may be associated with an increased risk of nephrotoxicity,** as reviewed in Chap. 21.

   b. **Beta-lactam antibiotic use** in one study was **associated with an increased risk of leukopenia** when standard doses of beta-lactam antibiotics were used in patients with underlying liver disease (12). The probable mechanism is impaired hepatic metabolism of the beta-lactam antibiotics, resulting in bone marrow suppression of white cell precursors from excessive antibiotic concentrations. The authors proposed a reduction in dosage of beta-lactam antibiotic when used in patients with significant hepatic dysfunction (12).

   c. **Drugs primarily excreted or detoxified by the liver** (e.g., chloramphenicol, clindamycin) **need dose adjustments**. Other drugs that should be used with caution or for which serum levels should be monitored include fluconazole, itraconazole, nitrofurantoin, and pyrazinamide (6). (See **Table 14.4** and individual chapter discussions.)

   d. When selecting a dose for a potentially nephrotoxic drug, creatinine clearance (glomerular filtration rate [GFR] should be estimated (just as in the elderly) even when the serum creatinine is normal (13). In patients with underlying liver disease a low GFR may overestimate the true GFR (two- to three-fold) as measured by the inulin clearance. This may be accounted for by underproduction of creatinine resulting from diminished muscle mass or by a decreased rate of hepatic production of creatine, the substrate for the production of creatinine in muscles (13). **In practice for those with an estimated low GFR and severe hepatic disease, we assume their estimated creatinine clearance may be approximately 50% of the calculated estimate using the formula in Sec. F.3.**

5. **In neutropenic patients,** bactericidal agents are preferred whenever possible.

6. Prosthetic device infections may be difficult to eradicate. (See Chaps. 8 and 9.)

G. **Question 7. What is the best route of administration?**

1. **IV antibiotics are usually preferred in serious infections,** to ensure adequate blood levels. Because of the pain associated with intramuscular injections these are often avoided. Often oral absorption is too unpredictable to trust in serious infections. Exceptions may exist (e.g., levofloxacin is 99% bioavailable). (See individual chapter discussions.)

2. **Continuous versus intermittent bolus intravenous infusion.** Whether intravenously administered antibiotics should be given by continuous infusion or by intermittent bolus remains controversial (6) and is undergoing serial evaluation. This is reviewed elsewhere (14,15).

    a. **Continuous** infusions may result in less vein irritation and phlebitis. Prior animal model studies suggested that concentrations of penicillins and cephalosporins in fibrin clots were related to peak serum levels achieved; therefore intermittent bolus therapy seemed appropriate for endocarditis and tissue infections (6).

    Recent data suggest that the clinical effectiveness of beta-lactam antibiotics is optimal when the concentration at the site of infection exceeds the minimum inhibitory concentration (MIC) of the infecting organism for a prolonged time (i.e., animal model data favors continuous infusion for serious systemic infections) (6). This is called **time-dependent bactericidal activity,** which has little relationship to the magnitude of drug concentration and includes the **beta-lactam antibiotics and vancomycin** (15). At this point, while awaiting other clinical data, **we generally do not advocate using continuous infusions** of time-dependent antibiotics (e.g., beta-lactams).

b. **Intermittent infusions** may be preferred for bactericidal antibiotics (agents where the MIC equals the minimal bactericidal concentration [MBC]) that exhibit **concentration-dependent bactericidal activity** over a wide range of drug concentrations. That is, the rate and extent of bactericidal action increase with increasing concentrations above the MBC up to a point of maximum effect, usually 5 to 10 times the MBC (15). The **aminoglycosides and fluoroquinolones** demonstrate this type of activity (6,15); the **higher the drug level, the greater the rate of bacterial clearance**, which slows as the drug level falls (15).

(1) **Potential implications.** Large, infrequently administered doses of concentration-dependent agents (e.g., aminoglycosides) that achieve maximal concentrations at peak at the site of infection should produce optimal bactericidal effect (15). This is in large part the **basis for once-daily regimens of aminoglycoside** dosing, which is discussed in detail in Chap. 21.

(2) However, clinical studies that clearly prove this approach (e.g., once-daily aminoglycoside dosing) superior to other dosing regimens are still not available.

Moellering emphasizes that "definitive clinical studies providing unequivocal support for these concepts remain to be carried out" (6). In his 1995 review, Levinson concludes: "The optimal dosing interval of concentration-dependent antimicrobial agents remains an unanswered question for any individual patient and type of infection, and is under study for aminoglycosides" (15). Therefore the long-term clinical implications of this dosing approach await further study.

3. **Oral therapy** is commonly used for mild to moderately severe outpatient infections and for completion of therapy of focal infections initially treated with IV antibiotics. In special circum-

Table 14-5.   Duration of antibiotic therapy for common infections

Diagnosis	Duration of Therapy (days)
Meningococcal meningitis	7–10
Pneumococcal meningitis	10–14
Haemophilus influenzae type b meningitis	10–14
Streptococcal group A pharyngitis	10
Otitis media	7–10
Bacterial sinusitis	10–14
Pneumococcal pneumonia	? optimal*
Gram-negative pneumonias (*Klebsiella, Enterobacter, Pseudomonas*)	? 21[†]
Mycoplasma pneumonia	14[‡]
Legionella pneumonia	21[‡]
Endocarditis (nonprosthetic)	
Viridans streptococci	28
Staphylococcal	28–42
Peritonitis	10–14
Septic arthritis (nongonococcal)	14–21[·]
Osteomyelitis	28–42[#]

* Most experts agree that therapy should be continued at least 3 days after the temperature returns to normal. Elderly patients may deserve 7 days of parenteral therapy.
[†] Difficult to eradicate; patients may require even longer courses.
[‡] To prevent relapse, a full therapeutic course should be given.
[·] Four weeks of therapy may be indicated in patients with gram-negative infections, slowly responding infections (despite adequate drainage), or infections with virulent organisms such as *S. aureus*.
[#] In vertebral osteomyelitis, patients often are treated for 6 weeks.

Part B: Antibiotic Resistance

Increasing bacterial resistance has been emphasized in recent reviews (2,18–23) as well as in the lay media (e.g., "War Against Microbes," *Business Week*, April 1998; "Super Bugs: The Bacteria Antibiotics Can't Kill," *New York Times Magazine,* Aug. 2, 1998; "Last Days of the Wonder Drugs," *Discover*, Nov. 1998; "Beware of the Superbugs," 20/20 ABC television June 4, 1999). **Although an extensive discussion of this topic is beyond the scope of this text, several issues deserve special emphasis.**

   I.   **Background.** After the introduction of sulfonamides in the middle to late 1930s and penicillin in the early 1940s, pharmaceutical companies introduced a series of antibiotics to combat resistant bacteria. These agents included, in the

3. **Invasive procedures** (including central venous catheters) **and foreign bodies** as a consequence of these procedures expose patients to nosocomial infectious complications.

4. **Resistant bacteria are as virulent as susceptible bacteria.** Because of the disproportionately high incidence of multidrug-resistant bacteria in hospitals, the argument has been made that resistant pathogens are dangerous only to severely ill patients (19) and overall may be less virulent, especially to "normal hosts." This does not appear to be the case. Both methicillin-resistant and methicillin-susceptible *S. aureus* can produce toxins, and the frequency and spectrum of staphylococcal diseases caused by susceptible and resistant strains appear to be the same (19).

IV. **Urgency of situation with multidrug-resistant bacteria.** In a 1994 Rockefeller University Workshop on multidrug-resistant bacteria, the participants concluded that the epidemiologic data in the United States suggest that we have already "reached the point that health agencies should be able to (and need to) take steps to avert a potential crisis. In particular, the acquisition of resistance to vancomycin, either by MRSA or resistant *S. pneumoniae*, would create highly invasive clones that could not be controlled by any currently available chemotherapeutic agent. Indeed, the transfer and expression of vancomycin resistance to staphylococci have already been demonstrated in the laboratory, and their emergence in clinical strains may only be a matter of time" (19). Recently, vancomycin intermediately resistant *S. aureus* (VISA) strains have been described clinically. (See Chap. 13, Part B.)

Kunin (18) writes, "We have now reached an unacceptable situation. Some hospital strains of invasive gram-negative enteric bacteria and enterococci are not susceptible to any available drug. Multiply resistant tubercle bacilli have appeared and spread rapidly. . . . [Furthermore] the situation has now reached a crisis stage worldwide and is predicted to worsen with the introduction of new quinolones, macrolides, and oral cephalosporins."

V. **Proposed solutions to the problem** (2,19–26,30)

A. **Awareness of the problem.** Special efforts should be made to bring the issue of antibiotic resistance to the attention of microbiologists, government health authorities, physicians (19), and especially lay public, in an appropriate manner.

B. **More prudent use of antibiotics in humans and animals is critical** in developing and developed countries (2,18–20,25,31). These are **global issues,** not ones applicable only to the United States.

1. Provider education, antibiotic control programs, shorter courses of antibiotics when feasible, and narrow-spectrum agents when feasible are all

late 1950s, the semisynthetic penicillins to treat pe［ ］it p
resistant *S. aureus* and, in the 1960s through the ［ ］
cephalosporins and aminoglycosides for hospital-a［ ］ant
organisms, especially gram-negative bacilli. Vanc ［ ］ents
(available in 1958) has been useful to treat increasin ［ ］voirs
lems associated with MRSA. **The concept of an u**
able bacterial disease is foreign to most physici ［ ］ism
the developing world, but if recent bacterial-res ［ ］re int
trends continue, it may become a reality. ［ ］d wh

II. **Current dilemma.** In the past decade, there has ［ ］se age
worrisome rise in resistant, often multidrug-resi ［ ］nd eve
bacteria—not only in hospital-acquired bacteria b
in community-acquired bacteria and *M. tuberculos* ［ ］anima
the United States and worldwide (2,18–23). ［ ］llow it t

  A. **Nosocomial infections.** In the past decade,
     positive bacteria have emerged as the most fre
     causes of nosocomial infection (2,19). ［ ］of many
     1. **Coagulase-negative staphylococci** comn ［ ］ly mem-
        cause prosthetic-device- and catheter-relate
        fections, and 60% to 90% of strains are methi ［ ］**ion,** and
        resistant (19). ［ ］ansmis-
     2. **Methicillin-resistant *S. aureus* (MRSA** ［ ］promote
        account for 5% to 40% of *S. aureus* infect ［ ］*tuber-*
        depending on the size and type of hospital.
        Chap. 13, Part B.) ［ ］tate the
     3. **Enterococci** are the third most common n ［ ］s.
        comial pathogen (after *S. aureus* and *E. coli*), ［ ］fect the
        in 1993 vancomycin-resistant enterococci v ［ ］mission
        reported in up to 14% of intensive care unit e ［ ］ intra-
        rococcal isolates, a 20-fold increase since 1
        (19). (See Chap. 13, Part B.) ［ ］**ucture**
     4. **Multidrug-resistant** *P. aeruginosa* and *P. ce* ［ ］ng poli-
        cia have become common in patients with cy ［ ］ health
        fibrosis. Multidrug-resistant *Acinetobacter* s ［ ］ubercu-
        can occur in intensive care units (19). ［ ］ous dis-
     5. Outbreaks of extended-spectrum beta-lactam ［ ］ance of
        Klebsiella spp. have been reported (20), prest ［ ］ntinued
        ably related to selection pressure from widespr ［ ］3. Sur-
        use of late-generation cephalosporins; they t ［ ］uate in
        ally are susceptible to imipenem. ［ ］ny out-
  B. **Community-acquired infections (2)** ［ ］ecently
     1. In recent years, *Neisseria gonorrhoeae* (see Cl ［ ］r short-
        10), *Salmonella*, and *Shigella* spp. (see Chap
        have shown increasing resistance. ［ ］**essing,**
     2. **Multidrug-resistant *M. tuberculosis*** is a s ［ ］ safety
        ous and increasing problem in the United St
        and worldwide. Case fatality rates of 40% to (
        occur in patients with normal immunity, and (［ ］veler to
        mortality occurs in the immunocompromised ［ ］ devel-
        ulation (19). ［ ］spread
     3. The increasing and ominous problem of **S. pn**
        moniae resistant to penicillin and other a ［ ］**more**
        biotics is discussed in detail in Chaps. 2 and ［ ］ion is at
     4. Ampicillin-resistant *H. influenzae* and *Bran* ［ ］nd anti-
        mella (Moraxella) catarrhalis are discusse(
        Chaps. 1 and 18.

appropriate approaches. The unrealistic demand for and, at times, poor compliance with antibiotic regimens by patients must also be dealt with. Targeting obvious areas of abuse (e.g., antibiotic abuse in URIs) is important. (See Chap. 1.)

2. **Appropriate pharmaceutical advertising and promotion is essential** (32,33).

3. Antimicrobial use in animals must be reviewed and improved (2,27–30).

C. **Improved surveillance.** Funding for, and interest in, surveillance systems at the state and national level declined in the 1970s and 1980s in the United States (5,6,19,34). This needs to be and is being rectified. In recent years there has been an improvement in tracking regional and national antibiotic-resistant organisms; more needs to be done. Better global surveillance has been suggested also (19).

D. **Increasing funding for basic research** in mechanisms of resistance, vaccine development, and development of novel interventions is needed. Unfortunately, by the early to mid-1990s the funding for research of bacterial disease had been reduced substantially by the National Institutes of Health (19).

E. **New antibacterial agents** (19,30,31). With initial success of the many antibiotic agents released in the late 1980s and early 1990s, many pharmaceutical companies reduced their antibacterial research efforts in the early to mid-1990s. As a result, fewer antibiotics are expected to be released in the immediate future. New research in this area is needed. It is hoped that development can be expedited, possibly even with a "fast track" for new antibiotics for multidrug-resistant bacteria.

F. **Prevention of transmission with infection control** practices, **improved sanitation** conditions in developing countries, and **improved care of the homeless,** those in crowded conditions, also is needed. Rapid diagnostic tests and rapid treatment with effective antimicrobials also will help reduce transmission.

G. **Hospital administrations** are encouraged to support and pursue a multidisciplinary systems-oriented approach to these problems, as emphasized in a 1996 report (35). Each hospital should establish its own strategies (a) to optimize the prophylactic, empiric, and therapeutic use of antimicrobials in the hospital, and (b) to detect, report, and prevent transmission of antimicrobial-resistant microorganisms (35).

VI. **Summary.** To deal with this increasing problem of multidrug-resistant bacteria and reverse this trend, we agree with Dr. Levy, who emphasizes, "The answer lies in efforts from all of us—physician, patient, microbiologist, public health official (and governmental policy officials), and manufacturer. No one can sit back and expect someone else to solve the problem. In the past, we have relied on the pharmaceutical companies to develop new drugs to deal with resistance—and they have largely succeeded. But, the ability to stay one step ahead of the bacteria has led to a complacency about the resistance problem. We can no longer maintain this attitude" (31).

Part C: End-of-Life Issues

End-of-life care issues are usually not well addressed in textbooks, as a recent report indicates (36). Although there are some excellent general discussions of end-of-life issues in textbooks (37), based on a literature search and recent conference on end-of-life issues (38), we are not aware of any such published discussions in terms of antibiotic use.

One report from Wales in 1989 indicated that on the basis of a questionnaire of a hypothetical case of a terminally ill patient, only 16% of respondents (72/448) indicated they would use antibiotics if the terminally ill patient became febrile (39).

Nevertheless, this remains an important topic and is an issue the clinician frequently faces. **We offer the following suggestions on this topic.**

I. **For patients designated "comfort care."**
   A. **We would not use broad-spectrum antibiotics** (e.g., imipenem, trovofloxacin, ceftriaxone, etc) for fear of selecting out a very resistant organism (e.g., MRSA, VRE, MDR gram negative), which may then pose a serious nosocomial threat.

   Since other therapeutic agents are stopped in "comfort-care-only" patients, we feel it is ethically reasonable to stop broad-spectrum antibiotics, and really ethically appropriate, in order to reduce resistance risks to the broader community of selecting out a totally resistant organism.
   B. **In special situations, directed antibiotic use with narrow-spectrum agents may be indicated for "comfort."**
      1. Therapy for a symptomatic UTI or cellulitis or pneumonia with a hacking cough may well be indicated, and whether to treat or not must be individualized.
      2. However, if the patient already had a very resistant organism, further treatment with very-broad-spectrum antibiotics, although potentially successful, may select for a totally resistant organism that would not be in the public's best interest. We would avoid such antibiotic therapy, as in Sec. A.
II. **For patients in whom broad-spectrum antibiotics may really be futile**, the issue is more complex and raises ethical issues beyond the scope of this handbook. We would offer a few considerations.
   A. **Broad-spectrum antibiotics are potent medicines.** It is easy for the clinician to write an order for

antibiotics. Consequently, hospitalized patients who are hopelessly ill and who are not candidates for surgical procedures and/or deep-line insertion and/or resuscitation and/or pacemakers and/or intubation, etc, nonetheless **are** often given broad-spectrum antibiotics for prolonged times.

- Again, we are concerned about the prolonged use of broad-spectrum antibiotics selecting out resistant pathogens, especially since many of these patients may have foreign bodies (tracheostomies, foley catheters), which makes eradication of bacteria difficult if not impossible.
- In these situations, we have found an awareness of the potential risks and open and candid discussions with families and the team to be helpful in terms of the pros and cons of prolonged antibiotics. An ethics consultation can be helpful.

B. **An ethics consultation,** if available, can help the care-giving team deal with the ethical issues raised by the question of whether to use a very-broad-spectrum antibiotic, especially if it is the last or one of the last available active agents (or experimental agents, as in VRE therapy) to help a single patient in whom therapy may be futile versus withholding therapy for the "public good" (i.e., other patients, family, to whom a fully resistant organism could spread and cause infection for which no commercially available antibiotics would be active).

Although the decision to withhold broad-spectrum antibiotics can be difficult, especially if the patient is young and competent, our ethics committee has felt it is ethically defensible (appropriate) when approached as a matter of justice.

References

1. Hager M. Antibiotics: the power of invention. *Newsweek* 1997; 130(24):70.
   See related discussion by Centers for Diseases Control. Control of infectious diseases. MMWR *1999;48:621.*
2. Reese RE, Betts RF. Principles of antibiotic use. In: Reese RE, Betts RF, eds. *A practical approach to infectious diseases*, 4th ed. Boston: Little, Brown, 1996:Chap. 28A.
   See a related general discussion by Thompson RL, Wright AJ. General principles of antimicrobial therapy. Mayo Clin Proc *1998; 73:995.*
3. Toshikawa TT. Unique aspects of infection in older adults. In: Toshikawa TT, Norman DC, eds. *Antimicrobial therapy in the elderly patient.* New York: Marcel Dekker, 1994:1–7.
   Useful textbook devoted to infections and antibiotic use in the elderly. See related papers by Yohikawa TT, Norman DC. Treatment of infections in elderly patients. Med Clin North Am

1995;79:651; and Crossley KB, Peterson PK. Infections in the elderly. Clin Infect Dis *1996;22:209.*

4. Medical Letter. The choice of antimicrobial drugs. *Med Lett Drugs Ther* 1998;40:33 and 1999;41:95.
   Excellent references updated every 2 years.

5. Foran RM, Brett JL, Wulf PH. Evaluating the cost impact of intravenous antibiotic dosing frequencies. *DICP Ann Pharmacother* 1991;25:546.
   Although cost estimates will vary from institution to institution, this study also estimated nursing time for administering each intravenous dose was about 4.6 minutes.

6. Moellering R Jr. Principles of anti-infective therapy. In: Mandell GL, Bennett JE, Dolin R, eds. *Principles and practice of infectious diseases*, 4th ed. New York: Churchill Livingstone, 1995:199–212.

7. Korzeniowski OM. Antibacterial agents in pregnancy. *Infect Dis Clin North Am* 1995;9:639.
   Includes a discussion of the fetal risk stratification system shown in Table 14.3.

8. Medical Letter. Safety of drugs in pregnancy. *Med Lett Drugs Ther* 1987;28:61.

9. Aronoff GR, et al. *Drug prescribing in renal failure: dosing guidelines for adults,* 4th ed. Philadelphia: American College of Physicians, 1999.
   Contains good summary tables of antibiotic dose reduction recommendations in renal failure. Also has tables of dose reduction of cardiovascular, psychotropic, and other agents. Useful handbook.

10. Cockcroft DW, Gault MH. Prediction of creatinine clearance for serum creatinine. *Nephron* 1976;16:31.
    An alternative approach has recently been advocated by A Levey et al: A more accurate method to estimate glomerular filtration rate from serum creatinine: a new prediction equation. Ann Intern Med *1999;130:461, but this is a cumbersome formula for ordinary use.*

11. Tschida SJ, et al. Anti-infective agents and hepatic disease. *Med Clin North Am* 1995;79:895.

12. Singh N, et al. B-lactam antibiotic-induced leukopenia in severe hepatic dysfunction: risk factors and implications for dosing in patients with liver disease. *Am J Med* 1993;94:251.

13. Westphal JF, Jehl F, Vetter D. Pharmacological, toxicologic, and microbiological considerations in the choice of initial antibiotic therapy for serious infections in patients with cirrhosis of the liver. *Clin Infect Dis* 1994;18:324.

14. Nightingale CH, Quintiliani R, Nicolau DP. Intelligent dosing of antimicrobials. *Curr Clin Top Infect Dis* 1994;14:252.
    Detailed discussion of concentration-dependent killing and concentration-independent killing of bacteria and possible clinical implications. For a related review by these same authors, see Nicolau DP, et al. Antibiotic kinetics and dynamics for the clinician. Med Clin North Am *1995;79:477.*

15. Levinson ME. Pharmacodynamics of antimicrobial agents: bactericidal and postantibiotic effects. *Infect Dis Clin North Am* 1995;9:483.

16. Tice AD, et al. Outpatient parenteral antibiotic therapy. *Infect Dis Clin North Am* 1998;12:827–1034.
    Symposium devoted to this topic.

17. Chow JW, et al. *Enterobacter* bacteremia: clinical features and emergence of antibiotic resistance during therapy. *Ann Intern Med* 1991;115:585.
    See related editorial comment in the same issue.
18. Kunin CM. Resistance to antimicrobial drugs: a worldwide calamity. *Ann Intern Med* 1993;118:557.
19. Tomasz A. Multiple-antibiotic-resistant pathogenic bacteria: a report of the Rockefeller University Workshop. *N Engl J Med* 1994;330:1247.
20. Tenover FC, et al. Antimicrobial resistance. *Infect Dis Clin North Am* 1997;11(4):757.
    This symposium has a series of articles by experts in their fields.
21. Moellering RC Jr, et al. Bacterial resistance: laboratory explanations and clinical consequences. *Clin Infect Dis* 1998;27:S1 (suppl 1).
22. Moellering RC, Jr, et al, eds. The specter of glycopeptide resistance: current trends and future considerations. *Am J Med* 1998;104(5A):1S.
23. Bartlett JG, et al. Attempting to avoid antibiotic resistance: lessons for the primary care physician. *Am J Med* 1999;106(5A):1S–52S.
23A. Kak V, Levine DP. Community-acquired methicillin-resistant *Staphylococcus aureus* infections: where do we go from here. *Clin Infect Dis* 1999;29:801.
    Editorial comment on this topic and two related articles in the same journal.
24. McCaig LF, Hughes JM. Trends in antimicrobial drug prescribing among office-based physicians in the United States. *JAMA* 1995;273:214.
    See related discussions in Chap. 1.
25. Winker MA, et al. Emerging and reemerging global microbial threats: call for papers. *JAMA* 1995;273:241.
    Editorial comment, in part, on reference 24.
26. Kunin CM. Problems in antibiotic usage. In: Mandell GL, Douglas RG Jr, Bennett JE, eds. *Principles and practice of infectious diseases*, 3rd ed. New York: Churchill Livingstone, 1990:427.
27. Smith KE, et al. Quinolone-resistant *Campylobacter jejuni* infections in Minnesota 1992–1998. *N Engl J Med* 1999;240:1525.
    Concludes that the use of quinolones in poultry, which began in the United States in 1995, has created a reservoir of resistant C. jejuni with human infections acquired from poultry. Also see reference 28.
28. Wegener HC. The consequences for food safety of the use of fluoroquinolones in food animals. *N Engl J Med* 1999;340:1581.
    Editorial on reference 27. Emphasizes that acquired campylobacter disease in humans should only be treated when severe, as unnecessary treatment in human disease also adds to the resistance problem. Also reviews experience in Denmark of decreasing quinolone use in animal feeds with no apparent adverse effects on the animals.
29. Wegener HC, et al. Use of antimicrobial growth promoters in food animals and *Enterococcus faecium* resistance to therapeutic antimicrobial drugs in Europe. *Emerg Infect Dis* 1999;5:329.
    VRE in hospitalized patients is linked to glycopeptide use in animals.
30. Moellering RC Jr. Antibiotic resistance: lessons for the future. *Clin Infect Dis* 1998;27:S135 (suppl 1).

Reviews options to improve antibiotic use and the importance of new agents.

31. Levy SB. Confronting multidrug resistance: a role for each of us. *JAMA* 1993;269:1840.
    Commentary by a physician with a long-term interest in this topic.

32. Waud DR. Pharmaceutical promotions: a free lunch? *N Engl J Med* 1992;327:351.
    A "sounding board" article.

33. Orlowski JP, et al. The efforts of pharmaceutical firm enticements on physician prescribing habits. *Chest* 1992;102:270.

34. Berkelmen RL, et al. Infectious disease surveillance: a crumbling foundation. *Science* 1994;264:368.
    Discussion impact of reduced financial support for surveillance studies.

35. Goldmann D, et al. Consensus statement: strategies to prevent and control the emergence and spread of antimicrobial-resistant microorganisms in hospitals—a challenge to hospital leadership. *JAMA* 1996;275:234.
    A multidisciplinary group of experts convened to provide hospital leaders with strategic goals and/or actions to help approach this problem at the hospital level.

36. Carron AT, Lynn J, Keaney P. End-of-life care in medical textbooks. *Ann Intern Med* 1999;130:82.

37. Rabow MW, Brody RV. Care at the end-of-life. *Current medical diagnosis and treatment 1999*, 38th ed. New York: Lange Medical Books/McGraw-Hill, 1999:Chap. 5.
    A very useful but concise discussion.

38. Improving end-of-life care: a conference of nursing and medical publishers. Sorros Center. New York, NY. March 12, 1999. Sponsored by the Robert Wood Johnson Foundation.

39. Marin PP, et al. Attitudes of hospital doctors in Wales to use of intravenous fluids and antibiotics in the terminally ill. *Postgrad Med J* 1989;65:650.

Prophylactic Antibiotics

I. **Basic principles**. In certain procedures, prophylactic antibiotics reduce the incidence of postoperative wound infections (1–3). However, there is ongoing discussion about whether prophylaxis should be used in clean procedures without foreign-body insertion. There is nearly uniform agreement about the value in clean contaminated procedures and reasonable agreement about use in clean procedures when foreign bodies are inserted. In the tables to follow, a variety of options are summarized.

   A. **Organisms involved. The major pathogen in postoperative clean surgery is *S. aureus*.** Potential resistant organisms (e.g., methicillin-resistant *S. aureus* [MRSA]) should be considered in clean procedures when MRSA is prevalent in an institution. Gram-negative bacteria cause wound infections following the surgery of colon, genitourinary, or gynecologic organs.

   B. **Timing of antibiotic administration.** Antibiotics must be given so that good tissue levels are present at the time of the procedure and for the first 3 to 4 hours after the surgical incision. Reviews suggest that the optimal time to give an antibiotic is **30 to 60 minutes before the incision is made** (1–4). For cesarean section it should be delayed until the umbilical cord is clamped.

   C. **Duration**
      1. Optimal duration remains as an area of discussion. For many surgical procedures, a single dose is adequate; some experts suggest antibiotics for up to 24 hours and for prosthetic device surgery, 24 to 48 hours.
      2. If the procedure lasts several hours, readministration is suggested if the antibiotic has a relatively short half-life. For example, based on serum half-life data, in a prolonged procedure (e.g., >6 hours), an additional intraoperative dose of cefazolin can be given at 4 hours; for cefoxitin, 2-hour intervals can be used (3). Since cefotetan requires one dose every 6 to 8 hours, it may be preferred, in a long gastrointestinal procedure, over cefoxitin, which should be given q2 hours to maintain high intraoperative levels.
      3. See **Table 15.1.**

   D. **Rationale for antibiotic choices.**
      1. Cephalosporins are widely favored because of their broad spectrum of activity and few side effects. Because first-generation agents are more active against *S. aureus*, are less expensive, and have a narrower spectrum of *in vitro* activity, these agents are preferred for most surgical procedures.

Table 15-1.   Recommended antimicrobial regimens

Surgical Procedure	Recommended Regimen
Biliary tract surgery	
High risk:	Cefazolin 1–2 g IV × 1 dose
>60 years	or gentamicin 1.7 mg/kg
Obstructive jaundice	IV q8h × 1 or 2 doses*
Acute cholecystitis	
Cholangitis	
Common duct stone	
Previous biliary surgery	
Nonfunctioning gall bladder	
Low risk	Not recommended
Gastrointestinal surgery	
Elective colorectal	**Oral GI prep;** Neomycin 1 g po and erythromycin base 1 g po given at 1 PM, 2 PM, 11 PM on day prior to surgery with or without cefoxitin 2 g IV q6h × 1 or 2 doses or cefotetan 2 g IV × 1 dose or metronidazole 500 mg IV and gentamicin 1.7 mg/kg IV q8h × 1 or 2 doses* (see text)
Nonelective colorectal	Cefoxitin or cefotetan or metronidazole and gentamicin* (at above doses)
Gastroduodenal procedures	
High risk: GI bleeding, obstruction, gastric ulcer or malignancy, decreased gastric acidity, obesity.	Cefazolin 1–2 g IV × 1 dose
Low risk	Not recommended
Appendectomy (Perforated appendix will need full therapeutic regimen.)	Cefoxitin 2 g IV q6h × 1–3 dose(s) or cefotetan 2 g IV q12h × 1 or 2 doses or metronidazole 500 mg IV q8h and gentamicin 1.7 mg/kg IV q8h × 1–3 dose(s)*
Gynecological surgery	
Hysterectomy (abdominal or vaginal)	Cefazolin 1 g IV × 1 dose or doxycycline 200 IV × 1 dose* or clindamycin 900 mg IV × 1 dose*
Cesarean section	
High-risk patients (i.e., premature membrane rupture, active labor)	Cefazolin 1 g IV × 1 dose or metronidazole 500 mg IV × 1 dose* (after cord clamping)
Low risk	Not recommended

Table 15-1. (*Continued*)

Surgical Procedure	Recommended Regimen
Therapeutic abortion First trimester with previous PID or Midtrimester	Cefazolin 1 g IV × 1 dose
Head and neck surgery Incision through oral or pharyn- geal mucosa	Clindamycin 600 mg IV and gentamicin 1.7 mg/kg IV × 1 dose or ampicillin- sulbactam
Uncontaminated	Not recommended
Neurosurgery CSF shunt	Not recommended
Craniotomy	Cefazolin 1 g IV × 1 dose or vancomycin**
Orthopedics Closed reduction of a fracture	Not recommended
Open reduction of a fracture	Cefazolin 1–2 g IV × 1 dose
Prosthetic joint replacement	Cefazolin 1–2 g IV q6h or vancomycin IV; either, up to 24h
Amputation	Cefoxitin 2 g IV × 1 dose
Laminectomy and spinal fusion Hardware implantation	Cefazolin 1–2 g IV × 1 dose
No hardware implantation	Not recommended
Urologic surgery If the urine is sterile	Not recommended
If the urine is infected	Sterilize urine before surgery
Transrectal prostate biopsy	Ciprofloxacin 500 mg po or 400 mg IV up to 48h
Vascular and cardiothoracic surgery Pulmonary resection	Cefazolin 1 IV q8h or cefuroxime 750 mg IV q8h up to 48h
Prosthetic valve, CABG, pacemaker or defibrillator implant	Cefazolin 1–2g IV q8h or cefuroxime 1.5g IV q8h or vancomycin IV**, doses given for up to 24–48h (see text)
Cardiac catheterization	Not recommended
Peripheral vascular surgery	Cefazolin 1–2 g IV × 1 dose

PID, pelvic inflammatory disease; CABG, coronary artery bypass grafts; CSF, cerebrospinal fluid.

Modified from Reese RE, Betts RF. Prophylactic antibiotics. In: Reese RE, Betts RF, eds. *A practical approach to infectious diseases,* 4th ed. Boston: Little, Brown 1996, Chap. 25; and from Medical Letter. Antimicrobial prophylaxis in surgery. *Med Lett Drugs Ther* 1999;41:75.

* Alternative in cephalosporin-allergic patient. (Gentamicin dose assumes normal renal function. See Chapter 21.)

** For hospitals in which MRSA commonly cause post-op wounds or in patients allergic to cephalosporins.

Of the first-generation cephalosporins, cefazolin has the added advantage of a moderately long serum half-life, which makes it the preferred agent. In colorectal surgery and appendectomy, cefoxitin or cefotetan is preferred because of their activity against bowel anaerobes. In prolonged procedures, cefotetan may be preferred, as discussed in Sec. C.

2. Vancomycin is often used for antistaphylococcal activity if the patient is allergic to cephalosporins or MRSA is a major hospital pathogen and prosthetic devices are being inserted.

3. When cephalosporins are contraindicated in the patient needing colon surgery, metronidazole and gentamicin have been used.

4. See **Table 15.1.**

Bacterial Endocarditis Prophylaxis

I. **Basic principles**. Although antimicrobial prophylaxis is commonly used in patients for endocarditis prophylaxis, **no adequate clinical trials in humans have been done**. The following are the 1997 guidelines published by American Heart Association to assist practitioners to help their decision making (5).

    A. **Cardiac conditions in which endocarditis prophylaxis is recommended**

        1. The **cardiac conditions** associated with endocarditis are summarized in **Table 15.2.**

        2. **In mitral valve prolapse,** the need for antibiotic prophylaxis is controversial and discussed in detail elsewhere (5). When a murmur of mitral regurgitation is present, prophylaxis is recommended. Also, if there is evidence of mitral regurgitation by Doppler echocardiography study, prophylaxis is suggested (5).

    B. **Dental procedures** that put patients at risk are summarized in **Table 15.3.**

    C. **Surgical procedures** that put patients at risk are summarized in **Table 15.4.**

II. **Recommended antimicrobial regimens** have been reviewed in detail elsewhere (5).

    A. **Dental, oral, upper airway procedures.** See **Table 15.5.**

    B. **Gastrointestinal and genitourinary procedures.** See **Table 15.6.**

    C. **A wallet card** summary of these recommendations is available for patient use. These cards are prepared and distributed by the American Heart Association (AHA).

III. **Unresolved issues.** The recent AHA recommendations acknowledge that there are currently no randomized and carefully controlled human trials in patients with underlying structural heart disease to definitively establish that

Table 15-2.   Cardiac conditions associated with endocarditis

Endocarditis Prophylaxis Recommended

High-risk category
  Prosthetic cardiac valves, including bioprosthetic and homograft valves
  Previous bacterial endocarditis
  Complex cyanotic congenital heart disease (e.g., single ventricle states, transposition of the great arteries, tetralogy of Fallot)
  Surgically constructed systemic pulmonary shunts or conduits
Moderate-risk category
  Most other congenital cardiac malformations (other than above and below)
  Acquired valvular dysfunction (e.g., rheumatic heart disease)
  Hypertrophic cardiomyopathy
  Mitral valve prolapse with valvar regurgitation and/or thickened leaflets*

Endocarditis Prophylaxis Not Recommended

Negligible-risk category (no greater risk than the general population)
  Isolated secundum atrial septal defect
  Surgical repair of atrial septal defect, ventricular septal defect, or patent ductus arteriosus (without residua beyond 6 mo)
  Previous coronary artery bypass graft surgery
  Mitral valve prolapse without valvular regurgitation*
  Physiologic, functional, or innocent heart murmurs*
  Previous Kawasaki disease without valvular dysfunction
  Previous rheumatic fever without valvular dysfunction
  Cardiac pacemakers (intravascular and epicardial) and implanted defibrillators

Source: Dajani AS, et al. Prevention of bacterial endocarditis: recommendations by the American Heart Association. *JAMA* 1997;277:1794.
* See reference (5) for further details.

antibiotic prophylaxis provides protection against development of endocarditis during bacteremic-inducing procedures (5). However, the practice is well entrenched in the United States, and failure to use proper prophylaxis has been associated with malpractice claims (6). Some studies present data that challenge the value of the invalidated practice of using antibiotics before dental procedures to prevent endocarditis, especially in low-risk patients. This issue has been discussed in a recent editorial by Durack (6).

Prophylaxis of Medical Conditions

I. **Influenza A.** Chemoprophylaxis with either amantadine or rimantadine to prevent the spread of influenza A in high-risk patients is reviewed in detail elsewhere (7). Since

Table 15-3.   Dental procedures and endocarditis prophylaxis

Endocarditis Prophylaxis Recommended*

Dental extractions

Periodontal procedures including surgery, scaling and root planing, probing, and recall maintenance

Dental implant placement and reimplantation of avulsed teeth

Endodontic (root canal) instrumentation or surgery only beyond the apex

Subgingival placement of antibiotic fibers or strips

Initial placement of orthodontic bands but not brackets

Intraligamentary local anesthetic injections

Prophylactic cleaning of teeth or implants where bleeding is anticipated

Endocarditis Prophylaxis Not Recommended

Restorative dentistry[†] (operative and prosthodontic) with or without retraction cord[‡]

Local anesthetic injections (nonintraligamentary)

Intracanal endodontic treatment; post placement and buildup

Placement of rubber dams

Postoperative suture removal

Placement of removable prosthodontic or orthodontic appliances

Taking of oral impressions

Fluoride treatments

Taking of oral radiographs

Orthodontic appliance adjustment

Shedding of primary teeth

Source: Dajani AS, et al. Prevention of bacterial endocarditis: recommendations by the American Heart Association. *JAMA* 1997;277:1794.
* Prophylaxis is recommended for patients with high- and moderate-risk cardiac conditions.
[†] This includes restoration of decayed teeth (filling cavities) and replacement of missing teeth.
[‡] Clinical judgment may indicate antibiotic use in selected circumstances that may create significant bleeding.

rimantadine has fewer side effects, it is often preferred. Elderly patients are typically given 100 mg daily; in younger patients a dose of 100 mg bid is used (7). (See related discussion of influenza in Chap. 1.)

II.   **Bacterial meningitis**

A.   **Meningococcal disease**. The risk of contracting invasive meningococcal disease among contacts of cases is the determining factor in the decision to give chemoprophylaxis. **Close contacts of all persons with invasive disease are at increased risk and**

Table 15-4. Other procedures and endocarditis prophylaxis

Endocarditis Prophylaxis Recommended

Respiratory tract
  Tonsillectomy and/or adenoidectomy
  Surgical operations that involve respiratory mucosa
  Bronchoscopy with a rigid bronchoscope

Gastrointestinal tract*
  Sclerotherapy for esophageal varices
  Esophageal stricture dilation
  Endoscopic retrograde cholangiography with biliary obstruction
  Biliary tract surgery
  Surgical operations that involve intestinal mucosa

Genitourinary tract
  Prostatic surgery
  Cystoscopy
  Urethral dilation

Endocarditis Prophylaxis Not Recommended

Respiratory tract
  Endotracheal intubation
  Bronchoscopy with a flexible bronchoscope, with or without biopsy[†]
  Tympanostomy tube insertion

Gastrointestinal tract
  Transesophageal echocardiography[†]
  Endoscopy with or without gastrointestinal biopsy[†]

Genitourinary tract
  Vaginal hysterectomy[†]
  Vaginal delivery[†]
  Cesarean section
  In uninfected tissue:
    Urethral catheterization
    Uterine dilatation and curettage
    Therapeutic abortion
    Sterilization procedures
    Insertion or removal of intrauterine devices

Other
  Cardiac catheterization, including balloon angioplasty
  Implanted cardiac pacemakers, implanted defibrillators, and coronary stents
  Incision or biopsy of surgically scrubbed skin
  Circumcision

Source: Dajani AS, et al. Prevention of bacterial endocarditis: recommendations by the American Heart Association. *JAMA* 1997;277:1794.
* **Prophylaxis is recommended for high-risk patients;** optional for medium-risk patients.
[†] **Prophylaxis is optional for high-risk patients.**

Table 15-5.   Prophylactic regimens for dental, oral, respiratory tract, or esophageal procedures

Situation	Agent	Regimen*
Standard general prophylaxis	Amoxicillin	Adults: 2.0 g; children: 50 mg/kg orally 1 h before procedure
Unable to take oral medications	Ampicillin	Adults: 2.0 g intramuscularly (IM) or intravenously (IV); children: 50 mg/kg IM or IV within 30 min before procedure
Allergic to penicillin	Clindamycin	Adults: 600 mg; children: 20 mg/kg orally 1 h before procedure
	or	
	Cephalexin[†] or cefadroxil[†]	Adults: 2.0 g; children; 50 mg/kg orally 1 h before procedure
	or	
	Azithromycin or clarithromycin	Adults: 500 mg; children: 15 mg/kg orally 1 h before procedure
Allergic to penicillin and unable to take oral medications	Clindamycin	Adults: 600 mg; children: 20 mg/kg IV within 30 min before procedure
	or	
	Cefazolin[†]	Adults: 1.0 g; children: 25 mg/kg IM or IV within 30 min before procedure

Source: Dajani AS, et al. Prevention of bacterial endocarditis: recommendations by the American Heart Association. *JAMA* 1997;277:1794.
* Total children's dose should not exceed adult dose.
† Cephalosporins should not be used in individuals with immediate-type hypersensitivity reaction (urticaria, angioedema, or anaphylaxis) to penicillins.

Table 15-6. Prophylactic regimens for genitourinary gastrointestinal (excluding esophageal) procedures

Situation	Agents*	Regimen[†]
High-risk patients	Ampicillin plus gentamicin	Adults: ampicillin 2.0 g intramuscularly (IM) or intravenously (IV) plus gentamicin 1.5 mg/kg (not to exceed 120 mg) within 30 min of starting the procedure; 6 h later, ampicillin 1 g IM/IV or amoxicillin 1 g orally Children: ampicillin 50 mg/kg IM or IV (not to exceed 2.0 g) plus gentamicin 1.5 mg/kg within 30 min of starting the procedure; 6 h later, ampicillin 25 mg/kg IM/IV or amoxicillin 25 mg/kg orally
High-risk patients allergic to ampicillin/amoxicillin	Vancomycin plus gentamicin	Adults: vancomycin 1.0 g IV over 1–2 h plus gentamicin 1.5 mg/kg IV/IM (not to exceed 120 mg); complete injection/infusion within 30 min of starting the procedure Children: vancomycin 20 mg/kg IV over 1–2 h plus gentamicin 1.5 mg/kg IV/IM; complete injection/infusion within 30 min of starting the procedure
Moderate-risk patients	Amoxicillin or ampicillin	Adults: amoxicillin 2.0 g orally 1 h before procedure, or ampicillin 2.0 g IM/IV within 30 min of starting the procedure Children: amoxicillin 50 mg/kg orally 1 h before procedure, or ampicillin 50 mg/kg IM/IV within 30 min of starting the procedure
Moderate-risk patients allergic to ampicillin/amoxicillin	Vancomycin	Adults: vancomycin 1.0 g IV over 1–2 h; complete infusion within 30 min of starting the procedure Children: vancomycin 20 mg/kg IV over 1–2 h; complete infusion within 30 min of starting the procedure

Source: Dajani AS, et al. Prevention of bacterial endocarditis: recommendations by the American Heart Association. *JAMA* 1997;277:1794.
* Total children's dose should not exceed adult dose.
[†] No second dose of vancomycin or gentamicin is recommended.

should receive prophylaxis as soon as possible, preferably within 24 hours of the diagnosis (8).
1. High-risk contacts need prophylaxis. **See Table 15.7.**
2. Note that low-risk contacts do not need prophylaxis (Table 15.7).
3. Confirmed cases of invasive meningococcal disease include *N. meningitidis* isolated from blood; cerebrospinal fluid; pleural, pericardial, synovial fluid; or petechial or purpuric lesions (8).
4. Throat and nasopharyngeal cultures are not of value in deciding who should get prophylaxis (8).
5. **Recommended regimens** for close contacts are shown in Table 15.8.
    The index case should receive chemoprophylaxis before hospital discharge unless the infection was treated with ceftriaxone or cefotaxime (8).
B. ***Haemophilus influenzae* b meningitis.** Transmission of *H. influenzae* from patients with meningitis to household contacts is well described. Secondary cases usually occur within 6 days of onset in the index case, but untreated household contacts remain at increased risk for at least 1 month after onset in the index case.
    1. The **rationale** for use of chemoprophylaxis to prevent secondary disease is eradication of nasopharyngeal colonization of *H. influenzae* type b,

Table 15-7. Disease risk for contacts of index cases of invasive meningococcal disease*

High risk: chemoprophylaxis recommended
Household contact: especially young children
Child care or nursery school contact in previous 7 days
Direct exposure to index patient's secretions through kissing or sharing toothbrushes or eating utensils
Mouth-to-mouth resuscitation, unprotected contact during endotracheal intubation in 7 days before onset of the illness
Frequently sleeps or eats in same dwelling as index patient

Low risk: chemoprophylaxis not recommended
Casual contact: no history of direct exposure to index patient's oral secretions (e.g., school or work mate)
Indirect contact: only contact is with a high-risk contact, no direct contact with the index patient
Medical personnel without direct exposure to patient's oral secretions

In outbreak or cluster
Chemoprophylaxis for persons other than those at high risk should be given only after consultation with the local public health authorities

Source: Peter G, et al, eds. *1997 Red Book: report of the Committee on Infectious Diseases,* 24th ed. Elk Grove Village, IL: American Academy of Pediatrics, 1997.
* Nasopharyngeal aspirate to throat swab cultures are **not** useful in determining risk.

Table 15-8. Recommended chemoprophylaxis regimens for high-risk contacts and index cases of invasive meningococcal disease*

Infants, Children, and Adults	Dose	Duration	% Efficacy	Cautions
Rifampin[†]				
≤1 mo	5 mg/kg orally every 12 h	2 days	72–90	May interfere with efficacy of oral contraceptives, some seizureprevention, and anticoagulant medications; may stain soft contact lenses
>1 mo	10 mg/kg (maximum 600 mg) orally every 12 h**	2 days		
	20 mg/kg (maximum, 600 mg) orally every 24 h	4 days		
Ceftriaxone				
≤12 yr	125 mg intramuscularly	Single dose	97	To decrease pain at injection site, dilute with 1% lidocaine
>12 yr	250 mg intramuscularly	Single dose		
Ciprofloxacin[†]				
≥18 yr	500 mg orally	Single dose	90–95	Not recommended for use in children

Source: Peter G, et al., eds. *1997 Red Book: report of the Committee on Infectious Diseases*, 24th ed. Elk Grove Village, IL: American Academy of Pediatrics, 1997.

* Oral sulfisoxazole may be used if the organism is known to be susceptible. The dosage is as follows: <1 year of age, 500 mg every 12 hours for 2 days; >12 years of age, 1 to 12 years of age, 500 mg a day for 2 days; and 1 to 12 years of age, 1 g every 12 hours for 2 days.

** Typical adult dose, 600 mg q12h for 2 days.

[†] **Not for use in pregnant women.**

thereby preventing transmission in young, susceptible contacts and the development of disease in those already colonized (9).

2. **Household contacts.** In those households with at least one contact* younger than 48 months whose immunization status against *H. influenzae* b is incomplete, rifampin prophylaxis is recommended for all household contacts irrespective of age (8). Based on the higher efficacy of the *H. influenzae* b vaccine, prophylaxis is not indicated when all household contacts younger than 48 months have completed their immunization series (8).

3. **Child care and nursery school** exposures are discussed elsewhere (8) and prophylaxis considerations should be supervised by public health officials.

4. **The index** patient with meningitis should also receive rifampin prophylaxis if treated with ampicillin or chloramphenicol. Prophylaxis is not needed for index cases treated with cefotaxime or ceftriaxone (8).

5. **Dosage.** Rifampin should be given orally once a day for 4 days in a dose of 20 mg/kg, with a maximum dose of 600 mg per day. The dose for infants younger than 1 month is not established; some experts recommend lowering the dose to 10 mg/kg/day. Patients unable to swallow the 150-mg or 600-mg capsules may be given aliquots of rifampin powder, preweighed by a trained individual (pharmacist). The rifampin can be mixed with a small amount of applesauce immediately before administration. Also, a liquid suspension can be made per package insert (8).

C. *S. pneumoniae* **meningitis.** At this point, prophylactic antibiotics are not recommended for contacts of sporadic cases of meningitis due to this pathogen.

III. **Recurrent otitis media.** The role of prophylactic antibiotics is discussed in Chap. 1.

IV. **Travelers' diarrhea.** Prophylactic antibiotics are not advised for healthy travelers. Travelers to risk areas typically carry a therapeutic course of antibiotics to be used if symptoms develop, as discussed in Chap. 5.

V. **Recurrent urinary tract infections** are discussed in Chap. 4.

VI. **Prevention of serious infections after splenectomy (1).** Overwhelming infection due to encapsulated organisms such as *S. pneumoniae*, *H. influenzae*, and, rarely, *Neisseria meningitidis* can occur after splenectomy. Methods of preventing these overwhelming infections, which can occur

---

* A household contact is defined in these circumstances as an individual residing with the index patient or a nonresident who spent 4 or more hours with the index patient for at least 5 of the 7 days preceding the day of hospital admission of the index patient (8).

months or years after splenectomy, remain unclear and controversial (1,10). Children may be at particularly high risk, but overwhelming infection can also occur in adults.

An adult splenectomized after trauma but otherwise healthy is at risk for overwhelming pneumococcal sepsis, although at a much lower incidence than young children (1,10,11), probably because of the adult's immune status, which supports the rest of the mononuclear-phagocytic system. Recognition that adults as well as children are at increased risk of infection years after splenectomy has led to consideration of spleen-sparing surgical approaches after trauma (1,10).

A. **Vaccines.** The **pneumococcal vaccine** usually is given to these patients, but its efficacy in this setting is unclear. If an elective splenectomy is performed, the pneumococcal vaccine should be administered at least 2 weeks before the elective splenectomy (10). The poly-saccharide *H. influenzae* **vaccine** is another useful agent, although efficacy data with this vaccine for this use are not available. The role of **meningococcal vaccine** in this setting has not been established, but it seems a reasonable consideration and has been suggested (11). (A single-dose vial of the quadrivalent vaccine is available now in the United States.)

B. **Prophylactic antibiotics.** Some experts recommend the use of oral penicillin daily (e.g., penicillin V, 125 mg bid in children and 250 mg bid in adults) in recently splenectomized patients. This is a particularly common practice in children (1,11), and we use penicillin prophylaxis in children for at least 2 to 4 years. Whether to use prophylactic penicillin routinely in adults who are not otherwise compromised is a controversial issue (1,10,11). We do not routinely treat adults with prophylactic antibiotics but use prophylactic antibiotics in adults with Hodgkin's disease who have undergone splenectomy, chemotherapy, or radiation therapy. Less frequently, ampicillin is used on a daily basis, as it is active against *H. influenzae* as well as *S. pneumoniae*, but it is more likely to cause side effects. Neither the optimal agent nor optimal duration of antibiotics in this setting has been established.

C. **Early therapeutic antibiotics.** Early empiric antibiotic therapy in patients who have undergone a splenectomy is an important consideration. Patients can be given a supply of antibiotics for use if an acute illness develops (11); they should also seek immediate medical attention. Oral penicillin and amoxicillin have been used. When these patients present with nonspecific febrile illnesses, often flulike, early antibiotic therapy is rational for unexplained fever or chills. Ideally, appropriate cultures should be obtained, but if facilities for culture analysis are not immediately available, starting antibiotics without cultures is reasonable (10). In community-acquired bacteremia of unclear primary focus of infection, therapy aimed at the likely pathogens should be instituted early while awaiting cultures. Cefuroxime and ceftriaxone are useful options. (See Chap. 7 for a related discussion.)

D. **Identification warning.** Because these patients are at risk of fulminant sepsis, we encourage each patient to have some form of personal identification (e.g., medical alert necklace or bracelet, or note in his or her wallet or purse) indicating that he or she has undergone splenectomy. The patients' families should be aware of this potential complication. The patient's medical record should clearly indicate the patient has undergone a splenectomy (1).

VII. **Miscellaneous**

A. **Prevention of recurrent rheumatic fever** is discussed in detail elsewhere (1,12).

B. **Prevention of recurrent cholangitis.** Selected patients with a compromised biliary system (e.g., an endoprosthesis *in situ,* history of choledochojejunostomy, hepaticojejunostomy, or sphincteroplasty) who are prone to develop recurrent bouts of cholangitis may benefit from chronic daily prophylactic antibiotics. The aim of suppressive antibiotic therapy is to prevent flare-ups of clinically overt cholangitis. Both TMP-SMX and fluoroquinolones have been used. This topic has been reviewed elsewhere (13).

C. **Oral antibiotics to prevent infection in the leukopenic host.** In general, we do not advocate their use unless as part of a special clinical study.

D. **Complicated diagnostic or therapeutic endoscopic retrograde cholangiopancreatography (ERCP).** Although antibiotics have often been given for this procedure because this seems reasonable, data now support prophylactic antibiotic use in this setting (14).

E. Prophylactic antibiotics for the prevention of opportunistic infections in HIV-positive patients (e.g., *Pneumocystis carinii*) is beyond the scope of this chapter but has recently been reviewed (14A).

F. **Prophylaxis against hematogenous infection after total joint replacement.** Whether patients with indwelling prosthetic joints need antibiotic prophylaxis when undergoing dental, gastrointestinal, or genitourinary procedures is **controversial** (15); some reviews of the data suggest that antibiotics usually add little except expense (16,17).

1. We agree with the Medical Letter recommendation that **most patients** with indwelling prosthetic joints generally **do not require** antimicrobial **prophylaxis** when undergoing dental, gastrointestinal, or genitourinary procedures (2).

2. **However, for procedures more than 45 minutes, surgery in an infected area** (including periodontal disease and drainage of abscess), and **procedures** with a **high inoculum of bacteria,** and possibly for selected patients at high risk

for infection, **prophylaxis may be advisable** (18–20).

G. **Prevention of recurrent episodes of sponta- neous bacterial peritonitis** (see Chap. 6.) is being evaluated. Norfloxacin (400 mg po daily) has reduced the 1 year recurrence rate from 68% to 20% (21). TMP- SMX has also been used in this setting (22). This topic has recently been reviewed (23).

References

1. Reese RE, Betts RF. Prophylactic antibiotics. In: Reese RE, Betts RF, eds. *A practical approach to infectious diseases*, 4th ed. Boston: Little, Brown 1996:Chap. 28B.

2. Medical Letter. Antimicrobial prophylaxis in surgery. *Med Lett Drugs Ther* 1999;41:75.
   This topic is periodically updated every 2 to 3 years.

3. Dellinger EP, et al. Quality standard for antimicrobial prophy- laxis in surgical procedures. *Clin Infect Dis* 1994;18:422.
   In this summary sponsored by the Infectious Disease Society of America, more than 50 experts in infectious diseases and 10 experts in surgical infectious diseases and surgical subspecialties reviewed the recommendations or suggested standards that might be applied without controversy in most hospitals. This is an excellent resource.

4. Classen DC, et al. The timing of prophylactic administration of antibiotics and the risk of surgical wound infection. *N Engl J Med* 1992;326:281.
   Prospective study of 2,847 patients undergoing elective clean or clean-contaminated surgery. When antibiotics were given 0 to 2 hours before surgery, wound infections were significantly reduced. See editorial comment by DR Wenzel in the same issue, emphasiz- ing the importance of preoperative administration.

5. Dajani AS, et al. Prevention of bacterial endocarditis: recommen- dations by the American Heart Association. *JAMA* 1997;277:1794.

6. Durack DT. Antibiotics for prevention of endocarditis during den- tistry: time to scale back? *Ann Intern Med* 1998;129:829.

7. Centers for Disease Control. Prevention and control of influenza: recommendations of the Advisory Committee on Immunization Practices (ACIP). *MMWR* 1999;48(RR-4):1–26.
   The role of the new antivirals (Relenza and Tamiflu), see Chap. 1, in prophylaxis awaits further clinical study.

8. Peter G, et al, eds. *1997 Red Book: Report of the Committee on Infectious Diseases*, 24th ed. Elk Grove Village, IL: American Academy of Pediatrics, 1997.

9. Lieberman JM, Greenberg DP, Ward JI. Prevention of bacterial meningitis: vaccine and chemoprophylaxis. *Infect Dis Clin North Am* 1990;4:703.

10. Styrt B. Infection associated with asplenia: risks, mechanisms, and prevention. *Am J Med* 1990;88:33N (suppl 5N).
    See a related editorial comment on this topic by Reid MM, Lancet 1994;344:970.

11. Buchanan CR. Chemoprophylaxis in asplenic adolescents and young adults. *Pediatr Infect Dis J* 1993;12:892.

12. Dajani A, et al. Treatment of acute streptococcal pharyngitis and prevention of rheumatic fever: a statement for health professionals. *Pediatrics* 1995;96:758.

13. Van der Hazel SJ, et al. Role of antibiotics in treatment and prevention of acute and recurrent cholangitis. *Clin Infect Dis* 1994; 19:279.
    Good clinical discussion of this topic. Optimal duration of maintenance preventive doses is unclear. Authors suggest treating the patient for 3 to 4 months and then evaluating whether the antibiotics can be stopped without recurrence of infection. If infection recurs, therapy can be restarted. Lower-than-therapeutic doses may be effective (e.g., one double-strength tablet of TMP-SMX daily rather than bid).

14. Byl B, et al. Antibiotic prophylaxis for infectious complications after therapeutic endoscopic retrograde cholangiopancreatography: a randomized, double-blind, placebo-controlled study. *Clin Infect Dis* 1995;20:1236.
    In this study, uninfected patients were assigned to receive piperacillin (4 g) or placebo tid; prophylaxis was started just before initial endoscopic retrograde cholangiopancreatography (ERCP) and was continued until biliary drainage was completely unobstructed. Authors concluded that antimicrobial prophylaxis significantly reduces the incidence of septic complications after therapeutic ERCP among patients presenting with cholestasis. No bacteremia was documented in the 30 patients receiving piperacillin. Seven of 32 (22%) patients receiving placebo had bacteremia.
    *   Nevertheless, the Medical Letter's antibiotic of choice for prophylaxis for biliary tract manipulation/surgery is cefazolin, and we also favor use of cefazolin in most cases of ERCP. The exception would be a patient who has a long hospitalization and/or has been treated with protracted antibiotics so that a broader-spectrum agent (e.g., piperacillin) aimed at hospital-acquired gram negatives may be reasonable; in this case we might also give a single dose of an aminoglycoside.*

14A. USPHS/IDSA Prevention of Opportunistic Infections Working Group. 1999 USPHS/IDSA Guidelines for the prevention of opportunistic infections in persons infected with human immunodeficiency virus. *Ann Intern Med* 1999;131:873

15. Haas DW, Kaiser AB. Antimicrobial prophylaxis of infections associated with foreign bodies. In: Bisno AL, Waldvogel FA, eds. *Infections associated with medical devices*, 2nd ed. Washington, DC: American Society for Microbiology, 1994.

16. Wahl MJ. Myths of dental-induced prosthetic device infections. *Clin Infect Dis* 1995;20:1420.
    Strong argument and review of data to stop the common practice of antibiotic prophylaxis for dental procedures to prevent late prosthetic joint infections, as this approach is not based on scientific evidence but rather on "myths."

17. Steckelberg JM, Osmon DR. Prosthetic Joint Infections. In: Bisno AL, Waldvogel FA, eds., *Infections associated with prosthetic indwelling medical devices*, 2nd ed. Washington, DC: American Society for Microbiology, 1994:259–290.
    Data from the Mayo Clinic: In 39,000 large-joint implants with approximately 275,000 joint-years of follow-up, the overall incidence of large-joint implant infections due to dental pathogens

(viridans streptococci) was 0.06 per 1,000 joint-years—a rate similar to that for endocarditis in the general population. Therefore routine prophylaxis is not warranted.

18. American Dental Association; American Academy of Orthopedic Surgeons. Advisory statement: antibiotic prophylaxis for dental patients with total joint replacement. *J Am Dent Assoc* 1997; 128:1004.

19. Waldman BJ, Mont MA, Hungerford DS. Total knee arthroplasty infections associated with dental procedures. *Clin Orthoped Related Res* 1997;343:164.
    Review of 3,490 patients at Johns Hopkins: Seven of 62 late infections were associated with a dental procedure temporally and bacteriologically. All dental procedures were extensive, average of 115 minutes.

20. LaPorte DM, Waldman BJ, Mont MA. Infections associated with dental procedures in total hip arthroplasty. *J Bone Joint Surg* (British) 1999;81:56.
    Another Johns Hopkins study: Retrospective review of 2,973 patients with three of 52 late infections strongly associated with a dental procedure. Dental operations lasted longer than 45 minutes.

21. Ginès P, et al. Norfloxacin prevents spontaneous bacterial peritonitis in cirrhosis: results of a double-blind, placebo-controlled trial. *Hepatology* 1990;12:716.

22. Singh N, et al. Trimethoprim-sulfamethoxazole for the prevention of spontaneous bacterial peritonitis in cirrhosis: a randomized trial. *Ann Intern Med* 1995;122:595.

23. Ginès P, Navasa M. Antibiotic prophylaxis for spontaneous bacterial peritonitis: how and whom? *J Hepatol* 1998;29:490.

16

Penicillin G and Penicillin-Resistant *Streptococcus pneumoniae*

The term **penicillin** is the generic term for a broad group of agents, including, but not limited to, penicillin G, penicillin V, oxacillin, dicloxacillin, nafcillin, ampicillin, amoxicillin, ticarcillin, and piperacillin. These agents are **bactericidal**. The precise mechanism of action of penicillins is unclear, but they interfere with the synthesis and promote lysis of bacterial cell walls.

Many, but not all, of the penicillins are excreted primarily by the kidney by both glomerular filtration and tubular secretion. Dose reductions in severe renal failure are discussed under the individual agents.

I. **Structure** (1,2). The penicillin nucleus and breakdown products are shown in **Fig. 16.1.**

  A. **Structural modifications.** Penicillins with differing antimicrobial activity can be made from 6-aminopenicillanic acid. Alteration of the side groups has resulted in compounds with a broader spectrum of activity, resistance to penicillinases, stability in acid pH (important in oral preparations), and other different pharmacokinetic characteristics.

  B. **Common nucleus.** The intact structural nucleus is necessary for biologic activities. In addition, as a result of the common nucleus in the structure of the penicillins, the **potential for allergic cross-sensitivity** among the penicillins presumably is high.

  C. **Penicillinase is a beta-lactamase enzyme that splits the beta-lactam ring** (see site 1, **Fig. 16.1**). The resulting penicilloic acid is inactive against bacteria. Penicillinase production is a principal mechanism of penicillin resistance in penicillin-resistant, coagulase-positive *Staphylococcus aureus, Pseudomonas* spp., and *Bacteroides fragilis*, and one of the mechanisms in *Escherichia coli* and *Proteus* spp. **When a penicillin is combined with a beta-lactamase inhibitor (clavulanic acid,** sulbactam, or tazobactam; see Chap. 18), **many bacterial beta-lactamases can be inhibited**.

II. **Spectrum of activity of penicillin G**

  A. **Gram-positive aerobic cocci**

    1. Penicillin is very active against *S. pyrogenes* (group A), viridans streptococci, *S. bovis*, and penicillin-susceptible *S. aureus*. As a single agent, penicillin G is not effective against serious enterococcal infections (e.g., endocarditis).

    2. **Resistance of *Streptococcus pneumoniae* to penicillin is being seen with increased frequency**. This topic is discussed in Chap. 2.

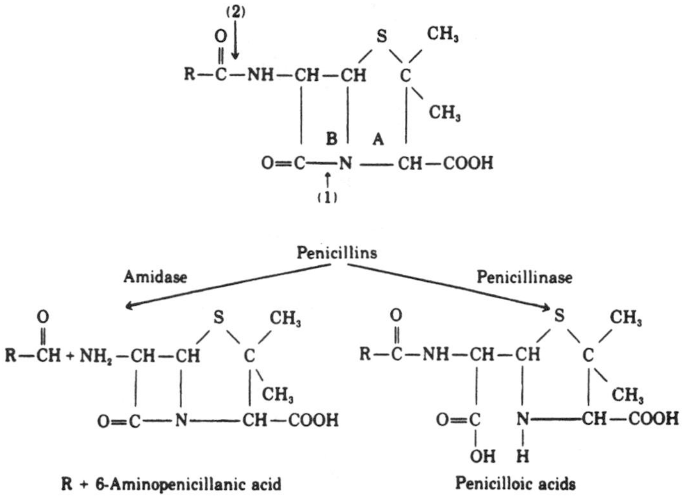

Figure 16.1.   Penicillin nucleus and breakdown products. (1) Site of beta-lactamase activity. (2) Site of amidase activity. (Amidase, an enzyme produced by microorganisms, cleaves penicillin at site 2.)

a. **Definitions in laboratory** (1,3).

(1) **Susceptible strains** have minimal inhibitory concentrations (MIC; see Chap. 13) to penicillin of ≤0.1 µg/ml.

(2) **Intermediate resistance** is defined as strains with MIC of 0.1 or 0.12 to 2 µg/ml.

(3) **Highly resistant (or fully resistant** strains) have a MIC of ≥2 µg/ml. These strains are more likely to be resistant to other antipneumococcal agents. Strains resistant to three or more agents are defined as multidrug-resistant strains (4).

(4) **Laboratory testing.** The National Committee for Clinical Laboratory Standards (NCCLS) recommends screening of pneumococci of at least blood and sterile fluid clinical isolates for penicillin resistance by disc diffusion, using a 1-µg oxacillin disc. For those organisms that are not susceptible by screening, another test is necessary to determine the MIC. One useful technique for this is the E test. (See Chap. 13.)

b. **Prevalence and frequency.** Penicillin resistance was uncommon in the United States at least through 1987, but in recent years, the incidence has increased significantly (3). Recent data from the United States suggested that 33% to 36% of *S. pneumoniae* are penicillin resistant, with the majority of isolates intermediately resistant. See summary table in Chapter 2, Table 2-4, on page 49.

c. **Mechanisms and spread** (1,2)

    (1) Pneumococcal resistance to penicillin results from **alterations in the genetic structure** of the organism, **giving rise to changes in one** or **more of its penicillin-binding proteins** (PBPs), thereby reducing affinity of the PBP for the drug.

    (2) Selective pressure exerted by antibiotic use is often presumed to be a chief factor responsible for the development of resistance, but young age, attendance at a day care center (especially a large center), and residence in a nursing home also contribute. Resistant strains may be transported to geographically distant areas, where they may spread rapidly, influenced by local risk factors noted earlier.

d. **Effect on presentation and severity of illness**. Antibiotic-resistant pneumococci per se are neither more nor less virulent than susceptible strains if proper therapy is not delayed.

e. **Susceptibility of penicillin-resistant *S. pneumoniae* to other antibiotics**.

    (1) **For intermediate-resistant strains of *S. pneumoniae***, the second- and third-generation cephalosporins often, but not always, are active. (See related discussions in Chap. 2 and Table 2-5, page 50.) The newer expanded-spectrum fluoroquinolones (e.g., levofloxacin) are typically active against these pathogens, as is vancomycin. **Also high serum levels of penicillin or ampicillin (amoxicillin) are clinically effective agents for non-CNS infections (5)**.

    (2) High-level resistant strains are resistant to ampicillin, ticarcillin, and piperacillin. Because resistance is not dependent on the production of beta-lactamase, these organisms are also resistant to amoxicillin-clavulanate and related beta-lactamase inhibitor combinations. (See Sec. c above.)

    (3) **Highly resistant strains of *S. pneumoniae*** often are resistant also to

erythromycin and clarithromycin, trimethoprim-sulfamethoxazole (TMP-SMX), and tetracycline. If these drugs are considered for use, **it is imperative that susceptibility testing be performed** (e.g., with the E test).

The currently available first-generation quinolones (e.g., ciprofloxacin, ofloxacin) are only modestly active against penicillin-susceptible *S. pneumoniae.* **The advanced, newer quinolones (e.g., levofloxacin) are very active against high-level resistant organisms** (see Chap. 32). **Vancomycin has been uniformly active against penicillin-resistant isolates;** imipenem is active against 90% to 100%.

f. **Serotypes involved and clinical implications.** Currently, the resistant isolates are of a few serotypes, most of which are present in the 23-valent pneumococcal capsular polysaccharide vaccine. Therefore **the pneumococcal vaccine should be aggressively promoted** and **routinely administered to appropriate candidates** (1).

g. **Clinical implications of penicillin-resistant *S. pneumoniae*** include the following:

(1) **Pneumococcal meningitis.** Because high-level penicillin-resistant *S. pneumoniae* should be considered resistant to third-generation cephalosporins (cefotaxime and ceftriaxone) until susceptibility data are known, **for possible or gram stain–confirmed** *S. pneumoniae* bacterial meningitis combination therapy with vancomycin and cefotaxime or ceftriaxone should be administered to all individuals older than 1 month (6). (See related discussions in Chap. 11.)

(2) **Sepsis and pneumonia**. High-dose penicillin (150,000 to 200,000 units/kg/day) presumably remains effective therapy against those strains at the intermediate level (5).

For patients who are severely ill when high-level penicillin resistance is a possibility (e.g., nosocomial pneumonia in debilitated patients or a grandparent in contact with children who attend day care), the newer, "second-generation" fluoroquinolones or vancomycin should be used. (See related discussions in Chap. 2.)

(3) **Otitis media**. Amoxicillin is still recommended for initial therapy. In dis-
cussing therapy of otitis media, the
1997 Red Book emphasizes the following (6): Based on concentrations in
middle ear fluid and *in vitro* activity, no currently available beta-lactam
antibiotic, including the oral cephalosporins, has better activity than amoxicillin against penicillin-**susceptible**
S. pneumoniae and against strains of
intermediate resistance. Cefuroxime
axetil, cefpodoxime, and cefprozil are
the only orally administered cephalosporins that have activity comparable
to but not better than the activity of
amoxicillin for highly resistant strains.

Recently, higher doses of amoxicillin (60 to 90 mg/kg/day) have been
suggested for acute otitis media to
achieve middle ear concentrations active against resistant strains (6,7). **(See
related discussions in Chap. 1.)**

h. **Methods to control** the rising incidence of
penicillin-resistant *S. pneumoniae* are being
evaluated. These include more careful use
of antibiotics, especially in the community;
shorter courses of antibiotics; and narrower-
spectrum antibiotics. In early 1996, a special
report was published on strategies to help
minimize and control the impact of drug-
resistant *S. pneumoniae* (8).

3. Resistance of group A streptococci to penicillin
has not been observed.

B. **Gram-negative aerobes.** Penicillin remains the
antibiotic of choice for *Neisseria meningitidis* and
Pasteurella multocida (9). Penicillin is no longer a
drug of choice for *N. gonorrhoeae.*

C. **Anaerobes.** Penicillin is very effective against anaerobic species (9), including *Clostridium* spp., *Fusobacterium* spp., and *Actinomyces israelii* (actinomy-
cosis). Although penicillin is active against many
Bacteroides spp. (particularly oropharyngeal strains),
it is not active against *B. fragilis* and some of the oral
gram-negative anaerobes. If *B. fragilis* infections are
suspected (e.g., intraabdominal or pelvic infections),
another agent should be selected.

D. **Spirochetes**. Penicillin is the drug of choice for *Treponema pallidum* (9) infection (see Chap. 10) and is
active against *Borrelia burgdorferi.*

III. **Parenteral preparations of penicillin G (benzylpenicillin).** There are three main forms of parenteral penicillin
G. The pharmacokinetics differ markedly (1).

A. **Aqueous penicillin G** is available in potassium and
   sodium salt forms. Ordinarily, the potassium salt form
   is used. Aqueous penicillin is given intravenously and
   therefore produces **high blood levels.** Excretion is rapid, yielding undetectable penicillin blood levels 4 hours
   after a dose. Therefore for serious infections, the aqueous form should be given at least every 4 hours.

   1. **High-dose therapy. In adults with normal
      renal function**, 3 to 4 million units q4h is
      used in serious infections such as meningitis
      due to susceptible organisms, in some forms of
      endocarditis due to mildly penicillin-resistant
      organisms, and in severe clostridial infections.
      A continuous infusion of 20 to 24 million units
      per day can be used (2).

   2. **Intermediate doses** of aqueous penicillin (9 to
      12 million units daily) are used in aspiration
      pneumonias or lung abscess and in moderate to
      severe soft-tissue infections due to group A strep-
      tococci. This dose of 9 to 12 million units/day is
      also used in conjunction with an aminoglycoside
      to provide synergy. For example, penicillin and
      gentamicin are used for synergy against entero-
      cocci (those without high-level resistance to gen-
      tamicin) and other resistant streptococci in
      endocarditis.
      This dose would also be active against inter-
      mediate-resistant *S. pneumoniae* causing pneu-
      monia. (See Chap. 2.)

   3. **Low doses.** When lower blood levels are ade-
      quate, procaine penicillin or oral penicillin is an
      option. If the aqueous intravenous form of peni-
      cillin is used in known **penicillin-susceptible**
      pneumococcal pneumonia, the dose can be kept
      at 2.4 million units per day. High doses of peni-
      cillin are not necessary for known penicillin-
      susceptible pneumococcal pneumonia and may
      only increase the chances of superinfection. In
      settings of known or suspected intermediate-
      resistant *S. pneumoniae*, higher doses of intra-
      venous penicillin (e.g., 9 to 12 million units per
      day) may be effective. For suspected or known
      high-level penicillin resistance, an alternative
      agent is indicated. (See prior discussion in Sec.
      II.A.2.)

   4. **Pediatric dose**. For children, 25,000 to 300,000
      units/kg/day is recommended, depending on the
      severity of the infection.

B. **Procaine penicillin G**. This repository form of penicillin has been developed to prolong the duration of
   penicillin in the blood. Peak levels (1 to 2 μg/ml) are
   reached in 2 to 4 hours, and detectable levels are present for 12 to 24 hours.

   1. **Doses** usually are given **every 12 hours intra-
      muscularly.** This preparation should not be

given intravenously because of the risk of procaine toxicity. To increase the peak serum levels, two separate intramuscular injections must be used.

2. **Uses**. This agent is **seldom used** now. Because of the increasing frequency of penicillinase-producing *Neisseria gonorrhoeae,* procaine penicillin regimens are no longer used for empiric gonococcal regimens. Some authorities may still recommend procaine penicillin G, 300,000 to 600,000 units intramuscularly q12h, as a regimen in penicillin-susceptible uncomplicated pneumococcal pneumonia once susceptibilities are known. However, oral agents are now often used in this setting (e.g., amoxicillin). Procaine penicillin is used in some of the alternative regimens for syphilis. (See Chap. 10.)

C. **Benzathine penicillin G** (long-acting) is an insoluble salt obtained by combining an ammonium base with penicillin G. **Very low blood levels** are achieved (approximately 0.10 to 0.15 units/ml), which persist for prolonged periods of time (i.e., 3 to 4 weeks). The major factor limiting use of this regimen is pain at the injection site. **Benzathine penicillin is used most commonly in the following conditions**:

1. **Syphilis** (primary, secondary, and latent), in which a prolonged blood level is necessary to kill the slowly dividing treponemal organisms, which are very sensitive to penicillin (MIC = 0.03 unit/ml). (See Chap. 10.)

2. **Rheumatic fever prophylaxis**. A monthly injection will provide a serum level above that necessary to inhibit group A beta-hemolytic streptococci (10).

3. **Streptococcal pharyngitis.** Many patients with group A beta-hemolytic streptococcal pharyngitis do not complete their oral antibiotic courses. In the high-risk patient (e.g., prior rheumatic fever) or the poorly compliant patient, use of benzathine penicillin will ensure maintenance of adequate levels (see Chap. 1). The highest cure rates for group A streptococcal pharyngitis are with a single dose of benzathine penicillin at a dose of 600,000 units in children less than 60 pounds and 1.2 million units in adults and children over 60 pounds (10). (See Chap. 1.)

IV. **Oral penicillin**. Oral penicillin G is partially inactivated by gastric acid. With a minor modification of the side chain, **penicillin V** (phenoxymethyl penicillin) is formed, and this oral congener **resists gastric acid breakdown and therefore provides acceptable serum levels**.

A. **Dosage**. The usual adult dosage is 1.6 to 3.2 million units/day divided into doses every 6 hours—that is, 400,000 units (250 mg) to 800,000 units (500 mg) q6h. In children, the usual dosage is 25,000 to 100,000 units/

kg/day divided into doses every 6 hours. A 500-mg dose results in a peak level of 3 to 5 μg/ml.

B. **Uses.** Oral therapy has been shown to be useful in pharyngitis, minor oral or dental infections, and minor soft-tissue infections due to susceptible organisms, as well as completion of courses of treatment after initial intravenous penicillin therapy. **Group A streptococci remain uniformly susceptible to all penicillins** and cephalosporins. No evidence of resistance has been identified. The American Heart Association (10) and the American Academy of Pediatrics recommend a single dose of intramuscular benzathine penicillin or a 10-day course of oral **penicillin V** (500 mg bid or tid in adults and children older than 12 years and 250 mg bid or tid for children younger than 12 years) as the **standard for therapy** for group A streptococcal pharyngitis. (See the related discussions in Chap. 1.)

C. **The spectrum of activity** of penicillin V is similar to that of penicillin G.

V. **Untoward and toxic reactions**

A. **Penicillin allergy and hypersensitivity reactions**. A detailed discussion of this topic is beyond the scope of this handbook; the reader is referred elsewhere (11). However, several comments deserve emphasis.

1. **Reactions to penicillin.** Adverse reactions to penicillin are estimated to occur in 1% to 10% of patients, with a fatal reaction occurring in 0.002% of patients (11).

2. **Classification of reactions** to penicillin are summarized in **Table 16-1.**

a. **Immediate reactions are the most dangerous**. Symptoms are related to the release of histamine and other vasoactive amines from the IgE-sensitized mast cells and basophils. Hypotension or bronchospasm can be severe and is fatal at times.

b. **Accelerated allergic reactions** are usually not life-threatening except for laryngeal edema, which may cause asphyxia. These reactions are also IgE mediated but not modified by IgG.

c. **Late reactions** are the **most frequent** type of reaction and account for 80% to 90% of penicillin reactions. They begin days to weeks after initiation of therapy. The most common reaction is a morbilliform eruption.

   (1) **Morbilliform rash.** No definite allergic mechanism has been demonstrated for this reaction. It is not IgE mediated (11). The occurrence of this rash cannot be predicted or diagnosed by skin tests.

   (2) Other delayed reactions are much less common.

Table 16-1. Allergic reactions to penicillin and semisynthetic penicillins

Immediate allergic reactions (2–30 min after penicillin)
  Erythema or pruritus
  Urticaria
  Angioedema
  Wheezing, rhinitis
  Hypotension or shock

Accelerated allergic reactions (1–72 h)
  Erythema or pruritus
  Urticaria
  Angioedema
  Laryngeal edema
  Wheezing, rhinitis

Late allergic reactions (more than 72 h)
  Morbilliform eruptions
  Urticaria—angioedema
  Urticaria—arthralgia
  Serum sickness

Less common reactions
  Immune hemolytic anemia
  Pulmonary infiltrates with eosinophilia
  Interstitial nephritis
  Granulocytopenia
  Thrombocytopenia
  Drug fever
  Hypersensitivity vasculitis
  Erythema multiforme
  Drug-induced systemic lupus erythematosus

Source: Condemi JJ, Sheehan MG, Allergy to penicillin and other antibiotics. In: Reese RE, Betts RF, eds., *A practical approach to infectious diseases,* 4th ed. Boston: Little, Brown, 1996.

   d. **Certain late reactions** occur infrequently to rarely. In many, an immunologic basis has not been established. **Fever** may be the only manifestation of a penicillin reaction. In such a case, penicillin or its derivatives can probably be administered in the future at no additional risk to the patient. However, because fever may accompany other, more severe reactions (e.g., vasculitis), patients with a history of drug fever need careful observation when they are reexposed to penicillin (11).

3. **Cross-reactions**
   a. **With other penicillin derivatives. Patients with a history of allergy to one penicillin should be presumed to be allergic to other penicillins unless appropriate skin tests prove otherwise.**

b. **With cephalosporins**. In penicillin-allergic patients, prior studies suggest the risk of allergic reactions to the cephalosporins is in the range of 5% to 15%, but this may be an overestimate; more recent estimates are as low as 1% (1,11,12). **In the patient with a history of an immediate reaction to penicillin, cephalosporins should be avoided unless careful skin testing can be performed.**

In the patient with a delayed mild reaction to penicillin (Table 16-1), cephalosporins are commonly used without difficulty (1,11,13).

c. **With aztreonam**. Studies have shown that patients allergic to penicillin can receive aztreonam without risk. (See Chap. 20.)

d. **With imipenem. Patients allergic to penicillin may cross-react with imipenem.** (See Chap. 20.)

4. **Documentation of allergic history.** Because the distinction between an immediate versus a delayed allergic reaction to any antibiotic is crucial in determining its implications for future antibiotic administration, it is important to elicit this history carefully and to document it in the patient's record.

B. **Drug fever** may be the only manifestation of a penicillin side effect. (See Chap. 12.)

C. **Eosinophilia** alone can occur with penicillin use. If the level exceeds 15% of the peripheral white blood cell count, it probably is reasonable to discontinue the drug, since these patients may go on to more serious drug reactions (1).

D. **Interstitial nephritis** may occur with high doses but is rare with oral penicillin G; it can occur with any penicillin (14), any age, and may be a hypersensitivity reaction.

1. **Signs and symptoms**. Signs and symptoms including hematuria, proteinuria, fever, morbilliform rash, at times a peripheral eosinophilia, and renal failure (50% of cases), which may be severe, are seen after several days of antibiotic therapy.

2. **Diagnosis**. A minority of patients have eosinophils in their urine sediments, which is a helpful diagnostic clue. A characteristic renal biopsy reveals an interstitial nephritis with eosinophilic aggregations. A nephrology consultation is advised.

3. **Therapeutic approach**. The offending agent should be discontinued. Whether cephalosporins can be used safely is debated, but we would be inclined not to use another beta-lactam antibiotic. Infectious disease consultation is advised for alternative antibiotics.

E. **Central nervous system toxicity**. An early clue to penicillin central nervous system (CNS) toxicity is **myoclonic twitching**. With very high blood levels and excessively high spinal fluid levels of penicillin, the patient may develop **seizures**. This is most likely to occur if the patient has renal failure and excessively high doses are used. (See Sec. VI.A.1.)

VI. **Special considerations**

A. **Dosage modification in renal failure**

1. **High doses of intravenous aqueous penicillin**. In moderate to severe renal failure, **especially when high-dose** aqueous penicillin G **therapy** is used, penicillin can reach very high blood levels. **To avoid CNS toxicity, penicillin G doses must be reduced in renal failure and in the elderly.** A useful **nomogram** is shown in **Table 16-2**.

2. When **moderate intravenous doses** (i.e., 10 to 12 million units/day) are to be used in patients with renal failure, we tend to reduce doses proportionately. (See suggestions given in Table 16-2.)

Table 16-2. Equivalent doses of aqueous penicillin G for high-dose therapy in renal failure*

Endogenous Creatinine Clearance (ml/min)	Penicillin G Dose[†] and Dose Interval[‡] (units)
125	1.7–2.0 million q2h or 2.6–3.0 million q3h
60	1.8–2.0 million q4h
40	1.3–1.5 million q4h
20	800,000–1 million q4h
10	800,000–1 million q6h
0	500,000–800,000 q6h or 700,000–1.1 million q8h
<10[§]	500,000 q8h

Source: Adapted from Bryan CS, Stone WJ, "Comparable massive" penicillin G therapy in renal failure. *Ann Intern Med* 1975;82:189.

* **To achieve mean blood levels equivalent to 24 million units per day** in the adult with normal renal function, the above doses and dose intervals can be used in patients with renal failure.

   A loading dose of 750,000–1,200,000 units is suggested in patients with a creatinine clearance of less than 20 ml/min, and then the above doses and intervals can be followed. In patients with a creatinine clearance exceeding 20 ml/min, no loading dose is suggested.

[†] The lower dose is calculated to provide a mean serum level of 20 µg/ml for the "average patient." The higher dose is an overestimate.

[‡] After hemodialysis, an additional 500,000 units should be given to replace expected losses for an average full 6-hour dialysis.

[§] Because the extrarenal clearance of penicillin is impaired by liver disease, in patients with hepatic and renal failure (creatinine clearance <10 ml/min), even lower doses of penicillin G are suggested.

3. When a **low-dose intravenous penicillin** or oral penicillin regimen is to be used, standard doses are employed.

B. **Dialysis**
   1. **Hemodialysis** removes penicillin, but the amounts removed vary. When the equivalent of high-dose therapy is used, an additional 500,000 units should be given after each 6-hour dialysis (Table 16.2). (A proportion of this supplemental dose could be given in a moderate- or low-dose regimen.)
   2. **Peritoneal dialysis** likewise removes a variable amount of penicillin. Usually, doses are not specifically supplemented after peritoneal dialysis.

C. **Probenecid use.** Penicillin G is eliminated primarily by the kidney, approximately 90% by tubular secretion, and 10% by glomerular filtration. Probenecid blocks the renal tubular secretory transport of penicillin, and this in turn results in higher (usually approximately twofold) and more prolonged blood levels of penicillin.
   1. **Dosage**. Probenecid 500 mg po qid has been recommended (in adults). Some patients may experience minor gastrointestinal symptoms with probenecid use.
   2. **Uses**. Because the addition of probenecid increases the frequency of side effects, **we seldom use probenecid with oral therapy.** Infectious disease consultation is advised if probenecid is used; amoxicillin may be preferred since this agent will provide higher serum levels. (See Chap. 18.)

References

1. Reese RE, Betts RF. Penicillin G and penicillin-resistant *Streptococcus pneumoniae*. In: Reese RE, Betts RF, eds. *A practical approach to infectious disease*, 4th ed. Boston: Little, Brown, 1996: Chap. 28C.
2. Wright AJ. The penicillins. *Mayo Clin Proc* 1999;74:290.
3. Breiman RF, et al. Emergence of drug-resistant pneumococcal infections in the United States. *JAMA* 1994;271:1831.
4. Clavo-Sanchez AJ, et al. Multivariate analysis of risk factors for infection due to penicillin-resistant and multidrug-resistant *Streptococcus pneumoniae:* a multicenter study. *Clin Infect Dis* 1997; 24:1052.
5. Tomasz A. The pneumococcus at the gates. *N Engl J Med* 1995; 333:514.
6. American Academy of Pediatrics. *1997 Red Book: report of the Committee on Infectious Diseases*, 24th ed. Elk Grove Village, IL: American Academy of Pediatrics, 1997:413.
7. Poole MD. Implications of drug-resistant *Streptococcus pneumoniae* for otitis media. *Pediatr Infect Dis J* 1998;17:953.

8. Jernigan DB, et al. Minimizing the impact of drug-resistant *Streptococcus pneumoniae* (DRSP): a strategy from the DRSP working group. *JAMA* 1996;275:206.
    See related report in MMWR *1996;45(RR):1.*
9. The Medical Letter. The choice of antibacterial drugs. *Med Lett Drugs Ther* 1999;41:95.
10. Dajani AS, et al. Treatment of streptococcal pharyngitis and prevention of rheumatic fever: a statement of health professionals on rheumatic fever, endocarditis, and Kawasaki disease of the Council on Cardiovascular Disease in the Young, the American Heart Association. *Pediatrics* 1995;96:758.
11. Condemi JJ, Sheehan MG. Allergy to penicillin and other antibiotics. In: Reese RE, Betts RF, eds. *A practical approach to infectious diseases*, 4th ed. Boston: Little, Brown, 1996: Chap. 27.
12. Donowitz GR. Third-generation cephalosporins. *Infect Dis Clin North Am* 1989;3:595.
13. Anne S, Reisman RE. Risk of administering cephalosporin antibiotics to patients with histories of penicillin allergy. *Ann Allergy Asthma Immunol* 1995;74:167.
14. Murray KM, Keane WR. Review of drug-induced acute interstitial nephritis. *Pharmacotherapy* 1992;12:462.

17

Penicillinase-Resistant Penicillins

Penicillinase-resistant penicillins are produced by modifying the side chain of the common penicillin nucleus structure, which inhibits the action of penicillinase (a beta-lactamase) by preventing opening of the beta-lactam ring. (See Fig. 16.1.) **These bactericidal agents are used primarily to treat penicillinase-producing *Staphylococcus aureus* (i.e., penicillin-resistant) but methicillin-susceptible *S. aureus* [MSSA]) (1,2).**

I. **Spectrum of activity**
   A. ***S. aureus* (MSSA)**
      1. **Initial therapy.** If infection in the non–penicillin-allergic patient is known or highly likely to be due to methicillin-susceptible *S. aureus*, these agents are preferred (3).
      2. **Penicillin-susceptible *S. aureus*. If susceptibility studies show that the *S. aureus* is susceptible to penicillin G,** penicillin G is the **preferred agent** (in the nonallergic patient) because it has a narrower spectrum of activity, has better *in vitro* activity than the penicillinase-resistant penicillins against susceptible *S. aureus* and is less expensive.
      3. **Methicillin-resistant *S. aureus* (MRSA)**, or oxacillin-resistant ***S. aureus* (ORSA)**, has emerged as an important nosocomial pathogen.*
         a. **Pathogenesis and transmission and infection control considerations are reviewed in Chap. 13, Part B.**
         b. **Treatment of MRSA infections. Intravenous vancomycin is the drug of choice** (3). (See Chap. 28.)

         Gentamicin is synergistic with vancomycin *in vitro* against many MRSA strains and can be combined for bacteremic and endovascular staphylococci. Rifampin plus vancomycin may be either synergistic or antagonistic *in vitro,* but ample clinical data demonstrate the usefulness of this combination, particularly where tissue penetration of vancomycin may be suboptimal (e.g., CSF) (4). Some strains are susceptible to TMP-SMZ and/or doxycycline (or minocycline) and/or the quinolones (3).
         c. **Eradication of the carrier state of MRSA**
            (1) **Topical treatment.** Bacitracin ointment has been used, but mupirocin

---

* Recent data in 1999 suggest MRSA is becoming more common as a community-acquired pathogen (4A); see related discussion in Chap. 13, Part B.

(Bactroban) applied to the anterior nares twice daily for 5 days is usually favored for eradication of nasal carriage. Unfortunately, some strains of MRSA are resistant to mupirocin.

(2) **Oral systemic therapy** is sometimes tried. Infectious disease consultation is advised. Rifampin and trimethoprim-sulfamethoxazole (TMP-SMX) have commonly been used. Minocycline and ciprofloxacin have been used if strains are susceptible.

(3) **Combination therapy** with topical therapy of the nares and oral antibiotics is often employed. Nasal colonization can be eradicated from a significant proportion of carriers.

B. **Other gram-positive aerobes.** These agents are active against penicillin-susceptible *Streptococcus pneumoniae* and *S. pyogenes*, but the minimum inhibitory concentrations for these organisms are higher for the penicillinase-resistant penicillins than for penicillin. Therefore if final culture reports show the pathogen to be either penicillin-susceptible *S. pneumoniae* or *S. pyogenes*, penicillin is preferred (1). They are not useful in penicillin-resistant *S. pneumoniae* infections. **The penicillinase-resistant penicillins are drugs of first choice only for penicillinase-producing MSSA *S. aureus* (3).**

C. **Gram-negative aerobes.** These agents are **not effective against** the Enterobacteriaceae (*Escherichia coli* and *Klebsiella* and *Enterobacter* spp.) or *Pseudomonas* spp. The penicillinase-resistant penicillins **are not recommended in the treatment of gonorrhea.** For patients with infections due to *Pasteurella multocida*, penicillin is the preferred agent (3). Tetracycline, cefuroxime or ciprofloxacin is recommended in the patient allergic to penicillin. In animal bite wounds with mixed flora, amoxicillin-clavulanate (or ampicillin-sulbactam) is suggested. (See Chap. 3.)

D. **Anaerobes.** Compared with penicillin, the penicillinase-resistant penicillins are less active against penicillin-susceptible anaerobes. These antistaphylococcal agents are not active against *Bacteroides fragilis*.

II. **Parenteral preparations.** There are no adequate studies to determine which antistaphylococcal agent is preferred (1,2). Overall, oxacillin and nafcillin are very similar and, except as noted later, are probably interchangeable. Methicillin was more commonly associated with interstitial nephritis, especially in adults; its use has therefore been discontinued in the United States (2).

A. **Oxacillin**

1. **Dose.** In adults, 6 g/day intravenously (IV) is recommended for moderate infections. For severe infections, 9 to 12 g/day IV has been suggested

but we prefer to limit the dose to 9 g/day to avoid excessive side effects. In children, the usual dose is 100 to 200 mg/kg/day in divided doses q4 to 6h. Because serum levels decline rapidly and are undetectable at 2.5 to 3.0 hours in severe infections, intravenous doses administered over 20 to 30 minutes, with a 4-hour dose interval, are preferred. Dosages for neonates are shown in Appendix A.

2. **In renal failure.** Because oxacillin is excreted both renally and hepatically, in renal failure, doses do not have to be modified. **Hemodialysis and peritoneal dialysis** do not remove oxacillin. Therefore no additional dose adjustments are necessary (5).

3. **Side effects.** Allergic reactions may occur as with other penicillins. Rarely, neutropenia has been observed. Interstitial nephritis appears to occur less frequently than with methicillin. Oxacillin-related **hepatitis** in prolonged intravenous use has been described (6). Therefore **weekly liver function tests are advisable for patients receiving prolonged therapy.** *Clostridium difficile* diarrhea may occur.

B. **Nafcillin**
   1. **Dosage** is similar to oxacillin in adults and older children. **Nafcillin should not be used in premature or young infants with jaundice**, as it is excreted primarily by hepatic mechanisms, which may be deficient in these neonates or infants (1).
   2. **In renal failure and dialysis, dosage modification is not necessary. Therefore nafcillin is an excellent choice in patients with renal impairment** who require an antistaphylococcal semisynthetic penicillin (5).
   3. **Central nervous system penetration.** Studies have shown adequate penetration of nafcillin into the spinal fluid, particularly when inflammation is present. Some authors suggest nafcillin is the **drug of choice in MSSA staphylococcal meningitis** (1).
   4. **Side effects** are similar to oxacillin. Interstitial nephritis may occur with nafcillin use, but it is less frequent than after methicillin use. Neutropenia can occur. Phlebitis and/or pain may occur at the infusion site and may be more common with nafcillin than with oxacillin (1).

III. **Oral preparations** (cloxacillin, dicloxacillin)
   A. **Indications for use.** Penicillinase-resistant penicillins in oral form often are considered the oral drugs of choice for known or highly suspected penicillin-resistant mild staphylococcal infections. They are useful in treating soft-tissue infections due to susceptible *S. aureus* or mixed *S. aureus* and *S. pyogenes* (group A streptococci). However, the first-generation oral cepha-

losporins are better tolerated, in terms of gastro-intestinal side effects, and are therefore often preferred over cloxacillin or dicloxacillin. (See Sec. C.)

B. **Agents available.** These are better absorbed in the fasting state.

1. **Cloxacillin** is available in an oral solution (125 mg/5 ml) and in 250-mg and 500-mg capsules. The usual dosage in children is 50 to 100 mg/kg/day, and in adults, 1 to 2 g/day divided into four equal doses.

2. **Dicloxacillin** is available as a suspension (62.5 mg/5 ml) and in 125-mg and 250-mg cap-sules. The usual dosage in children is 25 to 50 mg/kg/day; in adults, the usual dosage is 1 to 2 g/day divided into four equal doses. The higher dose range may be preferable for adequate anti-staphylococcal activity.

C. **Side effects.** These agents frequently cause mild **gastrointestinal symptoms;** often the standard oral dosages (e.g., 500 mg q6h in adults) cannot be toler-ated. Furthermore, the poor taste of the oral suspen-sion may adversely affect compliance in children (7). A first-generation oral cephalosporin is better toler-ated and therefore often preferred. If severe or persis-tent diarrhea occurs, antibiotic-related diarrhea must be considered.

References

1. Reese RE, Betts RF. Penicillinase-resistant penicillin. In: Reese RE, Betts RF, eds. *A practical approach to infectious diseases*, 4th ed. Boston: Little, Brown, 1996:Chap. 28D.

2. Wright AJ. The penicillins. *Mayo Clin Proc* 1999;74:290.

3. The Medical Letter. The choice of antibacterial drugs. *Med Lett Drug Ther* 1999;41:95.

4. Frainow HS, Abrutyn E. Pathogens resistant to antimicrobial agents: epidemiology, molecular mechanisms and clinical management. *Infect Dis Clin North Am* 1995;9:497.

4A. Kak V, Levine DP. Community-acquired methicillin-resistant *Staphylococcus aureus* infections: where do we go from here? *Clin Infect Dis* 1999;29:801.
    Careful editorial comment on two related articles in this October 1999 issue. Also see, CDC: four pediatric deaths from community-acquired methicillin-resistant Staphylococcus aureus. *MMWR 1999;48:707.*

5. Aronoff GR, et al. *Drug prescribing in renal failure: dosing guide-lines for adults,* 4th ed. Philadelphia: American College of Physi-cians, 1999.
    Also see 3rd edition, 1994, for oxacillin dose reduction.

6. Bruckstein AH, Attia AA. Oxacillin hepatitis. *Am J Med* 1978; 64:519.

7. Ruff ME, et al. Antimicrobial drug suspensions: a blind comparison of taste of fourteen common pediatric drugs. *Pediatr Infect Dis J* 1991;10:30.

Broad-Spectrum Penicillins and Beta-lactam/ Beta-lactamase Combinations

Several side-chain modifications of penicillin have been made to provide enhanced activity of the broad-spectrum penicillins.

I. **Aminopenicillins: ampicillin** and **amoxicillin** (1,2).
   A. **Spectrum of activity.** In addition to being active against penicillin-susceptible organisms, **ampicillin is** more active against enterococci, *Listeria monocytogenes*, and beta-lactamase negative *Haemophilus influenzae* (about 70% to 90% of strains).

   - Ampicillin should not be used for penicillinase-producing *Staphylococcus aureus* or beta-lactamase-positive *H. influenzae* or *Moraxella catarrhalis*.
   - Although active against many strains, many *Escherichia coli*, *Salmonella* spp., and *Shigella* spp. are resistant, so that ampicillin is no longer a drug of choice for these infections (3).
   - **Ampicillin is a "drug of choice"** for group B streptococci (*S. agalactiae*), *Proteus mirabilis*, and *Eikenella corrodens* (3).

   B. **Amoxicillin** is **only** available for **oral** use. It is closely related to ampicillin in both chemical structure and antibacterial activity. Amoxicillin has more complete absorption than ampicillin and for comparable doses provides twice the serum level (1,2). Amoxicillin is given tid rather than the qid dosing of ampicillin. Consequently, **amoxicillin has essentially replaced the use of oral ampicillin** (1,2), except ampicillin is still preferred for susceptible *Shigella* spp. (1).

   N.B. The combination of amoxicillin-clavulanate (Augmentin) is discussed separately in Sec. III.B.
   C. **Uses**
      1. **Ampicillin is used intravenously** for certain carefully selected cases of community-acquired pneumonia (see Chap. 2), enterococcal infections, group B streptococcal infections, and at times for known susceptible urinary pathogens or in combination with an aminoglycoside for empiric therapy of community-acquired pyelonephritis (especially if enterococcus is a concern). (See Chap. 4.)
      2. **Amoxicillin** (available as an **oral** agent **only**) is used for the following:
         a. **Acute otitis media** for which amoxicillin is the initial agent of choice as discussed in Chap. 1.

b. **Acute sinusitis** and **exacerbations of chronic bronchitis** as discussed in Chap. 1.

c. **Susceptible** pathogens in **UTI**.

d. Completion of therapy in which intravenous (IV) ampicillin was initially used. See Sec. 1.

e. Because it is very well absorbed, it is used in oral prophylactic antibiotic regimens to prevent endocarditis after dental manipulations. (See Chap. 15.)

D. **Dosage**

1. **Ampicillin**

a. **Intravenous**. In adults, 4 to 12 g daily is given depending on the organism involved and the severity and site of the infection. In adults with moderately severe infections, 1 g q4 to 6h often is given; for more severe infections, 1.5 g q4h may be necessary and, in meningitis in the adult, 2 g q4h is used. **In children,** the usual dosage range is 100 to 200 mg/kg/day in divided doses q6h. Higher doses (up to 400 mg/kg/day) are used in meningitis caused by known susceptible *H. influenzae*. Neonatal doses are shown in the Appendix.

b. **Oral**. The usual adult dose is 250 to 500 mg q6h **on an empty stomach.** In children, 50 to 100 mg/kg/day in divided doses q6h is suggested. As discussed earlier, amoxicillin has pretty much replaced oral ampicillin.

c. **Intramuscular**. Ampicillin can be given intramuscularly, but the intravenous route generally is preferred.

d. **Renal failure**. Because ampicillin is excreted by the kidney, dosage is modified in patients with significant renal impairment, particularly when high-dose regimens are used. If the creatinine clearance is 10 to 50 ml/min, the standard dose can be given q6 to 12h. If the creatinine clearance is less than 10 ml/min, the standard dose can be given every 12 to 24 hours (4).

e. **Dialysis**. Ampicillin is partially removed by hemodialysis. After dialysis, a supplemental dose is required. Peritoneal dialysis does not significantly lower ampicillin serum levels. For oral therapy, 250 mg q12h has been used (4).

f. **Pregnancy.** Ampicillin does cross the placenta. As with other penicillins, it should be used conservatively in pregnant women.

g. **Nursing mothers.** Ampicillin is excreted in human milk. In theory, the neonate could be sensitized by ampicillin in the mother's milk, so this agent should be used conservatively in nursing mothers as neonates commonly are treated with ampicillin.

2. **Amoxicillin**

    a. **Oral**. The usual adult dose is 250 to 500 mg q8h, and the fasting state is not essential. In children, 20 to 40 mg/kg/day is given in divided doses q8h. An oral suspension is available with 250 mg/5 ml and 125 mg/5 ml. **For otitis media in children, the "conventional" doses and high-dose regimens are discussed in Chap. 1**.

    b. **Renal failure**. If the creatinine clearance is 10 to 50 ml/min, the standard dose can be given q8 to 12h. If the clearance is less than 10 ml/min, the standard dose can be given q24h (4).

    c. **Dialysis**. Dosage is as described for ampicillin; see the preceding discussion. In chronic ambulatory peritoneal dialysis (CAPD) patients, 250 mg q12h has been suggested (4).

    d. **Pregnancy**. The package insert notes that safety for use in pregnancy has not been established.

    e. **Nursing mothers**. Penicillins are excreted in human milk. See Sec. 1.g earlier.

E. **Adverse effects** of ampicillin (and amoxicillin)

    1. These are similar to those described under penicillin. (See Chap. 16.)

    2. Epstein-Barr virus infection (mononucleosis), acute lymphocytic leukemia, or cytomegalovirus infection increases the risk for an ampicillin (or amoxicillin) macular papular rash to 60% to 100%. The reason for this is unknown, but it does not appear to be mediated by IgE (5).

    3. Morbilliform rashes are more common with ampicillin (amoxicillin) than with penicillin for unclear reasons (5).

II. **The extended-spectrum penicillins:** The carboxypenicillins include **carbenicillin** and **piperacillin** and ureidopenicillins, **mezlocillin,** and **piperacillin.** To meet the needs of more resistant gram-negative bacteria, including activity against *Pseudomonas aeruginosa*, these derivatives of ampicillin were developed (1,2).

A. **Overview of uses**

    1. For susceptible pathogens, prospective comparative studies have failed to demonstrate clinical superiority of one of these agents over another (1,2).

    2. **Monotherapy** with these agents may be associated with the rapid emergence of resistance and therefore is **not advised.**

    3. Except against *P. aeruginosa*, these agents are not **"drugs of choice"** (3).

    4. For severe *P. aeruginosa* infection (e.g., pneumonia, sepsis, wound infection), one of these agents

is combined with an aminoglycoside to achieve synergy and decrease the likelihood of selecting resistant organisms.

5. To cover hospital-acquired gram negatives, including *P. aeruginosa*, one of these agents is commonly combined with an aminoglycoside that broadens the coverage and may allow the combination to achieve synergistic action against many gram negatives. (See related discussions in Chaps. 2 and 7.)

6. These agents are "second line" agents against anaerobes, including bowel anaerobes.

7. One of these agents combined with an aminoglycoside has historically been a useful combination for empiric therapy of the febrile neutropenic patient. (See Chap. 12.)

B. **Which agent?**

1. **Carbenicillin**. The IV formulation has not been available in the United States for several years. Because of the increased activity and fewer side effects of the other agents, demand decreased and it was taken off the market. An oral formulation (Geocillin) is still available, but since it provides low serum levels, it can only be used for susceptible UTI and has for the most part been replaced by the quinolones (1,2).

2. **Ticarcillin versus mezlocillin versus piperacillin**. Generally, the pharmacy and therapeutics committee of each hospital selects one of these agents for routine use.

    a. **Piperacillin and mezlocillin are usually preferred over ticarcillin** since piperacillin and mezlocillin have lower sodium loads per day, are more active *in vitro*, and presumably have less of a tendency to cause clinical bleeding with acquired platelet dysfunction after surgery and/or in patients with renal failure than ticarcillin (6).

    b. **Because piperacillin is the most active *in vitro* against *P. aeruginosa*** and overall is about four times more active against this pathogen than is mezlocillin or ticarcillin (2), **we overall prefer piperacillin** since one of these agents is often used for *P. aeruginosa* therapy and/or hospital-acquired infection.

C. **Piperacillin (Piperacil)**

1. ***In vitro* activity.** See preceding discussions. Piperacillin is active against streptococci, including many enterococci, 60% to 80% of Enterobacteriaceae, *P. aeruginosa*, and most *Bacteroides fragilis* (2).

    N.B. Beta-lactamase producing *S. aureus* and *H. influenzae* are resistant to piperacillin, as are MRSA and penicillin-resistant *S. pneumoniae* and vancomycin-resistant enterococci.

2. **Dosages**
   a. **Adults**. The usual dose for serious infection is 3 to 4 g q4 to 6h in adults with normal renal function. For ease of administration, we commonly use 4 g q6h in adults. For serious infections, up to 18 g/day can be used.
   b. **Children**. In children 12 years of age or older, 200 to 300 mg/kg/day IV (not to exceed the adult daily dose) in divided doses q4 to 6h is suggested. Dosages for children younger than 12 years have not been established, and the safety of this agent in neonates is not known.
   c. **Renal failure**. If the creatinine clearance is more than 50 ml/min, no dose reduction is necessary. If the creatinine clearance is 10 to 50 ml/min, 3 to 4 g can be given q6 to 8h. If the creatinine clearance is less than 10 ml/min, 3 to 4 g can be given q8h (4).
      (1) **With hemodialysis,** the package insert suggests 2 g q8h with a supplemental 1-g dose after hemodialysis since dialysis removes 30% to 50%. Also, 3 to 4 g per dose q8h with a dose after dialysis has been used (4).
      (2) **With peritoneal dialysis** the doses for renal failure less than 10 ml/min can be used (4).
         Ideally, if patients have both hepatic failure and renal insufficiency, serum levels should be monitored.
   d. **Pregnancy**. This is a category B agent. (See Chap. 14.) Because there are no well-controlled studies in pregnant women, the package insert suggests this drug should be used during pregnancy only if clearly needed.
   e. **Nursing mothers**. Piperacillin is excreted in low concentrations in milk; therefore the package insert suggests that caution should be exercised if this agent is administered to nursing mothers.
2. **Cost** data are shown in the Appendix, Table B.

D. **Side effects**
   1. The side effects seen with penicillin may occur with these agents. (See Chap. 16.)
   2. Hypokalemia may occur but is less common with the newer agents than with carbenicillin (1,2).
   3. Platelet dysfunction is uncommon and is minimized by using piperacillin (1,2).

III. **Beta-lactam and beta-lactamase combinations:** an overview
   A. **Background**. Because structural modification of the penicillin side chain has limitations, new strategies of extending the antibacterial spectrum of the penicillin

family were explored. Since the primary mechanism of bacterial resistance to penicillins is through beta-lactamase (enzyme) production, inactivation of these enzymes was the next logical step (1,2). Therefore a beta-lactamase inhibitor (e.g., clavulanate, sulbactam, or tazobactam) was combined with certain extended penicillins.

1. See **Table 18-1.**
2. These beta-lactamase inhibitors bind **irreversibly to the beta-lactamase.** The bound beta-lactamase cannot hydrolyze the penicillin. Hence, the penicillin is free to bind to the penicillin binding protein and exerts its antibacterial effect (2).
3. These beta-lactamase inhibitors increase the antibacterial activity of their companion penicillin only when the bacterial resistance is primarily the result of beta-lactamase production (1).
   a. The inhibitors are effective against beta-lactamases produced by *S. aureus, H. influenzae, M. catarrhalis, Bacteroides* spp., many *E. coli,* and Enterobacteriaceae.
   b. **Some bacteria produce beta-lactamases that are not inhibited by these beta-lactamase inhibitors**, and therefore the bacteria remain resistant to the combination of beta-lactam/beta-lactamase inhibitor. Examples include certain species of *Enterobacter, Citrobacter, Serratia, Morganella,* and *Pseudomonas* (2).
4. **An important determinant of the effectiveness of these combinations is the *in vitro* activity of the active antibiotic. The overall intrinsic activity of piperacillin against gram negatives is greater than that of ticarcillin or ampicillin (7).**

B. **Amoxicillin-clavulanate (Augmentin)** is the **only oral combination agent available.**
   1. **Spectrum of activity.** Clavulanic acid inhibits the beta-lactamases of *S. aureus* (found in 80% of

Table 18-1. Available beta-lactamase inhibitors and beta-lactam antibiotic combinations

Active Antibiotics	Beta-Lactamase Inhibitor	Trade Name	Comment
Amoxicillin	Clavulanate	Augmentin	Only as oral agent
Ticarcillin	Clavulanate	Timentin	Only parenteral
Ampicillin	Sulbactam	Unasyn	Only parenteral
Piperacillin	Tazobactam	Zosyn	Only parenteral; most active antibiotic *in vitro*

these organisms), *H. influenzae* (found in 10% to 30% or more of these organisms), and *N. gonorrhoeae, H. ducreyi,* and *M. catarrhalis.* In addition, clavulanic acid inhibits beta-lactamases produced by many gram-negative bacilli, including *E. coli, Klebsiella,* and *Proteus* spp. Therefore the combination of amoxicillin-clavulanate is active against amoxicillin-susceptible as well as many previously amoxicillin-resistant organisms, including 97% to 100% of *S. aureus.* Most streptococci (including most enterococci), *N. gonorrhoeae, H. influenzae, E. coli,* and *Klebsiella* spp. are susceptible. It is not active against the beta-lactamases produced by *Enterobacter* or *Pseudomonas* spp. *Serratia* spp. also are resistant. *S. pneumoniae* with high-level resistance to penicillin will be resistant to amoxicillin-clavulanate.

Separate disc or broth testing with the combination must be performed.

2. **Pharmacokinetics**
   a. Both components are **well absorbed orally,** with peak levels at 1 hour, independent of meals, antacids, or milk.
   b. The drugs penetrate peritoneal and pleural fluids well. **Very high urine levels** are achieved compared with modest serum levels. There is only fair penetration into pulmonary secretions; therefore higher doses are necessary in pulmonary infections.
3. **Clinical uses**
   a. **Human and animal bite wounds.** Because of the polymicrobial nature of these infections, **this agent is the drug of choice** in this setting. (See detailed discussion in Chap. 3.)
   b. **Alternate therapy in acute otitis media.** Although amoxicillin remains the drug of choice in this setting, for patients who fail amoxicillin or as initial therapy in areas with very high resistant rates of *H. influenzae.* (See related discussions in Chap.1.)
   c. **Acute bacterial sinusitis** can often be managed with amoxicillin, but amoxicillin-clavulanate is preferred in some situations. (See Chap. 1.)
   d. **Urinary tract infection.** Although the fluoroquinolones and trimethoprim-sulfamethoxazole (TMP-SMX) are commonly used in UTI, for susceptible pathogens, amoxicillin-clavulanate provides another possible oral agent; it is not for uncomplicated UTI caused by amoxicillin-susceptible organisms.
   e. **Pulmonary infections.** This agent has been used in acute exacerbations of chronic bronchitis and early mild community-acquired

pneumonia in children and adults. (See Chap. 2.) (N.B. It is not active against mycoplasma or *Legionella*.)

 f. **Other considerations** include therapy for mild diverticulitis (see Chap. 6) and wound infections due to susceptible pathogens.

4. **Dosages**. This agent **should be administered with food** (e.g., at the start of a meal) to decrease the incidence of gastrointestinal (GI) side effects.

 a. **Availability.** An IV formulation is not available in the United States. Many oral formulations are available and include the following:

  (1) Oral **chewable tablets** in a **250-mg size** (250 mg amoxicillin and 62.5 mg clavulanate) and a **125-mg size** (125 mg amoxicillin and 31.25 mg clavulanate) for pediatric use.

  (2) An **oral suspension** with **125 mg/ 5 ml** (containing 125 mg amoxicillin and 31.25 mg clavulanate per 5 ml), one with **250 mg/5 ml** (containing 250 mg amoxicillin and 62.5 mg clavulanate per 5 ml), and **400 mg/5 ml** (containing 400 mg amoxicillin and 57 mg clavulanate) for pediatric use.

  (3) **Adult-sized tablets: 250 mg** (250 mg amoxicillin and 125 mg clavulanate), given **tid; 500 mg** (500 mg amoxicillin and 125 mg clavulanate), given **tid; 875 mg** (875 mg amoxicillin and 125 mg clavulanate) given **q12h**.

   Note: Two of the 250-mg amoxicillin/125-mg clavulanate tablets should not be taken at one time, as the double dose of clavulanate is more likely to cause GI toxicity. (A cost-effective method of giving the 500-mg dose is to give one 250-mg amoxicillin/125-mg clavulanate tablet along with one 250-mg generic tablet of amoxicillin.)

   The chewable tablets and adult tablets have different amoxicillin-clavulanate ratios, as just listed, and should not be interchanged.

 b. **For adults**

  (1) The usual dose is one 250-mg tablet q8h or one 500-mg tablet q12h.

  (2) For more severe infections and respiratory tract infections, one tablet of 875 mg q12h or one table of 500 mg q8h is advised by the package insert.

  (3) **N.B.** The bid (q12h) regimens are associated with less GI side effects. (See Sec. 5.)

c. **Children**
   (1) **Suspension or tablets for children:**
      (a) **For otitis media therapy of treatment failures,** higher doses of the amoxicillin component are being advised 80 to 90 mg/kg/day, using the new formulation to keep the dose of clavulanate at about 10 mg/kg/day (8). Prior doses were based on 40 to 45 mg/kg/day of the amoxicillin component (Chap. 1).
      (b) For sinusitis, lower respiratory tract infections, and more severe infections, based on the amoxicillin component, 45 mg/kg/day divided q12h or 40 mg/kg/day divided q8h has been used.
      (c) For less severe infection 25 mg/kg/day divided q12h or 20 mg/kg/day divided q8h has been suggested.
   (2) **Children weighing 40 kg or more can follow adult dose regimens**. The adult-sized 250-mg tablet should not be used unless the child weighs more than 40 kg.

d. **Renal failure.** The package insert does not suggest dose modification if renal failure is modest (i.e., a creatinine clearance of more than 30 ml/min).
   (1) Patients with a creatinine clearance of less than 30 ml/min should not receive the 875-mg tablet.
   (2) Patients with a creatinine clearance of 10 to 30 ml/min should receive 250 mg or 500 mg q12h, depending on the severity of infection.
   (3) Patients with creatinine clearance of less than 10 ml/min should receive 250 mg or 500 mg every 24 hours, depending on the severity of infection.
   (4) **Hemodialysis patients** should receive 250 mg or 500 mg q24h, depending on the severity of infection. Patients should receive an additional dose during and at the end of dialysis.

e. **Pregnancy.** This is a category B agent. (See Chap. 14.) The package insert indicates that because there are no adequate and well-controlled studies in pregnant women, this agent should be used during pregnancy only if clearly needed. The combination has been used safely in studies of pregnant women with bacteriuria or UTIs (9).

f. **Nursing mothers.** Because amoxicillin is excreted into milk, the package insert suggests caution should be exercised if this agent is administered to a nursing woman.

5. **Side effects**

   a. The usual side effects of penicillin can occur with amoxicillin-clavulanate. (See Chap. 16.)

   b. **GI side effects**—including nausea, vomiting, diarrhea, and abdominal cramps—are reported to occur in 10% or more of patients (9). These are related in part to the dose of clavulanate (i.e., more symptoms at higher doses) and can be **minimized if the drug is taken at the start of a meal** (1,9). **Also the bid regimens** are associated with fewer side effects than the tid regimens (Sec. 4a).

6. **Cost.** This is a relatively **expensive** agent. (See Appendix, Table C.)

IV. **Intravenous beta-lactam and beta-lactamase combinations.**

   A. **Ampicillin-sulbactam (Unasyn)** was approved in 1987.

      1. *In vitro* **activity.** Sulbactam inhibits many bacterial beta-lactamases, thereby extending the activity of ampicillin. The combination *in vitro* is active against beta-lactamase-producing strains of *H. influenzae, M. catarrhalis, N. gonorrhoeae,* many anaerobes (including *B. fragilis*), *E. coli, Proteus* spp., *Klebsiella* spp., *Acinetobacter calcoaceticus, S. aureus,* and *S. epidermidis.*

         a. **Ampicillin-sulbactam is not active against MRSA, *P. aeruginosa* and certain Enterobacteriaceae strains (*Serratia, Enterobacter,* and *Citrobacter* spp.)** (as discussed in Sec. III.A.3).

         b. **In addition, approximately 20% to 25% or more of *E. coli*** (including community-acquired) **are resistant** to this combination (9). Most of these *E. coli* strains have minimal inhibitory concentrations (MICs) that are very close to the breakpoint concentration for determining susceptibility (≤ 8 μg/ml). Although the clinical significance of this laboratory observation is unknown, a study in an animal model of infection caused by an ampicillin-sulbactam-resistant isolates of *E. coli* found the agent to be ineffective (10).

         c. Overall, not as many gram-negative bacilli are inhibited by ampicillin-sulbactam *in vitro* as by other intravenous beta-lactam/beta-lactamase combinations or with many cephalosporins (**Table 18-2**).

      2. **Pharmacokinetics.** The pharmacokinetics of ampicillin are not altered by the coadministration of sulbactam. **Excretion**, of both components, is primarily in the urine. **Tissue levels** are achieved

Table 18-2. Comparison of *in vitro* susceptibility data

Organism	Number Tested	Antimicrobial	% Susceptible
Escherichia coli	10,942	Piperacillin-tazobactam	91.5
		Ticarcillin-clavulanate	88.8
		Ampicillin-sulbactam	65.4
		Cefoxitin	96.1
		Cefotetan	99.3
		Ceftriaxone	99.2
		Imipenem	99.7
		Aztreonam	98.1
		Ciprofloxacin	99.0
Klebsiella pneumoniae	4,405	Piperacillin-tazobactam	90.9
		Ticarcillin-clavulanate	91.3
		Ampicillin-sulbactam	75.2
		Cefoxitin	90.3
		Cefotetan	97.4
		Ceftriaxone	95.2
		Imipenem	99.6
		Aztreonam	94.1
		Ciprofloxacin	94.5
Proteus mirabilis	3,822	Piperacillin-tazobactam	96.2
		Ticarcillin-clavulanate	95.0
		Ampicillin-sulbactam	90.4
		Cefoxitin	94.7
		Cefotetan	97.7
		Ceftriaxone	98.5
		Imipenem	82.9
		Aztreonam	91.7
		Ciprofloxacin	96.6
Serratia marcescens	1,392	Piperacillin-tazobactam	86.9
		Ticarcillin-clavulanate	84.3
		Ampicillin-sulbactam	9.1
		Cefoxitin	16.7
		Cefotetan	94.3
		Ceftriaxone	85.8
		Imipenem	90.5
		Aztreonam	86.0
		Ciprofloxacin	86.0

continued

Table 18-2. *(Continued)*

Organism	Number Tested	Antimicrobial	% Susceptible
Pseudomonas aeruginosa	2,941	Piperacillin	88.6
		Piperacillin-tazobactam	91.5
		Ticarcillin-clavulanate	86.3
		Ampicillin-sulbactam	2.1
		Cefoxitin	1.5
		Cefotetan	3.2
		Ceftriaxone	17.5
		Imipenem	88.0
		Ciprofloxacin	79.4
Staphylococcus aureus	4,454	Piperacillin-tazobactam	96.6
		Ticarcillin-clavulanate	98.1
		Ampicillin-sulbactam	98.0
		Cefoxitin	98.1
		Ceftriaxone	98.4
		Imipenem	98.7
		Ciprofloxacin	91.7
Streptococcus agalactiae (group B)	701	Piperacillin-tazobactam	98.2
		Ticarcillin-clavulanate	97.0
		Ampicillin-sulbactam	99.6
		Cefoxitin	96.6
		Ceftriaxone	97.0
		Imipenem	99.4
		Ciprofloxacin	92.9
Streptococcus faecalis	2,624	Piperacillin-tazobactam	94.7
		Ticarcillin-clavulanate	23.2
		Ampicillin-sulbactam	97.0
		Cefoxitin	2.1
		Ceftriaxone	7.0
		Imipenem	95.5
		Ciprofloxacin	62.5

Source: Adapted from Murray PR, et al. and the In Vitro Susceptibility Surveillance Group. Multicenter evaluation of the in vitro activity of piperacillin-tazobactam compared with eleven selected β-lactam antibiotics and ciprofloxacin against more than 42,000 aerobic gram-positive and gram-negative bacteria. *Diagn Microbiol Infect Dis* 1994;19:111.

in extravascular fluids, bile, and peritoneal and cerebrospinal fluid.

3. **Clinical uses** (1,2). This agent has been very useful, especially in the mixed aerobic and anaerobic infections, including mild to moderately severe community-acquired intraabdominal infections, aspiration pneumonias, community-acquired pneumonia (although it does not cover *Legionella* or *Mycoplasma*), UTIs, pelvic infections, deep neck infections, and soft-tissue infections, including diabetic foot infections.

4. **Dosage**
   a. **Adults.** The **usual dose** for mild to moderate infection is **1.5 g** (1 g ampicillin plus 0.5 g sulbactam) **q6h** if renal function is normal.

   - **In severe infection and/or most intraabdominal infections**, 3 g (2 g ampicillin and 1 g sulbactam) q6h is used.
   - **It is important to adjust doses in the elderly and those with renal dysfunction** to avoid excess serum levels (with potentially more side effects) and to provide cost-effective dosing (**Table 18-3**).

   b. **Pediatrics.** The package insert notes that the safety and effectiveness of ampicillin-sulbactam has been established for pediatric patients 1 year of age and older for skin and soft-tissue infections. The dose used in children is 300 mg/kg/day divided up q6h.
   c. **In renal failure,** the elimination of ampicillin and sulbactam is similarly affected and dose modification is necessary (**Table 18-3**).
   d. **Pregnancy.** This is a category B agent. (See Chap. 14.) Because there are no adequate studies in pregnant women, the package insert suggests this drug should be used during pregnancy only if clearly indicated.

Table 18-3. Ampicillin-sulbactam dosages in patients with renal impairment*

Creatinine Clearance (ml/min)	Recommended Dosage
>50	1.5–3.0 g q6h
30–50	1.5–3.0 g q6–8h
15–29	1.5–3.0 g q12h
5–14	1.5–3.0 g q24h

* In patients undergoing hemodialysis, preliminary data suggest the ampicillin will be partially removed (approximately 60%) but not the sulbactam. One could therefore give a supplemental dose of ampicillin after dialysis or time the daily dose of ampicillin-sulbactam so that it is given after dialysis.

   e. **Nursing mothers.** Low concentrations of
      this combination are excreted into milk.
      Therefore the package insert suggests cau-
      tion should be exercised when ampicillin-sul-
      bactam is administered to a nursing woman.
   f. **Contraindicated in ampicillin-allergic
      patients.** Because this agent contains ampi-
      cillin, it is contraindicated in patients aller-
      gic to ampicillin or other penicillins (unless
      skin testing is performed). This seems obvi-
      ous but is **a concern if physicians order
      antibiotics by a trade name (Unasyn)
      rather than its generic name.** This concern
      also applied to the combination of ticarcillin-
      clavulanate (Timentin) and piperacillin-
      tazobactam (Zosyn), discussed later.
5. **Side effects.** These are the same as those known
   to occur with ampicillin (9).
   a. Ampicillin **allergic reactions,** commonly
      rashes, can occur.
   b. **Minor enzyme elevations** (serum aspar-
      tate aminotransferase and alanine amino-
      transferase) occur in approximately 6% of
      recipients.
   c. Ampicillin-sulbactam may have a marked
      effect on oral flora, leading to colonization
      with gram-negative rods and fungi.
6. **Cost.** See Table B in the Appendix.
7. **Conclusion.** The role of this combination continues to evolve. Since its introduction in 1987, it
   has been a very popular agent for polymicrobial
   infections, diabetic foot ulcer infections, mild to
   moderate community-acquired intraabdominal
   and pelvic infections, mixed aerobic/anaerobic
   soft-tissue infections, selected cases of aspiration
   pneumonia, and severe UTI.
      In a survey we did in 1995, many infectious
   disease specialists believed this agent was often
   overused at their institutions; many were also
   changing to piperacillin-tazobactam.
   a. **See Sec. D for how this agent compares
      with similar** beta-lactam/beta-lactamase
      combinations; piperacillin-tazobactam may
      be preferred.
   b. We **would not use** ampicillin-sulbactam
      as monotherapy in patients with severe or
      life-threatening intraabdominal infection or
      mixed aerobic/anaerobic soft-tissue infections
      but prefer a combination of antibiotics in this
      setting (e.g., a third-generation cephalosporin
      and metronidazole or ampicillin-sulbactam
      and gentamicin). In addition, we would not
      use this agent alone for severe nosocomial
      infections, as many hospital-acquired gram-
      negative bacteria, including *E. coli* and *Kleb-*

siella spp., may be resistant; *Pseudomonas* spp. are also resistant. An aminoglycoside could be combined with it. It should not be used to treat methicillin-resistant staphylococcal infections.

   c. Ampicillin-sulbactam has not been studied extensively for treatment of infections in immunocompromised patients (9).

B. **Ticarcillin-clavulanate (Timentin)** (1,2)

   1. **Spectrum of activity.** This is very similar to that discussed for ampicillin-sulbactam under Sec. A.1 except for the following:

- The concerns with *E. coli in vitro* susceptibilities are not as prominent with ticarcillin-clavulanate. Nevertheless, many hospital-acquired *E. coli* are resistant.
- Enterococci are less susceptible to this agent than ampicillin-sulbactam or piperacillin-tazobactam.
- This agent is active against many strains of *P. aeruginosa* but is not as active as piperacillin-tazobactam against this organism (**Table 18-2**).

   2. **Pharmacokinetics.** Ticarcillin is excreted primarily by the kidney, with very high urine levels achieved. The half-life of both agents is approximately 1 hour, necessitating a 4- to 6-hour dose interval. Dosage adjustments are necessary in significant renal failure. The combination penetrates tissues well.

   3. **Clinical uses** indicate that this combination is effective for a variety of polymicrobial infections with susceptible pathogens (similar to ampicillin-sulbactam), including intraabdominal infections, pelvic infections, osteomyelitis, pneumonia, bacteremias, UTI, and skin and soft-tissue infections.

   4. **Dosages**

     a. **Adults.** Ticarcillin-clavulanate is available in 3.1-g vials containing 3 g ticarcillin and 0.1 g clavulanic acid as the potassium salt. The usual dosage in the average adult (60 kg) for systemic infections is one 3.1-g vial every 4 to 6 hours if the creatinine clearance is more than 60 ml/min. For gynecologic infections, in moderate infection 200 mg/kg/day in divided doses q6h and for severe infection 300 mg/kg/day (based on the ticarcillin content) in divided doses q4h is suggested by the package insert. For patients weighing less than 60 kg, the recommended dosage is 200 to 300 mg/kg/day (based on the ticarcillin content) divided every 4 to 6 hours.

       A vial containing 3 g ticarcillin and 0.2 g clavulanic acid is also available. This has been used in UTI, with a dosage of 3.2 g given q8h, per the package insert, when renal function is normal.

b. **Children** (≥3 months)

(1) In patients weighing less than 60 kg, 50 mg/kg/dose based on the ticarcillin component administered as follows:

- For mild to moderate infections, a dose q6h
- For severe infections, a dose q4h

(2) In patients weighing more than 60 kg,

- For mild to moderate infections, 3.1 g q6h
- For severe infections, 3.1 g q4h

c. **In renal failure,** in adults, use a normal loading dose. Thereafter, for a creatinine clearance of 10 to 50 ml/min 2 g q6 to 8h can be used and for a clearance of less than 10 ml/min, 2 g q12h is suggested.

d. **Prior penicillin allergy precludes the use of this agent** unless skin testing is done.

e. **Pregnancy**. This is a category B agent. Because there are no adequate and well-controlled studies in pregnant women, the package insert suggests this agent should be used during pregnancy only if clearly indicated.

f. **Nursing mothers.** The package insert suggests caution should be exercised when this agent is administered to a nursing woman.

5. **Side effects** are similar to those for penicillin, ampicillin, and/or ticarcillin. See prior discussions. The potential for hypokalemia and the potential for platelet abnormalities exist.

6. **Cost.** See Appendix Table B.

7. **Conclusion**

a. The main indication for the use of ticarcillin-clavulanate is for polymicrobial infections with susceptible aerobic and anaerobic infections. Traditionally, this agent has been popular on ob-gyn services for pelvic and intraabdominal infections.

b. In a survey we did in 1995, many infectious disease subspecialists had replaced this agent with one of the newer beta-lactam/betalactamase agents (e.g., piperacillin-tazobactam) and saw no special niche for this agent.

c. **We would not use it** as monotherapy in severe or life-threatening infections and prefer a combination of antibiotics. We would also not use it as monotherapy for severe nosocomial infections, because many hospital-acquired gram-negative bacteria may be resistant to it. Finally, it should not be used to treat MRSA infections.

In febrile, granulocytopenic cancer patients, ticarcillin-clavulanate has been evaluated primarily in combination with an aminoglycoside (9), and other options are available in this setting. (See Chap. 12.)

d. **See Sec. D for** a comparison of beta-lactam/beta-lactamase combinations; **piperacillin-tazobactam may be preferred.**

C. **Piperacillin-tazobactam (Zosyn)** became available in the United States in 1993 (11–13).

1. **Spectrum of activity.** Of the available beta-lactam/beta-lactamase antibiotics, piperacillin-tazobactam is the most active *in vitro*, in large part reflecting the enhanced *in vitro* activity of piperacillin over ampicillin and ticarcillin. (See Sec. III.A.4.) This agent has an *in vitro* spectrum of activity comparable to that of imipenem-cilastatin and superior to that of ceftazidime, ticarcillin-clavulanate, and ampicillin-sulbactam (9) (**Table 18-3**).

a. **Gram-positive aerobes.** This combination is active against methicillin-susceptible *S. aureus, S. pyogenes, S. agalactiae*, and *S. pneumoniae* (but not highly penicillin-resistant strains). Although it is active against *Enterococcus faecalis*, piperacillin-tazobactam is not active against *E. faecium* and MRSA (11).

b. **Enterobacteriaceae.** Most community-acquired Enterobacteriaceae (e.g., *E. coli, Klebsiella* spp.) are susceptible, but because of poor activity of piperacillin-tazobactam against many of the class 1 beta-lactamases, *E. aerogenes, E. cloacae, Citrobacter* spp., *Serratia* spp., and *P. aeruginosa* may be resistant (**Table 18-3**). (See Sec. III.A.3.)

c. Piperacillin-tazobactam has excellent activity against *H. influenzae, M. catarrhalis, Yersinia enterocolitica,* and *Plesiomonas shigelloides* but **not** *Salmonella* spp. or *Xanthomonas maltophilia*.

d. **Anaerobes.** Piperacillin-tazobactam has good activity against *B. fragilis* (but less than that of imipenem), *Bacteroides* spp., and *Clostridium perfringens* (11). Mouth anaerobes are typically susceptible to penicillin and piperacillin. Although some reviewers conclude there are no significant differences between the activity against anaerobes of piperacillin-tazobactam and other beta-lactamase inhibitor combination agents (9), other reviewers have concluded that piperacillin-tazobactam inhibits a broader spectrum of anaerobes than does ampicillin-sulbactam and ticarcillin-clavulanate (13) after review of the literature.

2. **Pharmacokinetics**. Preparations contain an 8:1 ratio of piperacillin to tazobactam; tazobactam does not interfere with the pharmacokinetics of piperacillin. Renal excretion accounts for 50% to 60% of the administered dose. Doses must be reduced in patients with a creatinine clearance of less than 40 ml/min (11).

3. **Clinical use.** Piperacillin-tazobactam has been used in **polymicrobial infections**. Early clinical studies have recently been summarized (11–13). The combination has been approved for use for moderate to severe infections with susceptible pathogens and appears effective in the following situations:

   a. **Intraabdominal infections** (especially appendicitis, including cases complicated by rupture or abscess). The combination appears as effective as imipenem or therapy with clindamycin and gentamicin (2).

   b. **Pelvic infections** in women.

   c. **Mixed** aerobic **skin and soft-tissue** infections, including diabetic foot infections.

   d. **Community-acquired pneumonia**, including beta-lactamase-producing *H. influenzae*. However, this agent is not active against *Mycoplasma* or *Legionella* (11). In addition, although it is an appealing agent for nosocomial pneumonia, it should not be used as monotherapy for suspected or known *P. aeruginosa* nosocomial pneumonia, for failures in this setting have been reported if piperacillin-tazobactam is used. Piperacillin-tazobactam has been combined with an aminoglycoside for nosocomial pneumonia therapy (11).

   e. **Clinical investigation.** Piperacillin-tazobactam with an aminoglycoside has been used for empiric therapy of the febrile, leukopenic patient without a focal infection (11).

4. **Dosages**

   a. **Adults**

      (1) The **usual dose** of piperacillin-tazobactam is **3 g/0.375 g q6h** if the creatinine clearance is higher than 40 ml/min (i.e., 12 g piperacillin per day).

      (2) For empiric therapy nosocomial pneumonia, the package insert suggests the 3.375 g dose q4h along with an aminoglycoside to ensure activity against *P. aeruginosa*.

      • If no *P. aeruginosa* is isolated, then the aminoglycoside can be stopped.

- If *P. aeruginosa* is isolated, then piperacillin alone can be used with an aminoglycoside since in documented pseudomonas infection, tazobactam does not enhance the activity of piperacillin against this pathogen (11), but will increase the cost of therapy.

(3) **An alternate approach for high-dose** therapy is to use a 4.5-g vial (piperacillin 4 g and tazobactam 0.5 g) q6h, along with an aminoglycoside for empiric therapy of nosocomial infections and possible pseudomonas infection (13).

b. **Children.** As of 2000, the package insert indicates the safety and efficacy in pediatric patients has not been established.

c. **In renal failure dose reductions** are shown in Table 18-4.

(1) For patients receiving **hemodialysis**, the package insert suggests the maximum dose of piperacillin-tazobactam is 2 g/0.25 g q8h. Because hemodialysis will remove 30% to 40% of the dose in a 4-hour dialysis, one additional dose of 0.75 g can be given after dialysis.

(2) **In chronic ambulatory peritoneal dialysis** (CAPD), approximately 10% of the piperacillin dose is recovered (11). Until further guidelines are available, in CAPD patients select the dose as if the creatinine clearance is less than 10 ml/min (**Table 18-4**).

d. In **cirrhosis** or other hepatic disease, no dosage modifications are required (13).

e. **Pregnancy.** This is a category B agent. (See Chap. 14.) There are no adequate and

Table 18-4. Piperacillin-tazobactam dosages in renal failure

Creatinine clearance (ml/min)	Recommended dosage regimen
>40	12 g/1.5 g/day in divided doses of 3.375 g q6h
20–40	8 g/1.0 g/day in divided doses of 2.25 g q6h
<20	6 g/0.75 g/day in divided doses of 2.25 g q8h

Source: From *Physician's Desk Reference,* 54th ed. Montvale, NJ: Medical Economics, 2000:1562.

well-controlled studies with piperacillin-tazobactam in pregnant women. Therefore the drug should be used during pregnancy only if clearly indicated (9).

f. **Nursing mothers.** Piperacillin is excreted in low concentrations in human milk; whether tazobactam is in human milk has not been studied. Therefore the package insert suggests that caution be used if this agent is administered to a nursing woman.

5. **Side effects.** The toxicity of piperacillin-tazobactam is similar to that of other penicillins and beta-lactam antibiotics (11–13). The most common side effects include the following:

   a. **Gastrointestinal** disorders, primarily diarrhea and nausea, occur in 4.6% of recipients.

   b. Skin reactions occur in 2.2% of recipients, with fewer than 1% having a rash.

   c. No significant hepatic or renal dysfunction has been noted in early reports.

   d. Mild hypokalemia can occur, presumably due to the nonresorbable anions presented to the distal tubules, which cause an increase in the pH and a secondary loss of potassium ions.

D. **Ticarcillin-clavulanate versus ampicillin-sulbactam versus piperacillin-tazobactam**. The optimal agent for selected polymicrobial infections has not been clearly delineated in the medical literature. None of these beta-lactam/beta-lactamase combinations is listed as the antibiotic of first choice for any specific pathogen (3). In a recent review (9), the authors concluded that "because of its broad spectrum of antibacterial activity, it (piperacillin-tazobactam) appears to be the best suited for treatment of mixed infections." In a 1996 summary of piperacillin-tazobactam, after an extensive review of the literature, the authors conclude, "The proven and theoretical advantages of piperacillin-tazobactam in comparison with those of ticarcillin-clavulanate appear to more than offset the modest difference in cost between the two compounds" (13).

   When one of these drugs is indicated, we would offer the following considerations:

   1. For situations in which *E. coli* is a likely pathogen, because 20% to 25% of *E. coli* strains are resistant to ampicillin-sulbactam, piperacillin-tazobactam is advised, although ticarcillin-clavulanate may be a reasonable alternative if one of these agents is to be used.

   2. Because cefazolin is effective against most community-acquired *E. coli* strains, the more expensive beta-lactam/beta-lactamase inhibitor combinations should be used selectively. For community-acquired intraabdominal or pelvic infections, we favor the most cost-effective cefazolin-metronidazole combination. (See Chap. 6.)

3. **Piperacillin-tazobactam can be used selectively** in the following situations:
   a. Severe (limb-threatening) diabetic foot ulcer infections, as discussed in Chap. 3.
   b. Selected patients with severe head and neck infections, complex sinusitis in the hospitalized patient.
   c. As monotherapy in nosocomial pneumonia not acquired in an intensive care unit (ICU) and where risk for *P. aeruginosa* infection is low and it is desirable to avoid an aminoglycoside.
   d. Selected ICU nosocomial pneumonias. If this drug is chosen, at least while awaiting cultures, it is advisable to combine it with an aminoglycoside. Usually, we would use piperacillin and an aminoglycoside combination as a more cost-effective regimen in this setting.
4. None of these agents should be used as monotherapy for known or highly suspected severe *P. aeruginosa* infection (e.g., pneumonia, sepsis) or as monotherapy in febrile episodes in neutropenic patients. This would preclude monotherapy with one of these agents for serious nosocomial infections, especially acquired in an ICU setting.
5. For the situation in which monotherapy is indicated and we are deciding between one of these beta-lactam/beta-lactamase combinations and imipenem, we tend to "save" imipenem for those patients who may have or develop resistant pathogens. (See Chap. 20.)

References

1. Reese RE, Betts RF. Broad spectrum penicillins and beta-lactam-beta-lactamase combinations. In: Reese RE, Betts RF, eds. *A practical approach to infectious diseases*, 4th ed. Boston: Little, Brown. 1996:Chap. 28E.
2. Wright AJ. The penicillins. *Mayo Clin Proc* 1999;74:290.
3. The Medical Letter. The choice of antimicrobial drugs. *Med Lett Drugs Ther* 1998;40:33 and 1999;41:95.
4. Aronoff GR, et al. *Drug prescribing in renal failure: dosage guidelines for adults,* 4th ed. Philadelphia: American College of Physicians, 1999.
5. Boguniewiez M, Leung YM. Hypersensitivity reactions to antibiotics commonly used in children. *Pediatr Infect Dis J* 1995;14:221.
6. Sattler FR, et al. Impaired hemostasis caused by beta-lactam antibiotics. *Am J Surg* 1988;155(5A):30.
7. Moellering RC Jr. Importance of beta-lactamase inhibitors in overcoming bacterial resistance. *Infect Dis Clin Pract* 1995;4:S1 (suppl 1).

8. Dowell SF, et al. Acute otitis media: management and surveillance in an era of pneumococcal resistance—a report from the drug-resistance *Streptococcus pneumoniae* Therapeutic Working Group. *Pediatr Infect Dis J* 1999;18:1.
   Treatment failures are defined as lack of clinical improvement after 3 days of therapy. Agents used for treatment failures should be active against beta-lactamase-producing H. influenzae *and* M. catarrhalis *and most penicillin-resistant* S. pneumoniae.

9. Bush LM, Calmon J, Johnson CC. Newer penicillins and beta-lactamase inhibitors. *Infect Dis Clin North Am* 1995;9:653.

10. Rice L, Carias L, Shlaes D. Efficacy of ampicillin-sulbactam versus that cefoxitin on treatment of *Escherichia coli* infections in a rat intra-abdominal model. *Antimicrob Agents Chemother* 1993; 37:610.

11. Bryson HM, Brogden RN. Piperacillin/tazobactam: a review of its antibacterial activity, pharmacokinetic properties, and therapeutic potential. *Drugs* 1994;47:506.
    Extensive review.

12. Moellering RC, et al. Piperacillin-tazobactam: a new dimension in antibiotic therapy. *Infect Dis Clin Pract* 1996;4:S1 (suppl 1).

13. Sanders WE Jr, Sanders CC. Piperacillin-tazobactam: a critical review of evolving clinical literature. *Clin Infect Dis* 1996;22:107.

The cephalosporins continue to be useful and popular antibiotics (1,2). They are **bactericidal** agents that inhibit bacterial cell wall synthesis. They remain appealing agents since they are safe, familiar to the clinician, active against penicillinase-producing *Staphylococcus aureus*, and possible to use in patients with delayed penicillin allergies. Unless special skin tests can be performed, **cephalosporins should be avoided in patients with a history of an immediate severe reaction to a penicillin** (or cephalosporin), such as anaphylaxis or angioedema. (See Sec. IV.A.)

I. **Introduction**

A. **Agents available**. The currently available cephalosporins are shown in **Table 19.1. The goal of this chapter is to summarize and to emphasize a limited number of agents that are particularly useful** and have withstood the test of time.

1. **From a historical standpoint,** it is useful to note that the different "generations" of parenteral cephalosporins had a logical sequence in terms of their development by the pharmaceutical industry.

a. **The first-generation** agents were active against methicillin-susceptible *S. aureus*, penicillin-susceptible *Streptococcus pneumoniae*, and other common gram-positive bacteria (e.g., streptococci group A and B, viridans streptococci) as well as many community-acquired gram negatives. These agents remain active and useful against these pathogens.

b. The **second-generation** agents cefamandole and later cefuroxime were developed because of their activity against ampicillin-susceptible and -resistant *Haemophilus influenzae* (and *Moraxella catarrhalis*), as well as many *S. pneumoniae*, while cefoxitin was the first cephalosporin to be active against anaerobes, especially *Bacteroides fragilis*; it was also active against *Neisseria gonorrhoeae*, including penicillinase-producing strains. Although still available and useful, these agents enjoy less popularity than in the past, for reasons to be discussed.

c. The **third-generation** agents were initially touted as having enhanced gram-negative activity, including activity against hospital-acquired pathogens and against *Pseudomonas aeruginosa* (e.g., ceftazidime). This still holds. In addition, the once-daily ceftriaxone agent has significant gram-positive

Table 19-1.   The major cephalosporins

First Generation	Second Generation	Third Generation
Parenteral	**Parenteral**	**Parenteral**
Cephalothin (Keflin)	Cefamandole (Mandol)	Cefotaxime (Claforan)
Cefazolin (Ancef, Kefzol)	Cefoxitin (Mefoxin)*	Cefoperazone‡ (Cefobid)
Cephapirin (Cefadyl)	Cefuroxime (Zinacef)	Ceftizoxime (Cefizox)‡
Cephradine (Velosef)	Cefotetan (Cefotan)*	Ceftriaxone (Rocephin)
		Ceftazidime (Fortaz, Tazidime, or Tazicef)
		Cefepime (Maxipime)†
Oral	**Oral**	**Oral**
Cephalexin (Keflex)	Cefuroxime axetil (Ceftin)	Cefixime (Suprax)
Cephradine (Velosef, Anspor)	Cefprozil (Cefzil)	Cefpodoxime (Vantin)‡
	Loracarbef (Lorabid)*‡	Ceftibuten (Cedax)‡
Cefadroxil (Duricef)‡	Cefaclor (Ceclor)‡	Cefdinir (Omnicef)‡

* A cephalosporin-like antibiotic.

† Some authors have referred to this agent as a fourth-generation cephalosporin; see text.

‡ We seldom use this agent. See text.

activity and has found many clinical roles in the hospital, emergency room, and home intravenous (IV) therapy.

    d. Cefepime has sometimes been called a **fourth-generation agent**, but it may be better summarized as a "hybrid" of cefotaxime and ceftazidime, two third-generation agents. The role of cefepime is still evolving.

  2. The cephalosporin "antibiotic market domination" of the late 1980s has been diminished somewhat by the advent of newer antibiotics, especially the newer quinolones released in the late 1980s and the newer macrolides (clarithromycin and azithromycin) released in the early 1990s.

  B. **Side effects**. These agents, overall are **well tolerated**. Their side effects are reviewed in Sec. IV unless there are special considerations with an individual agent, which are discussed under that agent.

  C. **Pharmacokinetic** data for the parenteral agents are summarized in **Table 19.2**. Like the penicillins, the antimicrobial effects of the cephalosporins depend on the presence of sustained concentrations of active

Table 19-2. Pharmacokinetic properties of parenteral cephalosporins (in adults)

	Half-Life (h)	Standard Dose (g)	Usual Dose Interval (h)	Half-Life (h) in End-Stage Renal Disease
Cephalothin	0.6	1.0–2.0	4	10
Cefoxitin	0.9	1.0–2.0	4–6–8	10–22
Cefotaxime	1.0*	1.0–2.0	6–8	3
Cefuroxime	1.0	0.75–1.5	6–8	15–20
Cefazolin	1.8	1.0	6–8	18–36
Cefoperazone	1.8	2.0	6–8	2
Ceftizoxime	1.8	2.0	8	25–35
Ceftazidime	1.8	1.0–2.0	8	16–25
Cefepime	2.0	1.0–2.0	12	14
Cefotetan	4.5	1.0–2.0	12	12–35
Ceftriaxone	7.0	1.0–2.0	24†	12–15

* Cefotaxime has a half-life of 1 hour in persons with normal renal function but is metabolized to a desacetyl derivative, which has a half-life of 1.6 hours and possesses significant antimicrobial activity and may interact synergistically with the parent compound (1).
† For non-CNS infections; for meningitis doses are given q12h. See text.

drug above the minimal inhibitory concentration of the infecting organism (**time-dependent killing**; see Chap. 14).

D. **Resistance issues**

1. **Intrinsic resistance**. Some organisms are always resistant to cephalosporins (e.g., all enterococci, *Listeria monocytogenes*, and the organisms of "atypical pneumonia" [*Legionella, Mycoplasma,* and *Chlamydia* spp.]) (2).

2. **Mechanisms of action and bacterial resistance**. The cephalosporins exert their antimicrobial effect by interfering with the synthesis of peptidoglycan, a major component of the bacterial cell wall; penicillin binding proteins (PBPs) are the targets of the cephalosporins (2). A detailed discussion of bacterial resistance of the cephalosporins is beyond the scope of this chapter. The three most common mechanisms by which bacteria can be resistant to cephalosporins include (a) production of enzymes, beta-lactamases, to inactivate drugs; (b) alteration of the drug target (essential PBPs); or (c) changes in the outer membrane that limit the ability of the drug to reach the target (2).

   a. **"Inducible beta-lactamase" production** can occur especially with certain species (*Enterobacter* spp., *Citrobacter* spp., *P. aeruginosa*). Clinically, this phenomenon manifests as treatment failure and emergence of drug-resistant organisms despite initial susceptibility to the cephalosporin used (1,2).

   b. **"Extended-spectrum beta-lactamases"** have recently been described, especially with nosocomial *Klebsiella pneumonia*. They confer high-level resistance to all beta-lactams. However, *in vitro* testing will indicate resistance mainly to ceftazidime, but suggest susceptibility to other cephalosporins which is erroneous (2).

3. **With unnecessary use of broad-spectrum cephalosporins** (e.g., especially with ceftazidime), resistance may develop. Prudent use of antibiotics is therefore important. (See Chap. 14.)

II. **Philosophy of use of IV preparations**

A. **First generation. Cefazolin (Ancef, Kefzol)** is the most commonly used agent, for it can be given IV (or intramuscularly) q6 to 8h rather than q4 to 6h, which other first-generation agents require.

1. **This first-generation agent is still the most active cephalosporin against methicillin-susceptible *S. aureus*** and is active against many gram-positive organisms. Therefore it is useful in the following:

   a. **Routine surgical prophylaxis.** (See Chap. 15 for details.)

    b. Known or suspected **methicillin-suscepti-ble S. *aureus*** (but not methicillin-resistant *S. aureus* [MRSA]) infections.

    c. An alternative agent for penicillin-suscep-tible *S. pneumoniae, S. pyogenes*, viridans streptococci, and *S. agalactiae* (streptococci group B).

2. **Still useful for community-acquired gram negatives** (e.g., *E. coli, K. pneumoniae*, etc).

    a. Cefazolin remains a useful agent for mild cholecystitis in patients under 70 years of age, and in initial cases of community-acquired pyelonephritis.

    b. The combination of cefazolin (active against gram negatives) and metronidazole (active against bowel anaerobes) is a very cost-effective regimen for community-acquired intraabdominal infections. (See related dis-cussion in Chap. 6.)

3. Cefazolin does not penetrate the cerebrospinal fluid (CSF) adequately.

4. **Cefazolin and other cephalosporins are not active against enterococci.** However, in most mixed aerobic and anaerobic intraabdom-inal infections, enterococci do not require spe-cific antimicrobial treatment. (See Chap. 6.)

5. **Pregnancy.** Since this agent is a category B agent (see Chap. 14), it should be used in pregnancy only if clearly indicated.

6. **In nursing mothers.** Cefazolin is present in very low concentrations in the milk; the package insert suggests caution should be exercised when cefazolin is used.

7. **Dosing.** See **Table 19.3.**

8. **Side effects.** See Sec. IV.

9. **Cost.** See Appendix Table B.

B. **Second-generation** cephalosporins.

1. **Cefamandole (Mandol)** use has largely been replaced by cefuroxime or third-generation ceph-alosporins. From a **historical standpoint**, it is important to emphasize that **this agent was associated with a significant risk of hypo-prothrombinemia** (more than 10% of recipients) **presumably related to the N-methylthio-tetrazole (NMTT) side chain**, which interferes with prothrombin synthesis. Although contro-versial, **similar concerns persist in newer agents (e.g., cefotetan) that have this same side chain.**

2. **Cefuroxime (Zinacef, Kefurox)** has been a pop-ular agent since the middle to late 1980s and has replaced cefamandole. Because of its spec-trum of activity (see Sec. a), it became and still is very popular for respiratory infections. In 1993,

Table 19-3. Typical dosages and summary of parenteral (IV) cephalosporins

Agent	Common Adult Single IV Dose*	Usual Dose Interval in Normal Renal Function[†] (h)	Typical Total Adult Daily Dose (g)	Pediatric Dose (d = day)	Dose Interval (h) with Decreased Creatinine Clearance				CSF Penetration	Potential for Bleeding Side Effects
					>50	30–49	10–29	<10		
First generation										
Cefazolin (Ancef, Kefzol)	0.5–1 g	8	1.5–3.0	25–100 mg/kg/d; divided into q6–8h equal doses	8	12	24	24–48	Poor	In renal failure
Second generation										
Cefoxitin (Mefoxin)	2 g	6–8	6–8	80–160 mg/kg/d; divided into q4–6h doses	6–8	8–12	12–24	24[‡]	Poor	
Cefuroxime (Zinacef)	750 mg–1.5 g	8	2.25–4.5	75–100 mg/kg/d; divided into q8h	8	8	12	24	Modest	No
Cefotetan (Cefotan)	1–2 g	12	2–4	Not advised	12	12	24	48	Poor	Yes
Third generation										
Cefotaxime (Claforan)	1–2 g	8[‡‡]	3–6	50–180 mg/kg/d; divided into q6h[§]	8[‡‡]	8–12	12	24	Excellent	No
Ceftriaxone (Rocephin)	1–2g[#]	24[#]	1–2	In meningitis, loading dose of 75 mg/kg and then 100 mg/kg/d (not	24[**]	24[**]	24[**]	See text	Excellent	No

Ceftazidime (Fortaz, Tazidime, Tazicef)	1–2 g	8	3–6	to exceed 4 g/d) divided q12h. In other infections, 50–75 mg/kg/d (not to exceed 2 g) divided q12h or once-daily doses 90–150 mg/kg/d; divided q8h (to maximum 6 g/d)	8	12–24*	24–48*	48–72*	Excellent	No
Expanded spectrum or fourth generation										
Cefepime (Maxipime)	1–2 g	12††	4	50 mg/kg/dose q12h†† if over 2 months of age	Usual	See text			Modest	

* Doses suggested for moderately severe infections; higher dose in severe infection.

† Or in patients with creatinine clearance >50 ml/min.

‡ Dose is also reduced 50%. See text.

§ Higher dose range of cefotaxime used in meningitis. Use adult dosages in children weighing >50 kg. Neonatal dosages shown in Appendix Table A.

‡‡ Dose interval for cefotaxime in children is usually q6h.

In meningitis, 2 g q12h is advised (see text). In less severe infections, 1 g daily may be used. See text.

** In CNS infections, a q12h regimen is preferred. See text.

†† In neutropenic patients, a higher-dose regimen is used: 2 g q8h in adults, and 50 mg/kg/dose q8h in children.

the American Thoracic Society (3) favored its use in empiric therapy of community-acquired pneumonia, especially in adults with comorbid illness. However, with the recent increased incidence of penicillin-resistant *S. pneumoniae* and the *in vitro* data suggesting cefuroxime is not an optimal agent for this pathogen, the role of cefuroxime as of early 2000 is undergoing considerable reassessment. (See Sec. a. below and Chaps. 2 and 16 for related discussions.)

a. ***In vitro* activity**

(1) **Gram-positive organisms**. Cefuroxime is very active against group A and B streptococci, viridans streptococci but not enterococci. Generally, cefuroxime is less active against methicillin-susceptible *S. aureus* than the first-generation cephalosporins (e.g., cefazolin), but cefuroxime is still active with a minimum inhibitory concentration $(MIC)_{90} \leq 1.6$ μg/ml.

In a recent *in vitro* study of more than 1,500 respiratory isolates of *S. pneumoniae*, cefuroxime was active against 99.1% of penicillin-susceptible strains, 53% of penicillin—intermediately susceptible strains, and no high-level penicillin-resistant strains (4). (See related discussions in Chap. 2.)

(2) **Gram-negative organisms.** Cefuroxime is very active against ampicillin-susceptible and ampicillin-resistant *H. influenzae* and *M. catarrhalis* as well as *Neisseria meningitidis*, *N. gonorrhoeae* (including penicillinase producers), and *Pasteurella multocida*. It is active against many community-acquired gram-negative bacteria (e.g., *E. coli, Klebsiella* spp., etc) but is less active *in vitro* than the third-generation cephalosporins against gram-negative bacteria.

Many hospital-acquired gram negatives and most *Pseudomonas* spp. and *Providencia* spp. are resistant.

(3) **Anaerobes**. Cefuroxime is not as active as cefoxitin or cefotetan against bowel anaerobes. Practically speaking, we would not rely on cefuroxime for anaerobic activity.

(4) ***Borrelia burgdorferi*** (agent of Lyme disease) are susceptible.

    b. **Pharmacokinetics**. See **Table 19.2.**

    c. **Clinical uses**. Although cefuroxime has commonly been used for community-acquired pneumonia (CAP), postinfluenza pneumonia, orbital cellulitis, complicated sinusitis, and epiglottitis, as of early 2000 it is less favored in these settings. (See Sec. a. above, Chaps. 2 and 16 for related discussions.)

        Oral cefuroxime (cefuroxime axetil, Ceftin) is considered one of the drugs of choice for early Lyme disease (i.e., erythema migrans) (5, 5A).

    d. **Doses**. See **Table 19.3.**

    e. **Pregnancy**. Since this is a category B agent, it should only be used if clearly indicated.

    f. **In nursing mothers,** since cefuroxime is excreted into milk, the package insert advises caution should be exercised when cefuroxime is administered to a nursing woman.

    g. **Cost**. See Appendix Table B.

    h. **Side effects**. See Sec. IV.

3. **Cefoxitin (Mefoxin)** is a cephamycin antibiotic (cephalosporin-like) that has enhanced anaerobic activity.

    a. *In vitro* **activity**

        (1) **Gram-positive bacteria**. Cefoxitin is slightly less active than the first-generation agents.

        (2) **Gram-negative bacteria**. Cefoxitin remains active against many community-acquired gram-negative bacteria but is not active against many hospital-acquired gram-negative bacteria (e.g., *Pseudomonas* spp., *Enterobacter cloacae*). It is active against *N. gonorrhoeae*, including penicillinase-producers.

        (3) **Anaerobes.** Cefoxitin is active *in vitro* against 80% to 90% of strains of *B. fragilis* at clinically achievable concentrations, although in well-established anaerobic infections, cefoxitin may not be as effective *in vivo*. **Generally, cefoxitin is viewed as the cephalosporin with the best activity *in vitro* against oral and bowel anaerobes.**

    b. **Pharmacokinetics**. See **Table 19.2.**

    c. **Clinical uses**

        (1) **Community-acquired mild to moderate intraabdominal infections**. For almost two decades, cefoxitin has been useful in these mixed gastrointestinal (GI) flora infections, especially before an abscess develops. Cefoxitin

remains a useful agent in diverticulitis, very early appendix rupture, and early to mild bowel perforation before *B. fragilis* has become established in high titers. However, the clinician has many antibiotic options for these infections, including ampicillin-sulbactam, ticarcilin-clavulanate, piperacillin-tazobactam. (See Chap. 6.) **Because cefoxitin and these beta-lactam and beta-lactamase inhibitor combinations are expensive, we often prefer a combination of cefazolin** (aimed at community-acquired gram negatives) **and metronidazole** (aimed at anaerobes) for mild to moderate community-acquired intraabdominal infections (see Chap. 6) and pelvic infections, see Sec. (2) below that do not involve *N. gonorrhoeae*.

(2)   **Pelvic infections**. Since cefoxitin is active against *N. gonorrhoeae*, many gram-negative bacilli, and most anaerobes, it has been clinically successful in a variety of pelvic infections, early pelvic abscesses, and pelvic inflammatory disease (PID) regimens. (See Chap. 10.)

(3)   **Mild to moderate mixed aerobic/anaerobic soft-tissue infections** may respond well to monotherapy with cefoxitin. The best results may occur when the duration of illness, prior to initiation of antibiotics, is short. Cefoxitin has been used in the mixed-flora foot infections in diabetic patients; it is not active against enterococci whose role in this setting is often unclear. (See Chap. 3.)

(4)   **Note. Cefoxitin should not be relied on as monotherapy in** the very ill patients with **bacteremia due to *B. fragilis*** (since cefoxitin may not be active against 5% to 15% of these isolates), **hospital-acquired intraabdominal sepsis** (since resistant gram-negative bacteria may be involved) **or a critically ill patient with intraabdominal sepsis or peritonitis**.

d.   **Dosing**. See **Table 19.3.**

e.   **Pregnancy**. Since cefoxitin is a category B agent, it should be used in pregnancy only if clearly indicated.

f.   **In nursing mothers**. Since low concentrations of cefoxitin are excreted in human milk, the package insert suggests caution should be exercised when this agent is administered to nursing mothers.

g. **Side effects**. See Sec. IV.

h. **Cost.** See Appendix Table B.

4. **Cefotetan** (**Cefotan**) has been promoted as a cost-effective cefoxitin-like agent with good anaerobic activity. Cefotetan can be given q12h, which is more cost-effective than the q6 to 8h cefoxitin regimens.

a. *In vitro* **activity**

(1) **Gram positives**. Overall, cefotetan is two to four times less active against gram-positive cocci than cefoxitin (6).

(2) **Gram-negative aerobes.** *In vitro,* cefotetan is more active than cefoxitin against enteric gram-negative bacilli but less active than the third-generation cephalosporins. It is active against gonococci but is inactive against many hospital-acquired gram negatives, including many strains of *Enterobacter* spp. and most strains of *P. aeruginosa* and *Acinetobacter* spp.

(3) **Anaerobes**. Cefotetan is considered comparable to cefoxitin *in vitro* against *B. fragilis* spp. but is less active against other *Bacteroides* spp. within the *B. fragilis* group (1).

b. **Potential side effect of hypoprothrombinemia. Cefotetan contains the NMTT side chain**, which may be related to an increased incidence of hypoprothrombinemia. (See Sec. II.B.1.) The exact incidence of this with cefotetan is unclear. Of interest, the package insert warning for cefotetan (but not cefoxitin) indicates that cefotetan "may be associated with a fall in prothrombin activity (i.e., a prolongation of protime) and, possibly, subsequent bleeding. Those at increased risk include patients with renal or hepatobiliary impairment or poor nutritional status, the elderly, and patients with cancer. **Prothrombin times should be monitored and exogenous vitamin K administered as indicated**" (7).

In his review of cefotetan's symposium, Barza concludes: "In my opinion, there is a higher risk of hypoprothrombinemia with cefotetan than with cefoxitin in patients who are vitamin K-deficient. However, if physicians are aware of this liability and provide vitamin K supplementation, the benefits of cefotetan, especially the cost savings, make it an attractive substitute for cefoxitin" (6).

We concur with Dr. Barza's conclusions but **suspect that many physicians who are using cefotetan in high-risk patients are not monitoring their patients as the literature and package inserts advise.**

c. **Clinical use** of cefotetan

(1) **For patients with underlying risk factors for hypoprothrombinemia (see Sec. b on p. 375), we do not recommend using cefotetan.**

(2) For young, otherwise healthy women with pelvic infections, endometritis, PID, or mild to moderate community-acquired intraabdominal infections, cefotetan for short courses is reasonable.

A similar view was presented in a publication of clinical practice guidelines. The Committee on Antimicrobial Agents of the Canadian Infectious Disease Society suggested that cefotetan could be considered an alternative single agent for prophylaxis of infection in patients undergoing elective bowel surgery, and it may be used to treat patients with acute PID and endometritis, but hypoprothrombinemia in debilitated patients is a concern (8).

(3) Cefotetan's role in **GI surgical prophylaxis** is reviewed in Chap. 15.

d. **Dosing.** See **Table 19.3.** As of early 2000, the safety and efficacy in children has not been established.

e. **Pregnancy.** Since this is a category B agent, it should be used only if clearly indicated.

f. **In nursing mothers**. Since cefoxitin is excreted into human milk, the package insert suggests caution should be used when administering to a nursing woman.

g. **Other side effects**. See Sec. IV.

h. **Cost.** See Appendix Table B.

5. **Cefonicid** (Monocid). As of 1999, this agent is no longer available in the United States.

C. **Third-generation cephalosporins** are **useful in several settings,** as shown in **Table 19.4.** Excessive use will select out for resistance, especially with ceftazidime. These agents are drugs of choice for only a limited number of organisms (**Table 19.4**).

1. **In vitro** activity

a. **Gram-positive aerobes** (9)

(1) **S. aureus.** The first- and some second-generation cephalosporins are at least two- to fourfold more active than cefotaxime, ceftizoxime, and ceftriaxone against penicillin-susceptible *S. aureus* and against some, but not all, beta-

Table 19-4. Common uses of third-generation cephalosporins

Setting	Agent Commonly Used	Comment
Gram-negative enteric meningitis (e.g., E. coli, Klebsiella spp.)	Cefotaxime,* Ceftriaxone, Ceftazidime	An unusual clinical problem. Seen in neonates, or post neurosurgery.
Bacterial meningitis	Cefotaxime,* ceftriaxone[†]	Excellent for H. influenzae,[†] N. meningitidis, and penicillin susceptible S. pneumoniae. For penicillin-resistant S. pneumoniae need vancomycin (see Chaps. 2, 11, and 16) and for Listeria monocytogenes need ampicillin or TMP-SMZ.
Febrile neutropenic patient without a focal source	Ceftazidime, cefepime[‡]	Ceftazidime not active against gram (+) cocci. If there is a Hickman catheter infection, would need to add IV vancomycin until culture data are available. Cefepime not active against MRSA. Also see Chapter 12.
S. viridans endocarditis	Ceftriaxone	Once-a-day dose.
P. aeruginosa activity	Ceftazidime, cefepime	For synergy (e.g., in pneumonia) combined with an aminoglycoside. Ceftazidime has little gram-positive activity. Ceftriaxone not active against P. aeruginosa.

continued

Table 19-4. (*Continued*)

Setting	Agent Commonly Used	Comment
Broad-spectrum activity (see text)	Ceftriaxone (cefepime also an option)	Ceftazidime has little gram-positive activity. Ceftriaxone not active against *P. aeruginosa*.
Gram-negative pathogens (e.g. *E. coli*, *K. pneumoniae*; indole-positive *Proteus*, *P. vulgaris*; *Morganella morganii*; *Providence stuartii*, *Serratia* spp.[†]	Ceftriaxone, cefotaxime, ceftazidime; cefepime	Active against most community-acquired gram negatives. Certain hospital-acquired gram negatives may be resistant.
N. gonorrhoeae infections	Ceftriaxone[†]	See Chap. 10.
Pseudomonas pseudomallei	Ceftazidime[†]	Rare problem.
Haemophilus ducreyi (chancroid)	Ceftriaxone[†]	Azithromycin is also an agent of choice.
Borrelia burgdorferi (Lyme disease)	Ceftriaxone	See *Med Lett Drugs Ther* 1997;39:47.

* For neonates, use cefotaxime, not ceftriaxone. See text.

[†] **Agent considered a "drug of choice"** (5).

[‡] In patients at high risk for severe infection (including patients with a history of recent bone marrow transplantation, with hypotension at presentation, with underlying hematologic malignancy or with severe or prolonged neutropenia) the package insert notes monotherapy may not be appropriate. Insufficient data exists to support efficacy in such patients.

lactamase-producing strains. When considering cefotaxime, ceftizoxime, or ceftriaxone in suspected sepsis in which staphylococci cannot be excluded, one of these three cephalosporins provides adequate initial activity against staphylococci (9). In patients with documented severe staphylococcal infections (e.g., *S. aureus* bacteremia), we would not use a third-generation cephalosporin as an agent of choice but would prefer an antistaphylococcal penicillin (e.g., oxacillin or nafcillin) or a first-generation cephalosporin (e.g., cefazolin).

(2) **Coagulase-negative staphylococci.** If the organisms are methicillin-resistant, a cephalosporin is not recommended, even if the *in vitro* data suggest that a cephalosporin may be active. If methicillin-susceptible, cephalosporins are potential agents, although vancomycin often is used.

(3) **Group A streptococci**. Some third-generation cephalosporins (cefotaxime, ceftizoxime, and ceftriaxone) are very active against these pathogens, with MICs typically less than 0.03 µg/ml, comparable to benzylpenicillin and, in fact, more active than cefazolin or cefoxitin.

(4) **Group B streptococci (*S. agalactiae*)** are also extremely susceptible to cefotaxime, ceftizoxime, and ceftriaxone, again with a MIC comparable to penicillin G and lower than cefazolin.

(5) **Groups C and G streptococci** are also very susceptible to the aforementioned third-generation agents.

(6) **Most viridans streptococci and *Streptococcus bovis*** have lower MICs for these third-generation agents than the first- or second-generation cephalosporins. This has implications in alternate endocarditis therapeutic regimens (e.g., ceftriaxone once daily).

(7) **_S. pneumoniae._** Cefotaxime, ceftizoxime, and ceftriaxone are very active against the usual highly susceptible organisms. *In vitro,* **in one large report ceftriaxone is active against 92% of intermediate-level penicillin-resistant strains but only 27% of high-level resistant strains** (4).

(8) These agents **are not active** against *L. monocytogenes*, enterococci, MRSA,

and most high-level penicillin-resistant *S. pneumoniae.*

b. **Gram-negative aerobes** (9)

(1) ***H. influenzae*** (and other *Haemophilus* spp.) and ***N. gonorrhoeae*** are extremely susceptible to the third-generation cephalosporins, including strains that produce beta-lactamases.

(2) ***N. meningitidis*** and ***M. catarrhalis*** are also very susceptible to the third-generation cephalosporins.

(3) **Enterobacteriaceae**. Resistance to cephalosporins has increased in some but not all species. In fact, **the excellent *in vitro* activity of the third-generation cephalosporins against gram negatives is a major advantage of these agents over the first- and second-generation cephalosporins.** Bacteria resistant to the older cephalosporins and, at times, even the aminoglycosides are often susceptible to the third-generation cephalosporins.

(a) ***E. coli***, both community-acquired and hospital-acquired, are usually very susceptible to the third-generation agents (i.e., cefotaxime, ceftizoxime, ceftriaxone, and ceftazidime [and cefepime]).

(b) **Most *Klebsiella*** spp. remain susceptible; occasionally, nosocomial strains isolated in the United States are resistant (and these usually are susceptible to imipenem). (See Sec. I.D.2. on p. 368)

(c) ***P. mirabilis, Providencia,*** **and** ***Citrobacter*** **spp., and** ***P. vulgaris*** generally are inhibited by very low concentrations.

(d) ***Enterobacter*** **spp., especially** ***E. cloacae,*** **have been a major weakness of the third-generation cephalosporins**, and these organisms are important nosocomial pathogens. Approximately 10% to 30% of *E. cloacae* may initially be resistant to the third-generation cephalosporins, but even the isolates of *E. cloacae* with MICs of 1 µg/ml or less contain subpopulations of organisms that are easily selected for resistance to the third-generation cephalosporins. (See Sec. I.D.2.) Presumably, the general use of cephalosporins, including the first- and second-generation cephalosporins, has caused the increase in isolation of this species over the last two decades. Also, *C. freundii* **similarly develops resistance,** although it has not become as prominent a nosocomial pathogen as *E. cloacae.*

  (e) **Because of the variability in** *in vitro* **susceptibility data, individual susceptibility testing must be performed for each third-generation cephalosporin that may be used by the clinician.**

 (4) **For** *P. aeruginosa,* **ceftazidime and cefoperazone can be considered potential agents.** Because cefoperazone is less active (and has the NMTT side chain), we believe that **ceftazidime is the better third-generation cephalosporin for** *P. aeruginosa* **activity.** Ceftazidime's MIC_{90} for *P. aeruginosa* is 8 µg/ml, signifying only modest activity. Some *Pseudomonas cepacia* strains are inhibited by ceftazidime.

  Cefepime, released in January 1996, **has similar** *in vitro* **activity** against *P. aeruginosa,* as does ceftazidime. (See Sec. D. on p. 384)

 c. **Anaerobes.** The activity of the third-generation cephalosporins against anaerobes was summarized elsewhere (4), but a few points deserve emphasis.

 (1) The anaerobic activity of cefotaxime, ceftizoxime, and ceftriaxone is suitable for respiratory pathogens (i.e., oral anaerobes).

 (2) None of the third-generation agents is considered a drug of first choice or even an alternate agent for bowel-related *B. fragilis* (5). **Cefoxitin** and **cefotetan,** second-generation agents, are **more active** *in vitro* **against anaerobes than any third-generation agent.**

 2. **Pharmacokinetics** are shown in **Table 19.2.**

 3. **Dosages** are shown in **Table 19.3,** including doses in renal failure.

 4. **Brief summary of individual agents**

 a. **Cefotaxime (Claforan)** was the first third-generation cephalosporin introduced and is still the **preferred agent in neonates** in part because we have the most experience with this agent and in part because it does not interfere with bilirubin metabolism in the neonate, as may ceftriaxone.

Otherwise, in adults, **ceftriaxone, which can be given once daily in most infections, and q12h in central nervous system infections, has often replaced cefotaxime in therapy of older children and adults because of its ease of administration.**

(1) **Pregnancy.** This is a category B agent. (See Chap. 14.)

(2) **Nursing.** Cefotaxime is excreted in human milk. The package insert suggests caution should be exercised when this agent is administered to a nursing woman.

(3) **Cost.** See Table B in the Appendix.

b. **Cefoperazone (Cefobid)** is not quite as active as ceftazidime against *P. aeruginosa* and contains the NMTT side chain, which appears associated with hypoprothrombinemia. (See Sec. II.B.1. on p. 369) **We do not favor the use of this agent.**

c. **Ceftizoxime (Cefizox)** must be given q8 to 12h for severe infections and q4h for life-threatening infections. **It has largely been replaced by ceftriaxone which is given q12 to 24h.**

d. **Ceftazidime (Fortaz, Tazidime, or Taxicef)** and cefepime are the most active cephalosporins against *P. aeruginosa.* **Ceftazidime has poor activity against gram-positive aerobes.** Its niche often involves therapy against known or potential *P. aeruginosa* infection, including the following:

(1) **Nonbacteremic, febrile, leukopenic patients** without an obvious source of infection and without a line-related infection (10,11). (See Chap. 12.)

(2) *P. aeruginosa* **meningitis.** In this rare problem, infectious disease consultation is advised.

(3) **In combination with an aminoglycoside for *P. aeruginosa* tissue or bloodstream infections in a patient with a delayed penicillin allergy.**

(4) **In nosocomial pneumonia** in which a gram stain or culture has ruled out *S. aureus*, ceftazidime has been used but in this setting resistance commonly occurs (e.g., with hospital-acquired *Enterobacter* spp).

(5) In malignant external otitis and early lower respiratory tract infections in cystic fibrosis patients.

(6) **Miscellaneous**

- **Pregnancy**. This is a category B agent. (See Chap. 14.)
- **Nursing**. Ceftazidime is excreted in human milk. The package insert advises it should be used with caution in a nursing woman.
- **Cost**. See Appendix Table B.
- **Resistance** will occur with excess use. (See Chap. 14 and Sec. I.D earlier.)

e. **Ceftriaxone (Rocephin)** is a **popular agent** both due to its broad spectrum of activity and its long half-life, allowing for q24h dosing in non–central nervous system (CNS) infections (Table 19.2).

(1) **See common uses in Table 19.4.** As monotherapy, it has been effective against serious infections.

It is **not advised in neonates** since ceftriaxone binds to serum proteins and may displace bilirubin. **Cefotaxime is preferred in neonates.**

(2) **Dosing. See Table 19.3.** For non-CNS infections, **in adults** a single dose given once daily is preferred, usually 1 g q24h. For CNS infections (e.g., meningitis, brain abscess), maximal doses are used, 2 g q12h in adults.

In children, with meningitis or severe infection, q12h regimen is used.

For neonates, cefotaxime is preferred; see Table A in the Appendix.

(3) **In renal failure.** Ceftriaxone has dual hepatic (40%) and renal (60%) excretion; in renal failure, the rate of hepatic excretion increases (2) so that dose adjustments are usually not necessary in renal failure (1,2).

If both hepatic and renal failure are present, the half-life of ceftriaxone is prolonged. If serum levels are not available and ceftriaxone is clearly the agent of choice, we have used a reduced dose (e.g., 500 mg q24h) for non-CNS infections in adults (1) though serum monitoring is preferred.

In patients on hemodialysis, the package insert suggests serum levels be monitored.

(4) **Pregnancy.** This is a category B agent. (See Chap. 14.)

(5) **Nursing.** Low concentrations of ceftriaxone are excreted in human milk. The package insert suggests that caution be exercised when ceftriaxone is administered to nursing women.

(6) **Cost.** See Appendix Table B.

(7) **Common side** effects are **discussed in Sec. IV. Rarely,** ceftriaxone may cause "sludge" to form in the gallbladder, especially in children, causing "**biliary pseudolithiasis.**" Associated symptoms may include nausea, epigastric distress, vomiting, and right upper quadrant abdominal pain. This topic is reviewed elsewhere (12).

Overall, we have found this agent to be very well tolerated.

D. **Cefepime (Maxipime)** is an expanded-spectrum cephalosporin released in 1996 (13–16).

1. *In vitro* **activity.** It has activity against gram-positive organisms comparable to cefotaxime and activity against gram-negative aerobic organisms comparable or superior to ceftazidime. Cefepime is less active against methicillin-susceptible *S. aureus* than cefazolin. It is active against many strains of *P. aeruginosa* similar to the *in vitro* activity of ceftazidime. It is not active against enterococci, methicillin-resistant *S. aureus* (MRSA), *B. fragilis*, or high-level penicillin-resistant *S. pneumoniae*.

2. **Pharmacokinetics.** See Table 19.2.

3. **Approved indications** include therapy of susceptible pathogens in (a) uncomplicated and complicated UTIs, (b) uncomplicated skin infections, (c) moderate to severe pneumonia, and (d) empiric therapy for the febrile neutropenic patient (16).

N.B. The package insert indicates this agent should not be used in meningitis.

4. **Dosages**

a. **For adults** usually 1 to 2 g intravenously (IV) (or intramuscularly [IM]) q12h, depending on the severity of infection.

In the febrile leukopenic patient, 2 g q8h is advised.

b. **For children** more than 2 months of age

(1) If weight is less than 40 kg, 50 mg/kg/dose q12h for most infections but q8h in the febrile neutropenic patient. Maximum dose/day should not exceed adult doses.

(2) If weight is more than 40 kg, adult doses can be used.

    c. **In renal failure** the package insert suggests normal doses for a creatinine clearance of more than 60 ml.

      (1) **If the interval selected is q12h**, and the clearance is 30 to 60 ml/min, give the usual dose q24h; for a clearance of 10 to 30 ml/min, give 50% of the usual dose q24h; for a clearance of less than 10 ml/min, give 25% of the usual dose q24h.

      (2) **If the interval selected is q8h**, and the clearance is 30 to 60 ml/min, give the usual dose q12h; for a clearance of 10 to 30 ml/ min give the usual dose q24h; and for a clearance of less than 10 ml/min, give 50% of the usual dose q24h.

    d. **Pregnancy.** Since this is a category B agent (Chap. 14), it should be used only if clearly indicated.

    e. **Nursing mothers**. Since cefepime is excreted into human milk, the package insert suggests that caution should be used before it is prescribed.

  5. **Side effects.** (See Sec. IV.)

  6. **Cost.** See Appendix Table B.

  7. **Summary.** The exact role for cefepime awaits further clinical study and experience. Some institutions have replaced ceftazidime with cefepime. As with other broad-spectrum agents (e.g., imipenem, piperacillin-tazobactam), if these agents are used excessively, bacterial resistance will presumably develop. This is especially true in difficult-to-treat infections (e.g., those associated with a foreign body).

III. **Oral cephalosporins.** See Table 19-5. Although **these are expensive agents** (see Appendix Table C), they are commonly used. Adults will have less GI upset with cephalexin or cephradine than with oral antistaphylococcal agents (dicloxacillin). In children, taste and aftertaste are important in compliance. In one report, oral cephalosporin suspensions were more "acceptable" than other agents (17). In general, these agents are rapidly and thoroughly absorbed (2).

    The indications and uses for these agents have been **summarized in** Tables 19-5 and 19-6. We have still found it helpful to summarize these agents as first-, second-, and third-generation agents.

  A. **First-generation oral agents** are useful for mild to moderately severe penicillin- and methicillin-susceptible *S. aureus* and group A streptococcal infections of the skin and soft tissue and susceptible urinary tract infection (UTI) pathogens.

    1. **Cephalexin (Keflex)** is well absorbed but because of the relatively high MICs of the susceptible gram-negative organisms, **this agent is**

Table 19-5.   Oral cephalosporins

Agent	Indication	Comment
First generation Cephalexin (Keflex), or Cephradine (Anspor, Velosef)	Mild/minor soft-tissue infections due to methicillin-susceptible *S. aureus* and/or *S. pyogenes* (strep A) Susceptible UTI Alternative in strep pharyngitis*	Use an adequate dose since activity against *S. aureus* is modest and excretion is rapid. See text. Probably prudent to use seven-day course for uncomplicated UTI rather than three-day course.
Second generation Cefuroxime (Ceftin), or Cefprozil (Cefzil), or Loracarbef (Lorabid)	Alternative therapy in otitis media, sinusitis, bronchitis. See Chap. 1. Cefuroxime axetil (Ceftin) has been used in Lyme disease. Alternate therapy in early selected cases of community-acquired pneumonia (CAP). See Chap. 2.	These are relatively expensive agents. See Appendix Table C. Cefaclor falling out of favor in children, for it may cause serum sickness. Oral cefuroxime has a poor taste vs "bubble-gum" flavored cefprozil, which is bid dosing.
Third generation Cefixime (Suprax)	Alternate therapy for *H. influenzae* and *M. catarrhalis* therapy in otitis media Susceptible UTI or mild soft-tissue infections due to susceptible pathogens Alternate for uncomplicated GC therapy.	Less active against *S. pneumonia* and not active for *S. aureus*. Do *in vitro* susceptibility data to show activity. See Chap. 10.
	No unique niche	
Cefpodoxime (Vantin)	No unique role	See text.
Ceftibuten (Cedax)	No unique role	See text.
Cefdinir (Omnicef)	Possible alternative in flares of bronchitis No unique role	See text.

UTI, urinary tract infection; GC, gonococcal infection.
* Although second- and third-generation cephalosporins have been used for strep pharyngitis, the first-generation agents are the most cost-effective.

Table 19-6. Common clinical uses of oral cephalosporins

Setting	Particularly Useful Agents	Comments
Soft-tissue infections, cellulitis	First-generation agent preferred (e.g., cephalexin, cephradine)	When *S. aureus* and streptococci activity is desired. Agents provide poor gram-negative tissue levels. (Cefixime and ceftibuten have poor *S. aureus* activity; good gram-negative activity.)
Otitis media	Cefprozil	Useful in delayed penicillin-allergic patients and when ampicillin-resistant *H. influenzae* are known or highly suspected. See Chap. 1.
	Cefixime, ceftibuten	Have less activity against *S. pneumoniae*, so do not use for initial empiric therapy; are used for possible *H. influenzae* and *M. catarrhalis* infections.
Sinusitis	Cefuroxime axetil (adults) Cefprozil (children or adults)	Especially if cannot use less expensive agents (i.e., TMP/SMZ, amoxicillin). See Chap. 1.
Bronchitis	Cefuroxime, cefprozil	Alternative agents for delayed penicillin-allergic patients or patients on rotating antibiotic regimens. See Chap. 1. Cefixime and ceftibuten are not as active against *S. pneumoniae*.

continued

Table 19-6. (*Continued*)

Setting	Particularly Useful Agents	Comments
Streptococcal pharyngitis	First-generation agent	Most cost-effective alternative in the penicillin-allergic patient when a macrolide is not used. See Chap. 1.
Urinary tract infection	Cephalexin, cephradine Cefaclor, cefuroxime Cefixime	When susceptibility data support use. For uncomplicated UTI, a 7-day (not 3-day) course is preferred. See Chap. 4.
Community-acquired pneumonia, mild and typically when >55 y.o.	Cefuroxime	For completion of therapy when intravenous cefuroxime has been used (see text); selected cases for oral therapy. (See Chap. 2.)

not useful in soft-tissue infections due to gram-negative bacteria. For UTI, even for uncomplicated UTI, a 7-day course, not 3-day course, is advised. (See Chap. 4.)

  a. **Dosage.** The usual suggested adult dose is 250 to 500 mg q6h. When treating significant *S. aureus* soft tissue infection in adults, a dose of 500 to 1,000 mg q6h is preferred (18). We do not use the regimen of 250 mg per dose for soft-tissue infections.

   In children, 25 to 50 mg/kg/day is divided into four equal doses. In streptococcal pharyngitis, a bid regimen can be used. (See Chap. 1.)

  b. **In renal failure** when the creatinine clearance is less than 10 ml/min, the dose interval is prolonged to q12h (19); when the creatinine clearance is 10 to 50 ml/min, a dose can be given q8 to 12h, depending on the severity of disease and renal failure.

  c. **Pregnancy.** Since this is a category B agent (see Chap. 14), cephalexin should be used in pregnancy only if clearly indicated.

  d. **Nursing mothers**. Since cephalexin is excreted into human milk, the package insert suggests that caution should be used when it is administered to a nursing woman.

  e. **Side effects.** Sec. IV.

  f. **Cost.** See Appendix Table C.

2. **Cephradine (Anspor, Velosef)** is considered equivalent to cephalexin and may be preferred if available locally at a lower cost than cephalexin.

  a. **Dosages:** same as for cephalexin.

  b. **In renal failure**, if the creatinine clearance is more than 50 ml/min, a normal dose is given q6h. If the clearance is 10 to 50 ml/min, 50% of the usual dose is given at normal intervals. With a creatinine clearance of less than 10 ml/min, 25% of the usual dose is given at usual intervals (19). A dose is advised after dialysis. In patients undergoing chronic ambulatory peritoneal dialysis (CAPD), doses similar to those with a creatinine clearance of less than 10 ml/min can be used (19).

  c. **Pregnancy.** Cephradine is a category B agent. (See Chap. 14.)

  d. **Nursing mothers.** Since cephradine is excreted into human milk, the package insert suggests caution when it is administered to a nursing woman.

  e. **Side effects.** See Sec. IV.

  f. **Cost.** See Appendix Table C.

3. **Cefadroxil (Duricef)** is a very expensive agent with no unique niches. **We do not advocate its use.**

B. **Second-generation oral cephalosporins** have enjoyed immense popularity primarily for upper respiratory (acute otitis media, sinusitis) and lower respiratory tract infections (acute exacerbations of chronic bronchitis, early community-acquired pneumonia). (See Chaps. 1 and 2.) They are active against penicillin-susceptible and some intermediate penicillin-resistant *S. pneumoniae* (but not high-level penicillin-resistant), *M. catarrhalis,* and *H. influenzae*—including beta-lactamase-positive pathogens, streptococci group A—and have modest activity against methicillin-susceptible *S. aureus.*

All these agents are relatively expensive. For streptococcal pharyngitis in the allergic patient, if a cephalosporin is indicated, a first-generation agent (e.g., cephalexin) is preferred. (See Chap. 1.)

1. **Cefuroxime axetil (Ceftin)** has a relatively unpalatable taste, including the suspensions, and therefore an **alternate similar agent (e.g., cefprozil) seems prudent in children** in an attempt to improve compliance. It is active against beta-lactamase-positive and -negative *M. catarrhalis, S. aureus,* group A and B streptococci, penicillin-susceptible *S. pneumoniae,* and some intermediate-level penicillin-resistant *S. pneumoniae.* (See Chaps. 2 and 16.) In adults, oral cefuroxime has been used to complete therapy initiated with parenteral cefuroxime (see Sec. II.B.2, p. 369) and as an alternative agent for sinusitis or bronchitis, especially in an allergic patient. (See Chap. 1.)

   a. **Dosage.** For children more than 13 years of age and adults 250 to 500 mg bid, depending on the severity of infection. In early Lyme disease (erythema migrans) 500 mg bid in children over 12 and adults has been used (5A).

   b. In **mild or moderate to even severe renal failure,** usual doses are given (19).

   c. **Pregnancy.** Since this is a category B agent, this drug should be used in pregnancy only if clearly indicated.

   d. **Nursing.** Cefuroxime is excreted in human milk; the package insert suggests consideration should be given to discontinuing nursing temporarily during treatment.

   e. **Cost.** This is an expensive agent to use. See Appendix Table C.

   f. **Side effects.** See Sec. IV.

2. **Cefprozil (Cefzil)** has similar *in vitro* activity as cefuroxime axetil. Because it is available in a bubble-gum-flavored suspension and can be **given bid,** it is commonly used in **otitis media** when amoxicillin has failed or is contraindicated in an allergic patient. It also can be used in

sinusitis and **acute exacerbations of chronic bronchitis.**

   a. **Dosage.** Cefprozil is available as a 250-mg or 500-mg tablet as well as a liquid bubble-gum-flavor oral suspension with 125 mg/5 ml and 250 mg/5 ml.

      (1) **In adults** with exacerbations of bronchitis, 500 mg po bid is given. In sinusitis, a similar dose could be used.

      (2) **In children** (6 months to 12 years) 15 mg/kg q12h is suggested per package insert.

   b. **In renal failure.** If the creatinine clearance is over 30 ml/min, standard doses can be used. For a clearance less than 30 ml/min, the package insert suggests 50% of the standard dose at normal intervals. Since cefprozil is partially removed after dialysis, cefprozil should be given after completion of dialysis. In CAPD, use doses as if creatinine clearance were less than 10 ml/min (19).

   c. **Pregnancy.** Category B.

   d. **Nursing mothers.** A small amount of cefprozil appears in human milk. The package insert suggests caution be used when cefprozil is administered to a nursing woman since the effect of cefprozil on nursing infants is unknown.

   e. **Cost.** See Appendix Table C.

   f. **Side effects.** See Sec. IV.

3. **Loracarbef (Lorabid)** has a cephalosporin-like structure. Its spectrum of activity is similar to cefuroxime axetil and cefprozil. Loracarbef has been used especially in acute otitis media, sinusitis, acute bronchitis, and selected cases of CAP similar to the indications for cefuroxime axetil and cefprozil. **It has no special niches and we seldom use it.**

   a. **Dosing.** The ingestion of food will decrease and delay the peak serum concentration; **doses should be given 1 hour before or 2 hours after meals.** The suspension is more rapidly absorbed than the capsules, and the **suspension is recommended for otitis media,** per the package insert.

    Loracarbef is available in 200-mg pulvules and an oral suspension (100 mg/5 ml and 200 mg/5 ml).

      (1) **In adults** and children 13 years of age or more, for acute exacerbations of chronic bronchitis, CAP, sinusitis, and uncomplicated pyelonephritis, 400 mg q12h has been suggested.

      (2) **In children** (6 months to 12 years of age), for otitis, the suspension prepa-

ration at 30 mg/kg/day in divided doses q12h.

b. **In renal failure.** When the creatinine clearance is 10 to 49 ml/min, a normal dose at twice the usual dose interval is given (i.e., q24h). In patients with a creatinine clearance of less than 10 ml/min who are not undergoing hemodialysis, the usual dose can be given every 3 to 5 days (19). Patients undergoing hemodialysis should receive a supplemental dose after dialysis. For patients with CAPD, there are no data, but patients have been dosed as if their creatinine clearances are less than 10 ml/min (19).

c. **Pregnancy.** This is a category B agent. (See Chap. 14.)

d. **Nursing.** The package insert notes it is not known as of 2000 whether this drug is secreted into human milk. Therefore caution should be exercised when this agent is given to a nursing woman.

e. **Side effects.** See Sec. IV.

f. **Cost.** See Table C in Appendix.

4. **Cefaclor (Ceclor)** is associated at times with serum-sickness in children (see Sec. IV); 10% to 15% or more of ampicillin resistant *H. influenzae* are resistant to cefaclor. Furthermore, its activity against *S. pneumoniae* is inferior. **Consequently, another second-generation cephalosporin is often chosen** (e.g., cefuroxime in adults and cefprozil in children and adults) (1).

C. **Third-generation oral cephalosporins** are expensive and occasionally useful in the allergic patient and in the special circumstances discussed later. Since most microbiology laboratories can only perform susceptibility data on a limited number of agents, the susceptibility data of these agents often are not available unless specifically requested. **We use these agents in a very limited fashion.**

1. **Cefixime (Suprax)** is more active than previously available oral cephalosporins against many gram negatives (*E. coli, Klebsiella* spp., *P. mirabilis*, and *S. marcescens*) but has no useful activity against *Pseudomonas* spp., many strains of *Enterobacter* spp., and *Acinetobacter* spp. It is very active against *N. gonorrhoeae, H. influenzae,* and *M. catarrhalis*, including beta-lactamase producers. However, **it is not active against S. aureus** and has decreased activity against *S. pneumoniae* when compared with other oral cephalosporins (1). Cefixime is not active against anaerobes.

a. **Clinical use.** The exact role for this agent introduced in 1989 is still evolving. It can be considered especially in the following (1):

(1) **Uncomplicated gonococcal infection** regimens (see Chap. 10).

(2) For *H. influenzae* or *M. catarrhalis* otitis media infections, **but** since cefixime is not as active against *S. pneumoniae* (a common pathogen in otitis), **cefixime is not a first-line agent for otitis**; it has been used when amoxicillin has failed. (See Chap. 1.)

(3) **In selected cases of UTI or gram-negative soft-tissue infections**, when susceptibility data allow, cefixime may occasionally be useful, especially when allergies preclude using more conventional, less expensive regimens.

(4) **In its review,** *Medical Letter* **concluded** that cefixime had no demonstrated advantage over previously available antibiotics that cost much less (20). This conclusion remains valid!

b. **Dosing. The oral suspension is absorbed more rapidly and completely than the tablets and is preferred in the treatment of otitis media.** Tablets are available in 200-mg and 400-mg sizes; the oral suspension contains 100 mg/5 ml.

(1) **In adults and children older than 12 years of age**, 200 mg bid or 400 mg once daily is suggested.

(2) **In children** more than 6 months of age, 8 mg/kg/day of the suspension once daily or two divided doses are suggested. For children weighing more than 50 kg or older than 12, adult doses can be used.

c. **In renal failure**, the dose can be reduced. If the creatinine clearance is 10 to 50 ml/min, 75% of the standard dosage at the standard interval is given. Patients whose clearance is less than 10 ml/min or patients on CAPD may be given half the standard dose at the standard interval. Patients on hemodialysis can be given 300 mg after dialysis (19).

d. **Pregnancy.** Since this agent is a category B agent, it should not be used unless clearly indicated.

e. **Nursing mothers.** The package insert indicates it is not known whether cefixime is excreted in human milk; consideration should be given to discontinuing nursing during treatment with this drug.

f. **Side effects**. See Sec. IV.

2. **Cefpodoxime (Vantin)** was approved for use in 1992. It is modestly active against *S. aureus* ($MIC_{90} = 2.0$ µg/ml) and is active against common

respiratory pathogens, including penicillin-susceptible *S. pneumoniae; H. influenzae,* and *M. catarrhalis*, including beta-lactamase producers; and *Streptococcus* groups A and B. It is active against many Enterobacteriaceae but not against *Enterobacter, Serratia* or *Morganella,* or *Pseudomonas* spp. It has been used in UTIs, CAP, acute otitis, bronchitis, and single-dose therapy of uncomplicated gonorrhea.

   a. **Dosing.** Both 100-mg and 200-mg tablets and an oral suspension (50 mg/5 ml and 100 mg/5 ml) are available.

      (1) **In adults** and children 13 years of age or more, 200 mg q12h for moderately severe infection is used.

      (2) **For children** (6 months to 12 years): 10 mg/kg/day divided q12h (maximum 400 mg/day) for 10 days for otitis media.

   b. **In renal failure**, the dose interval can be changed (19). If the creatinine clearance is 10 to 50 ml/min, a standard dose can be given q16h; if the clearance is less than 10 ml/min, a standard dose can be given q24 to 48h. In patients undergoing hemodialysis, 200 mg after dialysis only is suggested. For patients undergoing CAPD, dose as if the creatinine clearance is less than 10 ml/min (19).

   c. **Pregnancy**. Category B. (See Chap. 14.)

   d. **Nursing mothers**. Cefpodoxime is excreted into human milk. The package insert suggests that since there is a potential for a reaction in the nursing infant, a decision should be made whether to continue nursing or discontinue the drug, taking into consideration the importance of the drug to the mother.

   e. **Editorial comment.** Shortly after its release, **the *Medical Letter*** reviewed this agent and concluded: **"Cefpodoxime is a broad-spectrum oral cephalosporin that offers no clear advantage over previously available drugs for the treatment of any infection"** (21). We still concur with this and see no unique niche for this agent. We do not use it.

   In the woman with many antibiotic allergies, when susceptibility data allow, it may be useful in selected UTIs.

3. **Ceftibuten (Cedax)** was approved for use in late 1995. The *in vitro* activity of this "third-generation" oral agent is similar to that of cefixime in that it has **enhanced activity against many Enterobacteriaceae, but many gram-positive organisms are resistant** (including *S. aureus, S. agalactiae*, and viridans strepto-

cocci). Anaerobes are not susceptible. Ceftibuten is not active against *Acinetobacter* spp. and *Pseudomonas* spp. Susceptibility data are reviewed in detail elsewhere (22).

a. Although approved for pharyngitis and tonsillitis, less expensive agents are available. (See Chap. 1.) It should not be used for empiric therapy of otitis media since it is not active against many pneumococcal infections. Ceftibuten is a consideration for acute bacterial exacerbations of chronic bronchitis due to susceptible *H. influenzae* and *M. catarrhalis* especially.

b. **Dosages**. Ceftibuten is available in 400-mg capsules and a suspension (90 mg/5 ml and 180 mg/5 ml).

   (1) **Adults and children more than 12 years of age** 400 mg once daily.

   (2) **Children more than 6 months of age**. The recommended dose is 9 mg/kg/day as a single dose (up to a maximum of 400 mg/day). The package insert emphasizes that the **suspension must be administered 2 hours before or 1 hour after a meal.**

c. **In renal failure**, the dose can be modified. If the creatinine clearance is between 10 to 50 ml/min, 50% of the usual dose is given q24h; if the clearance is less than 10 ml/min, 25% of the usual dose is given q24h (19). In patients undergoing hemodialysis, a single 300-mg dose or 9 mg/kg (maximum of 300 mg) should be administered at the end of each hemodialysis session. There are no data for CAPD patients as of early 2000; use doses as if the creatinine clearance is less than 10 ml/min (19).

d. **Pregnancy**. Since this is a category B agent, it should not be used in pregnancy unless clearly indicated.

e. **Nursing mothers**. As of early 2000, the package insert indicates it is not known whether ceftibuten is excreted into human milk; caution should be exercised when ceftibuten is administered to a nursing woman.

f. **Editorial comment**. So far, this agent has no unique niches. In general, other cephalosporins or other agents are preferred. Ceftibuten is another agent that could be used for acute exacerbations of chronic bronchitis, especially when a once-daily regimen is highly desirable or as an agent to rotate with other antibiotics in this setting. (See Chap. 1.)

The *Medical Letter* did not give this agent a very good report in its review in 1996 when it concluded "ceftibuten is an expensive new oral cephalosporin that seems like a poor choice for the indications for which it is being marketed. In particular, recommending a drug for use in acute otitis media except when caused by pneumococci makes no sense; pneumococci are a frequent cause of otitis media and in clinical practice, the pathogen is usually not identified" (23).

4. **Cefdinir (Omnicef)** was recently approved for use in mid-1998 and reviewed (2,24).

   a. *In vitro* **activity** (24). Cefdinir is similar to cefpodoxime in antibacterial activity. Cefdinir is active against MSSA; penicillin-susceptible *S. pneumoniae, H. influenzae, M. catarrhalis, N. gonorrhoeae*; and many gram-negative bacteria but not against *Pseudomonas* spp.

      Cefdinir is not active against MRSA, atypical pathogens (*Legionella, Mycoplasma, Chlamydia*), enterococcus, and many anaerobes. It is not active against high-level penicillin-resistant *S. pneumoniae*, and we view its activity against intermediately penicillin-resistant *S. pneumoniae* as inadequate. In one report, the MIC_{90} of cefdinir against these strains was 3.1 ug/ml and the package insert suggests average peak serum levels after a 600 mg dose is only 2.9 μg/ml (25).

   b. **Pharmacokinetics.** Cefdinir is absorbed somewhat slowly from the GI tract with bioavailability of the capsules of only about 20% and 25% for the suspension. Food does not affect absorption. The drug is not metabolized and is excreted in the urine (25).

   c. **Approved uses** include therapy of susceptible pathogens in acute maxillary sinusitis, otitis media, acute exacerbations of chronic bronchitis, community-acquired pneumonia, and skin infections.

   d. **Dosages** per package insert are as follows:

      (1) **For adults:** 300 mg q12h or 600 mg q24h (the once-daily regimen is not advised in pneumonia or skin infections).

      (2) **For children** (6 months to 12 years of age): 7 mg/kg q12h or 14 mg/kg q24h.

      (3) **In renal failure,** for patients **with a creatinine clearance of less than 30 ml/min** the package insert suggests:

      - **In adults,** 300 mg once qd
      - **In children,** 7 mg/kg (up to 300 mg) given once qd
      - **In hemodialysis** patients, the above reduced doses can be given every other day, with doses initiated after dialysis, which can remove cefdinir.

(4) **Pregnancy.** Since this is a category B agent, this drug should be used only when clearly indicated.

(5) **Nursing mothers.** The 2000 package insert notes that following a single 600-mg dose, cefdinir was not found in breast milk.

e. **Side effects.** Like other oral cephalosporins, cefdinir is well tolerated. Diarrhea and vaginal candidiasis are the most common side effects (24).

f. **Cost.** Like other second- and third-generation cephalosporins, this is an expensive agent: cost to the pharmacist for 10 days in an adult is $67 (24) for the 300 mg q12h regimen. See Appendix Table C.

g. **Summary.** In its recent review, the *Medical Letter* concluded: "cefdinir is an oral third-generation cephalosporin similar to cefpodoxime. **Older, better established drugs are preferred**" (24). **We agree with this conclusion and see no special niche for this agent.**

IV. **Side effects of cephalosporins. In general,** these agents, both oral and IV formulations, are very **well tolerated.**

A. **Primary allergic reactions.** Prior data suggest there is approximately a **1% to 3% incidence** of primary allergic reactions to cephalosporins: urticarial and morbilliform rashes, fevers, eosinophilia, serum sickness, and anaphylaxis, which is extremely rare at less than 0.02% of recipients (2).

1. **In the patient with a history of an immediate reaction to penicillin** (i.e., anaphylaxis, bronchospasm, hypotension, etc.), **cephalosporins should be avoided** (26) unless careful skin testing can be performed.

2. **In the patient with a late or delayed mild reaction** (e.g., morbilliform rash) **to penicillins, cephalosporins can be and are commonly used with caution.**

   Although in the penicillin-allergic patient, the risk of cross-reaction to the cephalosporins was formerly believed in the 5% to 15% range (2); at least with the third-generation cephalosporins more recent estimates of cross-reactions are as low as 1% (27).

3. **Serum sickness has been observed more in recipients of cefaclor** (28). There is a concern that loracarbef may have an increased risk of serum sickness since its structure is similar to that of cefaclor. Serum sickness has been reported with cefprozil (29).

B. **Nephrotoxicity** is infrequent with cephalosporin monotherapy (1,2). Interstitial nephritis has occurred as a hypersensitivity response.

C. **Hematologic effects**
1. **Positive Coombs' reactions** are relatively common (3%) in patients on high-dose parenteral therapy (2), but hemolytic anemia is rare.
2. **Granulocytopenia** and/or **thrombocytopenia** are **rare** complications. However, in patients **with severe underlying hepatic dysfunction, various beta-lactam antibiotics, including the cephalosporins, have been associated with leukopenia; such patients should perhaps receive lower doses of beta-lactam antibiotics** (30).
3. **Hypoprothrombinemia** associated with NMTT side chain is discussed in Secs. II.B.1 and II.B.4. It has also been described with cefazolin use in patients with renal failure because of the side chain similar in structure to NMTT in cefazolin.
D. **Phlebitis** with IV use is reported in 1% to 2% and is related more to the known risks of IV catheters than to a particular thrombogenic potential of the cephalosporins (2).
E. **Ethanol intolerance.** Disulfiram-like reactions (flushing, tachycardia, nausea, vomiting, headache, hypotension) have been described with patients receiving **cefoperazone, cefotetan,** and cefazolin. The reaction may be related to the NMTT structure. Patients receiving these agents probably should be advised *not* to consume alcohol or alcohol-containing medications (1,2).
F. *Clostridium difficile* **diarrhea** may occur more often in recipients of second- and third-generation cephalosporins (31), including the oral third-generation agents.

References

1. Reese RE, Betts RF. Cephalosporins. In: Reese RE, Betts RF, eds. *A practical approach to infectious diseases,* 4th ed. Boston: Little, Brown, 1996:Chap. 28F.
2. Marshall WF, Blair JE. The cephalosporins. *Mayo Clin Proc* 1999;74:187.
3. Niederman MS, et al. Guidelines for the initial management of adults with community-acquired pneumonia: diagnosis, assessment of severity, and initial antimicrobial therapy. *Am Rev Resp Dis* 1993;148:1418.
4. Thornsberry C, et al. Surveillance of antimicrobial resistance in *Streptococcus pneumoniae, Haemophilus influenzae,* and *Moraxella catarrhalis* in the United States in the 1996–1997 respiratory season. *Diagn Microbiol Infect Dis* 1997;29:249.
   See detailed discussion of the clinical implications of this paper in Chap. 2.
5. Medical Letter. The choice of antibacterial drugs. *Med Lett Drugs Ther* 1999;41:95.

5A. Medical Letter. Treatment of Lyme disease. *Med Lett Drugs Ther* 2000;42:37.

6. Barza M. Cefotetan: summary of the symposium from an internists viewpoint. *Am J Surg* 1988;155(5A):103.
   Excellent summary from a symposium devoted to this agent.

7. *Physicians Desk Reference,* 53rd ed. Montvale, NJ: Medical Economics, 1999:3409.

8. Committee on Antimicrobial Agents, Canadian Infectious Disease Society. Cefotetan: a second-generation cephalosporin active against anaerobic bacteria. *Can Med Assoc J* 1994;151:537.

9. Neu H. Pathophysiologic basis for the use of third generation cephalosporins. *Am J Med* 1990;88:3S (suppl 4A).
   An update of these agents after almost one decade of use.

10. DePauw BE, et al. Ceftazidime compared with piperacillin and tobramycin for empiric treatment of fever in neutropenic patients with cancer: a multicenter randomized trial. *Ann Intern Med* 1994;120:834.
    Study of more than 870 patients, ceftazidime (2g q8h) was as effective as piperacillin and tobramycin.

11. Hughes WT, et al. 1997 Guidelines for the use of antimicrobial agents in neutropenic patients with unexplained fever. *Clin Infect Dis* 1997;25:551.

12. Lopez AJ, et al. Ceftriaxone-induced cholelithiasis. *Ann Intern Med* 1991;115:712.

13. Barradell LB, Bryson HM. Cefepime: a review of its antimicrobial activity, pharmacokinetic properties, and therapeutic uses. *Drugs* 1994;47:471.

14. Cunha BA, Gill MA. Cefepime. *Med Clin North Am* 1995;79:721.

15. Medical Letter. Cefepime (Maxipime): a new parenteral cephalosporin. *Med Lett Drugs Ther* 1996;38:84.

16. Biron P, et al. Cefepime versus imipenem: cilastatin as empirical monotherapy in 400 febrile patients with short duration neutropenia. *J Antimicrob Chemother* 1998;42:511.
    See related study by Yamamura D, et al. Open randomized study of cefepime versus piperacillin-gentamicin for the treatment of febrile neutropenic cancer patients. Antimicrob Agents Chemother *1997;41:1704.*

17. Ruff ME, et al. Antimicrobial drug suspensions: a blind comparison of taste of fourteen pediatric drugs. *Pediatr Infect Dis J* 1991;10:30.
    The oral cephalosporins ranked the best.

18. Baxter R, Chapman J, Drew WI. Comparison of bactericidal activity of five antibiotics against *Staphylococcus aureus. J Infect Dis* 1990;161:23.
    With high doses (1 g q6h) cephalexin could provide peak serum cidal levels of 1:8.

19. Aronoff GR, et al. *Drug prescribing in renal failure: dosage guidelines for adults,* 4th ed. Philadelphia: American College of Physicians, 1999.

20. Medical Letter. Cefixime: a new oral cephalosporin. *Med Lett Drugs Ther* 1989;31:73.

21. Medical Letter. Cefpodoxime proxetil: a new oral cephalosporin. *Med Lett Drugs Ther* 1992;34:107.

22. Jones R. Ceftibuten: a review of antimicrobial activity, spectrum and other microbiologic features. *Pediatr Infect Dis J* 1995;14:S77.
    This supplement deals with this agent.

23. Medical Letter. Ceftibuten: a new oral cephalosporin. *Med Lett Drugs Ther* 1996;38:23.

24. Medical Letter. Cefdinir: a new oral cephalosporin. *Med Lett Drugs Ther* 1998;40:85.

25. Fukuoka T, et al. *In vitro* and *in vivo* activities of CS-834, a novel oral carbapenem. *Antimicrob Agents Chemother* 1997;41:2652. *Data of this new agent is compared with many antibiotics, including cefdinir.*

26. Fekety FR. Safety of parenteral third-generation cephalosporins. *Am J Med* 1990;88:38S (suppl 4A).

27. Donowitz GR Third generation cephalosporins. *Infect Dis Clin North Am* 1989;3:595.

28. Heckbert SR, et al. Serum sickness in children after antibiotic exposure: estimates of occurrence and morbidity in a health maintenance organization population. *Am J Epidemiol* 1990;132:336. *Risk of serum sickness was significantly higher after cefaclor than after amoxicillin. See similar conclusion in Martin J, et al. Serum sickness-like illness and antimicrobials in children.* N Z Med J *1995;108:123.*

29. Lowery N, et al. Serum sickness-like reactions associated with cefprozil therapy. *J Pediatr* 1994;125:325.

30. Singh N, et al. B-lactam antibiotic-induced leukopenia in severe hepatic dysfunction: risk factors and implications for dosing patients with liver disease. *Am J Med* 1993;94:251.

31. Nelson DE, et al. Epidemic *Clostridium difficile*-associated diarrhea: role of second- and third-generation cephalosporins. *Infect Control Hosp Epidemiol* 1994;15:88.

20

Unique Beta-lactam Antibiotics: Monobactams and Carbapenems (Aztreonam, Imipenem, and Meropenem)

I. **Aztreonam (Azactam)** is the first clinically useful monobactam. It is active against most of the gram-negative aerobes without the nephrotoxicity of aminoglycosides (gentamicin or tobramycin) (1).

   A. **Mechanism of action.** Aztreonam interferes with the biosynthesis of **bacterial cell walls** by binding to penicillin-binding proteins.

   B. *In vitro* **activity.** Aztreonam is **unique among the beta-lactam antibiotics because it is active only against gram-negative aerobes**.

   1. **Gram-positive aerobes**: little or no activity.
   2. **Anaerobes**: little or no activity.
   3. **Gram-negative aerobes**
      a. **Highly susceptible organisms** include beta-lactamase and non–beta-lactamase-producing strains of *Haemophilus influenzae* and *Neisseria gonorrhoeae*, as well as *N. meningitidis*.
      b. **Most Enterobacteriaceae** are inhibited by less than 1 µg/ml (1) except for resistant strains shown in Sec. d. below.
      c. *P. aeruginosa.* Aztreonam inhibits 50% of *P. aeruginosa* at 4 µg/ml and 90% at 16 to 32 µg/ml; concentrations of aztreonam required to inhibit *P. aeruginosa* usually are twofold greater than those for ceftazidime (2). At least 12% of strains of *P. aeruginosa* are resistant (3). The combination of aztreonam and piperacillin (or mezlocillin) is synergistic against some strains of *P. aeruginosa* and *Enterobacter* spp. but not as frequently synergistic as the combination of piperacillin and an aminoglycoside (4,5).
      d. **Resistant strains** typically include *Citrobacter freundii, Enterobacter aerogenes,* some *E. cloacae, Legionella pneumophilia, Acinetobacter* spp. Cefoxitin antagonizes the activity of aztreonam against *Enterobacter* spp. (1).

   C. **Pharmacokinetics** (1,5).
   1. **Absorption.** Aztreonam is poorly absorbed after oral administration but can be given intramuscularly (IM) or intravenously (IV).
   2. **Excretion** is primarily by the **kidneys** and doses are reduced in renal failure.

3. **Penetration/distribution.** Aztreonam penetrates body fluids well but has limited penetration into the cerebrospinal fluid (CSF). After IV infusion of 0.5-g, 1-g, and 2-g doses, mean peak serum levels of more than 60 µg/ml, 160 µg/ml, and 250 µg/ml, respectively, are achieved (1). Urinary concentrations are very high with urinary concentrations of more than 250 µg/ml and more than 700 µg/ml achieved 4 to 6 hours after a single IV 500-mg or 1-g dose, respectively, in patients with normal renal function (1).

D. **Clinical role. Since aztreonam is active against gram-negative aerobes only, combination therapy is necessary for mixed infections with gram positives and/or anaerobes.** Aztreonam has been successfully used in the following (1,5):

1. **UTIs** as single agent for susceptible gram negatives.

2. **Intraabdominal** (including peritonitis) and/or **pelvic** infections **when combined with an anti-anaerobic agents** such as clindamycin or metronidazole.

3. **Bacteremias** due to susceptible gram-negative pathogens. For empiric, initial therapy, if gram-positive or an anaerobe infection is a concern, additional coverage will be necessary.

4. **Gram-negative pneumonias** due to susceptible pathogens. Since some nosocomially acquired *P. aeruginosa* may be resistant to aztreonam, an aminoglycoside is initially preferred until susceptibility data are available.

5. **Skin and soft-tissue** infections due to susceptible gram-negative pathogens. In mixed infections, a second agent will be necessary (e.g., clindamycin for anaerobes or streptococci group A and/or susceptible *S. aureus)*.

6. **Bone and joint** infections due to susceptible pathogens have been treated with aztreonam IV. Often an oral fluoroquinolone is preferred in this setting.

7. **Febrile neutropenic patients** have been treated with aztreonam combined with an aminoglycoside with or without vancomycin. (See Chap. 12.)

E. **Dosing.** Aztreonam may be administered **intravenously or intramuscularly.** The IV route is recommended for patients requiring more than 1 g per dose and in those patients with bacteremias, abscesses, peritonitis, or other severe or life-threatening infections.

1. **Adult and pediatric** (more than 9 months of age) **dosages are summarized in Table 20-1.**

2. **Renal failure** dose reduction is shown in **Table 20-2.**

a. **Doses for patients on hemodialysis** are similar to those whose clearance is <10 ml/min (see Table 20-2). Thereafter, per package

Table 20-1. Aztreonam intravenous dosage guidelines (normal renal function)

Type of Infection	Dose[‡]	Frequency (Hours)
Adults*		
Urinary tract infections	500 mg or 1 g	8 or 12
Moderately severe systemic infections	1 g	8
Severe systemic or life-threatening infections	2 g	6 or 8[§]
Pediatric patients[†]		
Mild-to-moderate infections	30 mg/kg	8
Moderate-to-severe infections	30 mg/kg	6 or 8

Source: Modified from *Physicians' Desk Reference 2000,* 54th ed. Montvale, NJ: Medical Economics Data, 2000.
* Maximum recommended dose is 8 g/day.
[†] Maximum recommended dose is 120 mg/kg/day.
[‡] Higher doses are used in more severe infection.
[§] In systemic or severe *P. aeruginosa* infections 2 g q6–8h is suggested.

insert, one-eighth of the initial dose should be given after each hemodialysis; 500 mg after dialysis has also been suggested (6).

    b. **In chronic ambulatory peritoneal dialysis (CAPD) patients** dosing guidelines followed for a clearance less than 10 ml/mm can be followed (6).

  3. **Use in penicillin-allergic or cephalosporin-allergic patients.** Patients with immunologically mediated reactions to penicillins and

Table 20-2. Dosing of aztreonam in renal failure

Estimated Creatinine Clearance	Adult Dose	Pediatric Dose
>30 ml/min	See Table 20-1	See Table 20-1
10–30 ml/min	Initial dose as in Table 20-1, then give half of the usual dose at the standard interval	Insufficient data*
<10 ml/min	Initial dose as in Table 20-1, then one quarter the usual dose at the usual fixed interval	Insufficient data*

* As per the 2000 package insert, there are insufficient data to support recommendations for dosing aztreonam in renally impaired pediatric patients.

cephalosporins are able to receive aztreonam with little risk of cross-sensitivity. In patients who may receive repetitive courses of aztreonam (e.g., cystic fibrosis patients), aztreonam may rarely provoke a hypersensitivity reaction (7).

4. **Pregnancy.** Aztreonam is a category B agent; it should be used during pregnancy only if clearly indicated.

5. **Nursing mothers**. Aztreonam is excreted in breast milk. The package insert suggests consideration should be given to temporary discontinuation of nursing and use of formula feedings while the mother receives aztreonam.

F. **Toxicity** (1,5). Aztreonam is a safe agent with side effects similar to those of other beta-lactams.

1. Serious **nephrotoxicity or ototoxicity has not been reported. Aztreonam has been promoted for the treatment of gram-negative aerobic infections as a safer agent than the aminoglycosides.**

2. **Adverse reactions** of rash, nausea, diarrhea, eosinophilia, and mild hepatic transaminase elevations have been seen as with other beta-lactam antibiotics.

G. **Cost**. See Appendix Table B. Although monotherapy costs compared with third-generation cephalosporins are competitive, aztreonam is much more expensive than gentamicin or tobramycin and combination therapy with aztreonam and an antianaerobic and/or antistaphylococcal agent raises costs.

H. **Summary. Guidelines for the optimal use of aztreonam are still evolving** (1,5).

1. Aztreonam is a **rational alternative for gram-negative bacillary infections in the penicillin- and cephalosporin-allergic patient,** in whom one might ordinarily use an extended penicillin or third-generation cephalosporin. Against susceptible pathogens, it is also an **efficacious and safe alternative to aminoglycosides,** especially in the elderly, in patients with hepatic insufficiency, and in patients with renal insufficiency.

2. Despite the higher initial costs of aztreonam versus the aminoglycosides, if one considers the potential costs of nephrotoxicity due to aminoglycosides and the cost of monitoring aminoglycosides, aztreonam becomes potentially cost-effective or at least competitive (5). Other potentially useful agents include the quinolones.

3. **In the *Medical Letter*'s listing of "The choice of antibacterial drugs" aztreonam is not listed as the "drug of first choice" for any pathogen** (8).

4. **We offer the following guidelines for consideration:**

a. In moderate to severe nosocomial infections, aminoglycoside therapy for gram-negative organisms for the initial 48 to 72 hours while awaiting cultures is prudent unless an aminoglycoside is contraindicated. Once susceptibility data are back, if the organism is broadly resistant but susceptible to aztreonam, azetreonam could be used. (See Chap. 21.) The development of resistance while on therapy is usually not a concern with aminoglycosides. The frequency with which bacteria develop resistance to aztreonam is not fully delineated. If the approach just outlined is used, the risk of resistance may be minimized.

b. There is a recognized potential of increasing bacterial resistance and possibly an increased incidence of *Clostridium difficile* diarrhea associated with the common use of advanced cephalosporins. Aztreonam appears to be associated less often with these problems and therefore may be an appealing alternative. Aztreonam probably is underutilized currently.

c. Because aztreonam is active only against gram-negative bacilli, when it is used empirically for mixed infections, combination therapy will be necessary, thereby increasing costs.

d. In some circumstances, an aminoglycoside may still be the preferred agent (see Chap. 21) as, for example, in combination therapy against enterococcus and *Listeria monocytogenes* and in combination with antipseudomonal penicillin in severe *P. aeruginosa* infections.

II. **Imipenem (Primaxin)**, a carbapenem released in 1985, has a very broad spectrum of activity. It is combined with cilastatin, a potent enzyme inhibitor, which prevents the inactivation of imipenem in the kidney (by inactivating enzymes in the brush border cells), ensuring good urinary concentrations. Cilastatin also appears to have a "nephroprotective" effect (1,5).

A. **Mechanism of action.** Imipenem binds with high affinity to penicillin-binding proteins, causing lysis of many gram-positive and gram-negative bacteria. This factor plus its ability to penetrate the cell membrane of multiple gram-negative bacilli and its resistance to a broad range of beta-lactamases from gram-positive and gram-negative bacilli help explain imipenem's broad spectrum of activity (1).

B. *In vitro* **activity.** Imipenem remains a potent antibiotic (9), although some resistance has developed over time (1,10).

1. **Gram-positive aerobes**
   a. **Very susceptible**, with a MIC_{90} typically of 0.1 µg/ml or less: penicillin-susceptible *Streptococcus pneumoniae*, group A and B streptococci, *Streptococcus bovis*, methicillin-susceptible *Staphylococcus aureus*, and *S. saprophyticus*. Imipenem is active against intermediate penicillin-resistant *S. pneumoniae* and most high-level resistant strains (1,5). (See Chap. 16 for a detailed discussion of penicillin-resistant *S. pneumoniae*.)
   b. **Moderately susceptible**. Amoxicillin-susceptible enterococci usually are susceptible, with the MIC_{90} of susceptible *Enterococcus faecalis* approximately 1 to 3 µg/ml. Imipenem is bacteriostatic against susceptible enterococci. Imipenem-aminoglycoside combinations may be synergistic against *E. faecalis*. However, many strains of *E. faecium* are resistant to imipenem.
   c. **Resistant.** Methicillin-resistant *S. aureus* (MRSA) or coagulase-negative species are **resistant**. *Corynebacterium JK* organisms are resistant, as are vancomycin-resistant enterococci (VRE).
2. **Gram-negative aerobic bacteria**
   a. **Nonenteric pathogens.** *N. meningitidis* and *N. gonorrhoeae* have a MIC_{90} of less than 0.20 µg/ml, and *H. influenzae* with a MIC_{90} of 0.6 µg/ml are very susceptible. The MICs for beta-lactamase-positive and -negative *N. gonorrhoeae* and *H. influenzae* are identical.
   b. **Enterobacteriaceae.** In an early review of more than 8,000 isolates, three levels of imipenem activity were recognized (11). A MIC_{90} of 1.0 µg or less (very susceptible) was seen with *E. coli*, *Klebsiella* spp., *Salmonella* and *Shigella* spp., *Citrobacter diversus*, *Hafniae alvei*, and *Yersinia enterocolitica*. A MIC_{90} of approximately 1 to 2 µg/ml (susceptible) was seen with *Enterobacter* spp., *C. freundii*, and *Serratia* spp. A MIC_{90} of 2 to 4 µg/ml (less susceptible) was seen, especially with the *Proteus* spp. Although some Enterobacteriaceae have developed resistance to imipenem over time, imipenem remains very active against most of these organisms and more active than noncarbapenem beta-lactam antibiotics (1,10).
   c. *Pseudomonas*
      (1) The MIC_{90} for *P. aeruginosa* is typically higher (e.g., 5 µg/ml in more than 1,600 strains in early testing) (11). Although some *P. aeruginosa* strains

have developed resistance to imipenem over time, in one 1996 report of more than 6,600 intensive care unit isolates, 87% of strains were susceptible to imipenem. Against these same strains, 89%, 93%, and 65% of strains were susceptible to amikacin, tobramycin, and gentamicin, respectively (10).

Similar MICs were noted for *P. fluorescens*. Imipenem may show synergism with tobramycin or other aminoglycosides against *P. aeruginosa* (1,5).

   (2) *Pseudomonas cepacia* and *P. maltophilia* (now called *Stenotrophomonas maltophilia*) strains are **resistant. S. maltophilia produces a beta-lactamase that easily hydrolyzes imipenem.**

 d. *Acinetobacter calcoaceticus* spp. are usually quite susceptible, but nosocomial infections due to resistant species can occur.

 e. *Legionella pneumophilia.* Although imipenem is active *in vitro;* it is not considered appropriate treatment for *Legionella* pneumonia because of the intracellular location of the organism (1,5).

C. **Pharmacokinetics**

   1. **Absorption.** Imipenem-cilastatin is poorly absorbed after oral administration but can be given IV or IM. Lower serum levels are reached after IM doses. In adults of average size with normal renal function, 500-mg and 1,000-mg doses IV provide peak serum levels of 30 to 40 µg/ml and 60 to 70 µg/ml, respectively (1).

   2. **Excretion** is primarily by the kidneys, and doses must be reduced in renal failure. Little of the drug is found in the feces, so there is relatively little impact on bowel flora; *C. difficile* diarrhea is not a common complication. (See Sec. F.3.)

   3. **Penetration/distribution.** Imipenem-cilastatin penetrates body fluids well, with at least modest penetration of the inflamed meninges.

D. **Clinical role.** Imipenem-cilastatin is **especially useful in infections caused by pathogens resistant to other agents or for infections that would otherwise require multiple antibiotics.** It is particularly useful in **complex nosocomial infections** (1,5).

   1. **See Table 20-3** for a summary.

   2. **Miscellaneous uses**

      a. **Eye infections.** Because of its broad spectrum of activity, it has been used in some eye infections (12).

      b. In **acute necrotizing pancreatitis**, imipenem has been used to try to prevent complex pancreatic infections. (See Chap. 6.)

Table 20-3. Clinical use of imipenem (or meropenem)

For **serious nosocomial infections** (e.g., bacteremia, pneumonia, complex UTI, severe perineal soft-tissue infection, osteomyelitis), **especially** those **involving resistant organisms,** or poly-microbial infections (mixed anaerobes, aerobic, gram-positive and -negative, especially for diabetics)*

Used as an alternative to combination therapy for complex **nosoco-mial intraabdominal infections,** thus avoiding ototoxic and nephrotoxic effects of aminoglycosides†

For *Pseudomonas* infections caused by organisms resistant to other antipseudomonal beta-lactam agents but, where possible, use in combination with an aminoglycoside.

Monotherapy in **febrile granulocytopenic patients.** (See Chap. 12.)

A **"drug of choice"** for severe nosocomial *Enterobacter* or *Serratia* or *Acinetobacter* spp., and *C. freundii* infections; also for *Campylobacter fetus* infections (8).

When *not* to use imipenem (or meropenem)
  Not alone in treatment of serious *Pseudomonas* infections‡ especially pneumonia
  Not for most community-acquired infections
  Not for surgical prophylaxis
  Not for methicillin-resistant staphylococcal infections or VRE
  Not alone in therapy for serious enterococcal infections (*E. faecalis*)
  Not in therapy for non–aeruginosa pseudomonal infections

Modified from Sobel JD. Imipenem and aztreonam. *Infect Dis Clin North Am* 1989;3:613.

* Editors' note: We "save for use" imipenem and meropenem for when cultures reveal or are likely to reveal resistant pathogens in someone usually already on antibiotics or who has recently received antibiotics. *C. freundii, Acinetobacter,* and *Enterobacter* spp. may be resistant to other antibiotics.

† Editors' note: Not for mild to moderate community-acquired infections where less broad agents are effective (e.g., cefazolin combined with metronidazole, cefoxitin, cefotetan, ampicillin-sulbactam, ticarcillin-clavulanate). See Chap. 6. Particularly useful in hospital-acquired intraabdominal infections in which resistant organisms may be involved.

‡ Editors' note: For susceptible *P. aeruginosa* infections, an antipseudomonal penicillin and an aminoglycoside are preferred. (See Chap. 21.)

---

  c. Because of minimal bile concentrations, we do not view this agent as optimal for biliary sepsis. (See Chap. 6.)

  d. Alternate agent for nocardial infections. It may be useful in selected infections due to high-level resistant *S. pneumoniae* (see Chaps. 2, 16), but other agents are usually available.

  e. Imipenem is not advised for prophylaxis because of the risks of promoting antimicro-bial resistance and because equally effective, less expensive agents with a narrower spec-trum are available (1). See Chap. 15.

 E. **Dosages**. For a given patient, the dose of imipenem **depends on** the **severity** of infection, **renal func-**

tion, and weight of the patient (with dose reductions if the patient weighs less than 70 kg). The prescribed dose of imipenem-cilastatin is understood to refer to the amount of the imipenem component being used (1).

1. **A detailed table for dosages for adults with weights of less than 70 kg and various levels of renal dysfunction is contained** in the package insert and current edition of *Physicians' Desk Reference*, which is readily available.

   We have used the following dose regimens.

   a. **For most serious infections in adults ≥70 kg,** an IV dose of 500 mg q6h is suggested (1,5) when renal function is normal. For life-threatening infections, doses of 1 g q6 to 8h have been used; infectious disease input is advised in this setting.

   b. **For adults weighing less than 70 kg,** an IV dose of 25 mg/kg/day has been suggested (1) and can be divided up every 6 hours.

   c. **In renal failure,** 50% of the usual dose can be given when the creatinine clearance is between 10 to 50 ml/min and 25% of the usual dose when the clearance is less than 10 ml/min (6). **Hemodialysis** removes 40% to 70% of the imipenem, so a supplemental dose can be given (reduced for renal dysfunction for a clearance of less than 10 ml/min) after dialysis. In patients undergoing **CAPD**, dosages are given as above in patients with a creatinine clearance of less than 10 ml/min (6).

2. **In children IV** imipenem use has recently been approved. **For patients more than 3 months of age,** the recommended dose is 15 to 25 mg/kg/dose IV every 6 h (to a maximum of 2 g daily). Higher doses have been used in children with pseudomonas infections and/or cystic fibrosis; infectious disease consultation is advised for high dose usage. See package insert for dosage in children less than 3 months of age. For neonates, see Appendix Table A.

   Imipenem is not advised for CNS infections because of the risk of seizures, per the package insert. It is also not recommended for pediatric patients weighing less than 30 kg with impaired renal function, since the package insert emphasizes there are no data in this setting.

   See related discussions of meropenem in Sec. III.

3. **Pregnancy.** Imipenem is a **category C** agent. (See Chap. 14.) The package insert indicates there are no adequate and well-controlled studies in pregnant women. Therefore this agent should be used during pregnancy only if the potential benefit justifies the potential risk to the mother and fetus.

4. **Nursing mothers.** The package insert indicates it is not known whether imipenem is excreted

in human milk. Because many drugs are excreted in human milk, caution should be exercised when this agent is administered to a nursing woman.

F. **Side effects and toxicity**. Overall, imipenem is well tolerated (1,5).

1. **Seizures** have occurred in imipenem recipients, especially if high doses and decreased renal function were present. Whether seizures actually occur at a higher frequency than other antibiotics, when proper doses are used, has not been clearly established (5). (See Sec. 5. below.)

   a. **To help minimize the risk of seizures, dosages of imipenem should be appropriately reduced in the elderly and in patients with renal insufficiency.** Recent data suggest seizures occur in significantly less than 1% of treated patients (1).

   b. If a seizure, tremor, or myoclonus occurs during imipenem therapy, antibiotic dosages or continued need of the antibiotic should be reassessed, and anticonvulsant therapy and neurologic evaluation should be considered. Meropenem would be preferred in this setting.

   c. **Imipenem use in meningitis is usually avoided, and if indicated, meropenem is preferred**. (See Sec. III.)

2. **Allergic reactions** such as drug fever, pruritus, rash, and urticaria are uncommon. Some experts feel **patients allergic to penicillin should be considered allergic to imipenem** (13) unless skin tests can be done. In addition, **imipenem should be avoided or administered under close monitoring to patients with a history of IgE-mediated hypersensitivity to other beta-lactam antibiotics** (14).

3. **Gastrointestinal symptoms** occasionally are seen. Nausea and vomiting may be decreased by decreasing the infusion rate or the dose (1). *C. difficile* diarrhea seems to be uncommon.

4. **Nephrotoxicity and hepatotoxicity do not seem to occur.**

5. **Drug interactions**. The package insert suggests that seizures have been reported in patients receiving **ganciclovir** and imipenem; therefore these drugs should not be used concomitantly unless the potential benefits outweigh the potential risks. Since **probenecid** may increase serum imipenem concentrations, these two drugs should not be used concomitantly.

   Imipenem may induce beta-lactamases, which can decrease the effectiveness of concomitantly used cephalosporins or expanded penicillins (1,5).

    G. **Resistance** can develop especially against *P. aerugi-nosa*. In severe infections due to this pathogen, mono-therapy with imipenem should be avoided.

    H. **Cost.** This is an expensive agent but may be competi-tive if it replaces multiple other agents. See Table B in the Appendix.

III. **Meropenem (Merrem)** is a new intravenous carbape-nem, approved in 1996, which is **very similar to impe-nem.** Meropenem has been reviewed elsewhere (1,5,15–19). Meropenem is stable to human renal dehydropeptidase and therefore can be given without cilastatin.

    A. *In vitro,* meropenem has broad antibacterial activity **similar to imipenem.** Meropenem is slightly more active against gram-negative organisms, whereas imipenem is slightly more active against gram-positives (1,16,18). Whether these minor *in vitro* differences have any clinical relevance remains to be seen, but no sig-nificant differences have been observed in compara-tive trials as of 1999 (1).

        1. Meropenem, like imipenem, is active *in vitro* against many penicillin-resistant *S. pneumoniae*, including many high-level resistant forms. (See Chaps. 2 and 16.)

        2. Meropenem is not active against MRSA, *E. fae-cium* and VRE strains of enterococci or *S. malto-philia*. Some strains of *P. aeruginosa* are resistant.

    B. **Pharmacokinetics.** The pharmacokinetics of mero-penem are similar to those of imipenem (1,5). Only an IV formulation is available. About 70% of each dose is recovered in the urine. Hemodialysis removes most of the drug. Its serum half-life is about 1 hour, so it is given q8h. Meropenem reaches therapeutic concen-trations in the CSF in patients with meningitis (18).

    C. **Clinical role**. Meropenem has been **approved for** IV therapy of (1,5,18):

        1. **Complicated intraabdominal infections in adults and children** over 3 months of age.

           a. The indications for use in this setting are similar for both imipenem (see Sec. II.D) and meropenem (i.e., complex mixed aerobic and anaerobic, nosocomial, infections). For mild-to-moderate community-acquired abdominal infections, other options are available. (See Chap. 6.)

           b. Since we have more experience in adults with imipenem, we would use imipenem in adults unless possibly in a patient with re-cent seizures, when meropenem would be preferred. Also in patients with renal failure, dose modification is easier with meropenem.

        2. **Bacterial meningitis in children** more than 3 months of age. Although meropenem has been used (20) and is approved for susceptible *H. in-fluenzae, S. pneumoniae*, and *N. meningitidis* in children, usually a third-generation cephalosporin

is preferred for meningitis due to cephalosporin-susceptible strains, since there is more experience with the cephalosporins in this setting. (See Chap. 11.)

For a case of known _S. pneumoniae_ resistant to penicillin, meropenem provides an alternative agent to vancomycin (see Chaps. 11, 16, and 28), and meropenem is preferred over imipenem, since meropenem seems unlikely to cause seizures even in meningitis therapy. (See Sec. II.F.1.) **Infectious disease consultation is advised** in these difficult cases.

3. Meropenem has been shown to be effective in a variety of clinical conditions, including pneumonia, febrile neutropenic patients, bacteremias, complex UTIs (i.e., for the same indications as imipenem) (1).

D. **Dosages**
   1. **In adults** the usual dose is 1 g IV q8h. In the management of febrile neutropenic adult patients 1 g q8h was as effective as 2 g q8h of ceftazidime alone and/or ceftazidime and amikacin (1). In bacterial meningitis, 2 g q8h has been effective (1).
      a. **In renal failure,** the package insert suggests that if the creatinine clearance is 26 to 50 ml/min, the regular dose is given q12h. If the creatinine clearance is 10 to 25 ml/min, one-half of the usual dose is given q12h. If the creatinine clearance is less than 10 ml/min, one-half of the usual dose is given q24h.
      b. **In dialysis.** As of early 2000, there is inadequate information regarding the dose of meropenem in patients on hemodialysis and peritoneal dialysis, per the package insert.
   2. **In pediatrics** for intraabdominal infections 20 mg/kg (maximum of 1 g) q8h and for meningitis 40 mg/kg (maximum 2 g) q8h is suggested by the package insert. Patients weighing more than 50 kg can be given adult doses.

      As of early 2000, the package insert indicates there are no dose recommendations for pediatric patients with renal failure (i.e., no experience).
   3. **In pregnancy.** The package insert notes this is a **category B** agent and should be used during pregnancy only if clearly needed. (See Chap. 14.)
   4. **In nursing mothers**. It is not known if this agent is excreted in human milk. The package insert suggests that caution should be exercised when IV meropenem is administered to a nursing woman.
   5. **In hepatic disease**, the package insert indicates no dosage adjustments are needed (in adults).

E. **Side effects. There are differences in the tolerability of imipenem and meropenem (1).**
   1. **Meropenem is unlikely to cause seizures** which have been reported with imipenem (18,21).

2. Meropenem has been less likely to cause nausea and vomiting as well as inflammation at the IV site compared to imipenem (1).
3. The frequency and severity of adverse events with meropenem does not seem to escalate at higher doses as with imipenem (1).
4. Rashes, diarrhea, and reversible increases in aminotransferase enzymes have occurred as with other beta-lactam antibiotics (1,5,18).

F. **Cost.** Meropenem is an **expensive** IV agent to use, even more so than imipenem (18). See Appendix Table B.

G. **Summary**. In their review, the *Medical Letter* concluded (18): "meropenem is an expensive new parenteral antibiotic similar to imipenem, possibly with less potential for causing seizures. Meropenem, like imipenem, could be used for treatment of hospital-acquired infections that may be resistant to other antibiotics. For treatment of intraabdominal infections or bacterial meningitis, meropenem generally offers no clear advantage over less costly older drugs."

We would add that except for very selected cases of meningitis in which meropenem may be useful (infectious disease consultation is advised in these difficult cases), the indications for meropenem are the same as those for imipenem. (See Sec. II.D.) In selected patients, the decreased side effects with meropenem may be important.

References

1. Hellinger WC, Brewer NS. Carbapenems and monobactams: imipenem, meropenem, and aztreonam. *Mayo Clin Proc* 1999; 74:420.
2. Neu HC. Aztreonam activity, pharmacology, and clinical uses. *Am J Med* 1990;88:2S (suppl 3C).
3. Ennis DM, Cobbs CG. The newer cephalosporins, aztreonam, and imipenem. *Infect Dis Clin North Am* 1995;9:687.
4. Greenberg RN, Meade DW, Danko LS. Comparison of the synergistic activity of aztreonam or tobramycin plus piperacillin or mezlocillin. *J Antimicrob Chemother* 1993;32:342.
   In vitro *90% of isolates (50 species of* P. aeruginosa *and 10 of* Enterobacter*) were synergistic or additive with piperacillin-tobramycin versus 65% tested against piperacillin-aztreonam.*
5. Reese R, Betts RF. Unique beta-lactam antibiotics: aztreonam and imipenem. In: Reese RE, Betts RF, eds. *A practical approach to infectious diseases*, 4th ed. Boston: Little, Brown, 1996:Chap. 28G.
6. Aronoff GR, et al, eds. *Drug prescribing in renal failure: dosing guidelines for adults*, 4th ed. Philadelphia: American College of Physicians, 1999.
7. Moss RB, et al. Evaluation of the immunologic cross-reactivity of aztreonam in patients with cystic fibrosis who are allergic to penicillin and/or cephalosporin antibiotics. *Rev Infect Dis* 1991;13:S598 (suppl 7).

Report from Johns Hopkins University that warns: Aztreonam should be administered cautiously to patients with cystic fibrosis who are allergic to other beta-lactam antibiotics because it is potentially allergenic with repeated use. See accompanying related articles in the same symposium issue.

8. Medical Letter. The choice of antibacterial drugs. *Med Lett Drugs Ther* 1999;41:95.
   Serially updated about every 2 years.

9. Hellinger WC, Brewer NS. Imipenem. *Mayo Clin Proc* 1991; 66:1074.

10. Itokazen GS, et al. Antimicrobial resistance rates among aerobic gram-negative bacilli recovered from patients in intensive care units: evaluation of a national post marketing surveillance program. *Clin Infect Dis* 1996;23:779.
    Amikacin and imipenem were the agents most active against more than 33,000 isolates tested.

11. Jones RN. Review of the *in vitro* spectrum of activity of imipenem. *Am J Med* 1985;78(6A):22.

12. Axelrod JL, et al. Penetration of imipenem in human aqueous and vitreous humor. *Am J Ophthalmol* 1987;104:649.
    After a 1-g IV dose, levels were well above the MIC_{90} of S. epidermidis, S. aureus, and the Enterobacteriaceae commonly involved in bacterial endophthalmitis.

13. Saxon A, et al. Immediate hypersensitivity reactions to beta-lactam antibiotics. *Ann Intern Med* 1987;127:204.

14. Sobel JD. Imipenem and aztreonam. *Infect Dis Clin North Am* 1989;3:613.

15. Finch RG, et al. Meropenem: focus on clinical performance. *J Antimicrob Chemother* 1995;36:1–223 (suppl A).
    Symposium covering in vitro activity update, pharmacokinetics, and emphasizing clinical trial data.

16. Wiseman LR, et al. Meropenem: a review of its antibacterial activity, pharmacokinetics and clinical efficacy. *Drugs* 1995;50:73–101.

17. Norrby SR, Carbapenems: efficacy and safety profiles—focus on meropenem. *Scand J Infect Dis* 1995;96:5–48 (suppl).

18. Medical Letter. Meropenem: a new parenteral broad spectrum antibiotic. *Med Lett Drugs Ther* 1996;38:88.

19. Norrby SR, Faulkner KL. Differentiating meropenem and imipenem/cilastatin. *Infect Dis Clin Pract* 1997;6:291.

20. Odio CM, et al. Prospective, randomized, investigator-blinded study of the efficacy and safety of meropenem vs. cefotaxime therapy in bacterial meningitis in children, Meropenem Meningitis Study Group. *Pediatr Infect Dis J* 1999;18:581.

21. Norrby SR, Gildon KM. Safety profile of meropenem: a review of nearly 5,000 patients treated with meropenem. *Scand J Infect* 1999;31:3.

21

Aminoglycosides

The role aminoglycosides play in clinical medicine continues to evolve as other classes of less toxic agents with expanded spectrum of activity (e.g., third-generation cephalosporins, aztreonam, fluoroquinolones) **have become available** (1). Nevertheless, because of cost considerations, the rare development of bacterial resistance, the reduced incidence of *Clostridium difficile* diarrhea, the low risk of allergic reactions, and the better understanding of their toxicity, the aminoglycosides remain very useful in selected settings. **These agents are, in most instances, bactericidal.** They penetrate the cell wall and membrane and bind irreversibly to the 30 S bacterial ribosomes. The precise mechanism through which the aminoglycosides cause bacterial cell death remains unclear (2). **The most commonly used aminoglycosides are gentamicin, tobramycin, and amikacin, and these agents will be emphasized** (1–3).

I. **Introduction: important principles of aminoglycoside use**
   A. **Aminoglycosides versus other classes of antibiotics. Aminoglycosides have excellent activity against almost all aerobic gram-negative rods.** If susceptibility data permit, it is preferable to **use ampicillin or a cephalosporin** or, in certain settings, aztreonam or the fluoroquinolones, as these agents are less toxic. However, **because of the potential for emergence of organisms resistant to these alternative agents, aminoglycosides retain their usefulness and, in some settings, may be preferred** (1).
      1. **Community versus nosocomial infections.** Aminoglycosides are active against community-acquired gram-negative bacteria but cephalosporins are preferred. **Aminoglycosides are particularly useful in hospital-acquired infections,** especially for *Pseudomonas* spp.
      2. **Modifying initial therapy.** Regardless of the circumstances under which the aminoglycoside was initiated, if the isolated pathogen is susceptible to a narrow-spectrum agent, appropriate modifications should be made.
   B. **Special problems with aminoglycoside use**
      1. **Toxicity. The aminoglycosides have considerable intrinsic toxicity.** This risk of toxicity must be considered, especially with use for any extended time (>7 days). (See Sec. VI.)
      2. **Narrow toxic-therapeutic ratio. The margin between effective and toxic concentrations is narrow.**
      3. **Monitoring of serum levels. Serum levels are measured to ensure effective levels and**

minimize toxicity. This topic is discussed in detail in Sec. V.

II. *In vitro* activity
   A. **Gram-negative aerobes. See Table 21-1.**
      1. **Community-acquired** gram-negative organisms. All aminoglycosides are equally active in proportion to achievable serum levels.
      2. **Hospital-acquired** (nosocomial) **gram-negative organisms.** In general, tobramycin *in vitro* is 2 to 4 times more active than gentamicin against *P. aeruginosa* (but the clinical implications of this are unclear). Netilmicin is less active than either tobramycin or gentamicin against susceptible *P. aeruginosa.* Against *Serratia* spp., gentamicin has 2 to 4 times the bactericidal activity of tobramycin. For other nosocomial organisms, the aminoglycosides are equally active in proportion to achievable serum levels (1).

      Against organisms resistant to one or more aminoglycosides, amikacin will be the most active, tobramycin will be the next most active, and gentamicin will be the least active.
   B. **Gram-positive aerobes.** The aminoglycosides have some activity against some organisms (e.g., staphylococci) but **alone are never the preferred agents** (3).

Table 21-1.   Aminoglycoside activity

Typically Active Against	Not Usually Active Against
Acinetobacter spp.*	
Citrobacter spp.*	
Enterobacter spp.*	
Escherichia coli[†]	*Pseudomonas (Burkholderia) cepacia*
Klebsiella spp.[†]	
Morganella morganii[†]	*Stenotrophomonas maltophilia*[§]
Proteus spp.[†]	
Providence spp.[†]	
Pseudomonas aeruginosa[‡]	
P. fluorescens	
Serratia spp.[†]	
Yersinia enterocolitica	

* Although aminoglycosides may be active *in vitro,* imipenem or meropenem are viewed as "drugs of choice" (3).
[†] Although aminoglycosides are active *in vitro,* cephalosporins usually preferred (3).
[‡] **Aminoglycosides,** often in combination with piperacillin, are **drugs of choice** for severe infections. For UTIs, ciprofloxacin (a quinolone) preferred (3).
[§] Formerly called *Pseudomonas maltophilia* or *Xanthomonas maltophilia.*

Gentamicin, together with ampicillin or penicillin, usually has the greatest activity against enterococci. However, in recent years, at major medical centers, there has been an increasing incidence of enterococci resistant to the combination of gentamicin-penicillin (so called high-level gentamicin resistance, with a minimum inhibitory concentration (MIC) to gentamicin of more than 2,000 µg/ml). In a recent report, 26% of enterococci demonstrated high-level resistance to gentamicin (2). The details of this problem and alternative therapeutic approaches are reviewed elsewhere (4) and discussed further in Sec. VII.B.

C. **Anaerobes** are not susceptible.

D. *Nocardia* is susceptible to amikacin (3).

E. *Mycobacterium.* Most *Mycobacterium tuberculosis* are susceptible to streptomycin and amikacin; most *M. avium-intracellulare* isolates are susceptible to amikacin (3).

III. **Pharmacokinetics**

A. **Gentamicin, tobramycin, and netilmicin have similar pharmacokinetics;** therefore standard doses, peak levels achieved, and serum half-lives are essentially the same (see **Table 21-2**). Amikacin is a semisynthetic kanamycin derivative with pharmacokinetics nearly identical to those of kanamycin. The **intravenous route is preferred**, but the intramuscular route can be used if there is no sepsis, hypotension, or thrombocytopenia.

B. **Excretion** of the aminoglycosides is **entirely renal, mandating dose reductions in renal failure**.

C. **Variation in pharmacokinetics.** There is **striking variation in the volume of distribution and rate**

Table 21-2. Expected peak and trough levels of respective aminoglycosides (in µg/ml) with conventional or individualized dosing

	Peak[*,†]	Trough[‡]	Toxic[†]
Gentamicin	6–10	1–2	>10
Tobramycin	6–10	1–2	>10
Amikacin	15–30	5–10	>35
Netilmicin	6–10	1–2	>10

Note: These ranges for peak and trough concentrations are used commonly, but their exact implications remain controversial, as reviewed by McCormack JP, Jewesson PJ. A critical reevaluation of the "therapeutic range" of aminoglycosides. *Clin Infect Dis* 1992;14:320.

[*] Drawn one-half hour after a half-hour IV infusion. See text. For pneumonia therapy, the higher levels of peaks are desirable.

[†] These peak toxic levels are with conventional dosage regimens. With once-a-day dosages, higher acceptable peak levels will routinely be achieved. See text.

[‡] Level just before next dose.

of excretion of aminoglycosides in individual patients with normal and abnormal renal function. **Thus it is usually important to monitor serum levels in all patients regardless of volume status or renal function**. (See Sec. V.)

Peak and trough level measures can be repeated every 3 to 4 days if the patient is stable. In a patient who has major changes in hydration status or renal function, levels have to be repeated more frequently (**Table 21-2**).

1. **Peak levels** (1) are the serum levels achieved 30 minutes after completion of an intravenous infusion. When the drug is given by the intramuscular route, peak levels occur at 45 to 60 minutes. In renal failure, the peak sample is drawn 120 to 150 minutes after the intramuscular dose, because the drug continues to be absorbed and not excreted. **Peak** serum **levels** are obtained to ensure that enough drug was administered for therapeutic efficacy. A peak level commonly is obtained after the first or second maintenance dose or after dosage adjustments.

2. **Trough levels** are obtained just before the next dose. If trough levels are elevated, the dose needs to be reduced or the dose interval needs to be prolonged. In renal failure, the trough level should ideally be obtained after the same dose in which the peak was measured.

D. **Tissue penetration.** Aminoglycosides achieve reasonable concentrations in bone, synovial fluid, and peritoneal fluid. Urinary concentrations are high and may exceed serum concentration by 100 times in patients with normal renal function (2). There is limited penetration into the central nervous system (CNS) and probably intraabdominal abscesses (1). Drug levels in bronchial secretions are poor (2).

IV. **Clinical use** (1,2)

A. **Aminoglycosides as drugs of choice** for specific pathogens (3)

1. **For *P. aeruginosa* infections other than urinary tract infections (UTIs)**, an aminoglycoside is combined with an extended-spectrum penicillin (e.g., piperacillin) for optimal therapy.

   • In the patient with a delayed penicillin allergy, ceftazidime is often substituted and used with an aminoglycoside.
   • In *P. aeruginosa* UTIs, ciprofloxacin is preferred (3).

2. **Gentamicin** is **used in combination** with another agent **to achieve synergy** against certain pathogens: (a) with penicillin, ampicillin, or vancomycin against gentamicin-susceptible enterococci or viridans streptococci; (b) with ampicillin against *Listeria monocytogenes*; (c) with an

extended-spectrum penicillin (e.g., piperacillin) against *P. aeruginosa* and susceptible *Enterobacter* spp. (Sec. 1 above); (d) with vancomycin and rifampin against *S. epidermidis* prosthetic valve infection; (e) in conjunction with ampicillin (or vancomycin) for endocarditis prophylaxis in high-risk patients before genitourinary (GU) or gastrointestinal (GI) procedures; (f) combined with an antistaphylococcal penicillin for right-sided endocarditis caused by *S. aureus*; and (g) in association with doxycycline for the treatment of brucellosis (1–3).

Gentamicin is the preferred aminoglycoside in combination therapy aimed at enterococci (1,2).

3. **Amikacin** has been used in some atypical mycobacterial infections. Amikacin (plus clarithromycin) is the drug of choice for *M. fortuitum* complex infections (3).

4. **Streptomycin (or gentamicin)** is an agent of choice for *Yersinia pestis* (plague); streptomycin remains a useful agent for *M. tuberculosis* therapy and for *M. kansasii* infections.

B. **Not the drugs of choice, but there are several situations in which the aminoglycosides are used.** Although netilmicin still is available, most institutions use gentamicin, tobramycin, or amikacin; netilmicin is no longer listed as an aminoglycoside of choice (3).

1. **As empiric therapy in life-threatening community-acquired gram-negative** infections. Gentamicin usually is preferred, because it is less expensive.

2. **Infections occurring in a hospital setting or in a patient who has recently been hospitalized;** an aminoglycoside is indicated while awaiting culture data.

   a. **In most community hospitals** where resistance to gentamicin is uncommon, we favor gentamicin because it is less expensive. An exception is the patient who has already received broad-spectrum antibiotics active against nosocomial pathogens and therefore may have been colonized and possibly infected with a relatively resistant gram-negative bacteria. Until susceptibility data are available, tobramycin or amikacin are the preferred agents.

   b. **Amikacin versus gentamicin (1). In large medical centers or specialized areas** (e.g., intensive care units, burn units) where the frequency of resistance to gentamicin, tobramycin, or netilmicin may be high, amikacin is preferred at least until susceptibility data are available. If gentamicin resistance is low (e.g., 1% to 5%), gentamicin remains the most rational cost-effective choice unless the patient has recently received gentamicin, in which case amikacin should be used while awaiting culture results in life-threatening infections. Amikacin is the aminoglycoside of choice for the treatment of gentamicin-resistant gram-negative bacteria (2).

If the gram-negative organism isolated is susceptible to all aminoglycosides, use gentamicin.

  c. **Note.** If a patient is potentially at high risk for aminoglycoside toxicity (e.g., a patient with hepatic failure or the frail elderly; see Sec. VI.C.4), an alternate agent can be used (e.g., aztreonam).

3. In **leukopenic, febrile patients** with no obvious focus of infection, an aminoglycoside and an extended-spectrum penicillin (e.g., piperacillin) have commonly been used. (See Chap. 12.)

4. **For susceptible pathogens in which a less toxic agent is unavailable,** aminoglycosides have been used effectively to treat susceptible gram negatives causing UTI, peritonitis, bone and joint infections, pneumonia, and sometimes gram-negative bacillary endocarditis.

5. **As alternative agents in nosocomial intra-abdominal infections.** (See Chap. 6.)

6. **For therapy for organisms that may develop resistance to monotherapy with a third-generation cephalosporin** (e.g., *E. cloacae, Citrobacter freundii,* and some *Acinetobacter* spp.) In this setting, an aminoglycoside is often combined with an extended-spectrum penicillin (e.g., piperacillin) for synergy. However, imipenem often is preferred for treatment of nosocomially acquired *Acinetobacter* spp. and some *Enterobacter* spp. (3).

C. **Aminoglycoside effectiveness** is not optimal in the following situations (1):

1. **In lower respiratory tract infections,** the low pH of bronchial secretions may decrease the activity of aminoglycosides. One cannot **rely on aminoglycosides alone** in major lower respiratory tract infections (e.g., pseudomonas pneumonia).

2. **Sterilization of abscesses** may be difficult with aminoglycosides because of poor activity in the chemical presence of bivalent cations, the low pH and anaerobic conditions.

3. **Prostatitis.** Aminoglycosides do not achieve useful levels in prostate tissue.

V. **Aminoglycoside dosing.** Numerous dosage regimens have been proposed, but studies showing that one method is clearly superior are not available. **What is widely accepted is that giving a routine conventional dose (e.g., 3 to 5 mg/kg/day** in divided doses q8h) **to adults**

with normal renal function is not an acceptable dose regimen in the very ill patient because of the variability in levels achieved. Zaske et al emphasized this when they studied more than 200 surgical patients and if this standard approach was used in patients with normal renal function, 47% of the patients were "underdosed" and 14% of patients were "overdosed" (5).

Three acceptable approaches are (a) single-daily dose regimens for short-use duration, (b) individualized dosing with a pharmacokinetic model, and (c) conventional dosing but with serial serum levels monitored and doses adjusted by someone skilled in the use of aminoglycosides.

A. **Single daily (once-daily) aminoglycoside dosing** (SDD) has been reviewed (6–11).
   1. **The underlying principles** of this approach include the following:
      a. **Concentration-dependent killing of bacteria.** The rate of bactericidal killing of aminoglycosides increases as the antibiotic concentration is increased. (See Chap. 14.) In theory, the higher serum levels with once-daily dosing will provide higher serum bactericidal levels and equivalent, or even enhanced, efficacy compared with conventional dosing. Transient high serum concentrations seem to be well tolerated.
      b. **Postantibiotics effect (PAE).** Aminoglycosides demonstrate a PAE against aerobic gram-negative bacilli both *in vitro* and in animal models. The PAE is the persistent suppression of bacterial growth after short antibiotic exposure. The duration of the PAE is greater the higher the peak and remains after the serum level falls below the MIC of the bacteria. In the animal model with normal neutrophils, the presence of neutrophils doubled the duration of the *in vivo* PAE (6). The importance of the PAE in humans has not been completely studied.
      c. Nephrotoxicity and probably ototoxicity are related to time-dependent drug accumulation. **SDD may be less toxic** than multiple daily doses because little or no tissue accumulation occurs during the several hours before the next infusion when serum levels are low or undetectable (10).
   2. **Clinical studies** have been summarized in detail elsewhere (6–11), SDDs appear to be comparable and in some cases superior in efficacy to traditional aminoglycoside dosage strategies. However, typically the studies with SDD have been for short duration of therapy and most have been carried out in patients under 55 years of age.
   3. **Exclusions. See Table 21-3.**

Table 21-3.   Exclusions for using SDD

SDD is not advised for:
Moderate to severe renal insufficiency (creatinine clearance
   <40 ml/min)
Serious burns (>20% body surface area)
Ascites
Severe sepsis syndrome
Cystic fibrosis
Fluid overload postoperatively
Dialysis
Neonates/children
Pregnant patients
Documented invasive *P. aeruginosa* infection in neutropenic
   patients
Patients receiving other nephrotoxic agents (amphotericin B,
   cis-platinum, radiocontrast material, nonsteroidal anti-
   inflammatory drugs)
Endocarditis
Mycobacterial disease
Patients needing protracted courses, >7 days*
Patients with significant underlying hepatic disease[†]

Source: Modified from Gerberding JL. Aminoglycoside dosing: timing is of
the essence. *Am J Med* 1998;105:256.
* For example, in *P. aeruginosa* pneumonia in which the patient may need
2–3 weeks of antibiotics.
[†] See text. We try to avoid aminoglycosides in these patients.

   a. In patients with a reduced creatinine clear-
       ance, high-dose aminoglycoside treatment
       will produce sustained serum concentra-
       tions, drug accumulation, and increased
       potential for toxicity. Therefore patients with
       significant renal insufficiency have been ex-
       cluded from published trials with variable
       criteria (10).
   b. Patients in whom the patient's volume of
       drug distribution or clearance is difficult to
       predict or markedly abnormal (e.g., ascites,
       severe sepsis syndrome, severe burns, cys-
       tic fibrosis, as well as recipients of large vol-
       umes of fluid infusion or those undergoing
       large fluid shifts) are not candidates (10).
   c. There are incomplete data on SDD for preg-
       nant women, children, and neonates, so SDD
       is not advised in these settings (10).
   d. In patients receiving synergistic antibiotics
       for endocarditis (e.g., enterococci), animal
       studies reveal SDD regimens are inferior (10).
   e. Since there are limited data on the toxicity of
       prolonged SDD regimens, we prefer individ-
       ualized dosing in patients needing protracted
       aminoglycosides (i.e., more than 7 days).

f. In general, **we try to avoid aminoglyco-sides in patients with significant under-lying hepatic disease (e.g., cirrhosis)** because of the risk of nephrotoxicity. If they must be used, infectious disease consultation and individualized dosing are suggested.

4. **Dosing regimens for gentamicin and tobra-mycin**. Although some studies have used 5 to 7.5 mg/kg/dose, generally, we favor the lower-dose regimen of **5 mg/kg/dose** (or 5.1 mg/kg/dose) as emphasized by others (6,7).

   The SDD is **infused over 60 minutes (11)**.

   a. **For "weight in kg" use ideal body weight (IBW) in kilograms, but if the patient weighs more than 20% to 30% over IBW, an obese dosing weight (ODW; see below) is used.**

      (1) **To estimate IBW**

      Women = 45 kg + 2.3 kg per inch of height over 5 ft

      Men = 50 kg + 2.3 kg per inch of height over 5 ft

      For example, for a male patient 5 ft 10 in. tall, an estimated IBW would be 50 + 2.3(10), or 50 + 23 = 73 kg

      (2) **For patients weighing more than 20% above IBW, an ODW is more reliable (12).**

      • **Obese dosing weight = IBW + 40% (of excess weight; i.e., actual wt minus IBW)**
      • **For example**, an obese woman has a wound infection requiring gentamicin or tobramycin. Her actual weight is 100 kg; her ideal weight is 60 kg.

      Obese dosing weight
      = IBW + 40% (100 – 60)
      = 60 + 40% (40) = 60 + 16
      = 76 kg, and this weight can be used in **Table 21-4.**

   b. **For estimating the creatinine clearance for doses** in Table 21.3, a modification of the equation of Cockcroft and Gault is used. (See pages 292–293 in Chap. 14.)

   c. **See Tables 21-4 and 21-5.**

5. **Single daily dosing versus "extended-inter-val dosing" in patients with renal dysfunc-tion.** There are insufficient data to determine which of the two main options for dose adjust-ment in renal dysfunction—daily doses, but with dose reduction versus standard dose, but extend-ing the dosing interval—is preferable (10).

Table 21-4.   Once-daily aminoglycoside maintenance dosing regimens for gentamicin and tobramycin

Estimated Creatinine Clearance (ml/min)	Dose in mg/kg (Given q24h) Over 60 Minutes
>80	5
60–80	4
50–60	3.5
40–50	2.5
<40	Individualized pharmacokinetics advised

Source: Modified from Gilbert DN. Aminoglycosides. In: Root RK, et al., eds. *Clinical infectious diseases: a practical approach.* New York: Oxford University Press, 1999:273–284.

    a. **Some centers favor prolonging the dose interval (i.e., extended interval dosing)** for various levels of decreased creatinine clearance, and this approach with detailed guidelines is reviewed elsewhere (7).
    b. **Other centers** (e.g., Gilbert et al. [10]) **favor single daily dose with lowering the total daily aminoglycoside dose** for patients with mild to moderate renal insufficiency. We tend to use this approach, which is less cumbersome.

    • **See Tables 21-4 and 21-5 showing dose modifications for different levels of renal function.**
    • With this approach, some experts feel it is important to document that the serum concentration 18 hours after an infusion is low (<2 µg/ml for gentamicin or tobra-

Table 21-5.   Once-daily aminoglycoside dosing regimen for amikacin

Estimated Creatinine Clearance (ml/min)	Dose in mg/kg (Given q24h) Over 60 Minutes
>90	15
70–90	12
50–70	7.5
40–50	4.0
<40	Individualized pharmacokinetics advised

Source: Modified from Gilbert DN. Aminoglycosides. In: Root RK, et al, eds. *Clinical infectious diseases: a practical approach.* New York: Oxford University Press, 1999:273–284.

mycin) or undetectable (10). Gilbert suggests that a serum level of more than 1 µg/ml at 18 hours for gentamicin or tobramycin suggests impairment of renal excretion. A repeat serum creatinine and recalculation of the estimated creatinine clearance and reassessment of the size of the daily dose are therefore indicated (11).

6. **Serum monitoring** in SDD continues to undergo evaluation.

   a. A **trough** level before the second or third dose is advised, and this level should be less than 1 µg/ml; if not, extend the dose interval. (See also Sec. 5.b earlier.)

   b. Peak levels are not necessary, except possibly in patients with rapid clearance (e.g., severe sepsis).

   c. Trough levels can be repeated every 48 to 72 hours.

   d. See trough level discussion in Sec. III.C.

7. **Summary.** Unless contraindicated (Table 21.3), we agree with a recent 1999 editorial that "the available data are sufficient to establish this strategy (i.e., SDD or extended dosing) as a standard approach for most serious infections where aminoglycoside treatment is indicated" (10).

B. **Pharmacokinetics model**

   1. Zaske and colleagues have devised a formula for the pharmacokinetics of aminoglycosides in individual patients with either normal or impaired renal function (5,13). Timed serum samples are used to determine the volume of distribution and the half-life of the aminoglycoside. Using a kinetic model, the appropriate dose needed to achieve a desired peak and trough is calculated. Acceptable peak and trough levels can be maintained by adjusting doses and dose intervals. (**See Table 21-2 for desirable peak and trough levels.**)

      a. Because of the **variations in the volume of drug distribution** and the patient's ability to excrete aminoglycosides, there is marked variation in levels achieved with conventional dosing techniques. (See Sec. C. below.) The patient's age, renal function, state of hydration, presence or absence of fever, and degree of obesity affect serum levels. **Individualized dosing allows adjustment for each patient** by measuring serum levels and calculating the aminoglycoside's half-life.

      b. When pharmacokinetic studies reveal shorter half-lives than average, patients need larger and more frequent doses to maintain adequate aminoglycoside peaks and to avoid prolonged periods of subtherapeutic levels.

The converse is true for those with longer half-lives (5).

c. **We believe that this is the ideal way to manage the dosage of aminoglycosides when protracted therapy (more than 5 to 7 days) is needed or in special settings** when single daily dosing is not appropriate. (See Table 21-3 and Sec. V.A.3.)

2. **A loading dose** is typically used for the initial dose. (See Sec. C.1. below.)

3. **Maintenance doses** are given **based on** serum levels and the **pharmacokinetic model.**

C. **Conventional dosing but with careful serum monitoring of levels and serial dose adjustments by someone experienced with aminoglycoside use** (1).

1. **Loading dose.** The purpose of this dose is to achieve therapeutic plasma levels rapidly. The loading dose is given independent of renal function.

a. **For adult patients** it is based on **ideal body weight** in kilograms. In the patient weighing 20% more than IBW, an ODW is calculated as per Sec. V.A.4. on p. 423.

(1) First calculate the IBW/ODW for the patient.

(2) **For gentamicin, tobramycin, and netilmicin,** a loading dose of 2 mg/kg is used.

(3) **For amikacin,** a dose of 7.5 mg/kg is suggested.

b. **For children** a loading dose of 2 to 2.5 mg/kg is suggested for gentamicin and tobramycin. For amikacin, 5 to 7.5 mg/kg has been used (maximum of 500 mg).

c. **For neonates.** See Appendix Table A.

2. For **maintenance doses**

a. **In adult patients with a normal serum creatinine**, gentamicin, tobramycin or net-ilmicin at 1.0 to 1.7 mg/kg/dose is given at an 8-hour interval in young to middle-aged patients and q12h in older patients. The low dose of 1 mg/kg/dose is used for UTIs and the higher dose of 1.5 to 1.7 mg/kg/dose is used for tissue or bloodstream infections.

For amikacin 5 mg/kg/dose is given at 8-hour intervals in the young to middle-aged, and at 12-hour intervals in older patients.

In children aminoglycosides are eliminated more rapidly, so the same loading dose (2 to 2.5 mg/kg/dose of gentamicin or tobramycin) is given q8h and 5 to 7.5 mg/kg/dose of amikacin (maximum of 500 mg/dose) can be given q8h.

b. **In patients with renal failure there are two options.** The optimal approach is unclear.

(1) **The usual dose interval can be prolonged.**

(a) **For gentamicin, tobramycin, and netilmicin.** To estimate the prolonged interval, the serum creatinine is multiplied by 8. Hence if the serum creatinine is 2.0, the maintenance dose can be given every 16 hours (serum creatinine of 2 × 8).

(b) **For amikacin**, multiply the serum creatinine by 9. If the creatinine level were 2.0, the adjusted interval would be 18 hours.

(2) **Give half the dose every half-life.** To avoid very prolonged intervals (e.g., more than 24 to 36 hours) that may be associated with prolonged low serum trough levels, half the dose can be given at the estimated half-life interval. For example, if the serum creatinine is 3.5, for gentamicin the estimated prolonged interval is 8 × 3.5 = 36 hours; 50% of the dose can be given q18h (i.e., at half the extended interval).

(3) **In renal failure we prefer "individualized dosing." See Sec. B. above.**

c. **Serum monitoring is essential; this dosing regimen is only an estimation**. These levels must be obtained after the first dose and then can be repeated in 48 hours. **Further dosing can be adjusted as needed by someone experienced in aminoglycoside use**, to maintain appropriate peaks and troughs (Table 21-2).

D. **Nomograms**. Dosing based on nomograms alone is **not advised**.

E. **Overview of methods of dosing aminoglycosides. Until further studies and clinical experience clarify this issue, we think a reasonable approach is for those patients in whom it is not clear they are infected with an aminoglycoside-requiring organism to dose aminoglycosides using a once-daily regimen for empiric short courses (e.g., 3 to 5 days), whereas if an aminoglycoside is genuinely required in the very ill patient and in certain complex patient settings where SDD is contraindicated (Table 21-3), individualized dosing is preferable. Individualized dosing may also be superior for prolonged courses (e.g., over 5 to 7 days).**

F. **Miscellaneous**
1. **In dialysis patients.** Predialysis levels are reduced by approximately 50% with a complete hemodialysis, so one-half of the usual single dose is given after dialysis. Because the duration of dialysis and type of dialysis machine affect the amount of drug removed, **monitoring serum aminoglycoside levels is necessary. After a complete peritoneal dialysis**, one-third to one-half of a usual single dose for a 24-hour period often is administered. Serum aminoglycoside levels are advised.
2. **Treating peritonitis related to chronic ambulatory peritoneal dialysis (CAPD). Aminoglycosides in peritoneal dialysis fluid** have been used to treat susceptible CAPD-associated infections. This topic is discussed in Chap. 6 and is reviewed elsewhere (14). This approach is not recommended for patients with systemic infections because therapeutic serum and tissue levels are not achieved.
3. **Pulmonary infections. Aerosolized aminoglycosides** have sometimes been used in special settings: in cystic fibrosis patients with *P. aeruginosa* in their sputum (15) and selected cases of purulent *P. aeruginosa* tracheobronchitis without pneumonia. An infectious disease consultation is advised for these special considerations.

VI. **Toxicity.** Hypersensitivity reactions are uncommon. Important side effects include the following (1,2,16):
A. **Neuromuscular paralysis,** though rare, has occurred after intraperitoneal lavage (no longer used or recommended) or after rapid intravenous bolus therapy, particularly in the setting of myasthenia gravis or concurrent use of succinylcholine or curare. This is usually reversible.
B. **Ototoxicity is frequently irreversible** (1,2,16). It may appear during or after therapy; repeated exposure engenders cumulative risk. A given patient may develop cochlear damage, vestibular damage or, rarely, both.
1. **Cochlear (auditory) toxicity.** Previous audiometric studies show that 2% to 14% of recipients demonstrate hearing loss, but clinically detected hearing loss is uncommon. Patients particularly at risk to develop clinical signs are those who have received a high cumulative dose or a protracted course of aminoglycosides. **In general, routine audiograms are not possible and are not recommended** if renal function is normal. In a cooperative patient who needs protracted aminoglycoside therapy (e.g., more than 2 weeks), serial audiograms are reasonable. **Serum levels should be monitored carefully and ad-**

**justed. Protracted courses of aminoglyco-
sides should be avoided whenever possible.**

2. **Vestibular** dysfunction manifested by **nausea,
   vomiting, vertigo, dizziness, and unsteady
   gait** with nystagmus is more difficult to evaluate
   in ill patients but presumably is related to the
   same predisposing factors that cause auditory toxicity. This appears to occur in 1% to 3% of patients.

3. **If a patient is receiving an aminoglycoside
   and develops symptoms of hearing loss,
   tinnitus, vertigo, or nystagmus, the aminoglycoside should be discontinued.**

C. **Nephrotoxicity** due to aminoglycoside use is a complicated topic. Toxicity occurs at the level of the proximal tubule. There is no agreement as to how injury
or death of proximal tubule cells results in a decrease
in the glomerular filtration rate. The overall incidence
of aminoglycoside nephrotoxicity is about 5% to 10%
of recipients (1,2).

1. Nephrotoxicity with aminoglycosides can manifest
   as rising BUN and creatinine, or proteinuria, or
   oliguria, or nonoliguric renal failure. The changes
   are **usually reversible when the drug is discontinued.** Progression to dialysis-dependent
   oliguric-anuric renal failure is uncommon.

2. **Commonly used definition of nephrotoxicity.**
   If the initial creatinine was normal, nephrotoxicity is either an increase in serum creatinine above
   1.5 or an increase of 0.4 mg/dl. If the initial serum
   creatinine is elevated but less than 3.0 mg/dl,
   nephrotoxicity is an increase of at least 0.5 mg/dl.
   A serum creatinine rise of more than 1.0 mg/dl
   defines nephrotoxicity if the initial creatinine
   exceeded 3.0 (16). **Serum creatinine levels
   should be obtained every 2 to 4 days in
   patients receiving aminoglycosides.**

3. There are no conclusive data that one aminoglycoside is more nephrotoxic than another (1,2).

4. **Risk factors associated with increased frequency of nephrotoxicity** are (1,2,16):
   a. **Concomitant liver disease.** In particular,
      **in patients with known hepatorenal syn-
      drome or at risk for it (e.g., patients with
      cirrhosis) or in patients with prothrom-
      bin time prolongation due to underlying
      liver disease, we would avoid aminogly-
      cosides** if other options exist.
   b. **Concomitant drug use** may be important.
      Vancomycin, amphotericin B, cyclosporine,
      furosemide, nonsteroidal antiinflammatory
      agents, and foscarnet appear to increase the
      frequency of nephrotoxicity.
   c. **Other risk factors.** Advanced age, previous
      courses of aminoglycosides (within 1 year),

greater total dose of aminoglycoside, and prior renal disease may be associated with toxicity.

5. **Prevention** of nephrotoxicity is not fully understood. Considerations include:

   a. Aminoglycosides **should be used only when indicated and for** the **shortest appropriate course.**

   b. Correction of hypovolemia, diminished renal perfusion, and congestive heart failure is appropriate.

   c. Aminoglycosides should be avoided in patients with underlying liver disease. (See Sec. 4. above.)

   d. For short courses of therapy SDD regimens and for longer courses individualized dosing may help reduce nephrotoxicity. (See Sec. V.A. and V.B.)

VII. **Cost.** The generic formulation of gentamicin is less expensive than all other aminoglycosides and cephalosporins. A single dose of gentamicin (in SDD) will typically cost under $5. Amikacin is the most expensive aminoglycoside (see Table B, Appendix).

Aminoglycoside therapy, however, has been associated with "hidden" costs such as the costs of measuring serum levels and cost of the occasional case of nephrotoxicity. A 1999 review emphasizes that SDD regimens have clearly been shown to decrease the cost of aminoglycoside administration. Hospitals have estimated that SDD administration may reduce hospital costs of aminoglycoside administration 50% to 60% (2).

VIII. **Resistance**

A. **Resistance of gram-negative bacilli to aminoglycosides,** with the exception of streptomycin, **evolves very slowly** (1,2). Nonetheless, excess use of an antibiotic may be followed eventually by the development of resistance. When gentamicin resistance is common, it is reasonable to use amikacin, especially if resistant blood isolates have been detected.

B. **High-level gentamicin-resistant enterococci** has increased significantly (2) in recent years.

   1. See laboratory definition in Sec. II.B.

   2. **Clinical significance.** Because of intrinsic cephalosporin resistance, these enterococci are potentially very important nosocomial pathogens. The epidemiology of nosocomial enterococcal infections is very similar to that of nosocomial infections caused by methicillin-resistant staphylococci and by multidrug-resistant gram-negative bacilli. **Therefore all enterococci isolated from normally sterile body fluids (e.g., blood) or serious wound infections should be tested in the microbiology laboratory for high-level aminoglycoside resistance,** as well as ampicillin and vancomycin susceptibility.

3. **Therapy.** If an organism is identified with high-level gentamicin resistance, optimal therapy is unclear; **infectious disease consultation is advised.**

IX. **Other aminoglycosides are used less frequently and will be discussed only briefly.**

A. **Streptomycin** was introduced in 1944 and was effective against many gram-negative bacteria and *M. tuberculosis*. However, resistance to streptomycin is now prevalent among gram-negative bacteria, so for these organisms, use is now limited.

The availability of streptomycin in the United States was limited in late 1991. However, by mid-1993, streptomycin became available from Roerig, a division of Pfizer. As of spring 2000, physicians and hospital pharmacies can order streptomycin by calling 1-800-254-4445 (Monday through Friday 8:30 A.M. to 5 P.M. EST).

1. **Current uses**

   a. **Tularemia.** Streptomycin (or gentamicin) is the drug of choice for susceptible strains of *Francisella tularensis* (3).

   b. **Antituberculous therapy.** Streptomycin in combination with other agents is still used (3). It requires parenteral administration, and with the availability of new oral antituberculous agents, streptomycin has assumed a lesser role in tuberculosis therapy.

   c. **Uncommon diseases** in which streptomycin is a drug of choice or alternative drug (3) are brucellosis (with tetracycline), glanders (*Pseudomonas mallei*), and plague (due to *Yersinia pestis*). Streptomycin in combination with penicillin, ampicillin, or vancomycin has been used for treatment of endocarditis due to those strains of enterococci exhibiting high-level resistance to gentamicin but preserved susceptibility to streptomycin (2).

   d. **Alternate agent.** Streptomycin may be used in granuloma inguinale or in rat bite fever due to *Streptobacillus moniliformis* or *Spirillum minus* (3).

2. **Dosage.** In adults with normal renal function, for tularemia or plague, a dose of 500 to 1,000 mg intramuscularly (IM) q12h can be used. In children, 20 to 30 mg/kg/day is given and divided into q12h doses.

   If renal failure is present, ototoxicity is the risk. Therefore, gentamicin for which levels can be monitored is an acceptable alternative in some situations or the dose of streptomycin must be reduced. One approach (17) is to give a 1-g loading dose of streptomycin and then to prolong the interval. If the creatinine clearance is 10 to 50 ml/min, a dose interval of 24 to 72 hours is used. If the creatinine clearance is less than

10 ml/min, a dose interval of 72 to 96 hours is used. Streptomycin is removed by hemodialysis and peritoneal dialysis. If streptomycin must be used in dialysis patients, monitoring of serum levels using the disc diffusion method is a possibility. Ototoxicity is the risk. Infectious disease consultation is advised.

In tuberculosis therapy, intermittent dosage schedules are used. The average adult dose is 15 mg/kg up to 1 g (500 to 750 mg/day for patients older than 60 years) IM once daily for the first 2 to 8 weeks of therapy; thereafter, 25 to 30 mg/kg (to a maximum of a 1.5-g dose) twice weekly is used. Dosages are reduced in renal failure. For children with tuberculosis, 20 to 40 mg/kg/day initially (up to a maximum of 1.0 g) and 25 to 30 mg/kg two or three times weekly (maximum of 1.5 g) has been advised, per the package insert.

3. **Toxicity. We tend to avoid using streptomycin in patients older than 55 years if an alternate agent is available.**
   a. **Ototoxicity.** When given 2 g daily for more than 60 days, the majority of patients develop vestibular toxicity. The incidence is reduced by half if the dosage is reduced to 1 g daily. Deafness can occur. Patients particularly at risk are those with impaired renal function, the elderly, and those receiving prolonged courses of therapy.
   b. **Nephrotoxicity** is much less common with streptomycin than with the other aminoglycosides.
   c. **Hypersensitivity** reactions include rash and drug fever.

B. **Paromomycin (Humatin).** Paromomycin sulfate is structurally related to streptomycin and is an amorphous powder with a saline taste (18). It is too toxic for parenteral administration. Because it is not absorbed from the intestinal tract, it can be used safely as alternative therapy for asymptomatic infections due to *Entamoeba histolytica* (19) and has been used in AIDS patients infected with the protozoa *Cryptosporidium parvum* (19).

1. **Pharmacokinetics.** Paromomycin is poorly absorbed from the GI tract. However, impaired GI motility or ulcerations of the intestine may facilitate absorption of the drug. Therefore paromomycin must be administered with caution to patients with ulcerative intestinal lesions. Accumulation may occur in patients with impaired renal function and the drug may be contraindicated in this setting.

2. **Uses**
   a. **Parasitic infections.** Paromomycin is a drug of choice for asymptomatic carriers of

> *E. histolytica* and *Dientamoeba fragilis* infections. It is also an alternative agent for infections due to *Giardia lamblia* (19).

   b. **Cryptosporidiosis in patients with AIDS.**
For cryptosporidiosis, paromomycin is considered the agent of choice (19) with a dose of 25 to 35 mg/kg/day in three or four divided doses. Paromomycin (sulfate) is available in 250-mg tablets that can be given with or after meals (18).

  3. **Adverse side effects** (18)

    a. Anorexia, nausea, vomiting, epigastric burning, cramps, and diarrhea are the most frequent.

    b. Rash, eosinophilia, and headache may occur.

    c. Overgrowth of nonsusceptible organisms (e.g., *Candida*) may occur.

References

1. Reese RE, Betts RF. Aminoglycosides. In: Reese RE, Betts RF, eds. *A practical approach to infectious diseases*, 4th ed. Boston: Little, Brown, 1996:Chap. 28H.

2. Edson RS, Terrell CL. The aminoglycosides. *Mayo Clin Proc* 1999; 74:519.

3. Medical Letter. The choice of antibacterial drugs. *Med Lett Drugs Ther* 1999;41:95.

4. Wells VD, et al. Infections due to beta-lactamase-producing, high-level gentamicin-resistant *Enterococcus faecalis*. *Ann Intern Med* 1992;116:285.

5. Zaske DE, Cipolle RJ, Strate RJ. Gentamicin dosage requirements: wide interpatient variations in 242 surgery patients with normal renal function, *Surgery* 1980;87:164.

6. Urban AW, Craig WA. Daily dosing of aminoglycosides. *Curr Clin Top Infect Dis* 1997;17:236.

7. Bailey TC, et al. A meta-analysis of extended-interval dosing versus multiple daily dosing of aminoglycosides. *Clin Infect Dis* 1997;24:786.
   Concludes that for many indications extended-spectrum dosing (single daily dose in those with normal renal function) appears to be as effective but more convenient than conventional dosing, with similar toxicity. Provides details of program used at Barnes and Jewish Hospitals at Washington University Medical Center.

8. Gilbert DN. Editorial response: Meta-analyses are no longer required for determining the efficacy of single daily dosing of aminoglycosides. *Clin Infect Dis* 1997;24:816.
   Favors single daily dosing concluding it is simpler, less time-consuming, and intuitively more cost-effective than traditional multiple doses per day.

9. Bertino JS Jr, Rotschafer JC. Editorial response: single daily dosing of aminoglycosides: a concept whose time has not come. *Clin Infect Dis* 1997;34:820.

Authors feel final data still not in as to whether single daily dosing is equivalent or superior to multiple divided doses.

See related discussion by Beringer PM, et al. Pharmacokinetics of tobramycin in adults with cystic fibrosis: implications for once-daily administration. Antimicrob Agents Chemother *2000;44:809.*

10. Gerberding JL. Aminoglycoside dosing: timing is of the essence. *Am J Med* 1998;105:256.
    Nice editorial comment on SDD/extended dosing of aminoglycosides. See related clinical article in same issue by Gilbert et al.

11. Gilbert DN. Aminoglycosides. In: Root RK, et al, eds. *Clinical infectious diseases: a practical approach.* New York: Oxford University Press, 1999:273–284.

12. Traynor AM, Nafziger AN, Bertino JS Jr. Aminoglycoside dosing weight correction factors for patients with various body sizes. *Antimicrob Agents Chemother* 1995;39:545.

13. Cipolle RJ, et al. Systemically individualized tobramycin dosage regimens. *J Clin Pharmacol* 1980;20(10):570.

14. Keane WF, et al. Peritoneal dialysis-related peritonitis treatment recommendations: 1996 update. *Perit Dial Int* 1996;16:557.
    These recommendations are serially updated every 3 to 5 years.

15. Ramsey BW, et al. Efficacy of aerosolized tobramycin in patients with cystic fibrosis. *N Engl J Med* 1993;328:1740.
    Authors conclude that the short-term (e.g., 4 weeks) aerosol administration of a high dose of tobramycin in patients with clinically stable cystic fibrosis is efficacious and safe for treating endobronchial infection with P. aeruginosa. *By prolonging optimal pulmonary status in these patients, this approach may help decrease the frequency of courses of intravenous antibiotics for pulmonary exacerbations. Whether longer-term administration of aerosolized tobramycin would increase the frequency of colonization by tobramycin-resistant bacteria is unknown.*

    See related article by Fiel SB. Aerosol delivery of antibiotics to the lower airways of patients with cystic fibrosis. Chest *1995;107:61S (suppl 2), for a review of this topic.*

16. Gilbert D. Aminoglycosides. In: Mandell GL, Bennett JE, Dolin R, eds. *Principles and practice of infectious diseases*, 5th ed. New York: Churchill Livingstone, 2000:Chap. 23.

17. Aronoff GR, et al, eds. *Drug prescribing in renal failure: dosing guidelines for adults*, 4th ed. Philadelphia: American College of Physicians, 1999.

18. McEvoy GK, et al. *Drug information.* American Society of Hospital Pharmacists. Bethesda, MD: American Hospital Formulary Service, 1999:52.

19. Medical Letter. Drugs for parasitic infections. *Med Lett Drugs Ther* 1998;40:1.

Clindamycin

Clindamycin, introduced in 1966, is an important antibiotic for intraabdominal or pelvic infections involving anaerobes (1,2). In addition, it is a second-line alternative agent in penicillin-allergic patients for the treatment of susceptible gram-positive infections. Clindamycin is bactericidal for some organisms but generally is bacteriostatic, depending on the bacterial species, inoculum of bacteria, and concentration of antibiotic available. Clindamycin inhibits protein synthesis at the ribosomal level.

I. **Spectrum of activity**
   A. **Gram-positive aerobes.** Clindamycin is effective against group A streptococci and most *Staphylococcus aureus* strains. **Of hospital isolates, 5% to 20% or more of strains of S. *aureus* may be resistant to clindamycin** (1,3,4). The emergence of clindamycin-resistant *S. aureus* has been noted in clindamycin-treated patients, especially when the organisms initially had erythromycin resistance at the onset of treatment. **Clindamycin-sensitive but erythromycin-resistant organisms should be considered resistant to clindamycin. Most methicillin-resistant strains of S. *aureus* are resistant to clindamycin.** Clindamycin is not active against enterococci but is active against penicillin-susceptible *Streptococcus pneumoniae*. Penicillin-resistant strains of *S. pneumoniae* are typically resistant to clindamycin. (See Chap. 2.)
   B. **Gram-negative aerobes.** Clindamycin has **no useful activity** against gram-negative aerobes.
   C. **Anaerobes.** Clindamycin is active against gram-positive and gram-negative anaerobes, including most *Bacteroides fragilis* and *Clostridium perfringens* strains. In the past decade, susceptibility data have shown increasing resistance of *Bacteroides* spp. to clindamycin at many but not all institutions. For example in a report from six hospitals in Chicago, rates of resistance against *B. fragilis* within this one city varied from 0 to 20% (5). Other data suggest that 6% to 11% or more of *B. fragilis* isolates are resistant to clindamycin (1–3,5A).
   Approximately 10% to 20% of clostridial species, other than *C. perfringens* and 10% to 20% of peptococci strains are resistant to clindamycin (1,2).
   D. Clindamycin is not effective against *Mycoplasma pneumoniae*, but certain strains of *Toxoplasma gondii* are susceptible, as are *Babesia microti, Pneumocystis carinii*, and some malarial species (1,2,4).
II. **Pharmacokinetics**
   A. **Route and levels. Clindamycin is well absorbed from the gastrointestinal (GI) tract** (i.e., 90%), and food does not decrease its absorption. Therapeutic blood levels can be achieved by the oral, intramuscular, or intravenous route.

B. **Penetration.** Clindamycin penetrates most body tissues well, including sputum, bile, bone, prostate, and pleural fluid, but does not penetrate the cerebrospinal fluid well. It crosses the placenta.

C. **Metabolism and excretion.** Clindamycin is metabolized primarily by the liver. **In severe hepatic insufficiency, the half-life of clindamycin is prolonged** to 8 to 12 hours; **therefore doses of clindamycin should be reduced** in patients with severe liver failure or combined liver and renal failure (6).

Enterohepatic circulation of clindamycin and its metabolites can lead to a prolonged antimicrobial presence in stool with changes in gut flora lasting up to 2 weeks after discontinuation of clindamycin. Some have suggested that perhaps this accounts for clindamycin's causing *C. difficile* diarrhea (4).

III. **Indications for use** (1,2,4). **Except for *Bacteroides* spp. clindamycin is not the agent of choice for any specific pathogen** (7). It is a very useful alternative agent.

A. ***Bacteroides fragilis* infections and/or intraabdominal/pelvic infections.** Although clindamycin is listed as a drug of choice (7) for *Bacteroides* spp., many infectious disease experts feel metronidazole is the drug of choice, especially for severe *B. fragilis* infections. (See Chap. 29.)

1. For very severe and/or life-threatening intraabdominal infection, bacteremia with *B. fragilis*, and/or well-established intraabdominal abscess, we prefer metronidazole.

In endocarditis or other intravascular infection due to *B. fragilis*, metronidazole, a consistently bactericidal agent, is preferred.

2. For moderate to severe infections without *B. fragilis* bacteremia, clindamycin is very effective for intraabdominal and pelvic infections when combined with an agent active against gram-negatives (such as gentamicin).

B. **For mixed aerobic and anaerobic soft-tissue infections** (e.g., perineum), clindamycin has an advantage over metronidazole in that clindamycin is also active against group A streptococci and *S. aureus* as well as anaerobes, whereas metronidazole is not active against streptococci and is not active against *S. aureus*.

C. **Alternative drug in allergic patients**

1. In patients allergic to both penicillin and cephalosporins, clindamycin is an effective alternative for susceptible aerobic gram-positive cocci (e.g., *S. aureus, Streptococcus pyogenes*). Clindamycin is considered a second-line alternative agent for penicillin-susceptible *S. pneumoniae*.

2. Clindamycin is not a reliable agent in patients with known *S. aureus* endocarditis or a staphylococcal bacteremia; a bactericidal agent such as a cephalosporin or vancomycin is preferable. In

other staphylococcal infections (e.g., soft-tissue infections and bone infections), clindamycin is very useful.

D. **Osteomyelitis.** Clindamycin penetrates bone very well, so it is a useful alternative for susceptible organisms in the allergic patient and has been used in carefully monitored oral programs. Some pediatric infectious disease experts use it as a first-line agent in childhood osteomyelitis due to susceptible pathogens.

   In polymicrobial infections in adults, it may be combined with another agent active against gram-negatives, e.g., ciprofloxacin.

E. **Severe aspiration pneumonia or lung abscess.** When these infections are believed to be related to poor oral or dental hygiene and aspiration of oral anaerobes, penicillin has historically been the drug of choice, although clindamycin is also favored. Some experts favor clindamycin in patients who are seriously ill with this problem, to ensure coverage for anaerobes that may be resistant to penicillin.

F. **Diabetic foot infections.** Clindamycin, combined with an agent with good activity against aerobic gram-negative rods (e.g., ciprofloxacin), is commonly used.

G. **Miscellaneous uses**
   1. **Invasive group A streptococcal infections** such as severe necrotizing fasciitis, streptococcal myositis, streptococcal toxic shock syndrome, and bacteremias (8). Clindamycin may be more effective because of its activity against non-growing organisms against which penicillin appears to be less active. (See related discussions in Chap. 3.)
   2. **Severe cellulitis** of an extremity. For this problem clindamycin is favored by some clinicians. (See related discussions in Chap. 3.)
   3. **Alternative agent for endocarditis prophylaxis for oral/dental procedures**. (See Chap. 15.)
   4. **Odontogenic infections.** Orofacial infections may have a dental source that may lead to Ludwig's angina, maxillary sinusitis, and retropharyngeal and parapharyngeal abscesses with a major anaerobic infection component. Clindamycin is favored over penicillin or metronidazole in this setting.
   5. **Posttraumatic endophthalmitis** due to *Bacillus cereus*. Clindamycin has fairly good penetration into the eye.
   6. **Chronic sinusitis or chronic otitis.**
   7. **Bacterial vaginosis** usually is treated with oral metronidazole, but oral clindamycin (300 mg po bid for 7 days) or the 2% clindamycin **vaginal cream** daily for 7 days is an alternative. (See Chap. 10.)
   8. **Streptococcal group A pharyngitis.** Clindamycin has sometimes been used in patients with

recurrent streptococcal pharyngitis or in patients with multiple allergies. (See Chap. 1.)

9. **Acne vulgaris.** A 1% **topical** clindamycin **gel** and lotion has been used in this setting.

10. With **infectious disease consultation**, clindamycin has been used in special settings, including (a) central nervous system toxoplasmosis (in combination with pyrimethamine), (b) *Pneumocystis carinii* pneumonia in AIDS (with primaquine, when standard therapy has failed), and (c) babesiosis and malaria regimens.

IV. **Route and dosage**

A. **Oral. In children,** the recommended oral dosage is 10 to 25 mg/kg/day divided into q6h doses or for mild to moderately severe infections, 20 to 30 mg/kg/day in four divided doses has been used. In severe infections in children, such as osteomyelitis, 30 to 40 mg/kg/day (up to 50 kg of body weight) divided into q6h doses has been used. **In adults,** 300 to 450 mg q6 to 8h can be given, depending on the severity of the illness. However, some patients may have many GI side effects at the 450 mg/dose regimen.

B. **Parenteral**

1. **In adults** 600 mg q8h is usually recommended. For some gynecologic infections and possibly in the therapy of morbidly obese patients, 900 mg IV q8h is preferred.

2. **In children** older than 1 month, 20 to 40 mg/kg/day is suggested, divided into q6 to 8h doses.

3. **In neonates,** doses are summarized in Appendix A.

C. **Clindamycin 2% vaginal cream** is an alternative agent for bacterial vaginosis and is given at a dose of 5 g intravaginally once daily for 7 days. See Chap. 10.

D. **In renal failure, no change in the dosage** is required. Clindamycin is **not removed by either peritoneal dialysis or hemodialysis (9).**

E. **In hepatic insufficiency**, the half-life is prolonged. **Doses should be reduced** or the dosage interval prolonged or, if possible, an alternative agent should be used. (See discussion in Sec. II.C.) Patients with moderate to severe liver disease should be given about half the usual dose, and further reductions may be necessary if the patient also has renal disease (2).

F. **Pregnancy**. This is a category B drug. (See Chap. 14.) The package insert suggests that this drug should be used in pregnancy only if clearly indicated. Limited data have not revealed adverse effects on fetal development (4).

G. **Nursing mothers.** Clindamycin has been detected in breast milk. Because of the potential for adverse reactions to clindamycin in neonates, the package insert suggests that the decision to discontinue the drug should be made, taking into account the importance of the drug to the mother.

H. **Potential for antagonism** exists with the macrolides and chloramphenicol, which also act at the ribosomal level and may competitively inhibit the action of each other. These drugs **should not be used in combination** with clindamycin.

I. **Cost.** Clindamycin is a relatively expensive agent. See Appendix Tables B and C.

V. **Side effects**

A. **Gastrointestinal.** The most significant adverse reactions caused by clindamycin involve the GI system (4).

1. **Antibiotic-associated diarrhea** may occur in up to 20% of patients receiving clindamycin, presumably because of alternations of the bowel flora caused by the compound's activity against anaerobic bacteria (4).

2. *C. difficile* **diarrhea** can occur as a side effect of any antibiotic. (**See Chap. 5.**) It is much less common in outpatients receiving clindamycin, and the incidence of clindamycin-induced *C. difficile* diarrhea in hospitalized patients varies considerably by institution (4). The overall incidence is presumably less than 1%, unless there are nosocomial outbreaks or special problems within a given institution. When this occurs, restriction of clindamycin use has been beneficial (10).

3. Anorexia, nausea, vomiting, flatulence, bitter taste, and abdominal distention can occur (2).

B. **Allergic reactions** such as fever, eosinophilia, rashes, and rarely anaphylaxis can occur (1,2,4,11).

C. **Hepatotoxicity.** Minor, reversible elevations of hepatocellular enzymes are frequent.

D. **Nephrotoxicity.** Clindamycin does not cause significant renal toxicity.

E. **Bone marrow suppression.** Occasionally, cases of neutropenia and thrombocytopenia have been reported.

F. **A metallic taste** in the mouth when clindamycin is given parenterally occurs infrequently.

References

1. Reese RE, Betts RF, eds. Clindamycin. *A practical approach to infectious diseases*, 4th ed. Boston: Little, Brown, 1996:Chap. 28I.
2. Kasten MJ. Clindamycin, metronidazole, and chloramphenicol. *Mayo Clin Proc* 1999;74:825.
3. Steigbigel NH. Macrolides and clindamycin. In: Mandell GL, Bennett JE, Dolin R, eds. *Principles and practice of infectious diseases*, 5th ed. New York: Churchill Livingstone, 2000:366–382.
4. Gold HS, Moellering RC Jr. Macrolides and clindamycin. In: Root RK, et al. *Clinical infectious diseases: a practical approach*. New York: Oxford University Press, 1999:Chap. 32.
5. Hecht DW, Osmolski JR, O'Keefe JP. Variation in the susceptibility of *Bacteroides fragilis* group isolates from six Chicago hospitals. *Clin Infect Dis* 1993;16:S367 (suppl 4).

Authors conclude that variation in the antimicrobial susceptibility of these bacteria is hospital-based and not attributable to the geographic region and therefore for certain agents (e.g., clindamycin), in vitro susceptibility data cannot be assumed or predicted by large-scale surveys done elsewhere. Other agents are more predictably active against B. fragilis (e.g., metronidazole, imipenem, piperacillin-tazobactam). See related reference 5A.

5A. Snydman DR, et al. Multicenter study of in vitro susceptibility of the *Bacteroides fragilis* group, 1995 to 1996, with comparison of resistant trends from 1990 to 1996. *Antimicrob Agents Chemother* 1999;43:2417.

Although combined resistant rates from 1990–1996 revealed 11% resistance of B. fragilis strains against clindamycin, in 1995–1996, 16% of strains of B. fragilis were resistant to clindamycin.

Studies continue to show that clindamycin resistance to anaerobes shows significant variations among hospitals as well as geographic areas. See related discussions in references 1,3,5.

6. Falagas ME and Gorbach SL. Clindamycin and metronidazole. *Med Clin North Am* 1995;79:845.

7. Medical Letter. The choice of antibacterial drugs. *Med Lett Drugs Ther* 1999;41:95.

8. Stevens DL. The flesh-eating bacterium: what's next? *J Infect Dis* 1999;179:S366 (suppl 2).

See related paper by Zimbelman J, et al. Improved outcome of clindamycin compared with beta-lactam antibiotic treatment for invasive Streptococcus pyogenes infection. Pediatr Infect Dis J 1999;18:1096.

9. Aronoff GR, et al, eds. *Drug prescribing in renal failure: dosing guidelines for adults*, 4th ed. Philadelphia: American College of Physicians, 1999.

10. Climo MW, et al. Hospital-wide restriction on clindamycin: effect on the incidence of *Clostridium difficile*-associated diarrhea and cost. *Ann Intern Med* 1998;128:989.

During an outbreak of C. difficile diarrhea caused by a clonal isolate of clindamycin-resistant C. difficile, restrictions on the use of clindamycin resulted in a reduction of cases of C. difficile diarrhea and eventual increased susceptibility among C. difficile isolates.

See related papers by Pear SM, et al. Decrease in nosocomial Clostridium difficile-*associated diarrhea by restricting clindamycin use. Ann Intern Med 1994;130:272; Johnson S, et al. Epidemics of diarrhea caused by a clindamycin-resistant strain of* Clostridium difficile *in four hospitals. N Engl J Med 1999;341:1645 and the editorial by Dr. Gorbach in the same issue as paper by Johnson S, et al.*

11. Mazer N, Greenberger PA, Regaldo J. Clindamycin hypersensitivity appears to be rare. *Ann Allergy Asthma Immunol* 1999;82:443.

Chloramphenicol

Chloramphenicol has been available since 1949. Because of the irreversible fatal aplastic anemia that, on rare occasions, is associated with its use, chloramphenicol should be used only when clearly indicated. In the United States, chloramphenicol currently has limited indications, but it remains widely used in Third World countries because it is readily available, inexpensive, and efficacious in many serious infections (1,2).

I. **Mechanism of action.** Against *Staphylococcus aureus* and Enterobacteriaceae chloramphenicol is bacteriostatic. It inhibits protein synthesis at the ribosomal level. However, against common meningeal pathogens (*H. influenzae*, penicillin-susceptible *Streptococcus pneumoniae*, and *Neisseria meningitidis*, but not group B streptococci), chloramphenicol is bactericidal (3).

II. **Spectrum of activity** (1,2). Chloramphenicol is a broad-spectrum antibiotic active against many gram-positive and gram-negative bacteria, rickettsiae, chlamydiae, and mycoplasmas. However, **it is not listed as the drug of first choice for any common pathogen** (4) and alternative agents are available.

   A. **Gram-positive bacteria**. Many gram-positive cocci, both aerobic and anaerobic, are susceptible to chloramphenicol, although the minimum inhibitory concentrations (MICs) are relatively high. Alternate agents are preferred. Chloramphenicol is not considered a drug of choice against enterococci or staphylococci. Methicillin-resistant *S. aureus* (MRSA) usually is resistant to chloramphenicol.

   However, with the recent increase in vancomycin-resistant enterococci (VRE), which are resistant to most available antibiotics (Chap. 28), there is renewed interest in chloramphenicol, for it is active *in vitro* against many strains of VRE probably because of its previous infrequent use (5).

   B. **Gram-negative bacteria.** *N. meningitidis* and almost all *H. influenzae* strains are susceptible. Chloramphenicol has variable activity against other gram-negative bacilli; therefore susceptibility studies are necessary. *Pseudomonas* spp. are resistant.

   C. **Anaerobes**. Chloramphenicol has **excellent activity against gram-positive and gram-negative anaerobes**, including *B. fragilis* (1,2).

   D. **Miscellaneous.** Chloramphenicol is active against the rickettsiae that cause Rocky Mountain spotted fever, Q fever, and typhus, and it is active against *Ehrlichia caffaenis* (4).

III. **Pharmacokinetics** (1,2)

   A. **Absorption.** Chloramphenicol is rapidly absorbed orally, although variable absorption occurs in children.

It penetrates body tissues well, including the spinal fluid and the unobstructed biliary tree. **Approximately 30% to 50% of serum levels appear in the cerebrospinal fluid (CSF)** in both the inflamed and uninflamed meninges (1,2).

B. **Inactivation.** Chloramphenicol is metabolized and inactivated primarily in the **liver** by glucuronyl transferase.

C. **Excretion. In renal failure,** the plasma half-life of the biologically active free chloramphenicol is not prolonged. Consequently, chloramphenicol is given in normal doses in renal failure (6).

IV. **Toxicity**

A. **Dose-related bone marrow suppression may occur in any patient** on chloramphenicol. Anemia, reticulocytopenia, and neutropenia can occur. Bone marrow suppression is increased substantially in patients with ascites or jaundice (2). Occasionally, only thrombocytopenia is seen. This **reversible** bone marrow depression appears to be due to a direct pharmacologic effect of the antibiotic.

1. **Monitoring patients**

   a. **Serial blood counts. A complete blood cell count and platelet count or estimate every 2 or 3 days** while a patient is on chloramphenicol is suggested. If there is evidence of bone marrow suppression, the dose should be reduced and reassessment made of the need for this agent. If the bone marrow suppression worsens, usually the drug is discontinued.

   b. **Serum levels.** Direct bone marrow toxicity is related to levels of free chloramphenicol. **Therapeutic levels are between 10 and 20 μg/ml. The risk of direct bone marrow suppression increases when unconjugated (free drug) levels exceed 25 μg/ml (1). Serum should be monitored, especially in neonates and with prolonged use.**

2. **Recovery.** Complete recovery occurs approximately 2 weeks after stopping the chloramphenicol **in this reversible form.**

B. **Aplastic anemia** is rare, occurring only 1 in 25,000 to 40,000 courses of chloramphenicol, **and usually is fatal**. The precise mechanism is unknown, but there is a genetic predisposition. The aplasia is not dose related and can become manifest weeks to months after the use of chloramphenicol.

Whether topical ophthalmic use of chloramphenicol can cause aplasia remains controversial (7).

C. **Gray-baby syndrome.** Premature infants and newborns younger than 2 weeks have immature hepatic and renal function. Chloramphenicol can accumulate in the blood of these infants, especially when higher doses of the drug are used, causing the so-called gray-baby syndrome, which can cause vasomotor collapse and death. **Therefore chloramphenicol should be avoided in the premature infant and in the first 2 weeks of newborn life except in extreme life-threatening situations, in which decreased doses should be used and serum levels monitored.**

D. **Glucose-6-phosphate dehydrogenase deficiency.** Chloramphenicol may precipitate hemolysis in patients with a severe deficit of glucose-6-phosphate dehydrogenase (1).

V. **Clinical indications. Since this agent is used so infrequently, discussion of its use with an infectious disease subspecialist is advised.** The package insert clearly notes the pharmaceutical manufacturer's warning that chloramphenicol **"must not be used when less potentially dangerous agents will be effective. . . . It must not be used in the treatment of trivial infections or where it is not indicated, as in colds, influenza, infections of the throat, or as a prophylactic agent to prevent bacterial infections." Because of the availability of less toxic antibiotics, chloramphenicol is** seldom used except in special settings or in the allergic patient. Chloramphenicol is not listed as the drug of first choice for any common pathogen (4).

A. **Potential indications for chloramphenicol use include the following:**

1. **Alternative for life-threatening *H. influenzae* infections. The third-generation cephalosporins are the drugs of choice in the empiric therapy of meningitis and acute epiglottitis in children (4).** If there is an allergy history that precludes the use of cephalosporins, chloramphenicol remains an acceptable alternative.

2. **Alternative for bacterial meningitis due to a susceptible organism in a penicillin-allergic patient. Chloramphenicol is an important alternate agent in the patient with bacterial meningitis and severe allergy to both penicillins and cephalosporins.**

3. **Brain abscess**. Chloramphenicol may be used in this setting while awaiting culture results or if no culture data are available.

4. **Alternative agent in severe anaerobic infection.**

5. **Alternative drug (4) in** *Salmonella typhi* infections, brucellosis, glanders (*P. pseudomallei*), plague, *Chlamydia psittaci* infections (psittacosis), tularemia, and intraocular infections due to susceptible pathogens.

6. **Rickettsial infections** (Rocky Mountain spotted fever, endemic typhus [murine], scrub typhus, epidemic typhus [louse-borne], Q fever). **Chloramphenicol may be the preferred agent when**

> the patients require parenteral therapy, in
> young children, and in pregnancy when a
> tetracycline cannot be used. Infectious disease
> consultation is advised.

7. **In susceptible** infections due to **vancomycin-
   resistant enterococci**, chloramphenicol may
   provide a possible alternative (5,8). (See related
   discussion in Chap. 28.)

VI. **Route and dosage**
   A. **Neonatal doses. Serum levels should be moni-
      tored in neonates. Infectious disease consulta-
      tion is advised in this setting.**
   B. **Children and adults**
      1. **Intravenous**. The usual dosage is 50 to 100 mg/
         kg/day in divided 6-hour doses; usually to a max-
         imum dose of 1 g q6h. Serial blood cell counts or
         serum levels should be monitored. (See Sec.
         IV.A.1.) Children vary greatly in their ability to
         metabolize the drug; thus monitoring of serum
         levels is important in young children and neo-
         nates (2).
         a. **In renal failure,** routine doses and dose
            intervals can be used (6).
         b. **In hemodialysis or peritoneal dialysis**,
            no dosage adjustments are required (6).
         c. **In hepatic failure.** If chloramphenicol must
            be used, serum levels should be monitored. In
            adults, an initial loading dose of 1 g followed
            by 500 mg q6h sometimes is suggested; the
            course should be limited to 10 to 14 days (1).
      2. **Oral chloramphenicol** is no longer available in
         the United States, although it is available in some
         countries (e.g., Mexico).
      3. **Drug interactions.** Chloramphenicol can pro-
         long the half-life of chlorpropamide, phenytoin,
         tolbutamide, and warfarin derivatives. The pro-
         thrombin time of patients receiving anticoagula-
         tion therapy must be closely monitored (2).

References

1. Reese RE, Betts RF. Chloramphenicol. In: Reese RE, Betts RF, eds.
   A practical approach to infectious diseases, 4th ed. Boston: Little,
   Brown, 1996:Chap. 28J.
2. Kasten MJ. Clindamycin, metronidazole, and chloramphenicol.
   Mayo Clin Proc 1999;74:825.
3. Rahal JJ Jr, Simberkoff MS. Bactericidal and bacteriostatic action
   of chloramphenicol against meningeal pathogens. *Antimicrob
   Agents Chemother* 1979;16:13.
4. Medical Letter. The choice of antibacterial drugs. *Med Lett Drugs
   Ther* 1999;41:95.
5. Lautenbach E, et al. The role of chloramphenicol in the treatment
   of bloodstream infection due to vancomycin-resistant enterococcus.
   Clin Infect Dis 1999;27:1259.

6. Aronoff, GR et al. *Drug prescribing in renal failure: dosing guidelines for adults*, 4th ed. Philadelphia: American College of Physicians, 1999.
7. Walker S, et al. Lack of evidence for systemic toxicity following topical chloramphenicol use. *Eye* 1998;12:875.
   This review concludes that topical use is not a risk factor for inducing dose-related bone marrow toxicity. See related articles by Smith JR, Wesselingh S, Coster DJ. It is time to stop using topical chloramphenicol. Aust N Z J Ophthalmol *1997;25:83; and Rayner SA, Buckley RJ. Ocular chloramphenicol and aplastic anemia: Is there a link?* Drug Saf *1996;14:273. This article tries to present arguments for and against its use.*
8. Norris AH, et al. Chloramphenicol for the treatment of vancomycin-resistant enterocococcal infections. *Clin Infect Dis* 1995;20:1137.
   See related paper by Perez MS, et al. Vancomycin-resistant Enterococcus faecium *meningitis successfully treated with chloramphenicol.* Pediatr Infect Dis J *1999;18:483.?*

Sulfonamides and Trimethoprim-Sulfamethoxazole

I. **Sulfonamides.** Sulfonamides were the first effective systemic antibacterial drugs used in humans and were initially introduced in the late 1930s. The sulfonamides, which are primarily **bacteriostatic,** act by interfering with bacterial synthesis of folic acid (1).

   A. **Pharmacokinetics.** Sulfonamides generally are used in the oral form, providing **bacteriostatic** blood levels. They are metabolized in the liver by acetylation and glucuronidation. Free drug and its metabolites are excreted by the kidney. Preparations less apt to become crystallized in urine have attained more widespread use. Sulfonamides compete for binding sites on plasma albumin and may increase blood levels of unconjugated bilirubin. (See Sec. I.E.)

   B. **Spectrum of activity.** Because **routine disk antibiotic susceptibility testing generally is unreliable, it is not used.** A minimum inhibitory concentration (MIC) can be performed if necessary. Many community-acquired *Escherichia coli* often are susceptible, particularly at levels achieved in the urine. The sulfonamides also are active against many strains of *Neisseria meningitidis, Chlamydia, Toxoplasma*, and some *Nocardia* spp. **A sulfonamide alone is not the drug of first choice for any bacterial pathogen** (2). Sulfonamides have *in vitro* activity against *Streptococcus pyogenes* and have been used in regimens to prevent recurrent attacks of rheumatic fever (3), but they are not advised for treatment of streptococcal pharyngitis.

   C. **Current clinical uses**

      1. **Situations in which sulfonamides are useful** include the following:

         a. *Toxoplasma gondii* infections (e.g., sulfadiazine or trisulfapyrimidine, with the drug pyrimethamine).

         b. *Nocardia asteroides* infections, which respond well to sulfonamides. Trimethoprim-sulfamethoxazole (TMP-SMX) often is listed as the agent of choice (2).

      2. **Miscellaneous indications** for sulfonamide use are the following:

         a. Rheumatic fever prophylaxis (3) (e.g., sulfadiazine, although this agent is not useful in established streptococcal pharyngitis infections).

         b. Alternate agent in *Chlamydia* pneumonia.

3. For initial uncomplicated urinary tract infection (UTI) due to *E. coli*, sulfonamides in the past were the empiric agents of choice. However, data suggest 25% to 35% or more of strains of *E. coli* that cause outpatient cystitis are resistant to sulfonamides (1). Therefore **alone sulfonamides are no longer the agents of choice for empiric therapy of initial uncomplicated UTI.** However, in combination with trimethoprim, sulfonamides (i.e., TMP-SMX) are useful empiric agents in UTI and prophylaxis of UTIs.

4. Sulfonamides have been used in selected patients to prevent recurrent otitis media. (See Chap. 1.)

D. **Preparations available and dosage regimens** (1–4). Sulfonamides are variably acetylated and glucuronated in the liver. The resulting inactive metabolites as well as free drug are filtered through the glomerulus and actively secreted into the urine (4).

Sulfonamide dosage should be altered for creatinine clearance of less than 50 ml/min; no dosage modification is necessary for patients with hepatic impairment (4).

Sulfonamides penetrate pleural, peritoneal, synovial, and cerebrospinal fluid (CSF); they cross the placenta and are detectable in breast milk.

1. **Short-acting** preparations usually are given four (and sometimes six) times daily.

a. **Sulfisoxazole** (e.g., Gantrisin, Azo Gantrisin) is excreted rapidly, is soluble in urine, and still is occasionally used in UTIs. Prior regimens for UTIs in adults involved a 2- to 4-g loading dose and then 1 g q6h. (In children, the initial dose is half the 24-hour dose, and the maintenance dose is 150 mg/kg/day divided into q6h doses.) We suspect this agent is now seldom used for UTI in adults.

b. **Sulfadiazine** (e.g., Microsulfon) is less soluble in urine and therefore less suitable for use in UTIs. It appears to be less protein-bound than sulfisoxazole, and one can achieve good blood and CSF levels with sulfadiazine. Therefore it often is used when a sulfonamide is indicated, **as in nocardial infection, toxoplasmosis, and rheumatic fever prophylaxis** in the penicillin-allergic patient. Although it has a longer half-life than sulfisoxazole, sulfadiazine is given four times daily. The usual therapeutic dose in adults is a 2-g loading dose with a maintenance dose of 1 g four times per day.

Various dose regimens for the treatment of toxoplasmosis and nocardiosis have been suggested, and infectious disease consultation is advisable.

    c. **Triple sulfa drug** (trisulfapyrimidines; e.g., triple sulfa tablets no. 2) usually is made up of sulfadiazine and two other sulfa preparations. Theoretically, each drug maintains its solubility in the urine to decrease the chances for crystalluria. In adults, the usual dose is 1 g four times daily.

  2. **Intermediate-acting** sulfonamides can be given two or three times daily. **Sulfamethoxazole** (Gantanol, Azo Gantanol) is less soluble than sulfisoxazole, is excreted more slowly, and therefore provides higher blood levels than sulfisoxazole. It can be given twice daily and has been used in UTIs, in which such a dose schedule helped with compliance. Because it has a greater tendency than short-acting sulfonamides to cause crystalluria, it is important to ensure a high urine output when it is used. The dose regimen in adults is a 2-g initial dose followed by 1 g bid. In children older than 2 months, the initial dose is 50 mg/kg; then 25 to 30 mg/kg per dose is given bid. **Sulfamethoxazole has been combined with trimethoprim and is available as cotrimoxazole (Bactrim, Septra), which is discussed in Sec. II and is used more than any sulfonamides alone.**

  3. **Long-acting sulfonamides** are **no longer recommended,** because these preparations have the capacity to produce hypersensitivity reactions (e.g., Stevens-Johnson syndrome), which then become a prolonged problem. An exception is sulfadoxine which is a component of Fansidar which is still used in some antimalarial regimens. (See Sec. III.)

  4. **Common topical sulfonamides** (5). Mafenide acetate (Sulfamylon) has been used topically on burns to help prevent bacterial colonization, particularly colonization with pseudomonads. Its use has been limited by the side effect of metabolic acidosis. Silver sulfadiazine (Flamazine) has fewer side effects and is used extensively for burns. Outbreaks of silver-resistant infections in burn units may ultimately limit its usefulness (5). Sulfonamides are used also in ophthalmic ointments and in vaginal suppositories and creams.

  5. **Sulfasalazine** (Azulfidine) is used in the treatment of ulcerative colitis.

E. **Toxicity**. Modern sulfonamides are more soluble, and crystalluria is much less of a problem, than in the past.

  1. **Pregnancy and neonates. Sulfonamides should not be used in the last trimester of pregnancy (especially the last month)** because they are transplacentally transmitted and compete for bilirubin-binding sites on plasma albumin, increasing the risk for kernicterus (5). Sulfonamides are **not recommended for ther-**

apy in neonatal infections or in nursing mothers because the neonate's hepatic enzyme system may be immature.

2. **Hematologic considerations.** Sulfonamides should be **avoided in patients with glucose-6-phosphate dehydrogenase (G-6-PD) deficiency,** because hemolysis can be precipitated. However, one study showed that G-6-PD-deficient patients who received TMP-SMX did not have hemolytic reactions during therapy (6). Bone marrow depression with anemia, leukopenia, or thrombocytopenia can occur with sulfonamide use, especially in those with folate deficiency.

3. **Hypersensitivity reactions** with rashes, vasculitis, erythema nodosum, erythema multiforme, and Stevens-Johnson syndrome can occur. These were particularly common with the long-acting compounds, which are no longer recommended.

4. **GI disturbances** with nausea, vomiting, and diarrhea can occur in 3% to 5% of patients (4).

5. Renal dysfunction due to tubular deposition of sulfonamide is now rare (4).

F. **Important drug interactions.** Sulfonamides may displace drugs from albumin-binding sites, increasing the clinical effect of the displaced drug (5).

1. **Oral anticoagulants.** The **doses of oral anticoagulants** (e.g., warfarin sodium) **should be reduced** and serial prothrombin times monitored carefully while patients receive sulfonamides, which compete for albumin-binding sites and, in effect, increase the activity of a given anticoagulant dose.

2. **Methotrexate** (MTX). Because sulfonamides displace methotrexate from its bound protein, **the risk of methotrexate toxicity increases if sulfonamides are used concurrently.** Consequently, sulfonamides should be avoided in patients receiving MTX.

3. **Oral hypoglycemic agents.** The hypoglycemic effect of sulfonylureas may be exaggerated by sulfonamides, although the precise mechanisms for this are unclear.

4. **Methenamine** compounds should not be given concomitantly with sulfonamides because there is an increased risk of insoluble urinary precipitate formation.

G. **Sulfonamide use in renal failure.** Because sulfonamides are excreted by way of the kidney, in renal failure **doses must be reduced or dose intervals prolonged** (7).

II. **Trimethoprim-sulfamethoxazole (TMP-SMX)** (1,5,8,9), formerly called *cotrimoxazole,* is available commercially as **Bactrim or Septra as well as in generic** preparations. This unique preparation was specifically formulated to include a combination of agents that would inhibit activity in two sequential steps of bacterial metabolism. It became available in the United States in 1973. The combination has two theoretic advantages: (a) It decreases the chances of bacterial resistance, and (b) the combination may act synergistically. The combination is available in oral and intravenous forms. The regular tablets contain 80 mg TMP and 400 mg SMX to provide an ideal blood ratio of 1:20 for optimal synergy. However, it is noteworthy that in different body fluids, the ratios of TMP to SMX are virtually never 1:20, so the value of the ideal ratio in the blood is uncertain. **Alone, each agent is bacteriostatic, but together they are bactericidal and synergistic *in vitro*.** Currently, sulfonamides are used most frequently in this combination (5)

A. **Mechanism of action.** TMP-SMX sequentially blocks two steps in the synthesis of folic acid by bacteria **(Fig. 24.1).**

B. **Pharmacokinetics** (1,4,5). **Oral TMP-SMX is well absorbed.** Peak serum levels occur 1 to 4 hours after ingestion. The intravenous preparation provides excellent blood levels. Serum half-lives of TMP and SMX are 8 to 10 hours and 10 hours, respectively (4). TMP-SMX is excreted primarily by the kidneys, so doses must be reduced in renal failure. Excretion occurs over several hours, and this permits twice-daily dosing. Each drug is distributed widely and can be detected in most tissues of the body. This agent penetrates the CSF well (20% to 40% of serum levels). Concentrations

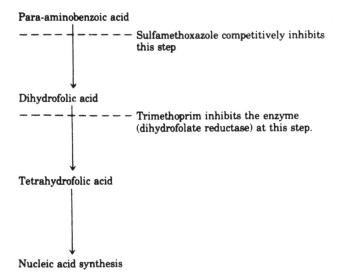

Para-aminobenzoic acid

— — — — — — — — — Sulfamethoxazole competitively inhibits this step

Dihydrofolic acid

— — — — — — — — — Trimethoprim inhibits the enzyme (dihydrofolate reductase) at this step.

Tetrahydrofolic acid

Nucleic acid synthesis

Figure 24.1.   Mechanism of action of trimethoprim-sulfamethoxazole. Most bacteria cannot use exogenous folate but must make their own folate for nucleic acid synthesis. Trimethoprim-sulfamethoxazole can sequentially block the formation of tetrahydrofolic acid and thereby interfere with cell replication.

of TMP in prostatic fluid usually are at least three times those of the serum concentration (1).

C. **Spectrum of activity.** Trimethoprim by itself has a wide spectrum of activity against gram-positive and gram-negative bacteria. (See Chap. 25.) Sulfamethoxazole is less active alone, but it enhances the activity of TMP when combined with it.

1. **Gram-positive cocci.** TMP-SMX is active against the majority of *Staphylococcus aureus, S. epidermidis,* penicillin-susceptible *S. pneumoniae* strains, and viridans streptococci. In a survey of penicillin-resistant strains of *S. pneumoniae* in Atlanta, Georgia, published in 1995, 75% of the isolates resistant to penicillin were resistant to TMP-SMX (10). (See related discussions in Chaps. 2 and 16.) It is not useful clinically against enterococci. This agent is active against many methicillin-resistant *S. aureus* (MRSA) species. Despite the apparent *in vitro* sensitivity of MRSA, some reviews emphasize that clinical success with TMP-SMX therapy for MRSA is extremely variable and unpredictable (8).

2. **Most Enterobacteriaceae, *Salmonella* and *Shigella* spp., *Haemophilus influenzae*** (ampicillin-susceptible and ampicillin-resistant), **and *Moraxella (Branhamella) catarrhalis*** are susceptible. TMP-SMX has activity against *Pasteurella multocida* (11), although it is usually not listed as an alternative agent for this pathogen (2).

3. TMP-SMX is **not active against** *Pseudomonas aeruginosa* or enterococci. However, *Burkholderia cepacia* (formerly *P. cepacia*) are usually susceptible and many *Stenotrophomonas* (formerly *Xanthomonas*) *maltophilia* are susceptible.

4. **Anaerobes.** TMP-SMX is not particularly active against anaerobes, including *Bacteroides fragilis* (1,9).

5. **Miscellaneous** (1,2,9).
   a. TMP-SMX is active against *Listeria monocytogenes, Yersinia enterocolitica, Aeromonas* species, *Legionella micdadei,* and *Legionella pneumophila.*
   b. *Pneumocystis carinii* (a parasite) is susceptible.
   c. Many *Nocardia* spp. are susceptible.
   d. *Treponema pallidum* is resistant.

6. **Resistance to TMP-SMX** has increased in recent years and is governed primarily by resistance to TMP. This is discussed in Chap. 25. Much of the resistance to TMP has been reported in developing countries, where TMP has been used extensively as monotherapy and where antibiotics are available without prescription (8). Increasing resistance of TMP-SMX against *Salmonella typhi, Shigella* spp., MRSA, and *S. pneumoniae* is noted.

Approximately **30% to 35% of nosocomial uropathogens are resistant** to TMP-SMX (8).

However, in a recent report of susceptibility studies in **community-acquired** (Seattle, WA) acute uncomplicated **cystitis** in women 18 to 50 years of age, the incidence of **resistance of *E. coli* to TMP-SMZ** rose from 9% in 1992 to more than **18% in 1996** (12).

D. **Current indications for use of TMP-SMX (1,2,8,9). For certain pathogens, TMP-SMX is considered the drug of first choice (2). These include** *M. catarrhalis, H. influenzae* causing upper respiratory infections and bronchitis, *Y. enterocolitica, Aeromonas* spp., *Burkholderia cepacia, S. maltophilia, Nocardia* spp., and *P. carinii.*

   1. **Urinary tract infections**

      a. **Acute initial uncomplicated UTI.** Because many strains of community-acquired *E. coli* are resistant to sulfonamides alone and amoxicillin (ampicillin), for empiric therapy of community-acquired uncomplicated UTIs, TMP-SMX is often preferred (2).

         However, with community-acquired *E. coli* beginning to become more resistant to TMP-SMX (see Sec. C.6. above) and up to 8% of strains of *S. saprophyticus* resistant to TMP-SMX (12), these resistance issues must be considered in empiric therapy of cystitis (12), and especially pyelonephritis. Although we still commonly use empiric TMP-SMX in the healthy young female with an uncomplicated UTI, if the patient has underlying diabetes or repetitive infections, or a possible early pyelonephritis, we would favor a quinolone.

      b. **Pyelonephritis. If the gram stain of unspun urine reveals gram-positive cocci, suggesting enterococci, TMP-SMX should not be used.** Because TMP-SMX penetrates tissue well, it is a useful agent in this setting **for susceptible pathogens,** especially since it can be given both intravenously and orally.

      c. **Recurrent UTI in adult women.** In women prone to recurrent UTI, TMP-SMX has helped decrease the rate of recurrence, presumably in part by decreasing colonization at the periurethral area (1). However, enterococcal colonization may result. An alternative regimen is a short course of self-administered antibiotic with a twice-daily dose of TMP-SMX for 3 days at the onset of symptoms. (See related discussions in Chap. 4.)

      d. **Prostatitis recurrent UTI in men.** In the absence of other genitourinary pathology, men with recurrent UTI often have chronic

bacterial prostatitis that seeds the genitourinary tract (13,14). Organisms in the prostate are extremely difficult to eradicate, because most antibiotics do not penetrate the prostate well. TMP-SMX penetrates the prostatic fluid and is very useful in these patients. (The fluoroquinolones also are useful in this setting.) (See Chap. 4 also.)

e. **Postcoital antibiotic prophylaxis for recurrent UTI** with TMP-SMX has been shown to be a safe, effective, and inexpensive approach to management in carefully selected young women with recurrent UTI (15). (See Chap. 4.)

2. **Respiratory infections.**

   a. *Pneumocystis carinii.* **TMP-SMX is considered the drug of choice in children and adults** for the treatment and prevention of *P. carinii* **pneumonia** (PCP) (16).

   A high incidence of adverse effects occurs in patients with AIDS who are treated with TMP-SMX, especially when maximal doses are used. (See related discussion in Sec. G.)

   b. **Acute exacerbations of chronic bronchitis.** Because TMP-SMX is active against penicillin-susceptible *S. pneumoniae, H. influenzae,* and *M. catarrhalis,* it is a useful agent in this setting (1,5) or as part of a rotating antibiotic regimen. (See Chap. 1.)

   c. **Pneumonia.** For susceptible gram-negative pathogens, intravenous TMP-SMX has been used for lower respiratory tract infections (5). TMP-SMX is an alternative agent for *L. micdadei* and *L. pneumophila* infections when erythromycin or a fluoroquinolone cannot be used (2).

   d. **Acute otitis media (AOM).** TMP-SMX has been used as an alternative agent for AOM, especially if ampicillin-resistant *H. influenzae* is a concern. (See Chap. 1.)

   e. **Sinusitis** has been treated effectively with TMP-SMX. With the advent of penicillin (and TMP-SMX) resistant *S. pneumoniae,* TMP-SMX may be less effective for sinusitis therapy. (See Chap. 1.)

3. **Gastrointestinal infections**

   a. **Shigellosis.** TMP-SMX is considered a useful alternative agent for enteritis caused by susceptible *Shigella* strains (2).

   b. **Salmonella.** Although ceftriaxone or a quinolone are drugs of choice for *S. typhi,* and cefotaxime or ceftriaxone or a quinolone are treatments of choice for other *Salmonella* spp. infections requiring treatment, TMP-SMX is often an excellent alternative agent (2). (See Chap. 5.)

    c. **Travelers' diarrhea.** A few years ago, TMP-SMX was the most common agent used to treat travelers' diarrhea. Now the fluoroquinolones often are preferred in adults since TMP resistance has become common. (See Chap. 5.)

    d. **Prevention of spontaneous bacterial peritonitis** in patients with underlying cirrhosis. The use of TMP-SMX and the quinolones in this setting is briefly discussed in Chap. 15.

4. **Some forms of meningitis. Gram-negative bacillary meningitis** caused by organisms only **moderately susceptible** to **third-generation cephalosporins** (e.g., *Enterobacter cloacae, Serratia marcescens*) or resistant to these antibiotics (*P. cepacia, Acinetobacter* spp.) may be candidates for TMP-SMX treatment if the organisms are susceptible (1,5,9,17). TMP-SMX is an alternate agent in meningitis due to *L. monocytogenes* (2), when ampicillin cannot be used.

5. **Prevention of infection in neutropenic patients.** Although TMP-SMX has been used in these patients, a recent panel of experts concluded that routine use of TMP-SMX should be avoided in this setting (9,18).

6. **Miscellaneous**

    a. **Endocarditis.** TMP-SMX has been used as an alternative agent for susceptible pathogens causing bacteremia or endocarditis (1,5). Infectious disease consultation is advised.

    b. **Nosocomial infections.** Gram-negative nosocomial infections due to bacteria resistant to many antibiotics may be susceptible to TMP-SMX (e.g., *Enterobacter, Klebsiella,* and *Proteus* spp.), and patients will respond to this therapy. *Burkholderia cepacia* (formerly *P. cepacia*) infections that have relapsed or failed other agents often have responded well to TMP-SMX. **Prior to using TMP-SMX for these types of infections,** *in vitro* **data should show that the organism to be treated is susceptible to TMP-SMX.**

    c. *Nocardia.* TMP-SMX is an important agent for *Nocardia* infections and sometimes is viewed as the agent of choice (2).

    d. *Y. enterocolitica* and *Aeromonas* spp. infections can be treated with TMP-SMX.

    e. **Brucellosis.** TMP-SMX is an alternative agent for brucellosis (2).

    f. **Prevention of infection in renal transplantation recipients.** Prophylaxis with TMP-SMX significantly reduces the incidence of bacterial infection following renal transplantation (especially infection of the urinary tract and bloodstream), can provide protection against PCP, and is cost-beneficial (19). Patients appear to tolerate this regimen well in this setting (19).

g. **Prevention of infection in patients with chronic granulomatous disease.** TMP-SMX prophylaxis is useful in the prevention of infectious complications (1,9).

h. *Mycobacterium marinum.* TMP-SMX is an alternative agent (2).

i. **GI infections with** cyclospora, isospora, and **coccidian parasites** in HIV-infected patients have been treated with TMP-SMX (20).

j. **Prevention of spontaneous bacterial peritonitis** in patients with underlying cirrhosis: In this setting, TMP-SMX appears useful. (See Chap. 15.)

E. **Forms available**

1. **Oral. Single-strength** (SS) tablets contain 80 mg TMP and 400 mg SMX. The **double-strength** (DS) tablets contain 160 mg of TMP and 800 mg SMX. There are unflavored and cherry-flavored **suspensions** containing 40 mg TMP and 200 mg SMX per 5 ml.

2. **Parenteral.** An intravenous form of TMP-SMX is supplied in 5-ml ampules* that contain 80 mg TMP and 400 mg SMX. The intravenous preparation is recommended for the following: (a) **severe UTIs** in patients who are vomiting or otherwise too ill to take an oral medication, (b) patients with severe **PCP**, (c) **severe** *Shigella* **infections,** and (d) certain serious multiresistant enteric gram-negative bacillary infections in which TMP-SMX is active *in vitro*. Infectious disease consultation is advisable in this setting. The intravenous form has also been used in the treatment of pneumonia, bacteremia, meningitis, and other serious infections.

   For severe or complicated UTI, 8 to 10 mg/kg/day (based on the TMP component) is recommended. The dose is divided into a q6h or q12h schedule until the patient improves enough to allow oral therapy. **See Table 24-1.**

F. **Dosage.** Since TMP-SMX is well absorbed, **the oral route is usually preferred** unless the patient has nausea, is vomiting, is NPO, or is critically ill. If intra-

---

* Each 5-ml ampule usually is added to 125 ml of 5% dextrose in water by the pharmacy for intravenous administration. In some patients, this may represent a significant fluid load. The package insert suggests that for patients on fluid restriction, each ampule may be added to 75 ml of 5% dextrose in water. (Also, the daily dose can be divided up into a q6h regimen rather than the q12h regimen. Supplemental diuretics may be needed in some patients.)

Table 24-1.   Dosing of TMP-SMX

Indication	Dosage*/Day (Normal Renal Function)	Duration and Comments
Uncomplicated cystitis in women	1 DS bid	For 3 days
Conventional therapy in UTI, UTI in elderly	1 DS bid	For 7–10 days
Pyelonephritis	IV or po, 1 DS bid po	For at least 14 days. See text for IV doses. For children use dose as in acute otitis media.
Prophylaxis of recurrent UTI in women	½ or 1 SS* every other night or ½ SS tab nightly qhs	Typically for at least 6–12 months; the urine should be sterilized first. See Chap. 4.
Prostatitis	1 DS bid	For 3–4 weeks or more. See Chap. 4.
Acute exacerbations of COPD	1 DS bid	Usually for 5–7 days. See Chap. 1.
Acute otitis media (AOM)	In children >2 months, TMP 8 mg/kg/day and SMX 40 mg/kg/day given in divided doses q12h **See Table 24-2**	5 days to 10 days. See Chap. 1.
Sinusitis	1 DS bid in adults. In children, see AOM doses	Usually for 10 days. See Chap. 1.
Pneumonia	IV initially (see text)	After improvement, switch to po, 1 DS bid in adults, duration must be individualized. See Chap. 2.
Salmonella, Shigella when susceptible	Dosages used for UTI	For 5 days
Traveler's diarrhea	1 DS bid	For 3 days in adults. Many *E. coli* now resistant to TMP-SMX. See text and Chap. 5. Quinolones usually preferred unless contraindicated.

continued

Table 24-1. (*Continued*)

Indication	Dosage*/Day (Normal Renal Function)	Duration and Comments
Susceptible, gram-negative meningitis[†]	10 mg/kg/day (based on TMP component) IV divided q6h[†]	Probably for 2 weeks. Infectious disease consultation advised.
Bacteremias and nosocomial infections	IV 8–10 mg/kg/day (based on TMP component) divided q6 or q12h schedule.	Go to oral doses when patient improves.
Prevention of *Pneumocystis carinii* pneumonia (PCP) in immuno-compromised e.g., AIDS[‡]	1 DS po qd or 1 SS po qd	While CD4 count is <200/μL or oropha-ryngeal candidiasis
Therapy of PCP	Initially, begin at 5 mg/kg of TMP component q6h for 3–5 days, then q8h for another 3–5 days, then 4 mg/kg of TMP q8h component until course completed.	Total course of 21 days. By tapering doses, side effects may be minimized. In very ill patients, IV therapy is initially used and converted to oral therapy as the patient improves.

* DS, double-strength tablet; SS, single-strength tablet. The DS tablet of TMP-SMX is a large tablet; some patients may prefer two of the smaller SS tablets.
[†] See Levitz AE, Quintiliani R. Trimethoprim-sulfamethoxazole for bacterial meningitis. *Ann Intern Med* 1984;100:881.
[‡] 1999 USPHS/IDSA guidelines for the prevention of opportunistic infections in persons infected with human immunodeficiency virus. *MMWR* 1999; 48(RR-10):1 and *Ann Intern Med* 1999;131:873.

venous (IV) therapy is initially used, one can often switch to oral therapy when the patient improves.

Adequate fluid intake should be encouraged to prevent sulfonamide crystalluria (1).

1. **See Table 24-1.**
2. **In children,** TMP-SMX is **not recommended for infants less than 2 months** of age because of the risk of kernicterus. For otitis media and other infections 8 mg/kg TMP (and 40 mg/kg SMX) per 24 hours given in two divided doses every 12 hours for 10 days. (See Chap. 1.) See **Table 24-2.** An identical dosage is given for 5 days for shigellosis.

Table 24-2. Pediatric dosages of TMP-SMX for UTI, otitis media, shigellosis, and the like* (pediatric suspension)

Weight		Dose (q12h)	
lbs.	kg	Teaspoonfuls	Tablets
22	10	1 tsp. (5 ml)	—
44	20	2 tsp. (10 ml)	1 tablet[†]
66	30	3 tsp. (15 ml)	1½ tablets
88	40	4 tsp. (20 ml)	2 tablets or 1 DS tablet

Abbreviation: DS, double strength.
Source: *Physicians' Desk Reference 1999,* 53rd ed. Montvale, NJ: Medical Economics Data, 1999. Copyright by Medical Economics Data. Reprinted by permission. All rights reserved.
* For children 2 months of age or older.
[†] Author's note: tablet = single strength.

3. **In pregnancy**
   a. TMP-SMX is **not recommended at term** as sulfonamides cross the placenta and may cause kernicterus.
   b. TMP-SMX is a **category C** drug. (See Chap. 14.) It is generally not recommended for use in pregnancy unless the benefits justify the risks to the fetus (5). (See Sec. G.4. below.)
4. **Nursing mothers.** Because sulfonamides are excreted in human milk and may cause kernicterus, the package insert does **not** advise the **use** of TMP-SMX for nursing mothers. (See Sec. **G.4.**)
5. **In renal failure, dosages** must be **modified**. The optimal approach is not well defined.
   a. The package insert suggests that standard doses can be used for a creatinine clearance of more than 30 ml/min. For a creatinine clearance of 15 to 30 ml/min, half the usual dose is suggested. For a creatinine clearance of less than 15 ml/min, use is not recommended.
   b. In a recent review (9), the authors suggest (a) usual doses for a creatinine clearance of more than 50 ml/min, (b) 50% of the standard dose be given q12h or the standard dose of 18 to 24 hours if the creatinine clearance is 10 to 50 ml/min, (c) a standard dose q24h if the creatinine clearance is less than 10 ml/min.
      Since TMP-SMX is removed by hemodialysis, standard doses can be administered after dialysis, with perhaps a supplemental fractional dosing provided on nondialysis days (9). Infectious disease input is advised. Adult

patients on chronic ambulatory peritoneal dialysis (CAPD) have been given the equivalent of one DS tablet of TMP-SMX q48h (5).

6. In **significant hepatic failure,** TMP-SMX should be avoided.

G. **Toxicity and side effects.** This combination **usually is well tolerated**, even for prolonged periods. Reactions can occur either to the TMP (see Chap. 25) or, more commonly, to the sulfonamide component. (See Sec. **I.E.**) Adverse reactions have been reviewed (1,4,9,21). **In patients with AIDS, drug toxicity** (rash, fever, neutropenia, thrombocytopenia, and transaminase elevation) **occur more frequently** (22), but dose reduction and the use of corticosteroids, commonly used in PCP, may help reduce these reactions. **In non-AIDS patients:**

1. **Mild GI symptoms,** including nausea, vomiting, diarrhea, cramps, and similar symptoms, occur in 3% to 3.5% of patients (21) and are the most frequent adverse effects (8).

2. **Skin rashes are relatively common,** occurring in 3% to 5% (1,9). They are usually typical drug eruptions with a **diffuse maculopapular** rash **or mild toxic erythema.** Most rashes are benign and resolve with discontinuation of therapy. However, exfoliative dermatitis, Stevens-Johnson syndrome, or toxic epidermal necrolysis occur rarely. An increased frequency of rashes occurs in AIDS patients receiving TMP-SMX (22). In HIV-infected patients with a history of cutaneous sensitivity or other TMP-SMX intolerance, desensitization has been successful with oral desensitization protocols (9,23,24).

3. **Bone marrow.** Except for bone marrow transplant recipients in whom engraftment may be delayed, occasionally in pediatric patients, and in AIDS patients, severe hematologic reactions to TMP-SMX are rare (21).

   Thrombocytopenia can occur as with sulfonamide use. Although neutropenia has been attributed to TMP-SMX, the precise relationship to drug therapy is difficult to determine, as neutropenia (a) is common in randomly sampled young children (controls); (b) is seen with viral illnesses for which the patient, especially children, may receive antibiotics; and (c) in reviews has been seen with similar frequency in patients receiving amoxicillin therapy (1). Further studies are necessary to clarify this question. If neutropenia occurs in a patient receiving TMP-SMX, it is prudent to discontinue the TMP-SMX and use an alternative agent.

   Megaloblastic bone marrow changes are uncommon except in those patients with preexisting depleted folate stores (e.g., alcoholics, the elderly, pregnant women, malnourished patients, and patients receiving phenytoin). It has been suggested that concomitant administration of folinic acid may reverse the antifolate effects of TMP-SMX, especially in patients not infected with HIV, without interfering with its antimicrobial effect. (See Sec. **VI.B.4** in Chap. 25, p. 465.) In one report, adjunctive folinic acid with TMP-SMX for PCP in AIDS patients was associated with an increased risk of therapeutic failure and death (25). Therefore empiric addition of folinic acid in this setting is not advised (25).

Rarely, in patients with G-6-PD deficiency, hemolysis may be precipitated with TMP-SMX use. (See Sec. **I.E.2**.) However, in one study, G-6-PD-deficient patients who received TMP-SMX did not have hemolytic reactions during therapy (6). In patients with AIDS who receive TMP-SMX for PCP, dose reduction may help reduce bone marrow suppression.

4. **Potential for teratogenesis and kernicterus. Because of the teratogenic effect seen in animal studies, TMP-SMX is generally contraindicated in pregnant** (5) **or lactating women.** Furthermore, because the sulfonamide component displaces bilirubin from albumin-binding sites and may therefore increase the risk of kernicterus, **TMP-SMX is contraindicated in infants younger than 2 months and during lactation and pregnancy, especially at term.**

5. **Drug/drug interactions.** The **sulfonamide-related interactions are reviewed in Sec. I.F.** and include interactions with oral anticoagulants and oral hypoglycemic agents. We try to avoid using sulfonamides, including TMP-SMX, in patients receiving **warfarin**. If TMP-SMX is used, prothrombin times should be monitored and, typically, the dose of warfarin should be reduced. TMP-SMX may prolong the half-life of phenytoin.

    Methotrexate concentrations can be increased and toxicity may ensue as a result of displacement from plasma-binding sites (9). A review of drug interactions has recently been published (26).

6. **Nephrotoxicity** does not appear to be a significant side effect (1). Clinically insignificant elevations of creatinine can occur with TMP. (See Chap. 25.)

7. **Hyperkalemia** may occur in patients with AIDS during treatment for PCP with TMP-SMX. (This is discussed in Chap. 25, Sec. **VI.B.3**, p. 465.)

8. **Local thrombophlebitis** uncommonly occurs with IV administration.

9. **Acquisition of resistance** is discussed in Chap. 25.

H. **Cost.** See Appendix Tables B and C.

III. **Fansidar** tablets are a combination of pyrimethamine (25 mg), a folate antagonist, and sulfadoxine (500 mg), a long-acting sulfonamide. This combination is still used in some antimalarial treatment regimens (16).

References

1. Reese RE, Betts RF. Sulfonamides and trimethoprim-sulfamethoxazole. In: Reese RE, Betts RF, eds. *A practical approach to infectious diseases,* 4th ed. Boston: Little, Brown, 1996:Chap. 28K.
2. Medical Letter. The choice of antibacterial drugs. *Med Lett Drugs Ther* 1999;41:95.
3. Dajani A, et al. Treatment of acute streptococcal pharyngitis and prevention of rheumatic fever: a statement for health professionals. *Pediatrics* 1995;96:758.
4. Sanche SE, Ronald AR. Sulfonamides and trimethoprim. In: Root RK, et al. *Clinical infectious diseases: a practical approach.* New York: Oxford University Press, 1999:Chap. 35.
5. Zinner SH, Mayer KH. Sulfonamides and Trimethoprim. In: Mandell GL, Bennett JE, Dolin R, eds. *Principles and practice of infectious diseases*, 5th ed. New York: Churchill Livingstone, 2000; 394–404.
6. Markowitz N, Saravolatz LD. Use of trimethoprim-sulfamethoxazole in a glucose-6-phosphate dehydrogenase-deficient population. *Rev Infect Dis* 1987;9:S218.
7. Aronoff GR, et al. *Drug prescribing in renal failure: dosing guidelines for adults*, 4th ed. Philadelphia: American College of Physicians, 1999.
8. Lundstrom TS, Sobel JD. Vancomycin, trimethoprim-sulfamethoxazole, and rifampin. *Infect Dis Clin North Am* 1995;9:747.
9. Smilack JD. Trimethoprim-sulfamethoxazole. *Mayo Clin Proc* 1999;74:730.
10. Hofman J, et al. The prevalence of drug-resistant *Streptococcus pneumoniae* in Atlanta. *N Engl J Med* 1995;333:481.
11. Sands M, et al. Trimethoprim-sulfamethoxazole therapy of *Pasteurella multocida* infection. *J Infect Dis* 1989;160:354.
    In vitro *activity suggests TMP-SMX may be a reasonable alternative agent for those who cannot take penicillin or amoxicillin, cefuroxime, or tetracycline.*
12. Gupta K, Scholes D, Stamm WE. Increasing prevalence of antimicrobial resistance among uropathogens causing acute uncomplicated cystitis in women. *JAMA* 1999;281:736.
    Serial studies of uropathogen resistance will be necessary. See related discussions in Chap. 32.
13. Smith JW, et al. Recurrent urinary tract infections in men: characteristics and response to therapy. *Ann Intern Med* 1980;91:544.
    Emphasizes the importance of the prostate as the source of relapsing UTIs in men. In prostatitis, prolonged courses of therapy (12 weeks) with trimethoprim-sulfamethoxazole result in higher cure rates than conventional 10-day courses. A classic article. See related discussions in Chap. 4.
14. Lipsky BA. Prostatitis and urinary tract infections: What's new; what's true? *Am J Med* 1999;106:327.

Still favors TMP-SMZ or a quinolone for therapy, typically 4 weeks for acute bacterial prostatitis.

15. Stapleton A, et al. Postcoital antimicrobial prophylaxis for recurrent urinary tract infection: a randomized, double-blind, placebo-controlled trial. *JAMA* 1990;264:703.
    The dose of postcoital TMP-SMX used was half a regular-strength tablet (i.e., 40 mg TMP, 200 mg SMX).

16. Medical Letter. Drugs for parasitic infection. *Med Lett Drugs Ther* 1998;40:1.
    See related editorial comment by KA Sepkowitz. Pneumocystis carinii *pneumonia without acquired immunodeficiency syndrome: who should receive prophylaxis?* Mayo Clin Proc *1996;71:102.*

17. Levitz AE, Quintiliani, R. Trimethoprim-sulfamethoxazole for bacterial meningitis. *Ann Intern Med* 1984;100:881.

18. Hughes WT, et al. 1997 Guidelines for the use of antimicrobial agents in neutropenic patients with unexplained fever. *Clin Infect Dis* 1997;25:551.

19. Fox BC, et al. A prospective, randomized, double-blind study of trimethoprim-sulfamethoxazole for prophylaxis of infection in renal transplantation: clinical efficacy, absorption of trimethoprim-sulfamethoxazole, effects on microflora, and the cost-benefit of prophylaxis. *Am J Med* 1990;89:225.
    During the hospitalization after the transplantation surgery, 160 mg TMP and 800 mg SMX bid was given if creatinine clearance exceeded 30 ml/min. After discharge, a single daily dose of 160 mg TMP and 800 mg SMX was used. (If creatinine clearance was less than 30 ml/min, one-half the usual dose per day was used.)

20. Goodgame RW. Understanding intestinal spore forming protozoa: cryptosporidia, microsporidia, isospora, and cyclospora. *Ann Intern Med* 1996;124:429.

21. Gutman, LT. The use of trimethoprim-sulfamethoxazole in children: a review of adverse reactions and indications. *Pediatr Infect Dis J* 1984;3:349.

22. Lee BL. Drug interactions and toxicities in patients with AIDS. In: Sande MA, Volberding PA, eds. *The medical management of AIDS*, 5th ed. Philadelphia: WB Saunders, 1997:125–142.

23. Gluckstein D, Ruskin J. Rapid oral desensitization to trimethoprim-sulfamethoxazole (TMP-SMX): use in prophylaxis for *Pneumocystis carinii* pneumonia in patients with AIDS who were previously intolerant to TMP-SMX. *Clin Infect Dis* 1995;20:849.

24. Caumes E, et al. Efficacy and safety of desensitization with sulfamethoxazole and trimethoprim in 48 previously hypersensitive patients infected with human immunodeficiency virus. *Arch Dermatol* 1997;133:465.

25. Safrin S, Lee BL, Sande MA. Adjunctive folinic acid with trimethoprim-sulfamethoxazole for *Pneumocystis carinii* in AIDS patients is associated with an increased risk of therapeutic failure and death. *J Infect Dis* 1994;170:912.

26. Gregg CR. Drug interactions and anti-infective therapies. *Am J Med* 1999;106:227..

25

Trimethoprim

Trimethoprim (TMP) not in combination with sulfamethoxazole (SMX) is available and is approved for use in uncomplicated urinary tract infections (UTIs) (1–3).

I. **Mechanism of action.** By inhibiting dihydrofolate reductase, TMP interferes with the production of tetrahydrofolic acid in bactericidal cells (Fig. 24.1).

II. **Spectrum of activity.** TMP is active and bactericidal against many gram-positive aerobic cocci and most gram-negative bacteria, except *Pseudomonas aeruginosa* and other *Pseudomonas* spp. (3). Enterococci usually are resistant. It is **active against common urinary tract pathogens** such as *Escherichia coli, Proteus mirabilis, Klebsiella pneumoniae,* and *Enterobacter* spp. Therefore its spectrum of activity is **very similar to that of the TMP-SMX combination.** Most anaerobes and *Chlamydia* spp. are resistant (2).

III. **Pharmacokinetics.** TMP is **well absorbed** from the gastrointestinal (GI) tract. The drug is excreted primarily unchanged by the kidneys, and urine concentrations are considerably higher than those in the blood. Dosage must be altered in renal failure. **TMP penetrates prostatic** and vaginal secretions well (1,3). TMP achieves high tissue levels in the kidney (3) and is excreted in breast milk. This drug increases the half-life of phenytoin.

IV. **Current clinical uses**

A. **Acute, uncomplicated UTI.** Some experts prefer TMP alone to TMP-SMX, as efficacy is nearly equal and adverse effects are less common (4). A 3-day dose regimen is preferred over a single-dose regimen. (See related discussions in Chap. 4.)

B. **Recurrent UTI suppression.** TMP has been used in suppressive regimens for recurrent UTI in women (1,2,4). The urine should be initially sterilized before chronic suppressive therapy is started. (See Chap. 4.)

C. **Prostatitis.** TMP has been used successfully in regimens for both acute and chronic prostatitis (1,2,4), especially in the sulfa-allergic patient. TMP-SMX and the oral fluoroquinolones are alternative agents in this setting. (See Chap. 4.)

D. TMP has been effective in the treatment of **travelers' diarrhea** (5); quinolones are preferred. (See Chap. 5 and Sec. VI.A.).

E. TMP alone cannot be substituted for the combination of TMP-SMX in the therapy for *Pneumocystis carinii* infections. For this purpose, a combination of **dapsone and TMP** is required, and this **combination is effective for mild to moderate *P. carinii* pneumonia** in patients with AIDS (6,7).

V. **Dosage**
  A. **Oral.** TMP is available as an oral agent in the form
     of scored 100-mg and 200-mg tablets. The effective-
     ness of TMP as a single agent in children younger
     than 12 years has not been established. The safety of
     TMP in infants younger than 2 months of age has not
     been demonstrated
       1. **For acute, uncomplicated UTI.** The usual adult
          dose is 100 mg q12h or 200 mg q24h for 10 days.
          Also, 100 mg q12h for 3 days has been used.
       2. **For recurrent UTI suppression** therapy in
          women, 100 mg at bedtime has been used.
       3. **For prostatitis,** 100 mg q12h or 200 mg q24h has
          been given for 4 to 12 weeks in patients allergic to
          sulfa in whom TMP-SMX could not be given. The
          oral fluoroquinolones are alternatives.
       4. **For travelers' diarrhea,** 100 mg bid for 3 to
          5 days has been used. A 3-day course usually is
          adequate.
       5. **For mild to moderate *P. carinii* pneumonia,**
          TMP and dapsone have been used (7,8).
  B. **In renal failure,** the dose interval is adjusted. Usually,
     a dose of TMP is given q12h. If the creatinine clearance
     is 10 to 50 ml/min, the usual dose can be given q18h.
     If the creatinine clearance is less than 10 ml/min, the
     usual dose can be given q24h (8).
  C. **Pregnancy.** TMP is a **category C agent** (see Chap.
     14) and should be used during pregnancy only if the
     potential benefit justifies the potential risk to the
     fetus. (See Sec. **VI.B.6.**)
  D. **Nursing mothers.** TMP is excreted in human milk.
     Because TMP may interfere with folic acid metabolism,
     the package insert in the past has suggested that cau-
     tion be exercised when TMP is administered to a nurs-
     ing woman. (See Sec. **VI.B.6.**)

VI. **Potential problems and adverse effects**
  A. **Resistance to TMP.** In a recent review of this agent,
     the authors emphasize that although there is a theo-
     retical concern that TMP resistance could develop more
     rapidly when used alone, this has not been observed in
     countries where TMP has been used as a single agent
     for many years (4). Resistance to TMP in individual
     patients is not reported when TMP has been used for
     short periods.
        Nevertheless, the global prevalence of TMP-resistant
     bacteria has increased in recent years. This is impor-
     tant, as resistance to TMP governs resistance to TMP-
     SMX. For example, from 1978 to 1981, *E. coli* resistance
     to TMP rose modestly from 2% to 6% in Boston, but
     from 8% to 30% in Paris, and to even higher rates (40%)
     in developing countries (9). The liberal use of TMP-
     SMX for both veterinary and human disorders has been
     implicated.
        Resistance rates of gram-negative pathogens in
     developing countries have been reported to be clearly

higher than those in the developed world. TMP resistance has been reported at high levels of 25% to 68% in South America, Asia, and Africa (10). In some developing countries, antibiotics may be more available without prescription and TMP may be used more often as monotherapy. Resistance to *Salmonella typhi* is worldwide. Also, resistance to TMP has become more common with *Shigella* spp., methicillin-resistant *Staphylococcus aureus* (MRSA), and recently, *S. pneumoniae* (3).

In countries in which TMP-resistant bacterial enteric pathogens are common, an agent other than TMP or TMP-SMX will be necessary (e.g., ciprofloxacin) for effective therapy of travelers' diarrhea.

B. **Adverse effects.** TMP is well tolerated in standard regimens.

1. **Skin rashes** have been noted in approximately 3% of patients, compared with 6% of patients receiving TMP-SMX (1) when conventional doses are used. In high-dose regimens, TMP is associated with a higher incidence of rashes and other adverse drug effects (11).

2. **Anaphylaxis** has been described after TMP use (12). **In someone with a delayed diffuse rash from TMP-SMX, it may be reasonable to use TMP alone in the future as sulfonamides cause rashes more commonly. If someone had an immediate or anaphylactic allergic reaction to TMP-SMX, we would avoid both TMP and sulfonamides in the future.**

3. **Hyperkalemia** is seen commonly in patients with AIDS who are treated with high doses of TMP-SMX or TMP and dapsone for *P. carinii* pneumonia. TMP is a sodium-channel inhibitor and functions as a potassium-sparing diuretic agent (13,14). Hyperkalemia can be seen in hospitalized patients without AIDS who are treated with TMP-SMX (15).

4. **Bone marrow effects.** TMP may interfere with folic acid metabolism, particularly in the folate-deficient patient (1,4) (e.g., elderly or alcoholic). Megaloblastic anemia, neutropenia, and thrombocytopenia have been described with prolonged use. The administration of folinic acid (e.g., 10 mg po daily in adults) prevents or treats this effectively without reducing the antibacterial activity of TMP, but folinic acid is expensive. However, because one report suggests that adjunctive folinic acid with TMP-SMX for *P. carinii* pneumonia in AIDS patients is associated with an increased risk of therapeutic failure and death (16), we do not add folinic acid in other regimens (e.g., TMP and dapsone for *P. carinii* pneumonia).

5. **Modest evaluations of serum creatinine** levels may occur in patients receiving TMP, but these are probably clinically insignificant (11).

6.   Teratogenicity of TMP in humans has not been clearly established. **It seems prudent to use an alternate agent in pregnancy and nursing women** (2).
7.   **Abnormal liver function tests** can occur (17).
8.   **Drug interaction.** TMP may predispose to **phenytoin** toxicity by increasing free levels of phenytoin (4).

C.   **Cost.** See Appendix Table C.

References

1.   Reese RE, Betts RF. Trimethoprim. In: Reese RE, Betts RF, eds. *A practical approach to infectious diseases*, 4th ed. Boston: Little, Brown, 1996:1285–88.
2.   Zinner SH, Mayer KH. Sulfonamides and trimethoprim. In: Mandell GL, Bennett JE, Dolin R, eds. *Principles and practice of infectious diseases*, 5th ed. New York: Churchill Livingstone, 2000;394–404.
3.   Lundstrom TS, Sobel JD. Vancomycin, trimethoprim-sulfamethoxazole, and rifampin. *Infect Dis Clin North Am* 1995;9:747.
4.   Sanche SE, Ronald AR. Sulfonamides and trimethoprim. In: Root RK, et al, eds., *Clinical infectious diseases: a practical approach*. New York: Oxford University Press, 1999:313–317.
5.   Dupont HL, et al. Treatment of traveler's diarrhea with trimethoprim/sulfamethoxazole and with trimethoprim alone. *N Engl J Med* 1982;20:841.
6.   Medina I, et al. Oral therapy for *Pneumocystis carinii* pneumonia in the acquired immunodeficiency syndrome: a controlled trial of trimethoprim-sulfamethoxazole versus trimethoprim-dapsone. *N Engl J Med* 1990;323:776.
     This study showed that in patients with AIDS, oral therapy with TMP-SMX or TMP (20 mg/kg/day) and dapsone (100 mg/day) are equally effective for mild to moderate first episodes, but there are fewer serious side effects with the TMP-dapsone.
7.   Medical Letter. Drugs for parasitic infection. *Med Lett Drugs Ther* 1998;40:1.
     TMP (5 mg/kg po tid × 21 days) and dapsone (100 mg po daily × 21 days) is listed as an alternative regimen for Pneumocystis carinii pneumonia therapy.
8.   Aronoff GR, et al. *Drug prescribing in renal failure: dosing guidelines for adults*, 4th ed. Philadelphia: American College of Physicians, 1999.
9.   Goldstein FW, et al. The changing pattern of trimethoprim resistance in Paris, with a review of worldwide experience. *Rev Infect Dis* 1986;8:725.
     See Jansson C, et al. Trimethoprim resistance arising in animal bacteria and transferred into human pathogens. J Infect Dis 1993; 167:785.
10.   Houvinen P, et al. Trimethoprim and sulfonamide resistance. *Antimicrob Agents Chemother* 1995;39:279.
11.   Naderer O, Nafziger AN, Bertino JS Jr. Effects of moderate-dose versus high-dose trimethoprim on serum creatinine and creatinine

clearance and adverse reactions. *Antimicrob Agents Chemother* 1997;41:2466.

12. Alonso MD, et al. Hypersensitivity to trimethoprim. *Allergy* 1992; 47:340.
    See related paper by Bijl AM, et al. Anaphylactic reactions associated with trimethoprim. Clin Exp Allergy *1998;28:510.*
    Anaphylaxis due to TMP-SMX is not always due to SMX (sulfamethoxazole). TMP can cause anaphylaxis rarely.

13. Choi MJ, et al. Brief report: trimethoprim-induced hyperkalemia in a patient with AIDS. *N Engl J Med* 1993;328:703.

14. Valazquez H, et al. Renal mechanism of trimethoprim-induced hyperkalemia. *Ann Intern Med* 1993;119:296.

15. Alappan R, et al. Hyperkalemia in hospitalized patients treated with trimethoprim-sulfamethoxazole. *Ann Intern Med* 1996; 124:316.

16. Safrin S, Lee BL, Sande MA. Adjunctive folinic acid with trimethoprim-sulfamethoxazole in *Pneumocystis carinii* in AIDS patients is associated with an increased risk of therapeutic failure and death. *J Infect Dis* 1994;170:912.

17. Lindgren A, Olsson, R. Liver reactions from trimethoprim. *J Intern Med* 1994;236:281.

Macrolides: Erythromycin, Clarithromycin, and Azithromycin

The commonly used macrolides in the United States are erythromycin and the semisynthetic derivatives of erythromycin, clarithromycin, and azithromycin, which have structural modifications to improve tissue penetration and broaden their spectrum of activity (1–3). The macrolides inhibit RNA-dependent protein synthesis by reversibly binding to the 50S ribosomal subunits of susceptible microorganisms. Although generally bacteriostatic, the macrolides may be bactericidal under certain conditions or against certain microorganisms (1,2). Since the structure of the macrolides is different from that of penicillin, penicillin derivatives, and cephalosporins, the macrolides have commonly been used in patients who have allergic reactions to beta-lactam antibiotics.

Erythromycin

I. **Spectrum of activity.** Erythromycin is broad spectrum in that it is active against many gram-positive and gram-negative bacteria, mycoplasmas, chlamydiae, treponemas, and rickettsiae.
   A. **See Table 26-1.**
   B. **Aerobic bacteria**. Certain points deserve emphasis.
      1. **Gram positives**
         a. Erythromycin is highly active against **group A streptococci** (GAS). Although resistance of GAS to erythromycin in some countries has been a problem (e.g., Finland), in the United States this has not been a problem. In the United States less than 5% of GAS are resistant to erythromycin (4).
         b. Penicillin-susceptible ***Streptococcus pneumoniae*** are susceptible to erythromycin, but many penicillin-resistant strains are also resistant *in vitro* to macrolides. The exact clinical significance of this remains debated (5) and this and related issues are discussed in Chaps. 2 and 16. Strains resistant to one macrolide are typically resistant to all macrolides (1).
         c. Many other streptococci are susceptible (groups B, C, G, etc), but group D (enterococci) is resistant.
         d. **Methicillin-sensitive *Staphylococcus aureus*** (MRSA) are often susceptible, but resistance may emerge during therapy in an

Table 26-1. *In vitro* activity of the macrolides

Organism	Erythromycin (≤0.5 mg/l)§	Mean MIC₉₀ (mg/l)*,†,‡ Clarithromycin (≤2 mg/l)§	Azithromycin (≤2 mg/l)§
Oral or respiratory			
Moraxella catarrhalis	0.25	0.25	0.06
Group A streptococci	0.03	<0.12	0.12
Streptococcus pneumoniae (1994/1997)			
Penicillin-sensitive	≤0.25/0.12	32	4.0/0.5
Intermediate resistance to penicillin	≤0.25/8	16	2.0/16
Penicillin-resistant	≤0.25/8	>32	8/16
Haemophilus influenzae			
Beta-lactamase-positive	4–16	8–16#	1–4**
Beta-lactamase-negative	.5–8	8–16	1–4**
Bordetella pertussis	0.03	0.03	0.06
Neisseria meningitidis	.5–4.0	1.0	0.12–2.0
Atypical respiratory			
Mycoplasma pneumoniae	≤0.01	0.0078–5	≤0.01
Legionella pneumophila	0.5	0.06	0.5
L. longbeachae	0.5	0.12	0.5
Chlamydia pneumoniae	0.5	0.25	0.25

continued

Table 26-1. (*Continued*)

| Organism | Erythromycin (≤0.5 mg/l)§ | Mean MIC₉₀ (mg/l)*,†,‡ | |
		Clarithromycin (≤2 mg/l)§	Azithromycin (≤2 mg/l)§
STD or GU			
N. gonorrhoeae (all)	0.5–4.0	0.5–2.0	0.06–0.5
C. trachomatis	≤0.125	...	≤0.125
H. ducreyi	0.03	...	0.004
M. hominis	≥128	64	4–32
Ureaplasma urealyticum	1–4	0.2	.5–4
Gardnerella vaginalis	≤0.03	...	≤0.03
Mobiluncus species	≤0.03	...	0.06
Other gram-positive			
Staphylococcus aureus			
MSSA	1–8	0.5	1.0
MRSA	>64	...	>128
S. epidermidis			
MSSE	>8, >64	>32	>32, >128
MRSE	>8, >64	>32	>32, >128
Streptococci			
Group B	≤0.12	0.06	0.12–0.1
Groups C, F, G	0.5	...	0.25
S. bovis	1.0–2.0	0.5	1.0–4.0

S. faecalis / S. faecium	>8	>32	>32
Viridans streptococci	0.06–2.0	0.03	0.12–16
Mycobacteria			
Mycobacterium avium complex	≥64	4–16	≥32
M. chelonae subsp chelonae	8.0	0.25	2.0
M. chelonae subsp abscessus	>8	0.5	8.0
Miscellaneous			
Borrelia burgdorferi	0.006–0.03	0.015–0.06	0.015–0.03
Helicobacter pylori	0.25	0.03	0.25

Abbreviations: GU, genitourinary; MIC, minimal inhibitory concentration; MIC$_{90}$, minimal concentration that will inhibit 90% of clinical isolates; MRSA, methicillin-resistant *Staphylococcus aureus*; MRSE, methicillin-resistant *Staphylococcus epidermidis*; MSSA, methicillin-sensitive *Staphylococcus aureus*; MSSE, methicillin-sensitive *Staphylococcus epidermidis*; STD, sexually transmitted disease; subsp, subspecies.

Source: Modified from Alvarez-Elcoro S, Enzler MJ. The macrolides: erythromycin, clarithromycin, and azithromycin. *Mayo Clin Proc* 1999;74:613.

* Values for MIC cutoff for susceptibility.

† MIC of clarithromycin alone; 14-hydroxy metabolite of clarithromycin may contribute to antimicrobial activity.

‡ All MICs broth dilution, inoculum 10^{-4}–10^{-6}; at least 10 strains from each source.

§ Recommended susceptibility breakpoints.

‖ Breakpoint ≤0.5 mg/L.

Recommended breakpoint ≤8 mg/L.

** Recommended breakpoint ≤4 mg/L.

individual patient (6). Interestingly, the *Medical Letter* does not list the macrolides as alternative agents for *S. aureus* (7).

MRSA strains are resistant to macrolides.

   e.   Erythromycin is the **drug of choice** for *Corynebacterium diphtheriae* and alternative agent for *Bacillus anthracis* (anthrax) (7).

2.   **Gram negatives**
   a.   Erythromycin is an **agent of first choice** for *Campylobacter jejuni, Bordetella pertussis* (whooping cough), *Legionella* spp. and the agent of bacillary angiomatosis (*Bartonella henselae* or *quintana*) (7).
   b.   Erythromycin is an **alternative agent** for *Haemophilus ducreyi* (chancroid), *Eikenella corrodens,* and *Moraxella catarrhalis* (7).
   c.   Erythromycin has weak activity against *H. influenzae* (2), and many (most) strains are resistant (1). Erythromycin is not viewed as an alternative agent for this pathogen, although clarithromycin and azithromycin are for respiratory isolates (7).
   d.   **Enterobacteriaceae** (e.g., *Escherichia coli, Klebsiella* spp., etc) are **resistant.**

C.   **Anaerobes.** Erythromycin has activity against some species of gram-negative anaerobes, but *Bacteroides fragilis* strains and *Fusobacterium* spp. usually are resistant (6).

D.   **Nonbacterial pathogens**
   1.   **Mycoplasmas.** Erythromycin is very active against *Mycoplasma pneumoniae* and is a **drug of choice** for this pathogen as well as the drug of choice for *Ureaplasma urealyticum* (7).
   2.   **Chlamydiae.** Erythromycin is active against *Chlamydia trachomatis* and *C. pneumoniae.*
   3.   **Spirochetes.** Erythromycin is active against *Borrelia burgdorferi*, the causative agent in Lyme disease. (Azithromycin and clarithromycin are alternative agents for this pathogen.) It also is active against *Treponema pallidum* but seldom is used for infections due to this pathogen.

II.   **Pharmacokinetics** (1–3,6,8)
A.   **Oral absorption.** Erythromycin is acid-labile. In the stomach, it rapidly decomposes to two inactive metabolites, one of which may contribute to gastrointestinal (GI) side effects. As a result of this instability and depending on the salt form, the rate of absorption may be unpredictable (35% ± 25%) (8). Pharmaceutical preparations for oral use have been made with an aim toward diminishing destruction by gastric acid and promoting better absorption (6).
   1.   Food in the stomach may decrease absorption of some forms.

2. Average serum levels achieved by the different oral preparations are similar; therefore no single oral formulation of erythromycin offers a clear advantage in adults (6).

3. In children, studies have suggested that erythromycin estolate has superior bioavailability over erythromycin ethylsuccinate (6).

4. Four hours after oral administration of a dose of 500 mg, peak serum concentrations are 1 to 2 µg/ml (1).

B. **Intravenous.** Serum concentrations 1 hour after 500 mg to 1 g intravenously (IV) are approximately 10 to 15 µg/ml (1). **Erythromycin should not be administered intramuscularly. Intravenous preparations achieve appreciably higher serum levels and should be used to treat serious infections requiring erythromycin.**

C. **Half-life and excretion.** The serum half-life of erythromycin is approximately 1 to 2 hours, and levels persist for approximately 6 hours (1,2). Because erythromycin is excreted primarily in the bile, it must be **used very carefully in patients with liver disease. Dose reduction is not necessary in mild to moderate renal failure.**

D. **Miscellaneous**

1. As a single agent, erythromycin provides adequate middle-ear levels against penicillin-susceptible *S. pneumoniae* and *S. pyogenes* but probably is not adequate to eradicate *H. influenzae* consistently (6).

2. Erythromycin crosses the placenta, but it is not known to be teratogenic. It is a category B agent. (See Chap. 14.) Also see Sec. IV.E. It also is excreted into breast milk (1).

3. Limited data from patients with septic arthritis suggest that erythromycin penetrates the synovial fluid poorly (6).

4. Because of limited preparation into brain tissue and cerebrospinal fluid (CSF), we would not use erythromycin in central nervous system (CNS) infections.

III. **Indications for use**

A. **Erythromycin** is considered **a drug of choice** (7) in the following infections:

1. *Mycoplasma pneumoniae* **pneumonia.** Tetracycline can also be used, but erythromycin is nearly 50 times more potent than tetracycline against *M. pneumoniae in vitro* (6).

2. *Legionella* **infections** (often combined with rifampin).

3. *Chlamydia* **trachomatis pneumonia,** which is more common in children than adults. Erythromycin is used also for *C. trachomatis* conjunctivitis

and chlamydial pelvic infections, especially during pregnancy (9).

4. **Miscellaneous.** Erythromycin is also used in *Bordetella pertussis* (whooping cough), for both therapy and prophylaxis; *Campylobacter jejuni* infections; *Corynebacterium diphtheriae* infections or carrier states; *Haemophilus ducreyi* (chancroid) genital lesions; *Bartonella (Rochalimaea) henselae*, the agent of bacillary angiomatosis (10); and *Ureaplasma urealyticum* infections (e.g., urethritis).

B. Erythromycin has also been used as an **alternative in the penicillin-allergic patient** for the following conditions:

1. Group A streptococcal upper respiratory infections. (See Chap. 1.)
2. *Streptococcus pneumoniae* pneumonia (penicillin-susceptible strains). (See Chap. 2.)
3. Superficial minor staphylococcal skin infections. Resistance to erythromycin may develop with its use over time, and erythromycin alone is not advised for deep-seated staphylococcal infections (6).
4. Rheumatic fever prophylaxis (11).
5. **Miscellaneous:** Erythromycin has been used in early syphilis, *Lymphogranuloma venereum*, and urethritis due to *C. trachomatis* (9). (See Chap. 10.)

C. **Miscellaneous**

1. Erythromycin, and especially azithromycin, has been commonly used in mild to moderate **community-acquired pneumonia,** especially of young to middle-aged adults. (See related discussions in Chap. 2 and under azithromycin later in this chapter.)
2. Oral erythromycin has been used with oral neomycin in surgical prophylaxis, prior to elective GI procedures. (See Chap. 15.)
3. Erythromycin is not recommended for therapy of meningitis or endocarditis.
4. **Erythromycin is no longer recommended as an alternative agent for dental/oral procedures for infective endocarditis prophylaxis** because of GI intolerance and unpredictable blood levels. (See Chap. 15.)

IV. **Preparations available and dosage**

A. **Oral forms.** Several oral preparations are available: erythromycin base, stearate salt, ethylsuccinate ester, and the estolate form. Although the blood levels achieved with these forms vary somewhat, when the agents are used against very sensitive organisms, these minor differences are not believed to be clinically significant (1). Also, no one formulation seems to cause substantially less GI upset than others (1), but overall the newer macrolides, clarithromycin and especially azithromycin, have less GI intolerance. See later.

1. Although current advertisements for various formulations of oral erythromycin stress differences in serum concentrations, any of the preparations is absorbed well enough to attain serum concentrations higher than those needed to inhibit growth of susceptible pathogens. No data are available revealing clinical failure in adults of any oral erythromycin formulation (generic or brand name, taken while fasting or with food) due to inadequate bioavailability. However, **in children, erythromycin estolate appears to be more bioavailable than erythromycin ethylsuccinate** (12), and absorption of the estolate is not affected by food (6).

2. **Erythromycin estolate is no longer recommended for use in adults** because of the associated incidence of cholestatic hepatitis. In children, however, erythromycin estolate rarely causes hepatitis, and it appears to be better absorbed, better tolerated, and more effective than ethylsuccinate (12).

3. **Oral dosages**
   a. **Adults.** The usual dosage recommended is 250 to 500 mg q6h. Patients may not tolerate the higher doses because of GI symptoms. **The estolate preparation is not recommended for use** in adults (6).
   b. **Children.** The usual amount is 30 to 50 mg/kg/day divided into q6h doses. In infants younger than 4 months, 20 to 40 mg/kg/day divided into q6h doses has been suggested. Erythromycin estolate and erythromycin ethylsuccinate are the most widely used preparations, as they are both tasteless and available in suspensions.

B. **Parenteral forms** of erythromycin are available (e.g., erythromycin lactobionate) for more serious infections requiring higher blood levels or for use when the patient cannot take oral medications.

   IV use may be associated with thrombophlebitis. This may be avoided in part by dilution of the dose in at least 250 ml of intravenous fluid (6) and careful infusion over 40 to 60 minutes into a large peripheral vein or, if necessary, through a central venous line. The usual adult dosage is 1 to 4 g/day, divided into q6h doses. A slow IV infusion may allow safe use. (See Sec. **V.A.**) For children, 50 mg/kg/day is recommended, divided into q6h doses. The high doses are used commonly in *Legionella*-caused pneumonias. Intramuscular use should be avoided.

   With the availability of IV azithromycin, which can be given once daily, often this IV macrolide is preferred for IV therapy in patients more than 16 years of age. See later discussion.

C. **Topical.** There is a 1.5% and 2% erythromycin gel or solution that can be applied twice daily for treatment of acne skin lesions. There is also an ophthalmic ointment, which is used for bacterial conjunctivitis.

D. **Renal failure.** In mild to moderate renal failure, dose modification is not necessary (6,13). **In severe renal failure,** with a creatinine clearance of 10 ml/min or less, **the drug may accumulate, and toxic side effects have been seen** in this setting (1) (e.g., transient hearing loss) (2). Therefore in severe renal failure, 50% to 75% of the usual dose can be given at the standard dose interval (13). **In dialysis** erythromycin is not removed by peritoneal dialysis or hemodialysis (13).

E. **Pregnancy. Erythromycin estolate should not be used in pregnancy.** (See Sec. IV.A.2.) Other erythromycin agents are safe in pregnancy, category B agents. (See Sec. II.D.)

F. **Nursing.** Erythromycin is excreted in breast milk; caution should be exercised when erythromycin is administered to a nursing woman.

G. **Hepatic insufficiency.** Because erythromycin is metabolized primarily by the liver, this agent should be avoided in patients with severe liver disease. If it is the agent of choice, dosages should be reduced and, ideally, serum levels should be monitored.

H. **Cost.** See Appendix Tables B and C.

V. **Toxicity and side effects.** Erythromycin is considered one of the least toxic commonly used antibiotics (1,2,6).

A. **Gastrointestinal symptoms.** With oral use, **epigastric distress is common,** as is diarrhea, but both can be diminished by taking the drug with meals.

Symptoms often improve if the dose is reduced. Gastrointestinal symptoms can occur with oral as well as intravenous therapy (6); a slow intravenous infusion (e.g., more than 60 minutes) may help to decrease the IV use associated nausea and vomiting, which may be seen more frequently in patients younger than 40 years (1).

1. **Because of these GI side effects, the newer macrolides are often preferred**, and of these, azithromycin appears to have the fewest GI side effects. See later.

2. Erythromycin may have therapeutic value in patients with severe diabetic gastroparesis (14). The cramps, nausea, vomiting, and diarrhea appear to be due to the GI motility-stimulating effect of the macrolides.

B. **Allergic reactions** (rash, fever, eosinophilia) are **uncommon,** generally mild, and dermatologic. Cutaneous reactions occur in approximately 0.5% to 2.0% of treated patients; rashes are usually maculopapular and sometimes urticarial. Fixed drug eruptions, contact dermatitis, and anaphylaxis occur rarely. The risk of erythromycin hypersensitivity appears to be higher in patients allergic to other antibiotics (15).

C. **Cholestatic hepatitis** is rare and, although formerly associated with the estolate preparation in adults, usually after approximately 10 days of therapy (1), can occur with other erythromycin preparations.

D. **Deafness** may occur with high-dose use but usually reverses several days after decreasing or discontinuing erythromycin. This may occur more in elderly patients with renal failure (6).

E. *Clostridium difficile* **diarrhea** occurs rarely with the use of erythromycin (6).

F. **Drug interactions**

1. Erythromycin inhibits the metabolism of numerous drugs presumably mediated by **interfering with the hepatic cytochrome P-450 enzyme system** (1,2). In this way **erythromycin can increase blood levels** (and therefore excess effect) of **theophylline, warfarin, carbamazine, cyclosporine, triazolam, alfentanil, and bromocriptine** (2,6).

    If theophylline must be used in patients receiving erythromycin, the dose of theophylline should be reduced by 25% to 40% to compensate; carbamazine doses may require a 50% reduction.

2. **Digoxin.** Erythromycin may improve digoxin absorption in some patients for it apparently inhibits one or more bacteria in the bowel that can break down some of the administered digoxin before it is absorbed (1).

3. **Drug-induced prolonged QT interval.** Since erythromycin, especially IV, may produce a long QT syndrome, erythromycin should probably be avoided in patients with a history of prolonged QT syndrome, especially drug induced (16). Rarely, IV erythromycin has caused cardiac rhythm disturbances in premature infants (17).

4. **Terfenadine (Seldane),** which is no longer available, **and astemizole (Hismanal) are contraindicated in patients taking erythromycin,** since they may be associated with increased terfenadine or astemizole levels. Rare cases of serious cardiovascular adverse events—including death, cardiac arrest, torsade de pointes, and other ventricular arrhythmias—have been observed when these agents have been given concomitantly with erythromycin. The increased terfenadine or astemizole levels lead to electrocardiographic QT prolongation. Similarly, erythromycin should not be taken with **cisapride (Propulsid).**

VI. **Overview of macrolides. See Sec. VII under "Azithromycin" on p. 487.**

Clarithromycin (Biaxin)

Clarithromycin differs chemically from erythromycin by having an O-methyl substitution at position 6 of the macrolide ring. Its spectrum of activity is similar to that of erythromycin, except for enhanced *H. influenzae* activity, and activity against atypical mycobacterium, but it has better pharmacokinetic properties, including a twice-daily dose regimen (18–20).

I. *In vitro* **activity.** This is similar to erythromycin except as noted later (**Table 26-1**).
   A. **Aerobes**
      1. **Gram-positive** bacteria resistant to erythromycin are resistant to clarithromycin (e.g., MRSA, high-level penicillin-resistant and many intermediate-level *S. pneumoniae*).
      2. **Gram-negative**
         a. *H. influenzae.* Clarithromycin is more active *in vitro* than erythromycin in part due to the additive effect of its active metabolite, 14-OH clarithromycin, which *in vitro* decreases the MIC against these organisms (1,2). The clinical significance of this is unclear (2).
         b. *M. catarrhalis* strains are susceptible.
         c. **Enterobacteriaceae.** Clarithromycin is not considered an active agent against these pathogens.
   B. **Anaerobes.** Clarithromycin's activity is similar to that of erythromycin (20) and therefore is only modest.
   C. **Miscellaneous**
      1. Clarithromycin has activity similar to that of erythromycin against *M. pneumoniae*.
      2. Clarithromycin is also active against *H. pylori*.
      3. *Mycobacteria.* Clarithromycin is active against *M. avium* complex, *M. chelonei, M. chelonei abscessus*, and other atypical mycobacteria (1,2).
         Clarithromycin **is considered a drug of choice for *M. avium* complex and an alternative agent** for *S. pyogenes, M. catarrhalis, H. pylori, H. influenzae* (upper respiratory strains), and *B. burgdorferi* (7).
      4. Clarithromycin is active against *U. urealyticum*.

II. **Pharmacokinetics**
   A. **Absorption. With or without food**, clarithromycin is acid-stable and **well absorbed orally** with an absolute bioavailability of about 50% (1,2); its absorption is better and more reliable than erythromycin's absorption (1,2). When taken with meals, bioavailability increases (19).
      After the oral suspension of clarithromycin, clarithromycin and its OH metabolite penetrate middle-ear effusions adequately, with antibiotic concentrations exceeding the MICs of the most susceptible otitis pathogens.
      An intravenous preparation is currently unavailable.
   B. **Half-life.** The half-life of oral clarithromycin and its 14-OH metabolite is approximately 3 to 4 hours. This longer half-life of clarithromycin **allows for a twice-daily dose schedule.**

C. **Distribution.** Clarithromycin penetrates tissue well, including lung, kidney, liver, nasal mucosa, and tonsils (20). Presumably, penetration of clarithromycin into the CSF of humans is inadequate.

D. **Metabolism and elimination.** Clarithromycin is metabolized extensively in the liver by the hepatic cytochrome P-450 enzyme system and the excretion of clarithromycin and the 14-OH metabolite is by renal mechanisms (2). See Sec. V.E.

III. **Indications for use** in adults

A. **Approved uses in adults**

1. **Upper respiratory tract infections.** Clarithromycin has been used to treat: (a) **GAS pharyngitis**, although penicillin is the agent of choice (see Chap. 1); (b) **acute maxillary sinusitis** (see Chap. 1); (c) **acute exacerbation of chronic bronchitis** (see Chap. 1); and (d) mild **community-acquired pneumonia,** especially in the young to middle-aged adult (see Chap. 2).

2. *Mycobacterium avium* **complex (MAC).** Clarithromycin has been useful in the prevention and treatment of MAC. This topic is reviewed in detail elsewhere (1,2,7,21–23).

3. *H. pylori* has been effectively treated with clarithromycin and omeprazole (1,2,7,23A).

4. **Uncomplicated skin and skin structure - infections** due to susceptible *S. pyogenes* or *S. aureus* (19). More conventional therapy (e.g., erythromycin, dicloxacillin, or oral first-generation cephalosporins) may be more cost-effective therapy. In the allergic patient or the patient who has GI side effects from erythromycin, clarithromycin provides a useful alternative but azithromycin may be even better tolerated.

B. **Approved uses in children** (24–27)

1. Clarithromycin has been approved for use in pharyngitis, tonsillitis, acute maxillary sinusitis, and mild CAP (due to mycoplasma, susceptible *S. pneumoniae*, or *C. pneumoniae*, TWAR), and skin and soft-tissue infections, with the same type of limitations as discussed under Sec. A. above.

2. It is approved for otitis media in children. Clinical trials in the treatment of otitis media have shown similar efficacy for clarithromycin, amoxicillin, amoxicillin-clavulanate, and cefaclor.

C. **Investigation** of the benefit of clarithromycin for rapidly growing atypical mycobacterial infections, Lyme disease, or toxoplasmosis is ongoing (1,2,28).

IV. **Dosages** may be given with or without meals.

A. **Adult dosages.** A dose of 250 mg to 500 mg bid is often used depending on the severity of infection.

B. **Pediatric use.** For children 6 months of age or older, 15 mg/kg/day divided q12h for 10 days is recommended in the package insert. Suspensions are available with 125 mg/5 ml and 250 mg/5 ml.

C. **Renal failure.** When the creatinine clearance is 10 to 50 ml/min, 75% of the usual dose is suggested. When the creatinine clearance is less than 10 ml, 50% to 75% of the usual dose is suggested (13).

   After **hemodialysis,** some sources suggest a dose, although data are limited. In CAPD, no dose adjustments are necessary (13).

D. **Hepatic failure.** Dosage adjustments are not necessary; there is an increase in renal clearance (6).

E. **Pregnancy. Clarithromycin is a category C drug** (i.e., used only **if there is no alternative).** (See Chap. 14.) Clarithromycin has demonstrated adverse effects on pregnancy, outcome, and embryofetal development in animals. High doses of clarithromycin during pregnancy have caused cardiovascular anomalies in rats, cleft palates in mice, and fetal growth retardation in monkeys (29). The package insert indicates there are no adequate and well-controlled studies in pregnant women. **Clarithromycin should be used in pregnancy only if the potential benefit justifies the potential risk to the fetus.** If pregnancy occurs while taking this drug, the patient should be apprised of the potential hazard to the fetus.

F. **Nursing mothers.** The package insert notes that it is not known whether clarithromycin is excreted in human breast milk, and caution should be exercised when administering clarithromycin to a nursing mother as clarithromycin is excreted in the milk of lactating animals and other drugs of this class are excreted in human milk.

V. **Toxicity and side effects.** As with other macrolides, clarithromycin is relatively nontoxic (2,30).

A. **Gastrointestinal.** Occasionally, clarithromycin in conventional doses causes nausea, diarrhea, abdominal pain, and metallic taste (2) but fewer GI side effects than recipients of erythromycin (31).

B. **No significant hepatic, renal, or hematologic toxicity** appears to occur (30) with clarithromycin use at conventional doses. Minor hepatic enzyme elevations can occur. In fewer than 1% of recipients, leukopenia and prothrombin time prolongation have been noted.

C. **Headache** may occur in up to 2% of recipients (30).

D. **With high-dose regimens** (e.g., therapy of MAC in AIDS patients or therapy of atypical mycobacterial infections in the elderly), more severe adverse reactions, including nausea, vomiting, metallic taste, abnormal liver function blood tests, and CNS side effects, may occur (2).

E. **Drug interactions** (1,2). **As with erythromycin, drug interactions with clarithromycin are extremely important** (2).

   1. **Because clarithromycin inhibits the hepatic P-450 system, it may result in increased lev-**

els of multiple medications metabolized by
the liver (2).
   a. Concomitant administration of clarithromy-
      cin and **carbamazepine** causes a major
      change in carbamazepine levels.
   b. Other potential interactions include those dis-
      cussed in Sec. V.F under "Erythromycin"; as
      well as caffeine, nicotine, and midazolam (2).
   c. Astemizole (Hismanal) concomitant use
      should be avoided; see earlier discussion
      under V.F.
2. **Antivirals.** Interactions of clarithromycin with
   zidovudine (AZT) resulting in lower AZT levels
   have been reported as well as similar interactions
   with other antiretroviral agents (2).
F. **Cost.** Oral clarithromycin is a relatively expensive
   agent. See Appendix Table C.
VI. **Overview of macrolides. See Sec. VI under "Azithromycin."**

Azithromycin (Zithromax)

Azithromycin is a newer macrolide developed to overcome some
of the shortcomings of erythromycin such as GI intolerance, low
bioavailability, and somewhat limited spectrum of activity (1,2).
It is really an azalide antibiotic, approved in 1991, and its nuclear
structure differs from that of erythromycin in that the lactone
ring contains a nitrogen atom. This molecular rearrangement has
resulted in a compound with **remarkable and unique properties** (32), including an expanded *in vitro* spectrum of activity,
high and **sustained tissue antibiotic levels**, which are much
greater than the serum antibiotic levels, and a **prolonged tissue
half-life, decreasing the doses per course of therapy and
duration** of therapy (1,2).
Azithromycin inhibits protein synthesis, similar to erythromycin.

I. **Spectrum of activity.** The broad-spectrum *in vitro* activity of azithromycin is summarized in **Table 26-1.** If erythromycin is active against pathogens, azithromycin is also,
   but azithromycin is also more active against some organisms (e.g., *H. influenzae*).
   A. **Gram-positive aerobes.** Azithromycin is active
      against erythromycin-susceptible *S. aureus* (approx-
      imately 80% of strains), *S. pyogenes*, many *S. pneumo-
      niae*, *S. agalactiae*, and coagulase-negative staphylo-
      cocci, but overall erythromycin and clarithromycin
      are more active against these gram-positive cocci.
      Enterococci usually are resistant (19). **Strains of
      these organisms resistant to erythromycin will
      be resistant to azithromycin,** including many
      intermediate- and most high-level penicillin-resistant
      S. pneumoniae. (See Chaps. 2 and 16.) MRSA strains
      are resistant to erythromycin and azithromycin.

In addition, **azithromycin is two- to eightfold less active than erythromycin against staphylococci** and streptococci but is more active against *H. influenzae* (29).

B. **Gram-negative aerobes.** Most gram-negative bacteria are intrinsically resistant to the macrolides because of the inability of the macrolide to penetrate the outer cell membrane effectively. **Azithromycin** appears to be able to penetrate the outer membrane better than erythromycin and therefore **has activity against some gram-negative organisms** normally resistant to erythromycin (33).

1. **Azithromycin is severalfold more active against *H. influenzae* than is erythromycin or clarithromycin.** It is more active than erythromycin against *M. catarrhalis* and *Neisseria* spp. It is very active against *Legionella* spp., probably the most active macrolide against *Legionella* spp. (2) (although the fluoroquinolones are viewed by some experts as the agents of choice for *Legionella* infections).

2. Azithromycin is **not active against Enterobacteriaceae** (e.g., *E. coli, Klebsiella* spp.), *Pseudomonas* spp., or *Salmonella* (34).

   Azithromycin is active against *H. pylori*, although not listed as an alternative agent for these infections (7). It is active against *Shigella* spp. and *C. jejuni* (7).

C. **Anaerobes.** Azithromycin inhibits some anaerobes similar to erythromycin but is not useful against bowel anaerobes (7).

D. **Miscellaneous**
1. Most ***B. burgdorferi*** strains are inhibited by 0.015 µg/ml, suggesting azithromycin is more active *in vitro* than erythromycin or clarithromycin (19).
2. ***Mycoplasma pneumoniae*** usually is very susceptible at 0.25 µg/ml (19) as are *C. pneumoniae*.
3. **Genitourinary pathogens** *C. trachomatis, U. urealyticum, N. gonorrhoeae,* and *T. pallidum* are susceptible to azithromycin (2).
4. Atypical mycobacterium are overall more susceptible to clarithromycin than azithromycin or erythromycin (2).

E. **Resistance to erythromycin implies cross-resistance with azithromycin** (19,34).

II. **Pharmacokinetics.** Compared with other available antimicrobial agents, azithromycin has unique pharmacokinetic properties. **It yields high and sustained tissue levels** in excess of serum levels. This involves active movement from the serum into the intracellular sites. Therefore for tissue infections, azithromycin can provide excellent antibiotic levels.

A. **Absorption.** Azithromycin is more stable than erythromycin at various pH ranges seen in the stomach, and approximately 37% of a single capsule dose is absorbed, compared with 25% absorption of erythromycin (35).

Although adsorption of the capsular formation of azithromycin was decreased in the presence of food, the new tablet formation is equally absorbed in the fasting or fed state (2).

B. **Tissue kinetics** (20,35). The unique pharmacokinetic profile of azithromycin reflects a rapid and extensive uptake from the circulation into intracellular compartments followed by slow release (2).

1. Higher peak serum concentrations will be achieved by erythromycin and clarithromycin (1,2).

2. But **azithromycin penetrates tissues rapidly and extensively to yield very high steady-state tissue concentrations that exceed serum levels by 10- to 100-fold** (1,2) (e.g., lung [100-fold], sputum [30-fold], cervix [70-fold], and skin [35-fold]) (2).

3. Azithromycin is rapidly and highly concentrated in a number of cell types, including polymorphonuclear leukocytes (PMNLs), monocytes, alveolar macrophages, and fibroblasts (35).

   a. The function of PMNLs is not affected by antibiotic uptake (35). **By migrating to sites of infection, these PMNLs may play a role in the transport of azithromycin to the actual site of infection.**

   Azithromycin is released spontaneously and slowly from phagocytes (and fibroblasts).

   b. Tissue concentrations do not peak until 48 hours after administration and persist for several days afterward (33).

4. The average tissue half-life is between 2 and 4 days.

5. With recommended dosages daily for 5 days, therapeutic concentrations of azithromycin persist at the tissue level for 5 days or more **after** the completion of therapy.

6. Very little or none of the drug is detectable in aqueous humor or CSF, although azithromycin is widely distributed in brain tissue (2).

C. **Metabolism and excretion** (1,2)

1. Most of the absorbed dose of azithromycin is eliminated unchanged principally in the feces (2). Urinary excretion of the unchanged drug is a minor elimination route.

2. No dosage modification is necessary for patients with class A or B cirrhosis (2).

III. **Indications for use.** For adults, both an oral and IV formulation are available. (See Sec. IV.) For children less than 16 years of age, only the oral formulation is approved as of early 2000.

A. **Approved uses in adults**

1. **Community-acquired pneumonia (CAP)** due to *S. pneumoniae, Mycoplasma, H. influenzae,* and

C. pneumonia. Mild to moderate CAP is commonly treated with oral regimens of azithromycin in young to middle-aged adults. For hospitalized patients, the IV formulation (approved for *S. pneumonia, M. pneumoniae, M. catarrhalis, S. aureus,* and *L. pneumophilia*) is used initially. (See related discussions in **Chap. 2.**)

N.B. For very ill hospitalized patients, since azithromycin often is not active against high-level penicillin-resistant *S. pneumoniae* and many intermediate-level resistant strains, monotherapy with azithromycin is not advised. (See Chap. 2.)

2. **Acute exacerbations of chronic bronchitis** have successfully been treated with azithromycin which is active against common pathogens, including most *S. pneumoniae, M. catarrhalis,* and *H. influenzae.* (See related discussions in Chap. 1.)

3. **Pharyngitis/tonsillitis due to GAS.** Azithromycin is an **alternative to first-line therapy (i.e., penicillin)** in individuals who cannot take first-line, preferred therapy (1,2). Erythromycin-resistant strains of GAS will be resistant to azithromycin. (Of note, the package insert suggests susceptibility tests with azithromycin for GAS should be performed in this setting. We suspect this is seldom done). This topic is discussed in detail in Chap. 1. When compliance is a major concern, the one dose daily for 5 days may be useful. Other alternative regimens are cheaper. (See Chap. 1, Tables 1-2 and 1-3.)

   Data establishing the efficacy of azithromycin in the prevention of subsequent rheumatic fever are not available (2).

   Overall, we believe that azithromycin will have a very limited role in this setting (1). (This topic is discussed in detail in Chap. 1.)

4. **Uncomplicated skin and soft-tissue infections** due to MSSA, GAS, or group B streptococci. Similar efficacy is achieved with 5 days of azithromycin or 10 days of cephalexin (19).

5. **STDs** (9). Also see Chap. 10.
   a. **Urethritis and cervicitis** due to *C. trachomatis* can be treated with azithromycin. For *N. gonorrhoeae,* other agents are preferred.
   b. **Genital ulcer disease** due to *H. ducreyi* (**chancroid**) has been treated with azithromycin.
   c. **Pelvic inflammatory disease (PID)** due to *N. gonorrhoeae, C. trachomatis,* and *M. hominis* can be treated initially with the IV formulation. (IV azithromycin 500 mg for 1 or 2 days followed by 250 mg po daily to complete a 7-day course.) If anaerobic microorganisms are suspected, an anti-anaerobic agent (e.g., metronidazole) is added (2). **However, there is considerably less experience with this regimen than other CDC regimens** for PID summarized in Chap. 10.

6. **Currently unapproved uses (as of early 2000) but conventional uses of azithromycin include** the following; the clinical studies supporting the use of azithromycin in these settings are reviewed elsewhere (2).

   a. **Sinusitis,** especially acute maxillary (19).
   b. **For MAC.** Azithromycin (1,200 mg once per week) is effective in **preventing** MAC in AIDS patients at risk (i.e., CD4 count <50). Since azithromycin does not have major drug interactions, it is preferred over clarithromycin (2,23).

      For therapy of established disseminated MAC in AIDS patients, studies suggest that combination regimens including clarithromycin convert blood cultures to negative more quickly and more often than azithromycin-containing regimens (2).
   c. **Infective endocarditis prophylaxis.** Either clarithromycin or azithromycin is an alternative in patients allergic to penicillin and who require antibiotic prophylaxis before oral, dental, esophageal, or respiratory procedures (2). (See Chap. 15.)
7. **For investigational uses, see Sec. C.**

B. **Approved uses in children.** The oral suspension for pediatric use was approved by the FDA in 1995; it is approved for children more than 6 months of age. (The IV preparation of azithromycin is approved, per the package insert, for children more than 16 years of age.)

   1. **Acute otitis media** caused by *S. pneumoniae, H. influenzae,* or *M. catarrhalis.* (See Chap. 1.)
   2. **Mild CAP** due to *S. pneumoniae, M. pneumoniae, C. pneumoniae*, and *H. influenzae.*

      N.B. Even the package insert emphasizes that azithromycin should not be used in moderate to severe pneumonia **or** in children with risk factors such as cystic fibrosis, nosocomial pneumonia, known or suspected bacteremia, immunodeficiency, or illness sufficiently severe to require hospitalization.
   3. **Pharyngitis/tonsillitis** due to group A streptococcal (GAS) infection as an alternative when first-line therapy cannot be used. (See related discussion Sec. III.A.3.)

C. **Investigational uses** have recently been reviewed (2,28).

   1. **Lyme disease** (*Borrelia burgdorferi*) in which azithromycin is listed as an alternative agent (7), although its precise role remains to be established (2).
   2. *Shigella* **infections.** Azithromycin has been shown to be very active *in vitro* against *Shigella* spp. and is a potential alternative agent (7).

   3. *H. pylori*. The role of **azithromycin** for the treatment of this pathogen remains to be determined; it is **not approved** (2) **or recommended** (7) even though clarithromycin is useful for *H. pylori* eradication. (See Sec. III.A.3 under Clarithromycin.)
   4. **Bartonella infections** (e.g., bacillary angiomatosis, cat scratch): azithromycin is listed as an alternate agent (7).
   5. **Miscellaneous areas** of clinical investigation (2) include the use of azithromycin in malaria prophylaxis, toxoplasmosis therapy, *Babesia microti* infection, and trachoma therapy.

IV. **Dosages**
   A. **See Table 26.2.**
      1. Azithromycin is available as a **250-mg tablet** (or capsule) commonly distributed in a **"Z-pack"** containing six tablets for a standard 5-day regimen in adults (two tablets [500 mg] day 1 and then one 250-mg tablet qd days 2 to 5). Tablets can be taken with or without food. Capsules should not be taken with food.
      2. The **flavored oral suspension** comes in 100 mg/5 ml and 200 mg/5 ml. The suspension should be given 1 hour before or 1 hour after meals.
      3. For MAC prophylaxis, **600-mg tablets** are available.
      4. A **1-g oral suspension** single-dose packet is also available and should be taken in the fasting state (e.g., for nongonococcal urethritis).
      5. For **IV azithromycin** 500 mg IV once daily is infused over at least 60 minutes in patients 16 years of age and older (36).
   B. **Pregnancy.** Azithromycin is a **category B** agent (i.e., used only if clearly needed). (See Chap. 14.) It does not produce abnormalities in pregnant animals.
   C. **Nursing mothers.** The package insert indicates that it is not known whether azithromycin is excreted in human breast milk and that caution should be exercised when azithromycin is administered to a nursing woman. However, it should be presumed that azithromycin is in human milk because it is present in the milk of lactating animals and because other macrolides are excreted into human milk (19).
   D. **Renal failure. No dosage adjustments** are necessary in mild to severe renal failure, including situations in which patients are on hemodialysis or chronic ambulatory peritoneal dialysis (CAPD) (13).
   E. In **patients allergic to erythromycin.** In the rare patient who has a history of a severe allergic reaction to erythromycin, until further data are available, **azithromycin should be avoided.**
   F. **Drug interactions** have been reviewed in detail elsewhere (37). Human clinical and pharmacokinetic **studies have shown no major drug/drug interactions between azithromycin and numerous**

other agents, including carbamazepine, theophylline, midazolam, terfenadine, zidovudine, or cimetidine (2). **This is a distinct advantage of azithromycin over erythromycin and clarithromycin.**

Coadministration of antacids does not affect absorption of azithromycin (2).

G. **Limitation.** Since azithromycin typically produces low serum levels, we feel this precludes its use as a potential alternative agent in the allergic prone patient with endocarditis, although little data exist on this topic.

V. **Toxicity and side effects.** Initial studies in about 4,000 adults and 2,000 children indicated **this is a very well-tolerated agent** (20,38), and continued extensive clinical experience supports this.

A. **GI** complaints are the most common, but far less so than erythromycin and less so than clarithromycin. Diarrhea, nausea, and mild abdominal discomfort can occur, more so if higher doses are used.

B. **CNS.** Mild headache and dizziness can occur.

C. Ototoxicity, severe liver toxicity, or nephrotoxicity do not seem to occur with conventional dosing (38). In high-dose regimens (e.g., for therapy of atypical mycobacterium), reversible, dose-related hearing loss has been described (1).

D. Rash appears to be uncommon.

VI. **Cost. See Appendix Tables B and C.**

A. Although a typical Z pack (actual wholesale price, AWP) is about $37, this is often competitive and at times less expensive than other conventional regimens. Also, the convenience of once-daily doses for only 5 days enhances compliance and often patient satisfaction.

B. **IV azithromycin,** at 500 mg daily, costs about $24 per day. This is about as much as IV generic erythromycin drug acquisition costs per day (i.e., for four 500-mg doses), but overall it is more cost-effective to give IV azithromycin in terms of nursing time and expenses, since only one dose of azithromycin is given daily versus the q6h regimen for IV generic erythromycin.

VII. **An overview of the macrolides**

A. **For IV use.** Since no IV formulation is available for clarithromycin, the choice is between IV generic erythromycin and IV azithromycin. Since IV azithromycin is more cost-effective to give per day (see Sec. V.B), is easier to give (requires a once-only dose per day), and lacks the drug interactions sometimes seen with erythromycin, **we favor IV azithromycin** when IV therapy is used in patients more than 16 years of age.

B. **For oral macrolide therapy**

1. **Generic oral erythromycin is still the most cost-effective regimen** and 250 mg qid for 10 days (AWP) is about $7.25 versus the $37 (AWP) of azithromycin Z pack.

However, the GI side effects of erythromycin, qid dosing schedule often for 10 to 14 days, and

Table 26-2.   Dosages of Azithromycin

Setting	Dose/Route	Duration
Adults		
CAP (community-acquired pneumonia)	IV 500 mg 1–3 days* then po 250 mg qd	Usually 5 days total
Legionellosis	IV 500 mg 1–7 days†	Usually 7 days
Acute bronchitis	Z pack	5 days total
Pharyngitis	Z pack	5 days total
Uncomplicated skin infections	Z pack	5 days total
STDs		
Urethritis	1 g po	Once only. See text and Chap. 10.
Cervicitis	1 g po	Once only. See text and Chap. 10.
Chancroid	1 g po	Once only. See Chap. 10.
PID	See text	
Sinusitis	Z pack	

MAC			
Prevention	1,200 mg once weekly		While CD4 counts depressed (<50 cells/UL)
Therapy		Infectious disease consult suggested	
SBE prophylaxis	See Chap. 15		
Children (over 6 months)			
Acute otitis media (AOM)	10 mg/kg day 1 followed by 5 mg/kg on days 2–5	5 days	
Mild CAP	Same as AOM	5 days	
Pharyngitis	12 mg/kg day 1–5 (not to exceed 500 mg daily)‡	5 days	

* For mild, early CAP, a standard Z pack is often used. See text.
† Precise guidelines not available. For moderate to severe cases, IV and/or oral therapy for 7 days presumably provides 21 days of tissue levels and therefore a 7-day course seems prudent. For patients doing very well, IV may be converted to oral, 250–500 mg qd to complete 7-day course.
‡ Failures at 10 mg/kg daily for 5 days have been reported. Therefore a higher dose is suggested. Penicillin is the preferred agent. See Chap. 1.

drug interactions must be balanced with the ease and fewer side effects of azithromycin.

2. **To maximize compliance and/or minimize GI side effects and/or minimize drug interactions, azithromycin is preferred.** Azithromycin can be used in pregnant women.

3. **Clarithromycin** can be given bid but still requires conventional durations of therapy and has the potential of multiple drug interactions. It must be avoided in pregnancy, if possible.

   It is the macrolide of choice for *H. pylori* eradication regimens and for combination therapy of MAC bacteremia in AIDS patients. See prior discussions.

References

1. Reese RE, Betts RF. Erythromycin, azithromycin, clarithromycin, and dirithromycin. In: Reese RE, Betts RF, eds. *A practical approach to infectious diseases*, 4th ed. Boston: Little, Brown, 1996: Chap. 28M.
2. Alvarez-Elcoro S, Enzler MJ. The macrolides: erythromycin, clarithromycin, and azithromycin. *Mayo Clin Proc* 1999;74:613.
3. Gold HS, Moellering RC Jr. Macrolides and clindamycin. In: Root RK, et al, eds. *Clinical infectious diseases: a practical approach*. New York. Oxford University Press, 1999:Chap. 32.
4. Bisno AL, et al. Diagnosis and management of group A streptococcal pharyngitis: a practice guideline. *Clin Infect Dis* 1997;25:574.
4A. Kaplan EL, et al. Susceptibility of group A beta-hemolytic streptococci to thirteen antibiotics: examination of 301 strains isolated in the United States between 1994 and 1997. *Pediatr Infect Dis J* 1999;18:1069.
    Only 2.6% of the isolates were resistant *to a macrolide.*
5. Amsden GW. Pneumococcal macrolide resistance: myth or reality. *J Antimicrob Chemother* 1999;44:1.
   Since very high tissue levels are achieved, in vitro *resistance to azithromycin may not predict* in vivo *failure as long as the MIC does not rise above 16 to 32 µg/ml for azithromycin.*
6. Steigbigel NH. Macrolides and clindamycin. In: Mandell GL, Bennett JE, Dolin R, eds. *Principles and practice of infectious diseases*, 5th ed. New York: Churchill Livingstone, 2000;366–382.
7. Medical Letter. The choice of antibacterial drugs. *Med Lett Drugs Ther* 1999;41:95.
8. Kanatani MS, Guglicimo BJ. The new macrolides: azithromycin and clarithromycin. *West J Med* 1994;160:31.
9. Medical Letter. Drugs for sexually transmitted diseases. *Med Lett Drugs Ther* 1999;41:85.
   Also see Chap. 10.
10. Tappero JW, et al. The epidemiology of bacillary angiomatosis and bacillary peliosis. *JAMA* 1993;269:770.
    Appears to be a new zoonosis assoaciated with both traumatic exposure to cats and infection with Rochalimaea *spp. or a closely related organism.*

11. Dajani A, et al. Treatment of acute streptococcal pharyngitis and prevention of rheumatic fever: a statement for health professionals. *Pediatrics* 1995;96:758.
12. Hoppe JE, the Erythromycin Study Group. Comparison of erythromycin estolate and erythromycin ethylsuccinate for treatment of pertussis. *Pediatr Infect Dis J* 1992;11:189.
    Erythromycin estolate in a lower dose administered twice daily was equivalent to erythromycin ethylsuccinate given three times daily.
13. Aronoff GR, et al. *Drug prescribing in renal failure: dosing guidelines for adults*, 4th ed. Philadelphia: American College of Physicians, 1999.
14. Janssens J, et al. Improvement of gastric emptying in diabetic gastroparesis by erythromycin. *N Engl J Med* 1990;322:1028.
    See editorial comment on this interesting use of erythromycin in the same issue.
15. Boguniewicz M, Leung DYM. Hypersensitivity reactions to antibiotics commonly used in children. *Pediatr Infect Dis J* 1995;14:221.
16. Nattel S, et al. Erythromycin-induced long QT syndrome: concordance with quinidine and underlying cellular electrophysiologic mechanism. *Am J Med* 1990;89:235.
    Authors conclude that erythromycin, especially intravenous use, should be avoided in patients with a history of drug-induced long QT syndrome.
17. Farrar HC, et al. Cardiac toxicity associated with intravenous erythromycin lactobionate: two case reports and a review of the literature. *Pediatr Infect Dis J* 1993;12:688.
    IV erythromycin may be associated with cardiac conduction abnormalities, typically presenting as QT prolongation and torsade de pointes. This may be related to a quinidine-like effect.
18. Neu HC. The development of macrolides: clarithromycin in perspective. *J Antimicrob Chemother* 1991;27:1 (suppl A).
19. Eisenberg E, Barza M. Azithromycin and clarithromycin. *Curr Clin Top Infect Dis* 1994;14:52.
    A good review.
20. Piscitelli SC, Danziger LH, Rodvold KA. Clarithromycin and azithromycin: new macrolide antibiotics. *Clin Pharmacol Ther* 1992;11:137.
    Extensive review.
21. Chaisson RE, et al. Clarithromycin therapy for bacteremic *Mycobacterium avium* complex disease: a randomized, double-blind, dose-ranging study in patients with AIDS. *Ann Intern Med* 1994;121:905.
    Clarithromycin monotherapy acutely decreased M. avium complex (MAC) bacteremia by 99% or more. Clarithromycin, 500 mg bid, was well tolerated and associated with better survival than other dosage regimens. Emergence of clarithromycin-resistant organisms was an important problem.
22. Benson CA, Elner JJ. *Mycobacterium avium complex* infection and AIDS. Advances in theory and practice. *Clin Infect Dis* 1993;17:7.
23. 1999 USPHS/IDSA guidelines for the prevention of opportunistic infections in persons infected with human immunodeficiency virus. *Ann Intern Med* 1999;131:873.
23A. Howden CW, Hunt RH. Guidelines for the management of *Helicobacter pylori* infection. *Am J Gastroenterol* 1998;93:2330.
    Practice guidelines from the American College of Gastroenterology.

24. Nelson JD, McCracken GH Jr, eds. Clinical perspectives on clarithromycin in pediatric infections. *Pediatr J Infect Dis* 1993;12: S98 (suppl 3).
    Symposium devoted to this topic, with several articles on otitis media and streptococcal pharyngitis and safety issues. See editorial comment at end by Dr JO Klem.

25. Aspin M, et al. Comparative study of the safety and efficacy of clarithromycin and amoxicillin-clavulanate in the treatment of acute otitis media in children. *J Pediatr* 1994;125:136.
    A randomized, multicenter, investigator-blinded study of 180 patients 6 months to 12 years of age. Compared clarithromycin (15 mg/kg in two divided doses) versus amoxicillin-clavulanate (40 mg/kg in three divided doses). Middle-ear samples were obtained by tympanocentesis in 175 patients. Clinical response was similar, and recipients of clarithromycin had fewer GI side effects.

26. Reed MD, Blumer JL. Azithromycin: a critical review of the first azalide antibiotic and its role in pediatric practice. *Pediatr Infect Dis J* 1997;16:1069.
    See related papers in this issue.

27. Langtry HD, Balfour JA. Azithromycin: a review of its use in pediatric infectious diseases. *Drugs* 1998;56:273.

28. Tarlow MJ, et al. Future indications for macrolides. *Pediatr Infect Dis J* 1997;16:457.

29. Medical Letter. Clarithromycin and azithromycin. *Med Lett Drugs Ther* 1992;34:45.

30. Wood MJ. The tolerance and toxicity of clarithromycin. *J Hosp Infect* 1991;19:39 (suppl A).

31. Anderson G, et al. A comparative safety and efficacy study of clarithromycin and erythromycin stearate in community-acquired pneumonia. *J Antimicrob Chemother* 1991;27:117 (suppl A).

32. Moellering RC, Jr. Introduction: revolutionary changes in the macrolide and azalide antibiotics. *Am J Med* 1991;91:1S (suppl 3A).
    Overview of a special supplement discussing azithromycin.

33. Zuckerman JM, Kaye KM. The newer macrolides: azithromycin and clarithromycin. *Infect Dis Clin North Am* 1995;9:731.
    Both agents are bactericidal against susceptible S. pyogenes, S. pneumoniae, and H. influenzae. Review of clinical uses. See related review by Schlossberg D. Azithromycin and clarithromycin. Med Clin North Am 1995;79:803.

34. Neu HC. Clinical microbiology of azithromycin. *Am J Med* 1991; 91:12S (suppl 3A).
    Contains good tables with MIC data.

35. Schentag JJ, Ballow CH. Tissue directed pharmacokinetics. *Am J Med* 1991;91:5S (suppl 3A).

36. Garey KW, Amsden GW. Intravenous azithromycin. *Ann Pharmacother* 1999;33:218.

37. Amsden GW. Macrolides versus azalides: a drug interaction update. *Ann Pharmacother* 1995;29:906.

38. Hopkins S. Clinical toleration and safety of azithromycin. *Am J Med* 1991;91:40S (suppl 3A).

27

Tetracyclines

Discovered more than 50 years ago, the tetracyclines (1,2) remain one of the most widely prescribed antibiotic classes in the world. Data collected in 1992 revealed that in the United States tetracyclines were prescribed by office-based physicians more often than were penicillin, ampicillin, ciprofloxacin, or TMP-SMZ (2).

The tetracyclines are **bacteriostatic** and act by interfering with protein synthesis at the ribosomal level.

The superior pharmacokinetic properties, lesser toxicity, enhanced compliance, and reasonable cost of doxycycline make it the tetracycline of choice. (See Sec. II.)

I. **Spectrum of activity**
   A. **Tetracyclines are active against a wide variety of pathogens. (3)**
      1. **See Table 27-1.**
      2. The tetracyclines, especially doxycycline, are active against many community-acquired respiratory tract pathogens, including penicillin-susceptible *Streptococcus pneumoniae* (see Sec. 3 below), *Haemophilus influenzae*, and *Moraxella catarrhalis* as well as many atypical pathogens, including *Mycoplasma*, *Legionella*, and *Chlamydia* spp. (4).
      3. Although any of the available agents (tetracycline, doxycycline, minocycline; see **Table 27-2**) can often be used **against some organisms, doxycycline or minocycline is more potent** (2).
         a. **Doxycycline** is more active against the following:
            (1) *S. pneumoniae* (4,5), including the majority of intermediate penicillin-resistant strains (5). Strains resistant to tetracycline are often susceptible to doxycycline (5).
            (2) *M. fortuitum* and *M. chelonei* (2).
         b. **Minocycline** is more active against:
            (1) *S. aureus*, including many strains of methicillin-resistant *S. aureus* (MRSA) and coagulase-negative staphylococci (e.g., *S. epidermidis*) (2).
            (2) *M. marinum* (2).
   B. Tetracyclines are no longer reliably active against *Neisseria gonorrhoeae* or *Bacteroides fragilis*.
II. **Pharmacokinetics.** Although intravenous preparations are available, **usually the oral route is used** when tetracyclines are administered. The intravenous preparations are used in the protocols for treatment of pelvic inflammatory disease (PID) (see Chap. 10) and, infrequently, in Lyme disease, where doxycycline is recommended.

Table 27-1. Broad-spectrum activity of tetracyclines (3,5)

Bacteria
  *S. pneumoniae**
    (penicillin-susceptible)
    (see text)
  *H. influenzae**
    (ampicillin-susceptible
    and resistant)
  *M. catarrhalis**
    (ampicillin-susceptible
    and resistant)
  Brucella spp.[†]
    (with rifampin)
  *Calymmatobacterium gra-
    nulomatis** (granuloma
    inguinale)
  Vibrio cholera[†] (cholera)
  Vibrio vulnificus[†]
  Helicobacter pylori[†]
  *Pasteurella multocida**
  *Bartonella henselae**
    (bacillary angiomatosis)
  Yersinia pestis
    (with streptomycin)
  *Francisella tularensis**

Ehrlichia[†]
  Ehrlichia chaffeenis
  Agent of human granulo-
    cytic ehrlichiosis

Chlamydiae
  C. psittaci (psittacosis)[†]
  C. trachomatis (trachoma)*
    (urethritis, cervicitis)[†]
    (lymphogranuloma
    venereum)[†]
  C. pneumoniae (TWAR)[†]

Spirochetes
  Borrelia burgdorferi[†]
    (Lyme disease)
  Borrelia recurrentis[†]
    (Relapsing fever)
  *Treponema pallidum**
    (syphilis)
  *Treponema pertenue**
    (yaws)
  Leptospire spp.*

Rickettsia[†]
  Rocky Mountain spotted fever
  Endemic typhus (murine)
  Epidemic typhus (louse-borne)
  Scrub typhus
  Trench fever
  Q fever

Mycoplasmas
  M. pneumoniae[†]
  *Ureaplasma urealyticum**

Mycobacterium
  M. marinum (minocycline)[†]
  *M. fortuitum complex**

Miscellaneous
  *Nocardia**
  *Actinomyces israeli**
  Malaria[‡]

---

* Alternative agent for (3).
[†] Drug of choice for (3).
[‡] See reference 7.

A. **Gastrointestinal (GI) absorption.** These agents are
    incompletely absorbed from the GI tract. **Absorption
    is impaired by milk, aluminum hydroxide, cal-
    cium, magnesium (e.g., in antacids), or iron pre-
    parations.** The tetracyclines combine with the metallic
    ion calcium or magnesium, forming inactive chelates.
    **Absorption is improved if the antibiotic is taken
    in the fasting state,** 1 hour before or 2 hours after
    meals. Although doxycycline is less affected by these
    cations, taking it 1 hour before or 2 hours after a meal
    may be prudent (2).

Table 27-2. Commonly used oral tetracyclines in adults

Name	Usual Capsule Dose (mg)	Usual Interval Between Doses (h)	Usual Total Daily Dose (mg) (See Text)	Approximate Cost (dollars) for 10 Days$
Short-acting				
Tetracycline hydrochloride*	250–500	6 (without food)**	1,000 mg–2,000 mg	$2.50–5.00
Long-acting				
Doxycycline hyclate†	100	12–24 (with or without food)	200 mg	$14.00 (generic form 100 mg bid)
Minocycline‡	100	12 (with or without food)	200 mg	—

* Trade names include Achromycin, Panmycin, Sumycin, Tetracyn.
† Trade names include Vibramycin, Doroyx, Doxycin.
‡ Trade name is Minocin.
§ Approximate actual wholesale price.
** No food in preceding 2h.

B. **Blood levels.** Therapeutic blood levels for susceptible organisms generally are achieved if recommended
doses are administered on an empty stomach. Because
the twice-daily dosing schedule of doxycycline improves
compliance, doxycycline is used commonly. **In renal
failure doxycycline is the preferred** agent for extrarenal infections. (See Sec. D.)

See Table 27.2.

1. **Short-acting agents.** Of the agents available
   (e.g., oxytetracycline and tetracycline), **tetracycline** frequently is used and is a cost-effective
   agent.
2. **Long-acting agents** can be given once or twice
   daily.
   a. **Doxycycline** has the longest half-life (15
      to 18 hours), which permits a dose interval
      of 12 to 24 hours, presumably improving
      compliance.
   b. **Minocycline** has a similar half-life.
   c. Both agents are dosed 200 mg initially, then
      100 mg once or twice daily.

C. **Distribution.** The tetracyclines diffuse reasonably
well into sputum, urine, and peritoneal and pleural
fluids. Good levels are achieved in synovial fluid and
sinuses, with levels approaching serum concentrations.
Because of its increased lipophilic properties, doxycycline gives higher concentrations in the brain and cerebrospinal fluid (CSF) than other tetracyclines. This
may be particularly important in options for oral therapy for Lyme disease (6).

D. **Excretion.** These antibiotics are excreted **in the urine**
except for doxycycline, which is excreted primarily
(90%) in the feces. Therefore **doxycycline is considered the tetracycline of choice for extrarenal
infections when the patient has underlying renal
failure.**

1. **Renal failure. Tetracycline should not be
   used in renal failure**; doxycycline is preferred.
2. **Hepatic failure** is not known to cause elevated
   serum levels of the tetracyclines. However, these
   drugs should be used very cautiously in such situations because they have been noted to cause
   hepatotoxicity.

E. **Drug interactions** (2)

1. **Anticonvulsants** (e.g., carbamazepine, barbi-
   turates, phenytoin) induce hepatic microsomal
   metabolism of tetracyclines, decreasing tetracycline serum concentrations.
2. **Cholestyramine and colestipol** if given concurrently with tetracycline can reduce GI absorption of tetracycline.
3. **Warfarin anticoagulation** may be potentiated
   by tetracyclines; serial prothrombin times should
   be carefully monitored.
4. **Oral contraceptive** efficacy may be decreased
   with concurrent use of tetracyclines.

III. **Indications for use.** Because of their broad-spectrum nature (Table 27-1), these agents are useful in several settings (1,2,7).
See Table 27-3.

IV. **Contraindications to use** (1,2)
  A. **Pregnancy and lactation.** Tetracyclines (including doxycycline) are **category D** agents. (See Chap. 14.) Tetracycline may cause hepatotoxicity in pregnant women. Furthermore, it is transferred across the placenta and has caused **dental deformities and dental discoloration in children** whose mothers received tetracycline while pregnant. Tetracycline is excreted in breast milk. Therefore the **tetracyclines should be avoided by pregnant or lactating women**.
  B. **Children younger than 8 years.** Except in patients suspected of having Rocky Mountain spotted fever or ehrlichiosis, there are **no indications for the use of tetracycline in children younger than 8 years** (1).

V. **Dosages.** With the availability of generic doxycycline and its bid dosing improving compliance, doxycycline is usually preferred (1,2) unless minocycline is needed for its unique susceptibility profile. (See Sec. I.A.)
  A. **Route.** Generic tetracycline or doxycycline **usually** is given **orally** as capsules or tablets, although most of the preparations are available also in the liquid form. Absorption is improved if the oral preparations are taken **while fasting**.
  B. **Dosage regimens**
    1. **Oral.** The common oral preparations available are shown in **Table 27-2.**
      a. **Generic tetracycline**
        (1) **In adults,** 250 to 500 mg of tetracycline hydrochloride q6h, or qid, can be used.
        (2) **In children more than 8 years of age,** 20 to 40 mg/kg/day is divided into q6h doses.
      b. **Doxycycline**
        (1) **In adults**, the usual first-day dosage is 200 mg administered as 200 mg initially or 100 mg q12h, and then 100 mg is given q12h to q24h, depending on the severity of the infection.
        (2) **In children older than 8 years* of age** who weigh less than 45 kg, 4.4 mg/kg is given on the first day, divided into two doses given at 12-hour intervals, followed by 2.2 mg/kg/day as a single dose or divided into q12h doses.
      c. **Minocycline** may be useful in **special settings** as in alternative therapy of *Nocardia* or MRSA infections. Infectious disease consultation is advised in these special settings. If renal function is normal, 100 mg bid has been used in adults.

* Adult regimens can be used in children weighing more than 45 kg.

Table 27-3.   Major clinical conditions for which tetracyclines may be used*

Respiratory infections
  Community-acquired pneumonia in an outpatient setting
  Atypical pneumonia (*Mycoplasma pneumoniae, Chlamydia pneumoniae,* psittacosis)
  Acute exacerbation of chronic bronchitis
  Legionellosis[†]

Genital infections
  ***Chlamydia trachomatis* (nongonococcal urethritis, pelvic inflammatory disease,** epididymitis, prostatitis, **lymphogranuloma venereum)**
  Granuloma inguinale[†]
  Syphilis[†]

Systemic infections
  Rickettsiae (Rocky Mountain spotted fever, endemic and epidemic typhus, Q fever)
  Brucellosis in combination with rifampin (or streptomycin)
  Lyme borreliosis
  Ehrlichiosis
  Relapsing fever (*Borrelia recurrentis*)
  ***Vibrio* (cholera, *V. vulnificus,* and *V. parahaemolyticus*)**
  Tularemia[†]
  Bacillary angiomatosis (bartonellosis)[†]
  Leptospirosis[†]

Other (local and systemic) infections
  Methicillin-resistant *Staphylococcus aureus* and *S. epidermidis*[†] (minocycline) when vancomycin or other agents are not considered appropriate
  Pasteurella multocida[†]
  Mycobacterium marinum[†]
  ***Helicobacter pylori* (in combination with bismuth subsalicylate and metronidazole or clarithromycin)**
  Yersinia pestis (combined with streptomycin)

Other conditions
  Acne vulgaris

Malaria (7)
  Prophylaxis of mefloquine resistant *Plasmodium falciparum* malaria (7)
  Therapy of certain forms of malaria

Source: Modified from Smilack JD. The tetracyclines. *Mayo Clin Proc* 1999; 74:727.
* Tetracyclines are the drug of choice for the infections that are in **boldface.**
[†] Infections for which a tetracycline is an acceptable alternative to standard agents.

    d. **In renal failure,** doxycycline is preferred and neither **peritoneal dialysis** nor **hemodialysis** alters the half-life of doxycycline. Therefore no dosage requirements are needed in renal failure and postdialysis dose adjustments for patients receiving doxycycline are unnecessary (8).

  2. **Parenteral**

    a. **Tetracycline hydrochloride** is no longer commercially available.

    b. **Doxycycline is used intravenously in PID regimens** (see Chap. 10), as an alternate agent in Lyme disease, and in renal failure for patients with extrarenal infections that require intravenous tetracycline. For adults and for children older than 8 years weighing more than 45 kg, standard therapy is 200 mg on the first day of therapy, given in one or two divided infusions, followed by 200 mg daily given in one infusion or usually two divided infusions at 12-hour intervals. In children older than 8 years who weigh less than 45 kg, 4.4 mg/kg is given on day 1 in two divided doses at 12-hour intervals, then 2.2 mg/kg/day once daily subsequently.

    Intravenous doxycycline is commonly used in PID regimens. In this setting, for adults, doxycycline 100 mg IV (or oral) q12h and cefoxitin 2.0 g IV q6h are recommended for at least 48 hours after the patient improves. Then oral doxycycline 100 mg bid is used to complete a 14-day course. (See Chap. 10.)

  3. **See Table 27-4.**

IV. **Toxicity and side effects** (1,2)

  A. **Teeth and bone**. Tetracycline can cause depression of bone growth, permanent gray-brown discoloration of the teeth, and enamel hypoplasia when given during tooth development.

  B. **Hypersensitivity** reactions such as anaphylaxis, urticaria, and rashes are uncommon. **Photosensitivity reactions consisting of a red rash on areas exposed to intense sunlight can occur with all tetracyclines;** these may be toxic rather than allergic reactions. **Patients receiving doxycycline, especially high-dose regimens, should either avoid intense sun exposure or use sunscreens with a reasonably high protection factor (18 or above).**

  C. **Gastrointestinal effects are usually minor. Epigastric distress and nausea can occur after oral administration**, and these symptoms are somewhat dose related. The tetracyclines are irritative substances to the GI tract.

  D. **Accentuated prerenal azotemia.** Tetracyclines appear to aggravate preexisting renal failure by inhibiting protein synthesis.

Table 27-4. Oral dosing regimens in adults**

Indication	Drug	Daily Dose (mg)	Duration in Days
Rickettsial infections	Doxycycline	200	7
(Rocky Mountain spotted fever, Ehrlichiosis)			
Lyme disease	Doxycycline	200	21
Chlamydial infections	Doxycycline	200	
Nongonococcal urethritis			7
PID**			14
Lymphogranuloma venereum			21
Psittacosis			10–21
Respiratory infections	Tetracycline or	2,000	
	Doxycycline	200	
M. pneumoniae			14
C. pneumoniae			14

Miscellaneous

Acne	Tetracycline	250	Chronically
Brucellosis	Doxycycline*	200	45
Cholera	Tetracycline	1,000	3–5
Granuloma inguinale	Doxycycline	200	At least 21 days
Malaria	Doxycycline	See Ref. 7	
MRSA	Minocycline	200	Variable[‡]
M. marinum	Minocycline	200	Variable[‡]
Nocardia	Minocycline	200–400	>90[‡]
Uncomplicated urinary tract (E. coli sensitive)	Tetracycline	2,000	3 (see Chap. 4)

* Plus streptomycin or rifampin.

** Doxycycline, tetracycline, and minocycline are usually given orally. See text. IV doxycycline is used in PID therapy.

[‡] For prolonged courses or use in unusual settings, ID (infectious disease) consultation is advised.

E. **Benign intracranial hypertension.** This entity
occurs only rarely in adults, but is seen in women on
tetracycline.

F. **Esophageal ulcerations have been reported with
doxycycline. To help minimize this, oral doses
should be given with adequate amounts of fluid.**

G. **Hepatitis** has been described after high doses of intravenous therapy or in pregnant women in whom acute
fatty necrosis can occur.

H. **Skin pigmentation changes and blue-black oral
pigmentation** changes can occur with prolonged
minocycline use.

I. **Thrombophlebitis** can occur with intravenous use.

J. **Vestibular** side effects, including dizziness, ataxia,
and vertigo, can occur with minocycline.

K. **Superinfections with** candida of the oral and anogenital region occurs.

References

1. Reese RE, Betts RF. Tetracyclines. In: Reese RE, Betts RF, eds.
    A practical approach to infectious diseases, 4th ed. Boston: Little,
    Brown, 1996:Chap. 28N.
2. Smilack JD. The tetracyclines. *Mayo Clin Proc* 1999;74:727.
3. Medical Letter. The choice of antibacterial drugs. *Med Lett Drugs
    Ther* 1999;41:95.
4. Bartlett JG, et al. Community-acquired pneumonia in adults:
    guidelines for management. *Clin Infect Dis* 1998;26:811.
5. Shea K, et al. Doxycycline activity against *Streptococcus pneumo-
    niae*. *Chest* 1995;106:1775.
    *Of more than 250 clinical isolates, 30% were resistant to penicillin
    but only 5% to 6% were resistant to doxycycline or minocycline; 74
    of 75 penicillin-resistant strains were "intermediately resistant."*
6. Dotevall L, Hagberg L. Penetration of doxycycline into cerebro-
    spinal fluid in patients treated for suspected Lyme neuroborre-
    liosis. *Antimicrob Agents Chemother* 1989;33:1078.
    *Small study from Sweden. Showed higher CSF levels of doxycycline
    in the 10 patients receiving 200 mg po bid compared with 12 patients
    receiving 100 mg bid. Because early central nervous system infection
    with acute infection may be more common than previously consid-
    ered, the higher doses of oral doxycycline may be prudent.*
7. Medical Letter. Drugs for parasitic infection. *Med Lett Drugs Ther*
    1998;40:1.
    *For further discussion of doxycycline in malaria prophylaxis, see
    Centers for Disease Control and Prevention.* Health Information
    for International Travel, *1999–2000. Atlanta: U.S. Department of
    Health and Human Resources, 1999.*
8. Aronoff GR, et al. *Drug prescribing in renal failure: dosing guide-
    lines for adults*, 4th ed. Philadelphia: American College of Phy-
    sicians, 1999.

Vancomycin, Linezolid, and Quinupristin/Dalfopristin

Vancomycin has become an extremely important agent for several circumstances, including (1–3) penicillin-resistant *S. pneumoniae* (see Chaps. 1, 2, and 16), methicillin-resistant *S. aureus* (MRSA) (see Chap. 17), and coagulase-negative staphylococci infections. Vancomycin is a **bactericidal** agent inhibiting bacterial cell wall synthesis. There is no competition between vancomycin and penicillin for binding sites, and cross-resistance between the two drugs does not occur (1).

I. **Spectrum of activity.** Vancomycin is usefully **active only against gram-positive bacteria**, particularly aerobes.

    A. **Gram-positive bacteria.** Vancomycin is bactericidal against susceptible pathogens. The exception is enterococci, against which it is only bacteriostatic. Vancomycin-resistant enterococci (**VRE**) have increased dramatically since 1991.

        1. ***Staphylococci.*** Vancomycin is active against methicillin-susceptible *Staphylococcus aureus* (MSSA) and MRSA and almost all strains of coagulase-negative staphylococci.

           Recently, *S. aureus* with intermediate levels of resistance of vancomycin (**VISA**), with minimum inhibitory concentration (MIC) of 6 µg/ml or more has been reported. Widespread use of vancomycin presumably contributes to the emergence of VISA. Patients with documented VISA need to be isolated to prevent nosocomial spread, and isolates should be reported through state and local health departments to the Centers for Disease Control (4,5). **Infectious disease consultation is advised for patients colonized or infected with VISA. (See infection control-related discussion in Chap. 13, Part B,** Sec. III.)

        2. **Enterococci.** Enterococci are not particularly pathogenic organisms in humans. They most frequently cause UTIs; are part of mixed aerobic/anaerobic flora in intraabdominal (see Chap. 6), pelvic, and surgical wound infections; and can cause bacteremias, although endocarditis due to enterococcus is relatively rare (6). Enterococci may be part of diabetic foot infections, especially established infections associated with ulcers. (See Chap. 3.) Enterococci are now the second or third most common nosocomial pathogens (1,6). This may be explained in part by selective pressure by frequent cephalosporin use and by spread from patient to patient or hospital personnel to patient. *Enterococcus faecalis* makes up the bulk of clinical isolates (85% to 90% in most laboratories). *E. faecium* accounts for 5% to 10% of clinical

isolates, and many of these strains are resistant to common antibiotics.

a. **Vancomycin is bacteriostatic against enterococci, and the combination of vancomycin and gentamicin is bactericidal** against enterococci, except for high-level gentamicin-resistant enterococci, which are discussed in Chap. 21.

b. **Vancomycin-resistant enterococci** are being isolated more frequently (6–9), especially in larger hospitals. Often these are strains of *E. faecium*. From January 1989 through March 1993, nosocomial VRE increased 20-fold, and during this time, intensive-care-unit (ICU) isolates increased from 0.4% to 13.9% (7). **Now about 15% of enterococci isolates from ICUs are VRE (6)**. The various phenotypes (van A, van B, etc) are discussed elsewhere (2,6).

   (1) Fortunately, colonization is often more common with VRE than actual infection, but bacteremia, urinary tract infections (UTIs), and wound infections can occur. Because VRE colonizes the gastrointestinal (GI) tract, **cultures of either stool or rectal swabs are the best way to identify carriers of VRE** (9).

   (2) Patients infected with VRE often are very debilitated, have had prolonged hospitalizations, and have often received multiple antibiotics, including vancomycin (1–3,6,8).

   (3) **Infection control of VRE** is reviewed in Chap. 13, Part B. Prudent use of vancomycin may help decrease the incidence of VRE. (See Sec. III. below.) Cohorting or private rooms, and contact isolation with gowns and gloves is advised (9).

   (4) **Therapy** for VRE. (See Sec. IX.)

3. *Streptococci.* Vancomycin is bactericidal against *Streptococcus pyogenes*, group C and G streptococci, viridans streptococci, and *S. pneumoniae* (including multidrug-resistant strains and high-level penicillin-resistant strains). (See Chaps. 2 and 16.) Thus far, all strains of *S. pneumoniae* are susceptible (2).

4. **Miscellaneous.** Vancomycin is active against *Corynebacterium JK* group, and *Clostridium difficile.*

B. **Gram-negative bacteria.** Vancomycin has no clinically useful activity against these organisms (1).

C. **Anaerobes.** Although vancomycin has some activity against *Clostridium* spp. and anaerobic streptococci, it is not used as an agent for anaerobic infections (1).

II. **Pharmacokinetics** (1,2). After intravenous (IV) doses, vancomycin is excreted primarily by glomerular filtration, and **the dose must be reduced in renal failure.** Vancomycin is not removed by dialysis. The liver may also be involved to a lesser extent in the disposition of vancomycin, and some evidence suggests that dose adjustments may be needed in patients with severe liver dysfunction (2). **Time-dependent killing** of bacteria is important (2). (See Chap. 14.)

A. **Oral preparation.** Vancomycin is poorly absorbed (1,2). Very high stool concentrations are achieved, making this agent useful in *C. difficile* diarrhea and staphylococcal enterocolitis.

B. **Intravenous preparation.** After intravenous administration, therapeutic levels are achieved in the serum and in synovial, ascitic, pericardial, and pleural fluids (1,2).

1. **Half-life.** The serum half-life in adults with normal renal function is 4 to 8 hours. In anuria, the half-life is prolonged to 7 to 12 days.

2. IV vancomycin produces inadequate bile levels and does not penetrate well into ocular tissue. **Vancomycin penetrates the inflamed meninges, but this penetration may be variable** (1,2). Adequate cerebrospinal fluid (CSF) concentrations cannot be consistently assured. This topic has recently been reviewed (10).

3. **Penetration** of vancomycin from serum **into peritoneal dialysis fluid** is variable and unpredictable. Therefore in peritonitis due to selected gram-positive organisms (e.g., MRSA peritonitis in patients receiving chronic intermittent peritoneal dialysis) necessitating vancomycin, the intraperitoneal route is recommended and convenient for the patient (11).

C. **Intramuscular administration is not advised** because of the pain on injection.

III. **Indications for use.** Vancomycin is used in serious infections in the allergic patient or in the patient with certain resistant organisms. **Because the administration of vancomycin is a frequently cited risk factor for subsequent colonization or infection with VRE, prudent use of vancomycin is emphasized** (12).

Guidelines for proper use of vancomycin should be a part of a hospital's quality improvement program and should include the participation of the pharmacy and therapeutics committee, infection control, and infectious disease, medical, and surgical staffs (12).

A. **Situations in which the use of vancomycin is appropriate or acceptable** (1,12,13).

1. **Treatment of serious infections due to beta-lactam-resistant gram-positive microorganisms. Clinicians should be aware that vancomycin may be less rapidly bactericidal and by many experts it is considered less**

effective than beta-lactam agents for beta-lactam-susceptible staphylococci.

a.   For **MRSA** (see Chap. 17), **Vancomycin is treatment of choice** (13). At times, gentamicin and/or rifampin are added for synergy (13). (See Chaps. 21 and 30.)

b.   **Staphylococcal coagulase-negative (SSCN) infections.** Surveys indicate that 35% to 65% of clinically important SSCN isolates are resistant to methicillin. Vancomycin, sometimes combined with gentamicin and/or rifampin for synergy, has become the treatment of choice for these infections (11). **Vancomycin appears to be effective in prosthetic device infections and CSF shunt infections, especially if combined with rifampin. It also is effective against SSCN nosocomial infections in intensive care nurseries** (1).

c.   **Serious diphtheroid infections** (e.g., endocarditis of prosthetic valves, CSF shunt infections, and infections in the compromised host) that are penicillin resistant (or that occur in the severely allergic patient) can be treated with vancomycin.

d.   **Penicillin-resistant *S. pneumoniae*.** Intermediate- and high-level resistant *S. pneumoniae* infections of the CNS (e.g., meningitis) may require vancomycin. Outside the central nervous system (CNS), high-dose beta-lactams or newer second-generation fluoroquinolones (e.g., levofloxacin) are alternatives for penicillin-resistant organisms. (See Chaps. 2 and 16.)

2.   **Treatment of the following additional infections or potential infections** due to gram-positive microorganisms when indicated.

a.   **In patients with a history of anaphylaxis or severe reactions to beta-lactam antimicrobials.** Patients with other types of allergic history ideally should be skin-tested for verification. Examples of such infections include the following:

(1)   **Serious *Staphylococcus aureus* (coagulase-positive) infections.**

(2)   **Endocarditis** due to viridans streptococci or susceptible streptococci, such as *Streptococcus bovis*, can be treated with vancomycin. Because vancomycin may be only bacteriostatic against some enterococci, most authorities recommend vancomycin plus an aminoglycoside as the treatment of choice for vancomycin-susceptible enterococcal endocarditis.

(3) **Central nervous system infections**. The penetration of vancomycin into the CSF may be variable when intravenous vancomycin is used. In the severely allergic patient with staphylococcal meningitis, infectious disease consultation is advisable to help adjust doses and monitor CSF drug levels if necessary.

b. **For bacterial meningitis (in children older than 1 month and adults) possibly or proven to be caused by *S. pneumoniae*** (13,14), IV vancomycin is combined with a third-generation cephalosporin (cefotaxime or ceftriaxone) until susceptibility data are available because of the increased prevalence of penicillin-, cephalosporin-resistant *S. pneumoniae*. Preliminary data suggest that adjunctive use of corticosteroids does not significantly reduce the penetration of vancomycin into the CSF in children. Since penetration of vancomycin in adult CSF may be compromised by steroid use, **some experts will also add rifampin** until susceptibility data are available (10,13,14). (See Chap. 11.)

c. **Antibiotic-associated colitis (AAC) that fails to respond to metronidazole therapy or AAC that is severe and potentially life-threatening**. Intravenous vancomycin produces low fecal concentrations; therefore oral vancomycin therapy is used. Because of the concern for selecting VRE, **vancomycin is no longer used for primary treatment of AAC.** (See Chap. 5 also.)

d. **Central catheter infections.** If a leukopenic patient has an inflamed exit site of Hickman catheter or if catheter-related infection is a major concern and the prevalence of MRSA in the hospital is substantial, empiric vancomycin while awaiting culture results is indicated. This topic is reviewed in reference 15 and in Chap. 12.

e. **Other settings in which empiric vancomycin therapy may be indicated for 72 hours while awaiting cultures in the febrile neutropenic patient are the following:** when beta-lactam-resistant viridans streptococci are suspected (e.g., in patients who have recently had intensive chemotherapy that produces substantial mucosal damage, as in high-dose cytarabine); when prior quinolones prophylaxis has been used; when there is colonization of MRSA; when a blood culture is positive for gram-positive bacteria but susceptibility data are pending; or when the situation is immediately life-threatening (15).

3. **Prophylaxis** is recommended by the American Heart Association for **preventing endocarditis** in patients at risk. Vancomycin is used in ampicillin- or amoxicillin-allergic patients who are undergoing GI or genitourinary manipulations, in patients with an artificial heart valve, or in other high-risk patients undergoing dental procedures. (See detailed discussion in **Chap. 15.**)

4. **Prophylaxis for implantation of prosthetic materials or devices at institutions with a high rate of infections due to MRSA or SSCN.** A single dose administered immediately preoperatively is sufficient unless the procedure lasts more than 6 hours, in which case the dose should be repeated. (See detailed discussion in Chap. 15.)

B. **Situations in which the use of vancomycin should be discouraged** (12,16)

1. **Routine surgical prophylaxis.** (See Chap. 15.)

2. **Routine empiric antimicrobial therapy for a febrile neutropenic patient** except as noted in Sec. A.2.d above. This remains a controversial topic (17).

3. Treatment in response to a single blood culture positive for coagulase-negative staphylococcus, if other blood cultures drawn in the same time frame are negative (i.e., if contamination of the blood culture is likely). Using this criterion, a single positive blood culture for SSCN is almost always either a contaminant or clinically unimportant bacteremia.

4. Continued empiric use for presumed infections in patients whose cultures are negative for beta-lactam-resistant gram-positive microorganisms.

5. Systemic or local (e.g., intravenous catheter or lock) prophylaxis for infection or colonization of indwelling central or peripheral intravascular catheters or vascular grafts.

6. Selective decontamination of the digestive tract.

7. Eradication of MRSA colonization.

8. Primary treatment of AAC. See Sec. A.2.c.

9. Routine prophylaxis for very-low-birth-weight infants.

10. Routine prophylaxis for patients on continuous ambulatory peritoneal dialysis.

11. Treatment (chosen for dosing convenience) of beta-lactam-sensitive gram-positive infections in patients who have renal failure.

12. Use of vancomycin solution for topical application or irrigation.

C. **Miscellaneous:** (a) MRSA **hemodialysis shunt infections** in patients undergoing hemodialysis have been effectively treated with vancomycin; (b) chronic ambulatory peritoneal dialysis (CAPD) can be associated with gram-positive coccal **peritonitis**. Vancomycin is a useful agent in carefully selected patients in this setting (11), see Chap. 6; and (c) **staphylococcal enterocolitis** rarely occurs, but if a case is documented, oral vancomycin is indicated.

D. **Despite these guidelines, vancomycin is often inappropriately used**. (See related discussion in Sec. VIII.)

IV. **Dosage**

A. **Oral**. An oral preparation is available but is very expensive. (See Appendix Table C.)

   1. **For *C. difficile* diarrhea** in adults (1), 125 mg q6h for 10 to 14 days is as effective a regimen as the previously used 500-mg po qid regimen. In children, the dose is 40 mg/kg/day in four divided doses. (Also see Chap. 5.)

   2. **For staphylococcal enterocolitis,** 500 mg q6h in adults has been suggested. (It is unclear whether this entity really exists.)

B. **Intravenous** (1,2)

   1. **Adults**

     a. **A common conventional dosage** suggested by the manufacturer in **adults with normal renal function** has been 500 mg (infused over 60 minutes) q6h. A more convenient and more cost-effective dosage regimen is 1 g q12h (given over 2 hours to avoid the so-called red man syndrome).

     b. **Mayo Medical Center vancomycin dosing nomogram.** In a recent 1999 review, the authors emphasize that conventional dosing (see above), does not take into account variability in patient's weight and renal function.

       (1) **See Table 28-1.**

       (2) **In obese** patients, ideal body weight can be used to determine the creatinine clearance (see Chap. 14, Part A, Sec. II. F.3., page 293), but actual total body weight is used in dose calculations (2).

     c. When vancomycin is given together with an aminoglycoside, some authorities recommend a reduced dose (e.g., 500 mg q8h [or, preferably, pharmacokinetic monitoring).

     d. When used for prophylaxis in cardiac surgery, some authors favor a single 15-mg/kg preoperative dose. (See Chap. 15.)

     e. **See Sec. IV.C. for dosages in renal failure.**

   2. **Children and neonates.** There is less experience with the use of vancomycin in children. For infants and children with non-CNS infections, 10-mg/kg doses IV over 60 minutes q6h (40 mg/kg/day) often are suggested. In CNS infections, 15 mg/kg doses IV over 60 minutes q6h are suggested to

**Table 28-1. Mayo Medical Center
IV vancomycin dosing nomogram*, †**

Creatinine Clearance	Dosing Interval
>80	Every 12 h
65–80	Every 12 to 18 h
50–64	Every 24 h
35–49	Every 24 to 36 h§
21–34	Every 48 h§

Source: Modified from Wilhelm MP, Estes L. Vancomycin. *Mayo Clin Proc* 1999;74:928.

* Use a dose of 15 mg/kg (actual body weight). The dosing interval is based on renal function. It can be estimated by using the estimated creatinine clearance. See Chap. 14 (p. 293) and the table above.

† If the estimated renal function is near the border of two dosing intervals, it may be reasonable to begin with the more aggressive interval; the dose can then be modified if necessary according to serum levels.

§ Patients with serious infection in whom the initial dosing interval is >24 h should have serum level monitoring performed before steady state to ensure that the levels are not subtherapeutic. It may be advisable to measure a random level about 24 h after the first dose. This level can be interpreted with respect to the seriousness of the infection to determine whether the dosage regimen needs to be modified.

attain peak serum concentrations between 30 and 40 µg/ml (10).

In neonates, close monitoring of vancomycin serum levels is important to ensure therapeutic efficacy without toxicity. (See Appendix Table A for dose regimens in neonates.)

C. **Doses in renal failure. In renal failure, maintenance doses must be reduced.**

1. **The Mayo Clinic Center vancomycin dosing nomogram*** can be used (**Table 28-1**).

2. **Matzke and colleagues published a very useful nomogram** designed to achieve peak and trough concentrations of 30 µg/ml and 7.5 µg/ml, respectively. After an **initial loading dose of 25 mg/kg** (infused at 500 mg/hr), the vancomycin **maintenance** dose remains constant at **19 mg/kg** (infused at 500 mg/hr), but the dosage interval depends on the creatinine clearance (**Fig. 28.1**). **Doses are based on actual total weight,** not ideal patient weight. (See Chap. 14 for instructions on how to estimate **creatinine clearance,** which is **based on ideal body weight.** See page 293.)

3. **Individualized dosing. Ideally, vancomycin dosage can be "individualized" based on se-**

* The nomograms may not work well in anuric patients or patients with rapidly changing renal function; serum drug level monitoring is useful in these patients (2). See Sec. V.

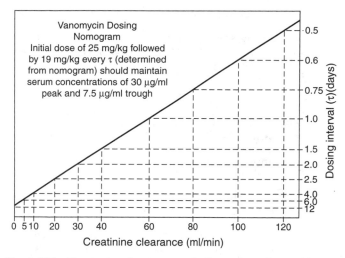

Figure 28.1. Nomogrtam for vancomycin dosage in patients with renal failure. (From Matzke GR, et al. Pharmacokinetics of vancomycin in patients with varying degrees of renal function. *Antimicrob Agents Chemother* 1984;25:433.)

rum concentrations, often with the help of pharmacokinetic consultation. Initial vancomycin dosage is calculated on a per-body-weight basis with the use of the nomogram (see Sec. 2 above) followed by adjustments to attain peak serum levels of 30 to 40 µg/ml and trough levels of 5 to 10 µg/ml.*

4. **Hemodialysis** or **peritoneal dialysis does not remove significant amounts of vancomycin**. Ideally, we prefer individualized dosing in this setting, with an initial loading dose of 25 mg/kg (infused at 500 mg/hr), and typically patients can be maintained on 19 mg/kg given every 5 to 7 days. If on day 5 after the prior dose, the serum level is less than 10 µg/ml, a maintenance dose is given. If on day 5 after the prior dose, the serum level is more than 10 µg/ml, the maintenance dose can be given usually in 48 hours (i.e., on day 7).

D. **Intraperitoneal administration**. In patients on CAPD, vancomycin dosage is discussed elsewhere (11).

E. **Vancomycin administration into the CSF**. Because of the somewhat variable penetration of intravenous vancomycin into the CSF, for inadequately responding meningitis, intrathecal injection is a

* For serious MRSA infection, it may be prudent to aim for a higher trough of 15 µg/ml in order to reduce the possibility of selecting out for resistant VISA organisms. (See Chap. 13, Part B.) Infectious disease consultation about this approach is suggested.

consideration. This topic has been reviewed elsewhere (10). **Infectious disease consultation is advised.**

V. **Monitoring serum vancomycin.** The theoretical dose range for vancomycin is commonly reported as peaks of 20 to 40 µg/ml and troughs of 5 to 10 µg/ml (2). Although monitoring serum vancomycin levels has often become a common practice in the last few years in the United States, in an excellent careful review of prior studies, the authors emphasize that **there are no data to support a cause-and-effect relationship between serum levels of the drug and either its efficacy or its presumed toxicities** (18).

A. Vancomycin pharmacokinetics are sufficiently predictable that adequate serum drug concentrations can be obtained by empiric dosing methods (e.g., see Sec. IV.C). These take into account the patient's age, weight, and renal function. This is especially true when renal function is normal. **Therefore routine vancomycin serum monitoring is not advised.**

B. In a thoughtful editorial comment of the preceding review, **Moellering** concurs. However, he **suggests a limited number of clinical settings in which following the vancomycin level in the serum or other body fluids may be prudent** (19).

1. **Patients receiving vancomycin/aminoglycoside combinations.**

2. **Anephric patients undergoing hemodialysis and receiving infrequent doses of vancomycin for serious systemic infections.**

3. **Patients receiving higher-than-usual doses of vancomycin** (e.g., patients being treated for high-level penicillin-resistant *S. pneumoniae* meningitis).

4. **Patients with rapidly changing renal function.**

C. In a recent review (2), the authors emphasize that **if monitoring is done only, trough levels** are needed. There are almost no data to suggest that peak levels are related to toxicity. Maintaining adequate trough levels may correlate with a better outcome. Furthermore, if nephrotoxicity is, in fact, related to trough levels, nephrotoxicity can be avoided.

Trough levels may be appropriate to consider in high-risk patients (see Sec. B above), those not responding well, or those with rapidly changing renal function (2).

VI. **Toxicity** (1–3). Currently available purified parenteral preparations are very well tolerated. **Only when another drug with nephrotoxic or ototoxic potential** (e.g. an aminoglycoside) **is used simultaneously is there significant risk of these toxicities.**

A. **Ototoxicity** is a potential side effect but is relatively **uncommon**; it appears to occur when very high serum levels (>80 µg/ml) are reached. The greatest risk of hearing loss occurs when vancomycin doses are not adequately adjusted or monitored in renal failure (1).

B. **Nephrotoxicity** is very **uncommon** if standard doses are used in the patient with normal renal function or if doses are appropriately reduced in the patient with renal failure. **When vancomycin is used with an aminoglycoside, it is important to monitor serum levels of both antibiotics to decrease the risk of toxicity.**

C. **Red man syndrome. If vancomycin is infused too rapidly, it may cause the so-called red man (red neck) syndrome,** which includes **flushing of the face, neck, or torso, pruritus, or hypotension** (20). This reaction is believed to result from nonimmunologically mediated **histamine release** secondary to hyperosmolarity associated with the rapid infusion of vancomycin. **Rapid bolus infusions also can cause pain and muscle spasms of the chest and back.**

   1. **Infusion rate. Most of these reactions can be avoided if vancomycin is infused slowly;** that is, each 500 mg is infused slowly over 1 hour (or 1.0 g over 2 hours, 1.5 g over 3 hours, etc).

   2. **Clinical implications.** Although the Red man syndrome resembles an allergic reaction, it is not immunologically mediated and such reactions do not preclude continued administration of vancomycin. **Bronchospasm and angioedema are not part of the Red man syndrome and, if seen, suggest a true allergic reaction to vancomycin.**

D. **Rashes** have been reported in approximately 5% of patients treated with vancomycin. Stevens-Johnson syndrome may occur rarely.

E. **Phlebitis** at the site of infusion **can be minimized if the vancomycin is diluted in 100 to 200 ml dextrose and saline water or saline solution and infused slowly** at a rate not exceeding 15 mg/min.

F. **Fever and chills** after intravenous administration occur much less frequently with the more recent preparations of vancomycin, which contain fewer impurities.

G. **Neutropenia** can occur, especially with prolonged use, and agranulocytosis has been described (21). Therefore **serial blood counts are indicated (at least weekly) for any patient on prolonged vancomycin therapy.**

H. **Anaphylaxis** has been described.

VII. **Cost. Oral** vancomycin is **expensive.** (See Tables B, C in the Appendix.)

VIII. **Continued inappropriate use of vancomycin**

A. Despite published CDC guidelines (see Sec. III), several investigators have reported that **30% to 80% of vancomycin used in hospitals is inappropriate** (22,23)!

1. This is in part due to the clinician's concerns about treating patients with known or potential multidrug-resistant coagulase-positive or -negative *Staphylococcus, Enterococcus*, and *S. pneumonia* (22,23).
2. **A variety of antimicrobial control practices have been tried** (e.g., automatic stop orders, vancomycin order sheets, an approval process before vancomycin is used), yet vancomycin use continues to increase (22).

B. **In a recent report, the authors noted that vancomycin use was heavily determined by rates of endemic MRSA and rates of line-associated bacteremia (23).**

1. The authors emphasized that if hospitals could recognize this link, then vancomycin use could be controlled better, not by classical antimicrobial control approaches (Sec. A.2) but by infection control measures to reduce MRSA rates and central-line infections (23) that create the concern and demand for vancomycin.
2. The editorial comment (24) on this study also stressed **infection control practices**, including the following:
    a. **Better handwashing** by health care workers to control MRSA and more use of the "user-friendly" soapless/waterless soaps.
    b. **New technology** (e.g., new IV catheters bonded with antibiotics) may help reduce catheter-related infections.
3. **With improved infection control practices, concerns for MRSA and line sepsis should decline; vancomycin use would also decline (24).** Also see Chap. 13, Part B.

IX. **Therapy for VRE**

A. The **optimal therapy for** documented infection with **VRE is not established. Infectious disease consultation is advised.**

B. **Several approaches have been utilized** (13).

1. **Chloramphenicol** may be useful in some patients with susceptible VRE (25). (See related discussions in Chapter 23.)
2. Antibiotic studies *in vitro* may at times suggest bactericidal combinations (26).
3. **Quinupristin/dalfopristin** (RP59500: **Synercid**) has been approved for use for the therapy of bloodstream infections due to VRE *E. faecium.* **See detailed discussion of this** agent at the end of this chapter. This agent is modestly successful against VRE but will not solve the problems of treating VRE.
4. **Linezolid (Zyvox)** is a **new antibiotic** anticipated to be available in April–May 2000 (26A) for the therapy of gram-positive infections, **especially multiresistant pathogens such as**

VRE and MRSA in adults. Linezolid belongs to a new class of synthetic antimicrobial agents, oxazolidinones. The precise mechanism of action is considered unknown at present, but it probably interferes with bacterial protein synthesis by binding at the 50s ribosomal level (27–30). **Infectious disease consultation is advised when using this drug.**

 a. Typically, adults have been treated with 600 mg IV or po bid. Linezolid is almost 100% bioavailable. Linezolid is undergoing evaluation in children and is available for compassionate use in children by callling 1-800-836-3535.

 b. Preliminary data suggest linezolid is well tolerated, with diarrhea, nausea, and headache the most common side effects (30).

 c. Linezolid is bacteriostatic and not advised for endocarditis.

 5. **Ignoring the VRE in polymicrobial surgical infections**. VRE may not persist when antibiotics are aimed at other susceptible organisms. (See Chaps. 3 and 5 for the potential role of enterococci in these mixed-infection settings.)

 6. Surgical replacement of the infected valve may be required in VRE endocarditis.

 7. Removal of the lines in bacteremia associated with intravenous lines may be associated with resolution of transient VRE bacteremia.

 8. Most VRE isolates remain susceptible to nitrofurantoin, which may be useful in selected cases of UTIs (2).

 C. **Infection control practices** are important to prevent the spread of this organism. (See Chap. 13, Part B.)

Teicoplanin

Teicoplanin (Targocid) is an antibiotic chemically similar to vancomycin but with important differences responsible for the unique physical and chemical properties of the complex. Although widely used in Europe for the treatment of gram-positive infections, teicoplanin was an investigational agent in the United States until late 1995, and at that point **clinical investigations were suspended.** As of early 2000, we are not aware of "compassionate-use" availability of this agent in the United States. This agent is discussed elsewhere (3).

Quinupristin/Dalfopristin (Synercid)

Quinupristin/dalfopristin (Synercid), a combination antibiotic, is the first agent from a new class of antibiotics called streptogramins. In September 1999, it was **approved by the FDA** for use in the United States **to treat bloodstream infections due to vancomycin-resistant** *Enterococcus faecium* **(VREF)** (31,32). This accelerated approval was based on a demonstrated effect on a surrogate end point that is likely to predict clinical benefit (i.e., the ability of Synercid to clear VREF from the bloodstream); clinical studies are still under way as of early 2000.

Synercid was **also approved** to treat patients with complicated skin and soft-tissue infections caused by methicillin-susceptible *S. aureus* (MSSA) or *Streptococcus pyogenes* (group A streptococci, GAS) (33). However, since there are many other agents active for these infections, at this time we do not advise using this agent to treat these infections. (See Chap. 3.)

I. **Introduction**
   A. **Mechanism of action.** The two antibiotics work synergistically by interfering with protein synthesis: Dalfopristin inhibits the early phase, whereas quinupristin interferes with the late phase of protein synthesis. Resistance is associated with resistance to both components.
   B. *In vitro* **activity.** Synercid is active only against gram-positive organisms.
      1. Synercid is active but bacteriostatic against vancomycin-resistant *E. faecium* (and bactericidal against MSSA, GAS) but the package insert emphasizes it is not active against *E. faecalis* strains. (See Sec. I.A.2 under "vancomycin").
      2. Preliminary data suggest Synercid may also be active against MRSA, *S. agalactiae*, *Corynebacterium jeikeium*, and *S. epidermidis*, but the package insert notes the clinical significance of this is unclear.
   C. **Pharmacokinetics.** Synercid is made up of 30% quinupristin and 70% of dalfopristin, each of which is converted into several active major metabolites.
      1. The elimination half-lives of quinupristin and dalforpristin are less than 1 hour.
      2. The package insert emphasizes fecal excretion constitutes the major elimination of both parent drugs and their metabolites, and biliary excretion is probably the principal route for fecal elimination. Doses do not require modification in renal failure.
      3. Synercid has been shown to be a major inhibitor of the activity of cytochrome P450 3A4 isoenzyme and can interfere with the metabolism of other drugs. (See Sec. III.G.)
II. **Indications for use** (31–34)
   A. Synercid is approved for use for therapy of **patients with serious or life-threatening infections associated with vancomycin-resistant** *E. faecium* **(VREF).**

      Because of the severity and difficulty in eradicating these infections, **infectious disease consultation is advised**.
   B. Although approved for use in complicated skin and skin structure infections caused by MSSA or GAS, other

very active agents are available for these infections (see Chap. 3) and we do not suggest using Synercid in this setting. In an unusual case of VREF bacteremia associated with a mixed VREF and MSSA or GAS wound infection, monotherapy with Synercid may be reasonable. Infectious disease consultation is advised.

III. **Dosages and administration.** Infectious disease consultation is advised.

   A. **Dose ranges**. The dose is diluted in at least 250 ml D5W and infused over 60 minutes.

   1. For vancomycin-resistant *E. faecium*, an IV dose (infused over 1 hour) of 7.5 mg/kg q8h is recommended with a duration dependent on clinical response.

   2. For complex skin and skin structure infections, 7.5 mg/kg q12h IV for 7 days is suggested.

   B. **Pediatric use.** The safety and efficacy of Synercid in patients under 16 has not been established.

   C. **Pregnancy.** Synercid is a **category B** agent. (See Chap. 14.) It should be used during pregnancy only if clearly needed.

   D. **Nursing.** Synercid is excreted in milk in animals; it is not known if it is excreted in human milk. Caution should be exercised administering Synercid to nursing women.

   E. **In renal failure** no dosage adjustment is required, including patients undergoing dialysis.

   F. **In hepatic failure**, no special dose changes are recommended at this time, but only preliminary data are available.

   G. **Drug interactions**

   1. Synercid significantly **inhibits cytochrome P450 3A4 metabolism** of **cyclosporin A, midazolam, nifedipime,** and **terfenidine**. Therefore concomitant administration of these or other drugs metabolized by this cytochrome P450 enzyme system (along with Synercid) may result in increased plasma concentrations of these drugs. This could increase or prolong their therapeutic effect and/or increase adverse reactions. Therefore **caution is advised using these drugs and monitoring levels** (e.g., cyclosporin) **when possible**.

   2. **Medications** metabolized by the cytochrome P450 3A4 enzyme system **that prolong the QTc interval should be avoided** when using Synercid. The latter does not seem to increase the QTc.

   3. **Examples of drugs whose concentrations may be raised by concomitant use of Synercid have been summarized in the package insert and include the following:** antihistamines **(astemizole, terfenidine)**, anti-HIV (NNRTI and protease inhibitors; e.g., delavirdine, nevirapine, indinavir, ritonavir); antineoplastic agents: vinca alkaloids (e.g., vinblastine), docetaxel, and paclitaxel; benzodiazepams (midazolam, diazepam); calcium channel block-

ers; HMG-CoA reductase inhibitor, cholesterol-lowering agents (statins); cisapride; cyclosporine, tacro-limus; methyprednisolone; carbamazine, quinidime, disopyramide, and lidocaine.

IV. **Side effects**

A. **IV site inflammation, pain, edema, and local reactions** are common and if severe may be reduced by increasing the infusion volume to 500 or 750 ml of D5W. (See III.A.)

B. **Arthralgias** and/or **myalgias** are common. Their etiology is unclear.

C. **Hyperbilirubinemia** is relatively common.

D. **GI side effects** (nausea, vomiting, diarrhea) occur in a small percent (<5%).

References

1. Reese RE, Betts RF. Vancomycin. In: Reese RE, Betts RF, eds. *A practical approach to infectious diseases*, 4th ed. Boston: Little, Brown, 1996:1319–1332.

2. Wilhelm MP, Estes L. Vancomycin. *Mayo Clin Proc* 1999;74:928.

3. Sulaiman AS, Rakita RM, Murray BE. Glycopeptides. In: Root RK, et al., eds. *Clinical infectious diseases: a practical approach.* New York: Oxford University Press, 1999:Chap. 31.

4. Centers for Disease Control. *Staphylococcus aureus* with reduced susceptibility to vancomycin—United States, 1997. *MMWR* 1997; 46:765.
   For an update see CDC report on **Staphylococcus aureus *with* reduced susceptibility to vancomycin.** MMWR *2000;48:1166. Report notes that* **instead of using VISA, a better acronym may be "GISA,"** *glycopeptide-intermediate S. aureus. Also see related companion article in this MMWR issue.*

5. Waldvogel FA. New resistance in *Staphylococcus aureus. N Engl J Med* 1999;340:556.
   Editorial comment on two reports in this same issue.

6. Moellering RC Jr. Vancomycin-resistant enterococci. *Clin Infect Dis* 1998;36:1196.
   See related paper by French GL. Enterococci and vancomycin-resistance. Clin Infect Dis *1998;27:S75 (suppl 1).*

7. Centers for Disease Control. Nosocomial enterococci resistant to vancomycin: United States, 1989–1993. *MMWR* 1993;30:597.

8. Lucas GM, et al. Vancomycin-resistant and vancomycin-susceptible enterococcal bacteremia: comparison of clinical features and outcomes. *Clin Infect Dis* 1998;26:1127.
   Risk factors for VRE bacteremia included central venous catheterization, hyperalimentation, prolonged hospitalization, and prior metronidazole use.

9. Fisher MC. Control of methicillin-resistant *Staphylococcus aureus* and vancomycin-resistant enterococcus in hospitalized children. *Pediatr Infect Dis J* 1998;17:823.
   Colonization with VRE may persist for months to years. There is no effective therapy to eliminate VRE carriage.

10. Ahmed A. A critical evaluation of vancomycin for treatment of bacterial meningitis. *Pediatr Infect Dis J* 1997;16:895.

11. Keane WF, et al. Peritoneal-dialysis related peritonitis treatment recommendations: 1996 update. *Perit Dial Int* 1996;16:557.
12. Centers for Disease Control. Preventing the spread of vancomycin resistance: report from the Hospital Infection Control Practice Advisory Committee. *MMWR* 1995;44(RR-12):1.
13. Medical Letter. The choice of antibacterial drugs. *Med Lett Drugs Ther* 1999;41:95.
14. Peter G, et al. *1997 red book: report of the Committee on Infectious Diseases*, 24th ed. Elk Grove, IL: American Academy of Pediatrics, 1997:413.
15. Hughes WT, et al. 1997 Guidelines for use of antimicrobial agents in neutropenic patients with unexplained fever. *Clin Infect Dis* 1997;25:551.
    Guidelines from infectious Disease Society of America.
16. Murray BE. What can we do about vancomycin-resistant enterococci? *Clin Infect Dis* 1995;20:1134.
    See related update by Murray BE. Vancomycin resistant enterococci infections. N Engl J Med *2000;342:710.*
17. Feld R. Vancomycin as part of initial empirical antibiotic therapy for febrile neutropenic patients with cancer: pros and cons. *Clin Infect Dis* 1999;29:503.
    Concludes that in 1999, most experts do not recommend vancomycin as part of initial empiric therapy for febrile neutropenic patients with cancer.
18. Cantu TG, Yamanaka-Yuen NA, Leitman PS. Serum vancomycin concentrations: reappraisal of their clinical value. *Clin Infect Dis* 1994;18:533.
    Review of literature emphasizing that there are no data clearly showing vancomycin serum level monitoring improves efficacy or reduces toxicity over careful conventional dosing regimens.
19. Moellering RC Jr. Monitoring serum vancomycin levels: climbing the mountain because it is there? *Clin Infect Dis* 1994;18:544.
    Routine monitoring of serum levels is not necessary. Editorial comment on reference 18.
20. Wallace MR, Mascola JR, Oldfield EC III. Red man syndrome: incidence, etiology, and prophylaxis. *J Infect Dis* 1991;164:1180.
    Good summary. Emphasizes that slow infusions (e.g., 1 g over 2 hours) reduces this side effect. If a patient has red man syndrome (RMS) after the first dose and vancomycin is the ideal agent to continue, the second dose should be given slowly (over longer than 2 hours) after pretreatment with an H_1-blocker (50 mg oral diphenhydramine 45 to 60 minutes before vancomycin infusion).
21. Adrouny A, et al. Agranulocytosis related to vancomycin therapy. *Am J Med* 1986;81:1059.
    A rare complication.
22. Fridkin SK, et al. Determinants of vancomycin use in adults intensive care units in 41 United States hospitals. *Clin Infect Dis* 1999;28:1119.
23. Jarvis WR. Epidemiology, appropriateness, and cost of vancomycin use. *Clin Infect Dis* 1998;26:1200.
    Vancomycin use is costly, increasing, and often not used appropriately per prior CDC guidelines for use. Further studies needed.
24. Wenzel RP, Wong MT. Editorial response: managing antibiotic use—impact of infection control. *Clin Infect Dis* 1999;28:1126.
    Editorial on reference 22.

25. Lautenbach E, et al. The role of chloramphenicol in the treatment of bloodstream infection due to vancomycin-resistant enterococcus. *Clin Infect Dis* 1999;27:1259.

26. Hayden MK, et al. Bactericidal activities of antibiotics against vancomycin-resistant *Enterococcus faecium* blood isolates and synergistic activities of combinations. *Antimicrob Agents Chemother* 1994;38:1225.
Using time-kill studies, bactericidal activity was attainable against 7 of 13 VRE isolates at 24 hours.

26A. Chien JW, Kucia ML, Salata RA. Use of linezolid, an oxazolidinone, in the treatment of multidrug-resistant gram-positive bacterial infection. *Clin Infect Dis* 2000;30:146.

27. Pharmacia and UpJohn Clinical Protocol (M/1260/0025), 1998.

28. Rybak MJ, et al. Comparative *in vitro* activities and postantibiotic effects of the oxazolidinone compounds eperezolid and linezolid versus vancomycin against *Staphylococcus aureus*, coagulase-negative staphylococci, *Enterococcus faecalis*, and *Enterococcus faecium*. *Antimicrob Agents Chemother* 1998;42:721.
See related study in Diagn Microbiol Infect Dis 1999;34:119.

29. Noskin GA, et al. Successful treatment of persistent vancomycin-resistant *Enterococcus faecium* bacteria with linezolid and gentamicin. *Clin Infect Dis* 1999;28:689.

30. Moellering RC Jr. A novel antimicrobial agent joins battle against resistant bacteria. *Ann Intern Med* 1999;130:155.
An editorial comment with a brief discussion of linezolid.

31. Dowzicky M, et al. Evaluation of *in vitro* activity of quinupristin/dalfopristin and comparator antimicrobial agents against worldwide clinical trial and other laboratory isolates. *Am J Med* 1998: 104:34S (suppl. 5A).

32. Moellering RC Jr, et al. The efficacy and safety of quinupristin/dalfopristin for the treatment of infections caused by vancomycin-resistant *Enterococcus faecium*. Synercid—Emergency Use Study Group. *J Antimicrob Chemother* 1999;44:251.

33. Nichols RL, et al. Treatment of hospitalized patients with complicated gram-positive skin and soft tissue structure infections: two randomized, multicenter studies of quinupristin/dalfopristin versus cefazolin, oxacillin, or vancomycin. Synercid Skin and Skin Structure Infection Group. *J Antimicrob Chemother* 1999;44:263.

34. Medical Letter. Quinupristin/dalfopristin. *Med Lett Drugs Ther* 1999;41:109.
In this November 1999 issue, it concludes that "quinupristin/dalfopristin appears to be modestly effective for treatment of vancomycin-resistant Enterococcus faecium *bacteremia, but that modest effect can be lifesaving. The drug has a high incidence of adverse effects, and a potential for serious adverse drug interactions. Its use to treat any other type of infection should be severely limited."*

bacterium stains, and cultures for bacteria, mycobacterium, and fungi are indicated if a pulmonary process/infiltrate is present. *Candida* species usually do not disseminate or cause pneumonia.

In the patient with unexplained fever and cough, *M. tuberculosis* needs to be excluded even if the chest x-ray is normal. N.B. These patients need to be placed on "airborne" isolation. (See Chap. 13, Part B.)

c. **Bronchoscopy** with bronchoalveolar lavage (BAL) may be necessary in patients with respiratory symptoms, hypoxemia, and chest x-ray abnormalities if routine sputums are not available and cannot exclude mycobacterium and *P. carinii*.

d. Urine and soft-tissue cultures as indicated.

e. **Stool** for bacteria cultures, for *C. difficile*, cryptosporidium, and ova and parasites, including acid-fast stains. *M. avium* can often be stained from a rectal swab.

f. **Serum cryptococcal antigen**

g. With focal central nervous system (CNS) findings, a serum *T. gondii* antibody test, if not already done. (See Chap. 11.)

h. In patients in whom the preceding studies are nondiagnostic, a **liver biopsy** is helpful for *M. avium* complex and less frequently for *H. capsulatum*, **and bone marrow biopsy** may yield a rapid diagnosis of *M. avium* or fungi such as *Histoplasma*.

i. If epidemiologic data suggest (e.g., international travel to endemic areas for leishmaniasis [tropical and subtropical areas, Spain]), screening should be done for visceral leishmaniasis (12). Infectious disease consultation is advised.

3. **Routine tests.** A complete blood count with differential, liver, and renal function tests are suggested.

4. **Radiographic tests.** Chest roentgenogram and CT scan of the abdomen and/or chest are dictated by results of initial tests and presence of organ-specific findings. If there are focal CNS findings on physical examination, a head CT and/or MRI will be necessary.

III. **Fever in the leukopenic patient is assumed to be infection**, although bacteriologic proof is often lacking. Infection secondary to the leukopenia that occurs in the course of disease or as a consequence of chemotherapy is the leading cause of death in leukemia and other malignancies. Early institution of empiric antibiotic therapy has decreased infection-related morbidity and mortality. A nice summary has recently been published (13).

A. **Setting**
   1. With **granulocyte counts of less than 500/mm³**, the risk of infection increases significantly. The risk of bacteremia is even greater if the granulocyte count is **less than 100/mm³**. The risk of infection is increased with prolonged granulocytopenia.
   2. **A fever** (oral temperature) of more than 38°C on more than one occasion or more than 38.5°C once usually **necessitates antibiotics**, at least until culture data are known.

B. **Initial approach. Leukopenic patients with fever need immediate evaluation and therapy.**
   1. **History.** Specific attention is directed toward prior surgery (e.g., splenectomy); recent therapy, including cytotoxic agents, radiation, and current medications (especially corticosteroids); and prior infectious episodes (and organisms). These data may influence decisions concerning empiric antibiotic therapy, including the likelihood of infection due to resistant pathogens.
   2. **Physical.** An obvious focus of infection that can be treated specifically should be sought. Remember that the **patient with leukopenia may not manifest the usual signs of infection (inflammation).** Those with soft-tissue infection may have little or no erythema or induration, although tenderness may be present. Careful inspection and palpation of any permanent catheter devices (e.g., Hickman catheter) is essential to help exclude an obvious tunnel or exit-site infection.
   3. **Baseline laboratory work-up** includes the following:
      a. **A chest x-ray**, even if pulmonary symptoms are absent. In leukopenic patients, purulent sputum often is not present.
      b. **A urine culture**, even if the urinalysis appears benign.
      c. **Blood cultures**. Two cultures at least 20 minutes apart.
      d. **Examination and culture of any exudates** (sputum, wound, or drainage).

C. **Empiric antibiotics are started** once cultures have been obtained. In the last decade infections due to *Pseudomonas* spp. have become less frequent and coagulase-negative staphylococci and other gram-positive infections are more frequent. *Enterobacter* and *Citrobacter* spp. are isolated more frequently and often produce beta-lactamases.
   1. **Common empiric parenteral regimens are shown in Table 12.5.**
      a. Simultaneous use of **two drugs** active against the identified infecting bloodstream organism in the leukopenic patient may be associated with improved clinical outcome.

Table 12-5. Febrile leukopenic patient without an obvious source of fever

Setting	Regimen (for adults, normal renal function)	Comment
Patient has no deep lines	Piperacillin (4 g IV q6h) plus aminoglycoside, or ceftazidime (2 g IV q8h) plus aminoglycoside, or	Time-honored combination. Risk of nephrotoxicity
	Ceftazidime alone, or	Significant experience. Avoids an aminoglycoside
	Imipenem alone, or	Cannot be used in patient with penicillin allergy
	Cefepime alone	Least amount of experience*
With a deep line, but no obvious line-related infection and **minimally ill**	Same as above	If patient has sustained fever or clinically declines, add empiric vancomycin until blood culture data are available
With a deep line but a sicker patient or with a focal line infection	One of above regimens 1–4, plus vancomycin	To cover gram-positive cocci, until blood culture data are available
Protracted leukopenia plus prior intensive antibiotics	One of above regimens 1–4, ? also add amphotericin B or fluconazole[†] and use amikacin for the aminoglycoside	To cover more resistant gram negatives and candidemia

* Approved for use in the febrile neutropenic patient as monotherapy in 1999. See Biron P, et al. Cefepime versus imipenem-cilastatin as empirical monotherapy in 400 febrile patients with short duration neutropenia. *J Antimicrob Chemother* 1998;42:511, in which cefepime was as effective and better tolerated than imipenem. (See Chap. 19.)

[†] See Malik IA, et al. A randomized comparison of fluconazole with amphotericin B as empiric anti-fungal agents in cancer patients with prolonged fever and neutropenia. *Am J Med* 1998;105:478, showing fluconazole is equally effective but less toxic in this setting.

    b. Monotherapy to reduce toxicity and IV administration dwell time is an important consideration in many patients.

  2. **Oral outpatient antibiotics** may be a consideration in carefully selected, compliant, and clin-

ically stable outpatients (13,14), but far more clinical experience is available with at least initial inpatient antibiotic administration (e.g., 24 to 48 hours) with serial observation. Recent studies (15,16) of oral antibiotics for the low-risk febrile leukopenic patient (usually in patients with solid tumors and anticipated short-term leukopenia) are hopeful, but these studies were carried out in the hospital setting. We agree with the study authors and editorial by Finberg and Talcott (17) that before oral antibiotics can be safely used for this problem in the outpatient setting, further large randomized studies need to be done.

D. **Duration of therapy is discussed elsewhere (13).**
   1. **Positive blood cultures.** Specific therapy is usually continued for 10 to 14 days; it may be extended if granulocytopenia persists.
   2. **Negative blood cultures.** In a patient who defervesces, antibiotic therapy is usually continued until the granulocyte count rises to more than 500/mm^3 or for 14 days, whichever is shorter if the patient becomes afebrile and is clinically stable.

E. Infectious disease consultation and/or **consultation** with someone experienced in infections in the leukopenic patient **is advised,** especially if the patient's fever persists despite empiric antibiotics. Options on the persistently febrile patient are reviewed elsewhere (13).

References

1. Speck EL, Roberts NJ Jr. Fever and fever of unknown etiology. In: Reese RE, Betts RF, eds. *A practical approach to infectious diseases*, 4th ed. Boston: Little, Brown, 1996:Chap. 1.
2. Hirschmann JW. Fever of unknown origin. *Clin Infect Dis* 1997; 24:291.
   Nice "state-of-the-art" review.
3. Amow PM, Flaherty JP. Fever of unknown origin. *Lancet* 1997; 350:575.
4. Knockaert DC, et al. Fever of unknown origin in elderly patients. *J Am Geriatr Soc* 1993;41:1187.
5. Lorin MI, Feigin RD. Fever without localizing signs and fever of unknown origin. In: Feigin RD, Cherry JD, eds. *Textbook of pediatric infectious diseases*, 4th ed. Philadelphia: WB Saunders, 1998:Chap. 73.
6. Tindall B, Carr A, Cooper DA. Primary HIV infection: clinical, immunologic, and serologic aspects. In: Sande MA, Volberding PA, eds. *The medical management of AIDS*, 4th ed. Philadelphia: WB Saunders, 1995:Chap. 6.
6A. Rich JD, et al. Misdiagnosis of HIV infection by HIV-1 plasma viral load testing: a case series. *Ann Intern Med* 1999;130:37.
   Only patients who have a high pretest probability of positive result should be evaluated for primary HIV infection by using plasma viral load testing.
7. Johnson DH, Cunha BA. Drug fever. *Infect Dis Clin North Am* 1996;10:85.

C. **In patients with significant hepatic impairment**, although data are limited, **doses** should be **reduced** by at least 50% (1,2).

D. **Pregnancy.** See related discussion in Sec. III. The package insert indicates metronidazole is a **Category B** agent (see Chap. 14); the drug should be used during pregnancy only if clearly needed.

The *Physician's Desk Reference* emphasizes that "metronidazole use in the second and third trimesters of pregnancy should be restricted to those patients in whom alternative treatment has been inadequate. The use of metronidazole in the first trimester should be carefully evaluated because metronidazole crosses the placenta barrier and its effects on human fetal organogenesis are not known" (10).

The **pros and cons of using metronidazole in pregnancy,** especially the first trimester, have **recently** been **reviewed** (11). In his commentary, the reviewer emphasizes that the "preponderance of published human experience does not support a teratogenic effect in any trimester" (11). He feels metronidazole should probably be avoided in the first trimester except for serious or life-threatening infections, pending further data. After organogenesis is complete, metronidazole should be considered for treating significant infections when other equally effective options are not available or are contraindicated (11).

E. **Nursing.** Metronidazole is secreted in human milk. (See Sec. III.)

F. **Pediatrics.** The safety and efficacy of metronidazole in pediatric patients has not been established except in the treatment of amebiasis (10).

VI. **Adverse effects.** In general, metronidazole is well tolerated (1,2).

A. **Carcinogenic potential.** (See Secs. III and V.D.)

B. **Alcohol intolerance. Alcoholic beverages should not be consumed by patients taking any formulation of metronidazole,** because of a disulfiram-like effect (i.e., nausea, vomiting, abdominal cramps, strange taste sensations, and headaches).

C. **Peripheral neuropathy,** manifested as numbness and tingling of the extremities, may be seen after therapy lasting a few months. This is usually reversible if the drug is stopped (2). **Seizures,** encephalopathy, or cerebellar dysfunction are rare. Some advise the drug be used with caution in patients with a history of central nervous system disorders. If neurologic symptoms develop while on therapy and there is no other obvious cause, metronidazole should be stopped (2).

D. **Anticoagulation interference.** Metronidazole can potentiate the effect of warfarin.

E. **Miscellaneous. Mild GI symptoms** of nausea, abdominal discomfort, and diarrhea can occur. Patients complain of a **metallic, unpleasant taste** while on oral therapy. Metronidazole may be a cause of **acute pancreatitis.**

VII.   **Cost.** Generic oral formulations are inexpensive. See Tables B and C in the Appendix.

References

1. Reese RE, Betts RF. Metronidazole. In: Reese RE, Betts RF, eds. *A practical approach to infectious diseases*, 4th ed. Boston: Little, Brown, 1996:Chap. 28P.

2. Kasten JJ. Clindamycin, metronidazole, and chloramphenicol. *Mayo Clin Proc* 1999;74:825.

3. Finegold SM. Metronidazole. In: GL Mandell, Bennett JE, Dolin R, eds. *Principles and practice of infectious diseases*, 5th ed. New York: Churchill Livingstone, 2000:361–366.

4. Dow G, Ronald AR. Miscellaneous and antibacterial drugs. In: Root RK, et al. *Clinical infectious diseases: a practical approach*. New York: Oxford University Press, 1999:Chap. 36.

5. Aronoff GR, et al, eds. *Drug prescribing in renal failure: dosing guidelines for adults*, 4th ed. Philadelphia: American College of Physicians, 1999.

6. Falagas ME, et al. Late incidence of cancer after metronidazole use: a matched metronidazole user/non-user study. *Clin Infect Dis* 1998;26:384.
    Although authors feel these data are reassuring after short-term use of metronidazole. Data with prolonged use are unavailable.

7. Medical Letter. The choice of antibacterial drugs. *Med Lett Drugs Ther* 1999;41:95.

8. Medical Letter. Drugs for parasitic infections. *Med Lett Drugs Ther* 1998;40:1.

9. Ahmadsyah I, Salim A. Treatment of tetanus: an open study to compare the efficacy of procaine penicillin and metronidazole. *Br Med J* 1985;291:648.
    In this trial, 76 patients received penicillin and 97 metronidazole. Patients in the metronidazole group had a significantly lower mortality, a shorter hospital stay, and improved response to treatment.

10. *Physician's Desk Reference*, 54th ed. Montvale, NJ: Medical Economics Data, 2000.

11. Coustan DR. Use of metronidazole in pregnancy. *Pediatr Infect Dis J* 1999;18:79.
    Author notes that in pregnant women with bacterial vaginosis, treatment with metronidazole may reduce the likelihood of preterm birth for those who are already at high risk for preterm delivery (previous preterm delivery, prepregnant weight less than 50 kg or both) and who are found to have bacterial vaginosis in the course of second-trimester pregnancy screening; therefore oral metronidazole is indicated and appropriate in this setting.

    However, in a recent report by JC Carey, et al., Metronidazole to prevent preterm delivery in pregnant women with asymptomatic bacterial vaginosis, N Engl J Med 2000;342:534, data showed treatment of asymptomatic bacterial vaginosis in pregnant women does not reduce the occurrence of preterm delivery or other adverse perinatal outcomes. See editorial on this topic in this same issue.

Rifampin, Rifapentine, and Rifabutin

Rifampin (Rifadin)

Rifampin was discovered in 1965. Its mechanism of action involves inhibiting DNA-dependent RNA polymerase by binding to the subunit of the enzyme in susceptible microorganisms, thus interfering with protein synthesis (1). Rifampin is bactericidal. Resistant strains of bacteria have altered RNA polymerase that is not inhibited by rifampin (1).

I. **Spectrum of activity.** Rifampin is a **broad-spectrum** agent, active against bacteria, mycobacteria, and chlamydiae (1,2)

A. **Bacteria.** The *in vitro* activity of rifampin as a single agent is summarized in **Table 30-1.**

B. **Mycobacteria.** Most strains of *Mycobacterium tuberculosis* are susceptible to rifampin, but **resistant strains have been isolated** with greater frequency in recent years (3). The susceptibility of other mycobacteria is variable: *M. kansasii* and *M. marinum* are susceptible, whereas *M. fortuitum* and *M. chelonei* are resistant (1).

C. **Chlamydiae.** Many species of *Chlamydia*, particularly *C. trachomatis*, are susceptible to rifampin.

II. **Resistance**

A. **Rapid emergence of resistant bacteria occurs with monotherapy** (1).

B. **Except for short-term prophylaxis, rifampin should not be used alone** (1).

III. **Pharmacokinetics and preparations.** Rifampin is red-orange in color in the crystalline state. The **oral** form is well absorbed from the gastrointestinal (GI) tract in the fasting state. In late 1989, an **intravenous preparation** of rifampin became available for use in patients for whom the oral route is not an option; this preparation should not be given intramuscularly (1,2).

A. **Distribution.** The drug is well distributed, with levels in body fluids and tissue similar to those observed in serum. Therapeutic concentrations are obtained in serum, urine, saliva, bone, pleura, pancreatic juice, and cerebrospinal fluid (CSF) (1,2).

B. **Metabolism.** Rifampin is cleared from the circulation primarily by hepatic metabolism and biliary excretion. Its half-life is 2 to 5 hours and is prolonged in hepatic disease. **In renal failure,** only modest dose adjustments are advised. (See Sec. VI.B.)

C. **Peak serum concentrations** after an oral dose of 600 mg or 10 mg/kg are variable but usually are in the range of 7 to 15 µg/ml (1).

Table 30-1. *In vitro* **activity of rifampin**

Organism	MIC$_{90}$ (µg/ml)*
Gram-positive	
Staphylococcus aureus[†]	0.015
S. epidermidis[†]	0.015
Streptococcus pyogenes	0.12
S. pneumoniae (*penicillin susceptible*)	4.0
Viridans streptococci	0.12
Enterococcus faecalis	16.0
J K diphtheroids	0.05
Listeria monocytogenes	0.25
Clostridium difficile	≤0.2
C. perfringens	≤0.1
Peptococcus, Peptostreptococcus spp.	1.6
Proprionibacterium acnes	≤0.1
Gram-negative	
Neisseria gonorrhoeae	0.5
N. meningitidis	0.12
Moraxella (*Branhamella*) *catarrhalis*	0.03
Haemophilus influenzae	0.5
H. ducreyi	0.03
Legionella pneumophila	0.03
Brucella spp.	1.25
Escherichia coli	16.0
Klebsiella pneumoniae	32.0
Enterobacter spp.	64.0
Pseudomonas aeruginosa	64.0
Bacteroides fragilis	0.8
B. melaninogenicus	0.2

Source: Modified from Craig WA. Rifampin and related drugs. In: Gorbach SL, Bartlett JG, Blacklow NR, eds. *Infectious diseases*. Philadelphia: WB Saunders, 1992:265–266.

* MIC$_{90}$ = concentration below which 90% of tested organisms are inhibited.

[†] In most cases, the MIC for methicillin-resistant strains is similar to those for methicillin-susceptible strains (1).

    D. **Patients taking rifampin often develop a harmless red-orange coloring of the urine, saliva, feces, sweat, and tears; they should be forewarned of this to prevent unnecessary anxiety.**

  IV. **Clinical use.** Rifampin is approved officially for use only in the treatment of patients with tuberculosis and carriers of *N. meningitidis* (4)

    A. **Tuberculosis.** Rifampin is an important agent in the treatment of *M. tuberculosis* and some of the atypical mycobacteria (5,6). Rifampin also is used as an alternative agent in multidrug regimens to treat *Mycobacterium avium* complex (MAC) infections in patients with AIDS (5). Rifampin has been used for chemoprophylaxis of tuberculosis in the rare isoniazid-allergic patient and for prophylactic therapy of contacts exposed to isoniazid-resistant organisms (6).

B. **Bacterial meningitis contacts.** Rifampin has been used successfully in eradicating the carrier state of close **contacts of meningococcal and *Haemophilus influenzae* meningitis**. This is one of the rare uses of rifampin as monotherapy but legitimate since it is used for a very short time. See the rationale and specific recommendations in Chap. 15.

C. **Investigational studies.** When rifampin is used alone for specific infections, resistance rapidly develops. Thus there has been increased interest in the **use of rifampin with other antibiotics to avoid this** and yet take advantage of rifampin's excellent *in vitro* activity (7–9).

1. **Therapy of methicillin-resistant *Staphylococcus aureus* (MRSA).**

a. **Rifampin in combination with a second agent (e.g., trimethoprim-sulfamethoxazole) has been used to try to eradicate nasal carriage of MRSA** (10). Topical nasal mupirocin has also been used to eradicate MRSA nasal carriers (11). See the related discussion in Chap. 17.

b. For **other MRSA infections,** vancomycin is the therapy of choice. (See Chap. 28.) There are no data to support the routine addition of rifampin to vancomycin, but if there is an inadequate response to vancomycin alone, then the addition of rifampin, gentamicin, or both should be considered (5). In his review, Farr emphasizes that rifampin resistance has been reported during therapy for MRSA infections with rifampin plus vancomycin, and the addition of gentamicin to the regimen may help prevent the development of rifampin resistance (9).

2. **Endocarditis and bacteremias.** Rifampin has been studied particularly in **endocarditis** due to *S. aureus* and *S. epidermidis* (9). For endocarditis due to *S. aureus*, there are conflicting *in vitro* data, as antagonism may be seen with combination therapy (12,13). Infectious disease consultation is advised before using rifampin in this setting. Bactericidal levels should be compared before and after adding rifampin.

   In the animal model of endocarditis caused by MRSA, the combination of vancomycin with rifampin was significantly more effective than vancomycin alone (10,12). In the experimental model of endocarditis caused by *S. epidermidis*, the addition of gentamicin or rifampin to vancomycin was beneficial, even though *in vitro* synergistic studies may not predict a beneficial effect (12). (See related discussions in Chap. 8.)

3. **Severe *Legionella* infections.** In treating severe infections due to *Legionella pneumophila* and other *Legionella* spp., rifampin has often been combined with a macrolide or a fluoroquinolone (5,7).

4. **Cerebrospinal fluid shunt infections.** In combination with another agent (e.g., vancomycin), rifampin has been used to treat staphylococcal coagulase-negative infections (14).

5. **Chronic osteomyelitis** due to *S. aureus* has been treated with a combination of nafcillin and rifampin (1,2). This complex and difficult problem is discussed elsewhere (9). In these difficult cases, infectious disease consultation is advised.

6. ***Brucella* infections.** Prolonged therapy with doxycycline plus rifampin has a clinical response similar to that of tetracycline plus streptomycin (1,5,7).

7. **Orthopedic implant infections.** Patients with prosthetic device infections have been treated with rifampin-containing antibiotic combinations (15,16). In a recent report, patients with stable implants, short duration of staphylococcal infection (<21 days), initial debridement, and IV antibiotics, if patients could tolerate long-term therapy with 3 to 6 months therapy of rifampin-ciprofloxacin, cure of the infection without device removal was commonly achieved (16,17). The authors of the editorial on this paper emphasize that only patients with a quinolone-susceptible staphylococci should be candidates for this form of therapy (17).

8. **High-level penicillin-resistant *S. pneumoniae* meningitis** often merits therapy with vancomycin. Some experts have suggested that rifampin may be added (5). If cefotaxime or ceftriaxone is used, rifampin in combination may improve results (18). (See related discussions in Chaps. 2, 11, and 16.)

9. **Miscellaneous uses** of rifampin include combination therapy with penicillin for eradication of group A streptococcal carrier states and in combination regimens to treat severe cat scratch disease (8).

V. **Adverse reactions. The most common side effect** observed with rifampin **is an orange-red discoloration of the urine.** (See Sec. III.D.) Permanent staining of soft contact lenses can occur during rifampin therapy (1). The adverse reactions of rifampin often are classified into the following four types (2):

A. **Immunosuppression.** In animal and *in vitro* studies, rifampin has been shown to suppress the secretion of migration inhibition factor by lymphocytes, the response of lymphocytes to stimulation by nonspecific mitogen, and the production of antibody by cultured lymph node cells (2). The precise implications of these studies for humans are unclear (9). In addition, tuberculin skin test reactivity may be diminished in patients receiving rifampin.

B. **Immunologic reactions**

1. **Allergic or hypersensitivity reactions** such as drug fever, skin rashes, and eosinophilia are uncommon.

2. **A flulike syndrome** with fever, malaise, and headache can occur, particularly with irregular administration. It is very infrequent with intermittent tuberculosis regimens (i.e., twice weekly on the same 2 days) and also infrequent with daily use. Renal failure, thrombocytopenia, hemolysis, and the hepatorenal syndrome can occur in this flulike syndrome (9). Interstitial nephritis is a rare complication. Most patients improve with supportive care and withdrawal of the agent. Presumably, the risk of these reactions can be reduced if the doses are given on a regular schedule.

C. **Toxic reactions**

1. **Hepatotoxicity** has been seen in patients with overdose, prior hepatic disease, and concurrent use of hepatotoxic agents (e.g., halothane anesthesia). In patients with mild liver function test abnormalities, rifampin must be used with caution, and liver function tests ideally should be monitored carefully if the drug is employed. For other uses of rifampin (i.e., when not treating mycobacterial infections) in patients without underlying hepatic dysfunction, serial liver function tests are not routinely recommended.

   There is some concern about whether the combined use of isoniazid and rifampin increases hepatotoxicity. In one review, Craig (1) emphasized that although elevated liver enzyme values are observed in approximately 5% to 10% of recipients of rifampin, "hepatitis occurs in 0.15% to 0.43% of persons treated with rifampin alone. The incidence of hepatitis rises to 2.5% in patients receiving multiple drug therapy for tuberculosis; however, most studies suggest that rifampin does not enhance the hepatotoxicity of isoniazid" (1).

2. **Renal injury** is uncommon (9).

3. **Exudative conjunctivitis,** which is reversible once the drug has been discontinued, has been reported.

D. **Drug interactions. By potentiating hepatic microsomal cytochrome P450-related enzymatic reactions, rifampin induces increased hepatic excretion of a number of drugs** and other compounds metabolized by the liver (1,2,9).

Table 30-2.   Previously described rifampin drug interactions*, part I

Drug	Comments
Anticoagulants, oral[†]	Increase anticoagulant dose based on monitoring of prothrombin time
Beta-blockers	May need to increase propranolol or metoprolol dose
Chloramphenicol	Monitor serum chloramphenicol concentrations; increase dose if needed
Contraceptives, oral[†]	Use other forms of birth control; document patient counseling in chart
Cyclosporine[†]	Monitor serum cyclosporine concentrations; increased dose will likely be needed
Digitoxin[†]	Monitor serum digitoxin concentrations; monitor for arrhythmia control and signs and symptoms of heart failure; increase dose if needed
Digoxin	Monitor serum digoxin concentrations; monitor for arrhythmia control and signs and symptoms of heart failure; clinically significant interaction most likely in patients with decreased renal function
Glucocorticoids[†]	Increase glucocorticoid dose twofold to threefold with concomitant rifampin therapy
Ketoconazole[†]	Avoid this combination if possible; monitor serum ketoconazole concentrations; increase dose if needed; space rifampin and ketoconazole doses by 12 hours
Methadone[†]	Increase methadone dose with concurrent rifampin therapy; control withdrawal symptoms
Phenytoin[†]	Monitor serum phenytoin concentrations; increase phenytoin dose if needed
Quinidine[†]	Monitor serum quinidine concentrations; monitor for arrhythmia control; increase dose if needed
Sulfonylureas	Increase sulfonylurea dose based on blood glucose control; monitor blood glucose with discontinuation of rifampin therapy
Theophylline[†]	Monitor serum theophylline concentrations; increased dose will likely be needed

Table 30-2. (*Continued*)

Drug	Comments
Verapamil[†]	Use alternative agent to verapamil if possible, because even very large increase in oral verapamil may not be sufficient; monitor serum verapamil concentrations; monitor patient for clinical response

Source: Borcherding SM, Baciewicz AM, Self TH. Update on rifampin drug interactions. *Arch Intern Med* 1992;152:711. Copyright 1992, American Medical Association.

* Carefully adjust doses when rifampin is discontinued; enzyme induction effect is gradually reduced over 1–2 weeks. For details see Borcherding SM, Baciewicz AM, Self TH. Update on rifampin drug interactions, II. *Arch Intern Med* 1992; 152:711.

[†] Major clinical significance is well established.

The interactions of rifampin have been reviewed in detail in a series of three papers appearing in 1987 (19), 1992 (20), and 1997 (21). The **drugs that may interact with rifampin are summarized from these reports in Tables 30-2, 30-3,** and **30-4,** respectively.

E. **Thrombophlebitis** can occur with the parenteral form (8).

VI. **Dosages and precautions**

A. **Dosages.** Capsules are available in 150-mg and 300-mg sizes. The oral regimen is preferred and is given 1 hour before or 2 hours after meals. For pediatric and adult patients in whom capsule swallowing is difficult or in whom lower doses are needed, but the oral route is desirable, a liquid suspension can be made according to the package insert. The same dose per day is given orally or intravenously.

1. **In tuberculosis,** the usual daily dose (as a single dose) is 10 mg/kg up to 600 mg for adults and 10 to 20 mg/kg, not to exceed 600 mg/day for children. The same doses are used in the intermittent regimens (2).

2. **In meningococcal meningitis and *H. influenzae* meningitis contacts,** dose regimens are discussed in Chap. 15.

3. **When used for nonapproved indications and for synergy**

a. For *S. epidermidis* prosthetic valve endocarditis, vancomycin given in combination with rifampin (300 mg q8h) and gentamicin (1.0 to 1.3 mg/kg q8h if renal function is normal) is advocated in adults (22). The vancomycin and rifampin are given for 6 weeks, and the gentamicin for the initial 2 weeks. (See Chap. 8.)

Table 30-3.   Rifampin drug interactions*, part II

Drug	Comments
Antacids	May need to space rifampin and aluminum hydroxide doses apart by several hours; more study needed
Haloperidol	Monitor serum haloperidol concentrations; alter dosing regimen if needed; limited initial study indicates serum concentrations and half-life are reduced by about 50%
Tocainide	Monitor arrhythmia control; increase dose if needed; 1 trial in healthy subjects found nearly 30% decrease in tocainide serum half-life
Disopyramide	Monitor arrhythmia control; increase dose if needed; initial study indicates decrease in disopyramide serum half-life of about 50%
Propafenone	Monitor plasma propafenone concentrations; monitor arrhythmia control; increase dose if needed
Ciprofloxacin	No interaction noted in humans to date; more study needed
Dapsone	Decrease serum concentrations; studies needed in patients with *Pneumocystis carinii* pneumonia
Fluconazole	May need to increase fluconazole dose; monitor signs and symptoms of infection; one trial in healthy subjects found 22% decrease in fluconazole serum half-life
Nifedipine	Monitor clinical response; may need to increase dose; controlled study needed
Diltiazem[†]	Consider alternative agent to diltiazem if possible, because even very large increase in oral diltiazem may not be sufficient; may monitor serum diltiazem concentrations (see Table 30-2 regarding similar interaction with verapamil); monitor clinical response
Diazepam	Monitor clinical response; may need to increase diazepam dose; 300% increase in diazepam oral clearance has been reported

Source: Borcherding SM, Baciewicz AM, Self TH. Update on rifampin drug interactions. *Arch Intern Med* 1992;152:711. Copyright 1992, American Medical Association.
* Agents available in the United States; for each interaction, carefully adjust doses when rifampin is discontinued; enzyme induction effect is reduced gradually over 1 to 2 weeks
[†] More study needed in patients; probably of major clinical significance.

Table 30-4. Rifampin drug interaction*, part III

Type of Drug	Comments
Clarithromycin	Monitor signs and symptoms of infection; more study needed.
Delavirdine	Avoid concomitant use if possible.
Doxycycline	Monitor clinical response and serum doxycycline concentrations; increased dosage may be needed.
Itraconazole	Monitor clinical response; increased dosage will likely be needed.
Midazolam	Monitor for decreased efficacy; increase dosage as necessary.
Nifedipine	Alternative class of agents should be considered; monitor clinical response; dosage increase may be needed.[†]
Nortriptyline	Monitor clinical response and serum nortriptyline concentrations.
Pefloxacin	Moderate rifampin induction effect; pending further research, no dosage adjustment recommended.
Protease inhibitors	Most significant decreases in serum concentrations seen with saquinavir mesylate, indinavir sulfate, and nelfinavir mesylate; ritonavir appears to have less reduction in serum concentrations; adjust dosage as necessary.
Tacrolimus	Monitor serum tacrolimus concentrations and clinical response; increased dosage may be needed.
Triazolam	Monitor for decreased efficacy; increase dosage as necessary.
Zidovudine	Monitor clinical response; increased dosage may be necessary.

Source: Stayhorn VA, Baciewicz AM, Self TH. Update on rifampin drug interactions, III. *Arch Intern Med* 1997;157:2453.
* Carefully adjust dosage when rifampin use is discontinued. Enzyme induction effect is gradually reduced during a 1- to 2-week period or longer. Based on small numbers of reports; further studies are needed for most of these agents.
[†] See also verapamil (Table 30.2) and diltiazem (Table 30.3).

    b. For prosthetic device infections, rifampin 450 mg q12h (16) and 300 mg q8 to 12h have been used.
B. **In renal failure,** dose modifications are suggested (23): for a creatinine clearance of 10 to 50 ml/min, 50% to 100% of the usual dose is suggested. For a creatinine clearance of less than 10 ml/min or the patient receiving chronic ambulatory peritoneal dialysis (CAPD), 50% of the usual dose is suggested (23).

C. **Pregnancy.** Rifampin is a **category C** agent. (See Chap. 14.) Rifampin crosses the placenta readily and is teratogenic in animals. There are no adequate and well-controlled studies in pregnant women in terms of the effects on the fetus. The package insert emphasizes that rifampin should be used during pregnancy only if the potential benefits justify the potential risks to the fetus (4). Rifampin has been used to treat severe cases of tuberculosis in pregnant women (1). Rifampin is not recommended for pregnant women who are contacts of infected patients with *H. influenzae* meningitis. Pregnant women in close contact with an index case of *N. meningitidis* can be treated with ceftriaxone if the woman is not allergic to cephalosporins. (See the related discussion in Chap. 15.)

D. **Nursing mothers.** The package insert suggests that because of the potential for tumorigenicity for rifampin in animal studies, a decision should be made whether to discontinue nursing or to discontinue the drug, taking into account the importance of the drug to the mother (4).

E. **Liver disease.** The use of rifampin in patients with liver disease is not recommended except in case of necessity; in such patients, the drug's half-life usually is doubled (1).

F. **Drug interactions.** See Sec. V.D.

Rifapentine (Priftin)

Rifapentine (Priftin) **is a long-acting analog of rifampin** that became available in late 1998 for oral use, with at least one other drug, in the treatment of pulmonary tuberculosis. It inhibits DNA-dependent RNA polymerase (24).

I. **Activity.** Rifapentine is active against *M. tuberculosis*, but strains resistant to rifampin are also resistant to rifapentine. Rifapentine is also active against *M. avium* and *Toxoplasma gondii* (24).

II. **Pharmacokinetics.** Rifapentine is well absorbed, especially when taken with food. It is excreted mostly in the feces (70%). It is metabolized to a desacetyl form that is microbiologically active, contributing 40% of the drug's overall activity (24).

III. **Clinical trials.** Only limited data are available so far about the clinical efficacy of this agent in pulmonary tuberculosis regimens (24). Further clinical studies are needed before the precise role of this agent is clarified.

IV. **Dosage.** The drug is available in 150-mg tablets. The recommended dosage of rifapentine in adults is 600 mg twice weekly (with at least 72 hours between doses) for the first 2 months of therapy and then 600 mg once a week, always in combination with other antituberculosis drugs (24).

V. **Adverse effects.** Like other rifamycins, rifapentine causes red-orange discoloration of body fluids and stains contact lenses. In clinical trials with isoniazid, rates of adverse reactions were similar to those with rifampin and rifapentine. The only adverse effect that occurred more often with rifapentine than with rifampin has been hyperuricemia when the drug was given twice weekly (24). (See related discussions under "Rifampin.")

VI. **Drug interactions.** Until further experience is available, it seems prudent to assume rifapentine can cause the same drug interactions as rifampin. (See prior discussion under "Rifampin.")

VII. **Conclusion.** In its February 1999 review of this agent, *Medical Letter* concluded: "rifapentine has the advantage over rifampin of requiring only twice-weekly doses for initial therapy of tuberculosis and once-weekly doses during the continuous phase of treatment. **It is not clear that rifapentine in the dosages currently recommended is as effective as rifampin. Until more data become available, rifampin is preferred" (24).** We concur with this conclusion.

Rifabutin (Ansamycin)

Rifabutin (Mycobutin) (25–31) is a semisynthetic ansamycin that was **approved for the prevention of disseminated *Mycobacterium avium* complex (MAC) in patients with advanced human immunodeficiency virus (HIV) infection** (28) in 1992. It **also is used** in regimens **to treat disseminated MAC** (5).

Rifabutin is active against most strains of MAC isolated from HIV-positive and HIV-negative people. The MIC_{90} of MAC is typically approximately 2 µg/ml (1). Rifabutin is also active against all rifampin-sensitive *M. tuberculosis* strains and about one-third of rifampin-resistant strains (9).

I. **Pharmacokinetics.** The drug is taken up by all tissues and is especially concentrated in the lungs, where levels may be 10 times higher than in the serum (9). Rifabutin has excellent solubility in lipids, which results in good intracellular penetration; CSF concentrations are about 50% of those in the serum (31).

   A. **Bioavailability.** Rifabutin is absorbed rapidly, and absolute bioavailability is in the range of approximately 20% (1).

   B. **Metabolism** is similar to that for rifampin. The elimination half-life is long (45 hours) and as a result of a very large volume of distribution, average plasma concentrations remain relatively low after repeated standard doses (25). Animal models suggest rifabutin has less of an effect on hepatic microsomal enzyme activity than rifampin.

II. **Clinical studies**

   A. Rifabutin also has been used **to prevent MAC** in patients with HIV infection. This topic has been reviewed elsewhere (28), but prophylaxis should be considered for HIV-infected adults and adolescents who have CD4+ lymphocyte counts of less than 50/mm³. **Clarithromycin or azithromycin are the pre-**

ferred prophylactic agents (see Chap. 26), but if these agents cannot be tolerated, rifabutin is an alternate prophylactic agent for MAC disease (28,31). Disseminated MAC should be ruled out before starting prophylaxis (i.e., with a negative blood culture for mycobacterium). Because treatment with rifabutin could result in the development of resistance to rifampin in persons who have active tuberculosis, tuberculosis should be excluded before rifabutin is used for prophylaxis (28).

B. Rifabutin has also been used **in therapeutic regimens** for disseminated MAI infections in patients with AIDS (5,26,27). Infectious disease consultation is advised.

III. **Dosages**. A 150-mg capsule is available.

A. **Prevention of MAC.** For the prevention of MAC in patients with advanced HIV infection who cannot tolerate clarithromycin or azithromycin, 300 mg po daily is recommended in adults (28) by the package insert. This can be administered as a once-daily dose or, in patients with a propensity to nausea, vomiting, or other GI upset, 150 mg bid with meals.

B. **For therapeutic regimens,** rifabutin 300 to 450 mg po daily has been suggested, along with clarithromycin or azithromycin, and/or ethambutol and/or ciprofloxacin (5,29,31). Because of the potential side effects at higher doses (Sec. IV), 300 mg/day of rifabutin may be a rational compromise (30). Infectious disease consultation is suggested.

C. **Pediatric use.** The safety and effectiveness of rifabutin for prophylaxis of MAC in children have not been established, per the package insert. However, preliminary recommendations suggest consideration for children infected with HIV and depressed CD4+ cell counts who cannot tolerate clarithromycin or azithromycin (28). Candidates for prophylaxis include the following CD4+ thresholds (cells/μl): children 6 years of age or more, less than 50; children aged 2 to 6 years, less than 75; children aged 1 to 2 years, less than 500; and children below 12 months of age, less than 750 (28). A liquid formulation of rifabutin is under development. The drug can be mixed with foods such as applesauce for administration to children (31). A dosage of 5 mg/kg of rifabutin has been used per package insert.

D. **Pregnancy.** Rifabutin is viewed as a **category B** agent. (See Chap. 14.) The package insert suggests that rifabutin should be used in pregnant women only if the potential benefit justifies the potential risk to the fetus. Chemoprophylaxis for MAC should be administered to pregnant women as well as other adults and adolescents (28). However, because of general concern about administering drugs during the first trimester of pregnancy, some providers may choose to withhold prophylaxis during the first trimester. **Azithromycin**

is the agent of choice for prevention of MAC in pregnancy. (See Chap. 26.) Experience with rifabutin in this setting is limited (28).

E. **Nursing mothers.** It is not known whether rifabutin is excreted in human milk. The package insert suggests that a decision should be made about whether to continue nursing or discontinue rifabutin, taking into account the importance of the drug to the mother.

F. **In renal failure** no dosage modifications are necessary. Neither hemodialysis nor CAPD requires dosage adjustment (23).

G. **In hepatic dysfunction,** the package insert does not currently advise any dosage modifications.

IV. **Side effects.** Rifabutin is generally well tolerated at the prophylaxis dose of 300 mg/day. Rash, GI intolerance, and neutropenia are seen in 2% to 4% of recipients (4). In therapeutic regimens for MAC and at higher doses (e.g., 600 mg/day or more), adverse effects can be seen in the majority of patients, especially leukopenia, GI intolerance, diffuse polyarthralgia syndrome (19%), and **anterior uveitis** (6%) (30). Use of rifabutin may cause an orange-brown discoloration of urine, feces, saliva, tears, and soft contact lenses (31).

Rifabutin is metabolized in the liver and induces activity of the hepatic cytochrome P450 enzyme group which may lead to pharmacokinetic interaction with other drugs administered concurrently (31). The extent to which this occurs, compared with rifampin, awaits further clinical experience. However, concurrent administration of fluconazole or clarithromycin can increase serum concentrations of rifabutin by 80% to 100% and potentially increase toxicity (e.g., increase the risk of uveitis) (31).

V. **Investigational uses.** Rifabutin continues to undergo clinical evaluation for therapy for MAC in patients with AIDS and in therapeutic regimens for *M. tuberculosis*. Rifabutin also is undergoing clinical investigation for the treatment of Crohn's disease (32).

References

1. Craig WA. Rifampin and related drugs. In: Gorbach SL, Bartlett JG, Blacklow NR, eds. *Infectious diseases*. Philadelphia: WB Saunders, 1992:265–271.
2. Reese RE, Betts RF. Rifampin and rifabutin. In: Reese RE, Betts RF eds., *A practical approach to infectious diseases*, 4th ed. Boston: Little, Brown, 1996:1338–1346.
3. Freiden TR, et al. The emergence of drug-resistant tuberculosis in New York City. *N Engl J Med* 1993;328:522.
   In April 1991, 19% of isolates were resistant to rifampin and INH!
4. *Physicians' Drug Reference*, 54th ed. Montvale, NJ: Medical Economics Data, 2000.
5. Medical Letter. The choice of antibacterial drugs. *Med Lett Drugs Ther* 1999;41:95.

6. American Thoracic Society and Centers for Disease Control. Treatment of tuberculosis and tuberculosis infection in adults and children. *Am J Resp Crit Care Med* 1994;149:1359.
   For a related paper, see Van Scoy RE, Wilkowske CJ. Antimycobacterial therapy. Mayo Clin Proc *1999;74:1038.*
7. Morris AB, et al. Use of rifampin in nonstaphylococcal, nonmycobacterial disease. *Antimicrob Agents Chemother* 1993;37:1.
8. Loeffler AM. Uses of rifampin for infections other than tuberculosis. *Pediatr Infect Dis J* 1999;18:631.
9. Farr BM. Rifamycins. In: Mandell GL, Bennett JE, Dolin R, eds. *Principles and practice of infectious diseases*, 5th ed. New York: Churchill Livingstone, 2000:348–361.
   Contains a good discussion of some of the therapeutic, though unapproved, uses of rifampin.
10. Mulligan ME, et al. Methicillin-resistant *Staphylococcus aureus*: a consensus review of the microbiology, pathogenesis, and epidemiology with implications for prevention and management. *Am J Med* 1993;94:313.
11. Wenzel RP, et al. Methicillin-resistant *Staphylococcus aureus* outbreak: a consensus panel's definition and management guidelines. *Am J Infect Control* 1998;26:102.
12. Fantin B, Carbon C. *In vivo* antibiotic synergism: contribution of animal models. *Antimicrob Agents Chemother* 1992;36:907.
13. Kaatz GW, et al. Ciprofloxacin and rifampin, alone and in combination, for therapy of experimental *Staphylococcus aureus* endocarditis. *Antimicrob Agents Chemother* 1989;33:1184.
   Although the combination may decrease the risk of acquisition of ciprofloxacin resistance, with respect to improved efficacy in this rabbit model the combination of ciprofloxacin and rifampin is unpredictable and strain-dependent and cannot be assumed to result in better therapeutic outcome than is achieved with ciprofloxacin alone.
14. Bisno AL, Sternau L. Infections of central nervous system shunts. In: Bisno AL, Waldvogel FA, eds. *Infections associated with indwelling devices*. Washington, DC: ASM Press, 1994:91–109.
15. Widner AF, et al. Antimicrobial treatment of orthopedic implant-related infections with rifampin combinations. *Clin Infect Dis* 1992;14:1251.
   Preliminary report from Switzerland in which nine of 11 patients with infected prosthetic implants (e.g., total knee, hip) that could not be removed were successfully treated with a protracted course of at least 2 months with oral rifampin in combination with a second agent (e.g., fluoroquinolones). See related paper by Drancourt M, et al. Oral rifampin plus ofloxacin for treatment of staphylococcal-infected orthopedic implants. Antimicrob Agents Chemother *1993; 37:1214.*
16. Zimmerli W, et al. Role of rifampin for treatment of orthopedic implant-related staphylococcal infections: a randomized controlled trial. *JAMA* 1998;279:1537.
   IV antibiotics were initially used for two weeks. See editorial comment in reference 17.
17. Zavasky DM, Sande MA. Reconsideration of rifampin: a unique drug for a unique infection. *JAMA* 1998;279:1575.
18. Bradley JS, Scheld WM. The challenge of penicillin-resistant *Streptococcus pneumoniae* meningitis: current antibiotic therapy in the 1990s. *Clin Infect Dis* 1997;24:S213 (suppl).

19. Baciewicz AM, et al. Update on rifampin drug interactions. *Arch Intern Med* 1987;147:565.
    First of a series of three articles. See references 20 and 21.
20. Borcherding SM, Baciewicz AM, Self TH. Update on rifampin drug interactions, II. *Arch Intern Med* 1992;152:711.
21. Stayhorn VA, Baciewicz AM, Self TH. Update on rifampin drug interactions, III. *Arch Intern Med* 1997;157:2453.
22. Wilson W, et al. Antibiotic treatment of adults with infective endocarditis due to streptococci, enterococci, staphylococci, and HACEK microorganisms. *JAMA* 1995;274:1706.
23. Aronoff GR, et al. *Drug prescribing in renal failure: dosing guidelines for adults*, 4th ed. Philadelphia: American College of Physicians, 1999.
24. Medical Letter. Rifapentine: a long-acting rifamycin for tuberculosis. *Med Lett Drugs Ther* 1999;41:21.
    For a more detailed review, see Jarvis B, Lamb HM. Rifapentine. Drugs *1998;56:607.*
25. Skinner MH, Blaschke TF. Clinical pharmacokinetics of rifabutin. *Clin Pharmacokinet* 1995;28:115.
    For a related paper, see Brogden RN, Fitton A. Rifabutin: a review of its antimicrobial activity, pharmacokinetic properties and therapeutic efficacy. Drugs *1994;47:983.*
26. Medical Letter. Rifabutin. *Med Lett Drugs Ther* 1993;35:36.
    See related symposium by Gordin FM, et al. Rifabutin: the research continues. Clin Infect Dis *1996;22:S1–S61 (suppl 1).*
27. Sullam PM, et al. Efficacy of rifabutin in the treatment of disseminated infection due to *Mycobacterium avium* complex. *Clin Infect Dis* 1994;19:84.
    See related paper by Dautzenberg B. Rifabutin in the treatment of Mycobacterium avium *complex infection: experience in Europe.* Clin Infect Dis *1996;23:S33 (suppl 1).*
28. 1999. USPHS/IDSA guidelines for the prevention of opportunistic infections in persons infected with human immunodeficiency virus. *Ann Intern Med* 1999;131:873. Or *MMWR* 1999;48(RR-10):1–66.
    For a related paper see Masio C, et al. Clinical and bacteriologic impact of rifabutin prophylaxis for Mycobacterium avium complex *infections in patients with human immunodeficiency virus infection.* Clin Infect Dis *1997;24:344.*
29. Medical Letter. Drugs for AIDS and associated infections. *Med Lett Drugs Ther* 1995;37:87.
30. Griffith DE, et al. Adverse events associated with high-dose rifabutin in macrolide-containing regimens for the treatment of *Mycobacterium avium* complex lung disease. *Clin Infect Dis* 1995; 21:594.
    Authors conclude that a rifabutin dose of 300 mg/day may be optimal in multidrug regimens for MAC that include macrolides.
    For a related paper see Petrowski JT. Uveitis associated with rifabutin therapy: a clinical alert. J Am Optometric Assoc *1996; 67:693.*
31. McFenson LM. Rifabutin. *Pediatr Clin Infect Dis J* 1998;17:71.
32. Gui GP, et al. Two-year outcomes analysis of Crohn's disease treated with rifabutin and macrolide antibiotics. *J Antimicrob Chemother* 1997;39:393.

Spectinomycin

Spectinomycin (Trobicin) was approved in 1971 for use in certain gonococcal infections. The structure of spectinomycin is similar, but not identical, to that of the aminoglycosides. Spectinomycin inhibits protein synthesis at the ribosomal level, and its activity against gonococci is bactericidal. **Spectinomycin is used only as an alternative agent for some infections caused by _Neisseria gonorrhoeae_** (1–4).

I. **Indications for use**
   A. **Alternative regimens for gonococcal infections**. (See Chap. 10.)
      1. **Uncomplicated urethral, endocervical, or rectal infections. When the drugs of choice (cephalosporin or quinolone) cannot be used,** spectinomycin is an alternative (1–4). It is active against penicillin-resistant strains of gonococci. In published trials, cure rates of 98.2% of uncomplicated urogenital and anorectal injections have been achieved with spectinomycin (2).
      2. **Treatment of gonococcal infections in pregnancy.** Pregnant women who cannot tolerate cephalosporins can be treated with spectinomycin (2).
      3. **Disseminated gonococcal infections.** Patients who are allergic to beta-lactams and quinolones (or for whom quinolones are contraindicated) can be treated with spectinomycin (2).
   B. **Actual or potential resistance.** Spectinomycin does not produce sustained, high bactericidal levels in blood, and resistant strains have been reported in the United States and elsewhere (4).

      Whether the drug should be used more often in initial infections has been reviewed in the past. Prior data suggest that extensive use of spectinomycin in initial gonococcal therapy might lead to the emergence of spectinomycin-resistant gonorrhea (5). The need for careful use of spectinomycin has also been emphasized in a report by Boslego and coworkers (6). After only 3 years of using spectinomycin as the primary treatment for uncomplicated gonococcal urethritis in U.S. military men in the Republic of Korea, more than 8% of recipients were treatment failures (6).

II. **Contraindications and limitations to use** (1–4)
   A. **Pharyngeal gonococcal infection.** Spectinomycin **is ineffective** against this infection, probably because the drug is not secreted in saliva in adequate concentrations.
   B. **Incubating syphilis. Spectinomycin will not abort incubating syphilis** and may actually prolong the incubation period. Thus **patients treated with spectinomycin should have a syphilis serology test** at

the time of treatment and again in 2 to 3 months to rule out this associated diagnosis.

C. **Nonspecific urethritis** (nongonococcal urethritis [NGU]). At least 50% of cases that are not susceptible to spectinomycin are due to *C. trachomatis*.

III. **Route and dosage.** Spectinomycin is given **intramuscularly** and is well absorbed by this route. In uncomplicated anogenital gonococcal infection, 2 g spectinomycin is given intramuscularly as a single dose in men or women and, in children, 40 mg/kg (maximum 2 g) IM is given once (2). For alternative treatment of inpatients with disseminated gonococcal infections who are allergic to or cannot be given beta-lactam agents (i.e., cephalosporins) and quinolones, spectinomycin, 2 g IM q12h, can be used (2); optimal duration is not well defined, but a 7-day course seems prudent (2).

In renal failure, no dose adjustment of spectinomycin is required. Neither hemodialysis nor chronic ambulatory peritoneal dialysis removes spectinomycin (7). Spectinomycin is relatively expensive. See Appendix Table B.

IV. **Toxicity** appears very limited, perhaps because the total dose is low. There are no known serious adverse reactions.

V. **Conclusions.** Spectinomycin has a **limited but useful role in gonococcal infections.** The best use of this agent is in the treatment of gonorrhea in persons who cannot tolerate or be treated with cephalosporins or quinolones (1,2,4).

References

1. Medical Letter. The choice of antibacterial drugs. *Med Lett Drugs Ther* 1999;41:95.
2. Centers for Disease Control. 1998 Sexually transmitted disease treatment guidelines. *MMWR* 1998;47(RR-1):59–69.
3. Gilbert DN. Aminoglycosides. In: Mandell GL, Bennett JE, Dolin R, eds. *Principles and practice of infectious diseases*, 5th ed. New York: Churchill Livingstone, 2000:Chap. 23.
4. Reese RE, Betts RF. Spectinomycin. In: Reese RE, Betts RF, eds. *A practical approach to infectious diseases*, 4th ed. Boston: Little, Brown, 1996:1346–1347.
5. Karney WW, et al. Spectinomycin versus tetracycline for the treatment of gonorrhea. *N Engl J Med* 1987;296:889.
6. Boslego JW, et al. Effect of spectinomycin use on the prevalence of spectinomycin-resistant and the penicillinase-producing *Neisseria gonorrhoeae*. *N Engl J Med* 1987;317:272.
7. Aronoff GR, et al. *Drug prescribing in renal failure*, 4th ed. Philadelphia: American College of Physicians, 1999.

Fluoroquinolones

Quinolone antibiotics have been available since the mid-1960s (1–3). Thousands of different quinolone structures have been synthesized, but fewer than 10 FDA-approved agents are clinically useful (2). Although there are a number of **ways to categorize quinolones,** a useful clinical approach based on potency and the newest spectrum of antibacterial activity against bacterial organisms is **shown in Table 32-1** (3). Sometimes the more recently introduced "third- and fourth-generation" fluoroquinolones may be referred to as "expanded-spectrum" fluoroquinolones, versus "conventional fluoroquinolones" (i.e., early "second-generation" agents such as ciprofloxacin).

Since bacterial resistance to the first-generation quinolones (nalidixic acid, oxolinic acid, cinoxacin) developed rapidly, they were little used and will not be mentioned further. More active fluoroquinolones, the "second-generation" agents (norfloxacin and ciprofloxacin, followed by ofloxacin, enoxacin, and lomefloxacin) were released from 1986 to 1992. These agents have been very useful clinically but typically lacked consistent activity against gram-positive cocci (including penicillin-resistant *Streptococcus pneumoniae*) and anaerobes. The recently introduced expanded-spectrum "third- and fourth-generation" fluoroquinolones, which include sparfloxacin, levofloxacin, trovafloxacin, gatifloxacin and moxifloxacin, were introduced after 1997 (Table 32-1). They have enhanced gram-positive and anaerobic activity as well as gram-negative and atypical organism activity.

The broad spectrum of antimicrobial activity, excellent bioavailability, good tissue penetration, long serum half-life (often allowing for once-daily dosing), and in general few side effects have made the fluoroquinolones very attractive agents. **The challenge for the health care provider is to use these agents prudently:** to limit their use to a particular clinical setting that calls for their enhanced spectrum, rather than in any and all infections. By doing so, the clinician **will reduce the consequence of excessive antibiotics** (e.g., *Clostridium difficile* diarrhea, *Candida* spp. overgrowth, colonization with broadly resistant organisms) for his/her specific patient **and** will **minimize** the development of **resistance**, thus lengthening the useful life of these agents for society.

I. **An overview of the fluoroquinolones**
   A. **Structure**. Many structural modifications can be made to the basic synthetic nucleus to achieve specific goals (e.g., enhanced gram-positive or anaerobic activity).
   B. **Mechanism of action** is reviewed in detail elsewhere (3). Fluoroquinolones inhibit DNA gyrase, a bacterial enzyme essential for DNA replication, and thus inhibit DNA supercoiling that is produced by DNA gyrase. They promote gyrase-mediated double-stranded DNA breakage at specific sites.

Table 32-1.   Classification of quinolones

First generation
  Nalidixic acid
  Oxolinic acid
  Cinoxacin

Second generation
  Norfloxacin
  Ciprofloxacin*
  Enoxacin
  Lomefloxacin
  Ofloxacin

Third generation[†]
  Levofloxacin[‡]
  Sparfloxacin
  Gatifloxacin[§]
  Grepafloxacin**

Fourth generation
  Trovafloxacin[‖]
  Moxifloxacin[§]

Source: Modified from Walker RC. The fluoroquinolones. *Mayo Clin Proc* 1999; 74:1030.

* Most potent against *Pseudomonas.*

[†] More potent against *Pneumococcus* and/or anaerobes than earlier compounds were.

[‡] Although classified by some as second-generation agent (2), because of its expanded spectrum against *S. pneumoniae,* including penicillin-resistant strains (see Chap. 2), it seems appropriate to view this as a third-generation agent.

[§] Most active *in vitro* against *S. pneumoniae.* See text.

[‖] More potent against anaerobes.

** Withdrawn in 1997. See text.

C. ***In vitro* activity. The *in vitro* activity of the fluoroquinolones** is summarized in **Table 32-2** (4).

1. **Gram-positive bacteria.** Compared with the earlier-generation quinolones, the third- and fourth-generation quinolones (levofloxacin, gatifloxacin, trovafloxacin, and moxifloxacin) have more activity against penicillin-susceptible and penicillin-resistant *S. pneumoniae* (5). (See related discussions in Chaps. 2 and 16.) Some strains of *S. aureus* are suceptible. However, against penicillin-susceptible *S. pneumoniae,* penicillin is as active *in vitro* and against nafcillin-(methicillin-) susceptible *S. aureus,* nafcillin is as active as the fluoroquinolones (6) (Table 32-2).

2. **Gram-negative bacteria.** All the fluoroquinolones are very active against gram-negative cocci and bacilli, which cause infections in community-residing individuals, including organisms like *Hemophilus influenzae* and *Moraxella catarrhalis.* However, against *Pseudomonas aeruginosa* and other hospital pathogens there are differences

Table 32-2. The minimum inhibitory concentrations (MIC₉₀) in vitro of quinolone antibiotics (measured in µg/ml)*

Organism (No. of Strains Tested)	Ciprofloxacin	Ofloxacin	Levofloxacin	Trovofloxacin
Gram-positive cocci				
S. pneumoniae				
penicillin-susceptible (1,500)	1–4	1–4	1*	0.12–0.25
penicillin-intermediate (221)	1–4	1–4	1*	0.12–0.25
penicillin-resistant (791)	1–4	1–4	1*	0.06–0.25
S. aureus				
methicillin-susceptible (422)	0.5–8	0.25–0.5	0.25	<0.015–0.125
MRSA (598)	1–64	16–32	8–16	0.03–4
Group A streptococci (52)	0.5	2	0.5	0.06–0.12
S. agalactiae (group B) (44)	0.5–1.0	2	1.0	0.25
Enterococci				
E. faecalis (187)	1–8	2–8	2	0.25–2
E. faecalis (VRE) (5)				8
E. faecium (10)	>16	>16	>16	>16
E. faecium (VRE) (35)				8
Viridans streptococci (301)	8	4–8	2	0.12–0.25
Gram-negative cocci				
Neisseria gonorrhoeae (112)	0.008	0.03		0.015
N. meningitidis (61)	0.008	0.03		0.008
Enteric gram-negative bacilli				
Escherichia coli (346)	<0.015–0.5	0.05–0.12	0.06–0.25	<0.015–4
Klebsiella pneumoniae (199)	0.06–4	1–2	0.5	0.12–1
Enterobacter cloacae (55)	1–2	0.06–4	0.6	1–2

E. aerogenes (77)	0.06–0.12	0.25–0.5	0.06	0.06–0.12
Citrobacter spp. (69)	<0.015–16	0.06–16	<0.015–0.12	0.03–16
Proteus mirabilis (107)	0.03–1	0.12–0.25	0.06	0.25–4
Stenotrophomonas maltophilia (132)	8–32	8–>16	8	1–>8
Serratia marcescens (180)	0.12–2	0.5–4	0.12	0.12–4
Salmonella typhi (30)	0.03	0.06	—	0.03
Salmonella spp. (72)	0.03	0.25	—	0.06
Shigella spp. (48)	0.015	0.06	—	0.03
Other gram-negative bacilli				
Acinetobacter spp. (64)	0.25–1.0	0.5	0.5	0.03–0.25
Haemophilus influenzae (483)	0.02–0.06	0.03–0.06	0.03	0.015–0.05
Pseudomonas aeruginosa (345)	0.25–>16	2–>16	0.5–8	0.25–>16
Legionella spp. (33)	0.015	0.015	—	0.008
Anaerobes				
Bacteroides fragilis (500)	4–64	4–64	2	0.25–2.0
Peptostreptococci (166)	0.25–8	0.5–8	0.25	0.125–1.0
Other				
Chlamydia trachomatis	2	1		
Mycoplasma hominis	1	1		
Mycoplasma pneumoniae	1	1		
Ureaplasma	16	2		
Mycobacterium tuberculosis	1	1		
M. avium				

Modified from reference (4).
* See also Table 2-5 on page 50.

(Table 32.2). Briefly against *Pseudomonas aeruginosa*, ciprofloxacin = trovofloxacin > levofloxacin = gatifloxacin = moxifloxacin > ofloxacin. Sparfloxacin is not approved for pseudomonas.

3. **Anaerobes. Trovofloxacin is the most active**, more so than gatifloxacin and moxifloxacin. The others have limited activity against anaerobes.

4. *Chlamydia/Mycoplasma.* The recently introduced fluoroquinolones are active against *Mycoplasma pneumoniae, Chlamydia pneumoniae,* and *C. trachomatis.* Ofloxacin is active against *C. trachomatis* **(Table 32-2)**.

5. *Legionella pneumophila.* Ciprofloxacin is quite active, as are the third- and fourth-generation fluoroquinolones. Ofloxacin, though active, is less so.

6. **Resistant organisms.** All fluoroquinolones lack significant activity against multiresistant organisms: methicillin-resistant *Staphylococcus aureus* (MRSA), vancomycin-resistant enterococci (VRE), and multidrug-resistant nosocomial gram negatives (e.g., *Stenotrophomonas maltophilia*).

D. **Pharmacokinetics**

1. **Oral absorption.** In general, the fluoroquinolones are **well absorbed. However, antacids, sucralfate, magnesium, aluminum, iron, zinc, calcium, enteral nutrition with these supplements, and didanosine can decrease absorption of the oral fluoroquinolones if they are taken closely together.**

2. **Intravenous preparations** are available for some of the fluoroquinolones: ciprofloxacin, ofloxacin, levofloxacin, trovofloxacin and gatifloxacin. **Oral regimens provide similar serum levels as the more expensive IV formulations. Therefore the IV formulations are indicated only when patients are NPO, have active nausea and vomiting, etc.** As enteral nutrition is possible, patients can be on oral therapy (1,2).

3. The **fluoroquinolones penetrate tissue well**, including lung, bronchial mucosa, kidney, prostate, bone, and the genital tract.

4. **Elimination via renal mechanisms varies** (2).

   a. Levofloxacin and ofloxacin depend entirely on renal elimination; dosage modifications are very important in renal failure.

   b. Trovofloxacin is eliminated entirely by the hepatic route. No dosage adjustment is necessary in renal failure, but in patients with hepatic insufficiency, doses of trovofloxacin must be reduced. About 50% of moxifloxacin is metabolized in the liver; dosage reduction is not necessary in renal failure.

   c. With ciprofloxacin, sparfloxacin, and gatifloxacin moderate dosage adjustments are necessary in renal failure.

5. **Pharmacodynamically,** the fluoroquinolones have been shown to have **"concentration-dependent killing"** rates and a postantibiotic effect against most gram-negative bacteria, similar to the aminoglycosides (2,7). (See Chap. 14.)
6. **Drug interactions** are discussed in Sec. F.5.

E. **Adverse reactions.** The fluoroquinolones are generally well tolerated (1,2,8). **A summary of side effects follows.**

1. **Gastrointestinal symptoms** (e.g., primarily nausea, but also anorexia, vomiting, and/or diarrhea) are the **most common**, seen in 5% or more. *Clostridium difficile* diarrhea can occur but is uncommon, perhaps because of the quinolones minimal effect on anaerobic flora (8).

2. **Allergic reactions** include nonspecific rashes, urticaria, and phototoxicity, which occur overall in 1% to 2% of patients. **Lomefloxacin** and **sparfloxacin** have **increased** rates of **phototoxicity** when compared with other fluoroquinolones. (See Sec. III.)

3. **Liver function test abnormalities and hepatic toxicity with trovofloxacin.** In early 1999, trovofloxacin was found to be associated with rare but fatal cases of liver toxicity. During the 18 months after FDA release of the drug, postmarketing reports identified 140 cases of severe liver toxicity (including 14 cases of acute liver failure) among 2.5 million prescriptions (2). The mid-1999 revised package insert (and the current 2000 insert) emphasizes that trovofloxacin "has been associated with **serious liver injury leading to transplantation and/ or death**" and that this "liver injury has been reported **with both short-term and long-term drug exposure.**" Trovofloxacin "use exceeding 2 weeks in duration is associated with a significantly increased risk of serious injury. Liver injury has also been reported following trovofloxacin re-exposure."

   Therefore the FDA recommended in June 1999 that trovofloxacin be used only for life-threatening or limb-threatening infection in patients with initial IV therapy started in an inpatient health care facility. **(See related discussion in Sec. III.)**

4. **Central nervous system (CNS) symptoms** can occur in 1% to 4% of patients. The most common symptoms have been headaches (mild), slight dizziness (more with trovofloxacin), mild sleep disturbance, and alteration of mood with agitation, anxiety, or depression. **Seizures** have rarely been reported and may be seen in patients receiving other medications simultaneously [e.g., nonsteroidal antiinflammatory agents (NSAID) with all; theophylline with ciprofloxacin or enoxacin].

5. **QT prolongation with torsades de pointes** has been described with sparfloxacin, grepafloxacin and moxifloxacin. (See Sec. III.)
6. **Tendon rupture** (8). Postmarketing data suggest that quinolone use may be associated with tendon rupture, which has been described primarily in the Achilles tendon (unilateral or bilateral) but also in the shoulder and hand. The pathogenesis is not understood. It is more common in men more than 50 years of age and in those who use steroids concomitantly. **Therefore at the first sign of tendon pain or inflammation, the quinolone should be discontinued** and exercise avoided until the tendinitis has subsided.
7. **Drug interactions.** See under **Sec. F.5.**
F. **Precautions in use**
1. **Do not use in patients allergic to the very early analogs** (e.g., nalidixic acid, oxolinic acid, or cinoxacin) or other fluoroquinolones.
2. **Avoid use in children**. Fluoroquinolones can produce cartilage erosions in young animals. **Fluoroquinolones are therefore not recommended for use in children (and pregnant women and nursing mothers).** CDC guidelines (9) indicate fluoroquinolones are not approved for use in children because of concerns about toxicity based on animal studies. **Exceptions include** (1,2,10–12).
   a. **Cystic fibrosis** patients, because the benefits are believed to outweigh the potential risks. Investigations of ciprofloxacin in this setting demonstrated no adverse effects (9).
   b. **In special circumstances** fluoroquinolones may be justified in children younger than 18 years when alternative safe therapy is not available (10–12). For children who weigh 45 kg or more, adult regimens are advised, if fluoroquinolones are used.
3. **Avoid in pregnancy and nursing mothers** because of the potential effect on developing cartilage of the fetus or infant. (See Sec. 2.) The fluoroquinolones are **category C** agents. (See Chap. 14.)
4. **Trovofloxacin.** The FDA has advised that it should not be initiated in the ambulatory setting. (See Sec. III.)
5. **Drug interactions**
   a. **Do not take with antacids** containing magnesium or aluminum, which can markedly diminish absorption of fluoroquinolones. This effect can be minimized if the antacid is taken 2 to 3 hours after the fluoroquinolone is taken. **Other multivalent metal cations** impair absorption. (See prior discussion in Sec. D.)

    b. **Monitor theophylline levels** or reduce doses when patients are on ciprofloxacin and enoxacin, since these fluoroquinolones can raise serum levels of theophylline. See individual agent discussions.

    c. **Caffeine.** Some fluoroquinolones, especially enoxacin and ciprofloxacin, can affect caffeine metabolism, raising caffeine levels. Patients should be warned to avoid the fluoroquinolones late in the evening with a heavy caffeine load.

    d. **Warfarin.** The question of whether a warfarin-fluoroquinolone interaction actually occurs in patients remains unanswered. While awaiting data, close monitoring of the prothrombin time of patients receiving warfarin and fluoroquinolones seems prudent (13).

    e. **Cyclosporine.** Whether there is a drug interaction of cyclosporine and fluoroquinolones is unclear. Careful monitoring of serum concentrations of cyclosporine and measures of renal function have been suggested (13).

G. **Cost.** In general, the fluoroquinolones are expensive agents. See Appendix Tables B and C.

II. **Clinical indications**

A. **Drugs of choice.** Although the fluoroquinolones have an FDA-approved indication for many different types of infections, they are listed as drugs of choice **for only a few infections** (14), including those due to the following:

1. *Salmonella* and *Shigella* spp.
2. *Legionella* spp. ± rifampin (macrolides also drugs of choice)
3. *Bartonella henselae* (cat scratch bacillus)
4. *Campylobacter jejuni*

    N.B. For the preceding indications, many fluoroquinolones would work, but we would be inclined to use ciprofloxacin, since an even broader- spectrum fluoroquinolone would not be necessary.

B. **Common uses,** but not antibiotic of choice. When the infecting organism is known or suspected to be resistant to other preferred agents (often less expensive or narrower spectrum) or if the clinical situation were so severe that an incorrect choice could not be tolerated by the patient, fluoroquinolones are very useful.

    See **summary Table 32-3.** Certain issues need special emphasis.

1. **Urinary tract infections (UTIs).** Although most community-acquired uncomplicated UTIs are due to pathogens susceptible to trimethoprim-sulfamethoxazole (TMP-SMX) and therefore this inexpensive agent is preferred (14) if not contraindicated, the incidence of community-acquired TMP-SMX-resistant pathogens is rising, so that in someone with possible early pyelonephritis or

Table 32-3. An overview of the fluoroquinolones

Setting	Suggested Agent*	Related Discussions
UTI	Ciprofloxacin	Chapter 4
Prostatitis	Ciprofloxacin	Chapter 4
Urethritis/PID	Ofloxacin	Chapter 10
Intraabdominal infection	Ciprofloxacin + metronidazole, rarely trovofloxacin[†]	Chapter 6
Travelers' diarrhea	Ciprofloxacin	Chapter 5
Bacterial diarrhea	Ciprofloxacin	Chapter 5
Diabetic foot infections	Ciprofloxacin and anaerobic therapy in advanced infections	Chapter 3
Sinusitis, refractory otitis, acute exacerbations of COPD	Levofloxacin[‡]	Chapter 1
CAP	Levofloxacin[‡]	Chapter 2
Nosocomial pneumonia	Ciprofloxacin or Levofloxacin[§]	Chapter 2
Septic arthritis, osteomyelitis[‖]	Ciprofloxacin	Chapter 9

* Seems prudent to use the narrowest-spectrum fluoroquinolone that will do the job.
[†] Special cases where a simple regimen (one dose daily) may be essential to ensure compliance. See text. Infectious disease consult advised.
[‡] An advanced-generation fluoroquinolone, with activity against penicillin-resistant *S. pneumoniae* is preferred. This agent is also active against common CAP pathogens and atypical pathogens.
[§] Depending on susceptibility data.
[‖] Primarily due to susceptible gram negatives. See Chap. 9.

underlying diabetes, we will use a fluoroquinolone, usually ciprofloxacin. (See related discussion in Chap. 24, page 452.)

Ciprofloxacin is preferred if *P. aeruginosa* is known or suspected. The fluoroquinolones are very useful for complex UTI due to susceptible pathogens. (See Chap. 4.)

2. **Prostatitis.** Although TMP, TMP-SMX, and the fluoroquinolones all penetrate the prostate well, the fluoroquinolones are often used in this setting (15) based on susceptibility data and/or side effect profile, although TMP and TMP-SMX are more cost-effective. (See Chaps. 4, 24, and 25.)

3. **Urethritis/cervicitis/PID. Ofloxacin** is currently the preferred fluoroquinolone (16) and the agent with which there is the most experience for this use. (See Chap. 10.)

4. **Intraabdominal infections.** Antibiotic options including piperacillin-tazobactam, cefazolin-metronidazole combination, ampicillin-sulbactam ± gentamicin are **discussed in Chap. 6.** We have often used ciprofloxacin plus metronidazole (or clindamycin) to provide good gram-negative and anaerobic activity, respectively. Trovofloxacin may be reasonable monotherapy in very carefully selected patients with infectious disease input. (See Sec. III.)

5. **Travelers' diarrhea.** The fluoroquinolones are preferred, and ciprofloxacin is commonly prescribed. (See Chap. 5.)

6. **Bacterial gastroenteritis** (e.g., *Salmonella, Shigella,* etc). When therapy is indicated, fluoroquinolones are preferred (14) and ciprofloxacin is commonly used. (See Chap. 5.)

7. **Diabetic foot infections** are discussed in **Chap. 3**, with Table 3-4 (page 83) summarizing therapeutic options. Ciprofloxacin has had the greatest clinical experience in this setting and remains the most active currently available fluoroquinolone against *P. aeruginosa.*

8. **Refractory sinusitis/otitis media (AOM).** Amoxicillin remains the agent of choice for acute sinusitis and AOM. When this agent fails or in the patient with multiple antibiotic allergies, an advanced-generation fluoroquinolone (e.g., levofloxacin) with activity against penicillin-resistant *S. pneumoniae* may be indicated. (See Chap. 1.)

9. **Acute exacerbations of chronic bronchitis** can usually be treated with less expensive and narrower spectrum antibiotics. **(See Chap. 1 and Table 1-5.)** Occasionally, in patients with multiple drug allergies, culture-proven resistant sputum pathogens, or the need to rotate a different class of antibiotics, a fluoroquinolone may be indicated. If so, a 5-day course of an advanced-generation agent (e.g., levofloxacin) that is active against most penicillin-resistant *S. pneumoniae* is reasonable.

10. **Community-acquired pneumonia** is **discussed** in great detail in **Chap. 2**. The appeal of the advanced-generation fluoroquinolones (e.g., levofloxacin) is that they are active against the common pathogens causing community-acquired pneumonia (CAP), including penicillin-susceptible and -resistant *S. pneumoniae, H. influenzae, M. catarrhalis*, and the atypical pathogens (*Mycoplasma, Legionella, Chlamydia* spp.) (17).

    a. **Macrolides** remain agents of choice for CAP in those under 50 years of age.

    b. Advanced fluoroquinolones are useful in patients with known or highly likely penicillin-resistant *S. pneumoniae* pneumonia and/or if very ill with pneumonia and multilobar disease, requiring intensive-care-unit level of care while awaiting susceptibility data and other information. (See Chap. 2.) These agents are also useful in CAP in selected cases, as reviewed in Chap. 2.

11. **Nosocomial pneumonia** is discussed in detail in **Chap. 2**.

   a. **Initial empiric therapy** often involves combination therapy (e.g., antipseudomonal penicillin and an aminoglycoside) until culture data are available. An advanced fluoroquinolone (± an aminoglycoside) may be useful in the allergic patient.

   b. **For completion of therapy** an oral fluoroquinolone can often be used; which agent will depend upon culture data, if available, and local susceptibility patterns and trends.

12. **Septic arthritis and osteomyelitis** due to susceptible pathogens, primarily gram negatives, have been treated with fluoroquinolones. (See Chap. 9.) Ciprofloxacin has been the most commonly used agent.

13. **Miscellaneous**

   a. **Meningococcal carrier state** has been treated with ciprofloxacin. (See Chap. 15.)

   b. Cat scratch disease, due to *Bartonella henselae*, has been treated in selected cases with ciprofloxacin (14).

   c. **Fever of unclear etiology in the leukopenic patient.** In an attempt to avoid hospitalization or minimize the hospital stay, oral antibiotics are being studied in these patients. The fluoroquinolones (especially active against gram negatives, e.g., ciprofloxacin) combined with an agent for gram positives (e.g., amoxicillin-clavulanate) have been particularly studied (18–20). The optimal patient setting, regimen, and dosage is still undergoing study. Infectious disease consultation is advised in this situation. (See Chap. 12.)

   d. **Mycobacterial infections** are sometimes treated with fluoroquinolones (14,21). Infectious disease and/or pulmonary consultation is advised.

   e. **Patients with cystic fibrosis** and pulmonary colonization/infection with *Pseudomonas* have been treated with ciprofloxacin. (See Sec. I.F.2.)

III. **Brief comment on individual agents.** Although several agents are available, in the past decade of using these antibiotics, **certain common practices and special niches have often evolved that have allowed the clinician to eliminate or effectively use some of these agents. See Table 32-3.** In addition to the general comments made in Sec. I, we emphasize the following:

A. **Norfloxacin (Noroxin)** became available in 1986. It provides good urinary and gastrointestinal levels but does not provide acceptable serum levels or nonrenal tissue levels. Although it is potentially a useful agent in UTI and travelers' diarrhea, we and many others have for the most part **replaced norfloxacin with ciprofloxacin.**

B. **Ciprofloxacin (Cipro)** was released in late 1987 and **remains a very useful agent (Table 32-3).** It remains as active against *P. aeruginosa* as any fluoroquinolone but is not as active against pneumococci, including penicillin-resistant strains and anaerobes, as are the "third-" and "fourth-generation" agents. Ciprofloxacin can raise theophylline and caffeine levels but overall is well tolerated. (See Sec. I.E.)

C. **Ofloxacin (Floxin)** was released in 1990. In its review *Medical Letter* concluded that ofloxacin "appears to be equivalent to ciprofloxacin" (for UTI, prostatitis, skin and soft-tissue infections, lower respiratory tract infections) and "it can be used for chlamydial infections" (22). **Ofloxacin is active against** *C. trachomatis*, and there is considerable clinical experience with its use for these infections. It has therefore achieved a **special niche in the therapy of nongonococcal urethritis, where it remains the quinolone of choice and is part of a regimen for PID (16).** (See Chap. 10.) Ofloxacin **does not interfere with theophylline or caffeine** metabolism as may ciprofloxacin. It is not approved for nor has it been used much in osteomyelitis.

D. **Lomefloxacin (Maxaquin)** was released in 1992 as a once-daily fluoroquinolone for the treatment of UTI and bronchitis caused by *H. influenzae* and *M. catarrhalis*. It has no unique *in vitro* activity compared with the other fluoroquinolones. With postmarketing experience it became apparent that **phototoxicity** is more common than initially appreciated. The package insert notes that moderate to severe phototoxic reactions have occurred in patients exposed to direct or indirect sunlight (including shaded or diffuse light through glass) during or following treatment. These phototoxic reactions have occurred with and without the use of sunscreens or sunblocks. Single doses have been associated with photosensitivity in which recovery may be prolonged for several weeks.

   Because lomefloxacin has no unique *in vitro* activity or unique niche, but has the phototoxicity concern, **we do not use or recommend it, since there are so many other fluoroquinolones to choose from.**

E. **Enoxacin (Penetrex)** was approved for use in the treatment of UTI and single-dose therapy of gonorrhea in 1991 and was marketed in 1992. It has no unique *in vitro* spectrum of activity. Since this agent has no special attributes or niche, **we do not use it.**

F. **Sparfloxacin (Zagam)** was introduced in late 1997 as a once-daily oral regimen (23). **Phototoxicity**, sometimes severe, has occurred in about 8% of recipients of sparfloxacin, including some who use sunscreens. The manufacturer advises cautioning patients to avoid direct sunlight and indirect sunlight while taking the drug and for 5 days afterward! **QT prolongation**, with torsades de pointes, has occurred. **At this time we are reluctant to use this agent until the extent of these two side effects has been clarified.**

G. **Grepafloxacin (Raxar)** was approved for use in late 1997 as a once-daily regimen (24). **Prolongation of the QTc interval was reported (24).** In late October 1999 grepafloxacin was voluntarily withdrawn from the market due to severe cardiovascular adverse reactions.

H. **Levofloxacin (Levaquin)** became available in late 1997 and has been summarized (25). This expanded-spectrum fluoroquinolone **has good activity against penicillin-resistant** S. pneumoniae (see Chap. 2, page 50) **and other CAP pathogens.** Therefore it is a useful agent in selected cases of CAP (see Sec. II.B.10 and Chap. 2) and selected cases of refractory sinusitis, otitis, in adults, and acute exacerbations of chronic obstructive pulmonary disease. (See Sec. II.B and Chap. 1.)

The oral formulation is extremely well absorbed and provides serum levels essentially the same as those provided by IV; the **oral and IV formulations are 99% bioequivalent.** With normal renal function, only one dose per day is needed; the dose interval is prolonged in renal failure.

I. **Trovofloxacin (Trovan)** was approved for use in early 1998 (4,26). Several issues deserve emphasis.

1. ***In vitro* activity (Table 32-2).** Similar to levofloxacin, trovofloxacin has good activity against respiratory pathogens involved in CAP, sinusitis, bronchitis, etc, including penicillin-resistant S. pneumoniae and atypical organisms. It is about as active as ciprofloxacin against P. aeruginosa. **Trovofloxacin is the most active available fluoroquinolone against anaerobes, including B. fragilis; its in vitro activity is similar to that of metronidazole (26)** against anaerobes.

2. **Pharmacokinetics.** Oral trovofloxacin is well absorbed, with and without food, with 88% bioavailability. Similar serum levels are achieved from oral and IV doses. The IV formulation contains the prodrug alatrofloxacin mesylate, which is rapidly hydrolyzed to yield trovofloxacin. It is **metabolized in the liver**, mostly by conjugation, and excreted mostly in the feces. No dose reductions are necessary in renal failure, but dose reductions are indicated for mild to moderate cirrhosis.

3. **Clinical use.** Although trovofloxacin was initially approved for more than 10 indications when it was first released in early 1998, **when the serious liver toxicity problems (Sec. I.E.3.) became apparent in postmarketing studies, in**

June 1999, the FDA-approved indications were dramatically scaled back. The mid-1999 revised package insert emphasizes that trovofloxacin "should be reserved for use in patients with serious, life- or limb-threatening infections who receive their initial therapy in an inpatient health care facility (i.e., hospital or long-term nursing care facility)"; in addition, trovofloxacin **"should not be used when safer, alternative antimicrobial therapy will be effective** (27)."

a. **Trovofloxacin has been approved for** hospitalized patients with nosocomial pneumonia, CAP, complex intraabdominal infections, gynecologic and pelvic infections (e.g., endomyometritis, septic abortion), and complicated skin and skin structure infections, including diabetic foot infections (27).

- Note that these are all complex problems in hospitalized patients.
- Even before the liver toxicity problems were recognized, the *Medical Letter* emphasized that trovofloxacin should be limited to the treatment of mixed infections in which anaerobes might be involved (26).

b. **Conventional combination antibiotic therapy can be used to provide the broad-spectrum coverage of trovofloxacin.**

- For intraabdominal infections, a cephalosporin and metronidazole, ciprofloxacin and metronidazole (or clindamycin), or TMP-SMX and metronidazole can be used to provide gram-negative and anaerobic coverage. (See Chap. 6.)
- Even the trovofloxacin package insert favors safer conventional combinations over trovofloxacin (see earlier).

c. **In summary,** despite the excellent *in vitro* activity of trovofloxacin, given its potential toxicity and the availability of other agents, **we rarely use this agent** and would do so only when a very simple regimen (once daily) was very important to ensure compliance. **We think it is prudent to enlist infectious-disease consultation/discussion before using this agent.**

4. **Miscellaneous considerations**
   a. See general overview in Sec. I.
   b. There are no apparent significant drug interactions with theophylline, warfarin, cyclosporine, or digoxin.

c. Trovofloxacin does not appear to cause excessive phototoxicity or QTc interval prolongation.

d. **Dizziness** has been reported in 3% to 11% of recipients and may be substantially reduced if trovofloxacin is taken at bedtime or with food. Patients should know how they react to trovofloxacin before they operate an automobile or machinery or engage in activities requiring mental alertness and coordination (27).

e. **Clinicians should monitor liver function tests** (AST, ALT, bilirubin) **in trovofloxacin recipients who develop signs or symptoms consistent with hepatitis.** Clinicians should consider discontinuing trovofloxacin in those patients who develop liver function test abnormalities (27).

f. **Trovofloxacin usually should not be given for more than 2 weeks** (27).

g. Doses do not need modification in renal failure but do need modification with underlying hepatic disease.

5. **Dosages. Infectious disease input is advised.**

a. For nosocomial pneumonia, complex intra-abdominal or pelvic infections, initially 300 mg IV/po once daily and decreased to 200 mg IV/po once daily as soon as clinically indicated; up to 14 days.

b. For severe skin and soft-tissue infection, including complicated diabetic foot infections, 200 mg IV or po once daily and change to oral 200 mg once daily (from IV) as soon as patient improves; up to 14 days.

c. For renal dysfunction, no dose adjustment.

d. For chronic hepatic disease, cirrhosis, see package insert dose modifications and consider alternate agent. Infectious disease consultation is advised.

J. **Recently approved agents.** In late December 1999 the two new agents below were approved for use in CAP, acute bacterial exacerbations of chronic bronchitis, or acute sinusitis (28–32). **Because of the potential for prolongation of the QT interval with both of these agents (28), while awaiting further clinical experience with these agents we think it is prudent to limit their use to cases of CAP due to documented penicillin-resistant *S. pneumoniae* and suggest infectious disease input before using either.** Both agents are active against *Legionella* spp. and *M. pneumoniae* and both are active against some anaerobes, but not as active as trovofloxacin is against anaerobes. Neither drug seems to affect the cytochrome P 450 enzyme system (28).

text continued on bottom of page 559

Table 32-4. Dosages in normal renal function

Ciprofloxacin po*
UTI

Acute, uncomplicated	100 mg po bid	× 3 days
Mild and moderate	250 mg po bid	10–14 days
Severe, complicated, pyelonephritis	500 mg po bid	14 days
Prostatitis	500 mg po bid	2–4 weeks. See text.
Intraabdominal infection[†]	500 mg po bid	10–14 days
Travelers' diarrhea	500 mg po bid	3 days
Bacterial diarrhea	500 mg po bid	5–7 days[‡]
Susceptible lower respiratory tract gram negatives (e.g., hospital-acquired pneumonia)	500–750 mg po bid	At least 14 days total treatment. See text.
Septic arthritis, osteomyelitis due to susceptible pathogens	500–750 mg po bid	See Chap. 9.

Ofloxacin (po/IV)

Acute, uncomplicated urethral and cervical gonorrhea	400 mg, single dose	1 day
Nongonococcal cervicitis/urethritis due to C. trachomatis	300 mg bid	7 days
Mixed infection of the urethra and cervix due to C. trachomatis and N. gonorrhoeae	300 mg bid	7 days
Acute pelvic inflammatory disease[§]	400 mg bid	14 days

Levofloxacin (po/IV)

CAP	500 mg q24h	10–14 days
Susceptible lower respiratory infections in hospitalized patients	500 mg q24h	10–14 days
Refractory sinusitis, bronchitis	500 mg q24h	5–7 days

Trovofloxacin, gatifloxacin, and moxifloxacin
See text.

* Ciprofloxacin can be given IV: for mild to moderate UTI 200 mg IV q12h; for severe or complicated UTI 400 mg q12h. Doses given over 60 minutes. A 500 mg po dose and a 400 mg IV dose provide similar serum levels.
† Needs to be combined with an anaerobic agent (e.g., metronidazole or clindamycin). See Chap. 6.
‡ Typhoid fever is treated with 10 days.
§ Ofloxacin is combined with metronidazole. See details of therapy of PID in Chap. 10, Table 10-5.

1. **Moxifloxacin (Avelox)** has improved gram-positive activity, including against penicillin-resistant *S. pneumoniae* over levofloxacin (28,29,31), but is a little less active against Enterobacteriaceae and *Pseudomonas* spp. than

Table 32-5. Dose adjustments in renal failure

	Creatinine Clearance (ml/min)			Hemodialysis (HD)	CAPD
	>50	10–50	<10		
Ciprofloxacin	100%*	50–75%*	50%*	250 mg po or 200 mg IV q12h	250 mg po q8h or 200 mg IV q8h
Ofloxacin	100%*	200–400 mg q24h	200 mg q24h	100–200 mg after HD	Same as for creatine clearance <10 ml/min
Levofloxacin	100%*	250 mg q24–48h after usual 500-mg initial dose	250 mg q48h after usual 500-mg initial dose	Same as for creatinine clearance <10 ml/min	
Trovofloxacin	See text.				
Gatifloxacin	See text				
Moxifloxacin	See text				

Modified from Aronoff GR, et al, eds. *Drug prescribing in renal failure: dosing guidelines for adults*, 4th ed. Philadelphia: American College of Physicians, 1999.

* Refers to % of usual dose, when renal function is normal.

ciprofloxacin. In adults, 400 mg orally is given once daily, and doses do not need to be adjusted in renal failure. It does not interfere with theophylline or warfarin, and has a low propensity for phototoxic and CNS side effects.

2. **Gatifloxacin (Tequin)** has similar in vitro activity (28,32) with enhanced activity against penicillin-resistant *S. pneumoniae* over levofloxacin (28). The usual adult dose of gatifloxacin is 400 mg po or IV every 24h. Doses must be reduced if the creatinine clearance is <40 ml/min.

IV. **Dosages of the fluoroqinolones.**
   A. **With normal renal function, see Table 32-4.**
   B. **In renal failure, see Table 32-5.**

V. **Miscellaneous**
   A. **Cost**. In general, the fluoroquinolones are **expensive** agents. See Appendix Tables B and C. Nevertheless, they may be cost-effective agents if they can shorten the hospital stay, avoid hospitalization for IV antibiotic administration, or can be used in the oral forms rather than in another IV preparation.
   B. **Resistance to fluoroquinolones** (2,33). With widespread use of the fluoroquinolones, selective pressure is exerted on patient populations, particularly those in intensive-care and specialized-care units in hospitals (2) and hospitalized patients in general, rather than in those with community-acquired pathogens. This selective pressure results in the emergence of quinolone-resistant bacteria (2). Quinolone resistance can also develop by mechanisms of reduced drug penetration and altered regulation of active efflux mechanisms (2).
      1. **Nosocomial pathogens**
         a. ***P. aeruginosa.*** Resistance is common with infections involving a foreign body (e.g., Foley catheter, tracheostomy) or with prolonged use (e.g., cystic fibrosis respiratory infections). At this time approximately 15% to 30% of *P. aeruginosa* are resistant to all the currently available fluoroquinolones.
         b. **MRSA** are now usually resistant to available fluoroquinolones.
         c. *Serratia marcescens*, other *Pseudomonas* spp., *Acinetobacter* spp., and *S. maltophilia* often are resistant.
      2. **Community-acquired** resistance of bacteria is uncommon, but there is concern that this may change in the future with more extensive use of fluoroquinolones in both humans and animal food (33). (See related discussions in Chap. 14.)

      Although fluoroquinolone-resistant *Neisseria gonorrhoeae* has been isolated in the Far East, such strains fortunately have only been rarely isolated in the United States (34).

      Recently, pneumococci with decreased susceptibility to quinolones has been described (35).

References

1. Reese RE, Betts RF. Fluoroquinolones. In: Reese RE, Betts RF, eds. *A practical approach to infectious diseases*, 4th ed. Boston: Little, Brown, 1996:Chap. 28S.
2. Walker RC. The fluoroquinolones. *Mayo Clin Proc* 1999;74:1030.
3. Andriole VT. The quinolones: prospects. In: Andriole VT, ed. *The quinolones*, 2nd ed. San Diego: Academic Press, 1998:Chap. 16.
4. Garey KW, Amsden GW. Trovofloxacin: an overview. *Pharmacotherapy* 1999;19:21.
   Contains several MIC tables comparing in vitro activity of the fluoroquinolones.
5. File TM, et al. A multicenter, randomized study comparing the efficacy and safety of intravenous and/or oral levofloxacin versus ceftriaxone and/or cefuroxime axetil in the treatment of adults with community-acquired pneumonia. *Antimicrob Agents Chemother* 1997;41:1965.
6. Akaniro JC, et al. *In vitro* activity of sparfloxacin (AT-4140), a new quinolone agent, against isolates from pediatric patients. *Antimicrob Agents Chemother* 1992;36:255.
7. Lode H, Borner K, Koeppe P. Pharmacodynamics of fluoroquinolones. *Clin Infect Dis* 1999;27:33.
8. Lipsky BA, Baker C. Fluoroquinolone toxicity profiles: a review focusing on newer agents. *Clin Infect Dis* 1999;28:352.
   For additional data, see related chapter in text cited in reference 3.
9. Centers for Disease Control. 1998. Guidelines for treatment of sexually transmitted diseases. *MMWR* 1998;47(RR-1):68.
10. Schaad UB. Use of quinolone in pediatrics. In: Andriole VT, ed. *The quinolones*, 2nd ed. San Diego: Academic Press, 1998:351–357.
11. *1997 Red Book: Report of the Committee on Infectious Diseases*, 24th ed. Elk Grove, IL: American Academy of Pediatrics, 1997:607–608.
12. Schaad UB, et al. Use of the fluoroquinolones in pediatrics: consensus report of an International Society of Chemotherapy Commission. *Pediatr Infect Dis J* 1995;14:1.
13. Radandt JM, Marchbanks CR, Dudley MN. Interactions of fluoroquinolones with other drugs: mechanisms, variability, clinical significance, and management. *Clin Infect Dis* 1992;14:272.
14. Medical Letter. The choice of antibacterial drugs. *Med Lett Drugs Ther* 1999;41:95.
15. Lipsky BA. Prostatitis and urinary tract infection in men: What's new, what's true? *Am J Med* 1999;106:327.
16. Medical Letter. Drugs for sexually transmitted infections. *Med Lett Drugs Ther* 1999;41:85.
   For related resource see the CDC's 1998 guidelines for treatment of sexually transmitted diseases. MMWR 1998;47(RR-1):1.
17. Hooper DC. Expanding use of fluoroquinolones: opportunities and challenges. *Ann Intern Med* 1998;129:908.
18. Freifeld A, et al. A double-blind comparison of empirical oral and intravenous antibiotic therapy for low risk febrile patients with neutropenia during cancer chemotherapy. *N Engl J Med* 1999; 341:305.
   Study from National Cancer Institute concludes in hospitalized low-risk patients who have fever and neutropenia during cancer chemotherapy; empirical therapy with oral ciprofloxacin and amoxicillin-calvulanate is safe and effective.

19. Kern WV, et al. for the International Antimicrobial Therapy Co-operative Group of the European Organization for Research and Treatment of Cancer. Oral versus intravenous empirical antimicrobial therapy for fever in patients with granulocytopenia who are receiving cancer chemotherapy. *N Engl J Med* 1999;341:312.
    Concludes in low-risk patients with cancer who have fever and granulocytopenia. Oral therapy with ciprofloxacin plus amoxicillin-clavulanate is as effective as IV therapy.
20. Talcott JA, Finberg RW. Fever and neutropenic: how to use a new strategy. *N Engl J Med* 1999;341:362.
    Editorial discussing references 18 and 19. **Concludes that optimal way to safely use outpatient oral antibiotics for the febrile neutropenic patient still needs study.**
21. Alangaden GJ, Lerner SA. The clinical use of fluoroquinolones for the treatment of mycobacterial disease. *Clin Infect Dis* 1997; 25:1213.
22. Medical Letter. Ofloxacin. *Med Lett Drugs Ther* 1991;33:71.
23. Medical Letter. Sparfloxacin. *Med Lett Drugs Ther* 1997; 39:41.
24. Medical Letter. Grepafloxacin: a new fluoroquinolone. *Med Lett Drugs Ther* 1998;40:17.
25. Medical Letter. Levofloxacin. *Med Lett Drugs Ther* 1997;39:41.
26. Medical Letter. Trovofloxacin. *Med Lett Drugs Ther* 1998;40:30.
27. Pfizer/Roerig Pharmaceutical. Trovan (trovofloxacin) tablet/IV package insert. June 1999.
    Similar concerns are summarized in Physicians Desk Reference, *54th ed. Montvale, N.J.: Medical Economics Co., 2000:2372.*
28. Medical Letter. Gatifloxacin and moxifloxacin: two new fluoroquinolones. *Med Lett Drugs Ther* 2000;42:15.
29. Barman-Balfour JA, Wiseman LR. Moxifloxacin. *Drugs* 1999; 57:363.
30. Perry CM, Balfour JA, Lamb HM. Gatifloxacin. *Drugs* 1999;58:683.
31. Felmingham D, Tesfaslasie Y, Robbins MJ. The *in vitro* activity of moxifloxacin against 817 isolates of *S. pneumoniae* collected from 27 centers throughout the U.K. and Ireland during the 1997–1998 cold season. *39th Interscience Conference on Antimicrobial Agents and Chemotherapy.* San Francisco, Abstract 379, Sept. 1999.
32. Huczko E, et al. Susceptibility of bacterial isolates to gatifloxacin and ciprofloxacin from the clinical trials during the 1997–1998 period. *39th Interscience Conference on Antimicrobial Agents and Chemotherapy.* San Francisco, Abstract 351, Sept. 1999.
    See series of related abstracts presented at the symposium indicating gatifloxacin is active against CAP pathogens, M. tuberculosis, *penicillin-resistant* S. pneumoniae. *It is undergoing IV and po dose evaluation and appears well tolerated as a once daily regimen.*
33. Kohler T, Pechere JC. Bacterial resistance to quinolones: mechanisms and clinical implications. In: Andriole VT, ed. The quinolones, 2nd ed. San Diego: Academic Press, 1998:Chap. 4.
    See related paper by Acar JF, Goldstein FW. Trends in bacterial resistance to fluoroquinolones. Clin Infect Dis *1997;24:S67 (suppl 1).*
34. Centers for Disease Control. Fluoroquinolone-resistant *Neisseria gonorrhoeae.* San Diego, California, 1997. *MMWR* 1997;47:405.
35. Chen DK, et al. Decreased susceptibility of *Streptococcus pneumoniae* to fluoroquinolones in Canada. *N Engl J Med* 1999; 341:233.

Urinary Antiseptics

Urinary antiseptics are agents that concentrate in the urine but do not produce adequate levels in the serum. Therefore these agents are **useful only in** the prevention or therapy of **lower urinary tract infections** (UTIs) but are not for severe pyelonephritis or associated systemic infection (1–3). In addition, this unique drug disposition has **advantages, including** reduced suppression of normal bacteria compared with other antimicrobials used for UTIs, decreased rates of resistance, low rates of yeast overgrowth syndromes, and minimization of teratogenic risk and fetal toxicity (3).

I. **Nitrofurantoin** inhibits various enzymes within bacteria and nitrofurantoin intermediates also damage DNA directly, leading to DNA strand breakage (2,3).

    A. **Spectrum of activity.** Nitrofurantoin is active against most *Escherichia coli* and a minority of *Enterobacter* and *Klebsiella* spp. *Pseudomonas* spp. are resistant, as are most *Proteus* spp. Nitrofurantoin also is active against gram-positive bacteria that sometimes produce a UTI, such as enterococcus, *Staphylococcus aureus*, and coagulase-negative staphylococci (1–3).

    B. **Pharmacokinetics.** Nitrofurantoin is well absorbed from the gastrointestinal (GI) tract, but nontherapeutic levels are achieved in the serum and body tissues. Bioavailability increases when taken with food. Therapeutic urinary concentrations of the drug are present for up to 6 hours. Tubular reabsorption provides levels in renal medullary tissue. The liver is the principal site of metabolic inactivation (2,3).

        The drug is contraindicated in renal failure (i.e., creatinine clearance of less than 50 ml/min) (4) because adequate urinary antibiotic levels may not be achieved and serum levels increase in renal failure, presumably increasing the toxicity of this agent.

        In alkaline urine, the antibacterial effect of nitrofurantoin is decreased; therefore the urine should not be alkalinized (2).

    C. **Resistance.** Nitrofurantoin's *in vitro* activity has remained stable despite four decades of use. This has been explained in part by its broad mechanisms of action, high oral bioavailability, and low concentrations at mucosal surfaces (i.e., absence of therapeutic concentrations outside the urinary tract) (3).

    D. **Preparations available**

        1. **Furadantin** is the **microcrystalline** form and has been available since 1953.

        2. **Macrodantin** is the **macrocrystalline** form, and it appears to be associated with a **lower incidence of GI side effects** (2). Macrodantin

has activity and pharmacokinetics similar to furadantin. **We use the macrodantin preparation.**

3. **Nitrofurantoin monohydrate (75 mg)/macro-crystals (25 mg) (Macrobid)** is a slow-release formulation, in a capsule, equivalent to 100 mg nitrofurantoin.

4. An intravenous preparation of nitrofurantoin is no longer available.

E. **Uses. Nitrofurantoin is used in the treatment of susceptible uncomplicated (lower) UTIs or the prophylaxis of recurrent UTI** (1–3,5). Cure rates for lower UTIs range from 70% to 95%. Although nitrofurantoin may be effective for asymptomatic upper UTI, it **should not be used for symptomatic upper UTIs or complex UTIs** in which therapeutic levels of antibiotic may not be attained at the site of infection (1–3).

1. **Therapy of uncomplicated UTIs** due to susceptible pathogens. A dose of **100 mg bid** with meals in adults with normal renal function **for 3 days** is adequate for short-course therapy (3), although a 7-day course may be used per the package insert.

   In children more than 1 month of age, 5 to 7 mg/kg/day is given in divided doses qid, commonly for 7 days. **Therapy in pregnancy** is discussed in Sec. 5.

   In lower UTI due to susceptible enterococci, nitrofurantoin may provide an alternative agent for the ampicillin-allergic patient (5).

2. **Prophylaxis of UTIs.** Macrodantin has been given at bedtime or after coitus as a single 50- or 100-mg dose to women with recurrent, uncomplicated UTI. (See Chap. 4.) In children more than 1 month of age, 1 to 2 mg/kg/day in one dose has been used.

   Prolonged therapy requires periodic clinical assessment for pulmonary and neurologic toxicity as well as complete blood count and transaminase determinations (3). (See Sec. F.)

3. **In renal failure** (i.e., creatinine clearance of less than 50 ml/min), **the drug is contraindicated** (4), as discussed in Sec. B.

4. **In hepatic failure,** the drug probably should be avoided because of its association with hepatotoxicity.

5. **In pregnancy,** caution should be used; this is a **category B agent.** (See Chap. 14.) This topic has been reviewed elsewhere (3,6). Nitrofurantoin is considered a safe and effective agent when ampicillin (amoxicillin) cannot be used because of allergies or resistance. A single 200-mg dose of nitrofurantoin for asymptomatic bacteriuria has been associated with a failure rate of 27%, similar

to other single-dose failure rates. Symptomatic bacteriuria (acute cystitis) or relapse after single dose has been treated with nitrofurantoin 100 mg bid-qid for 3 to 7 days (3,6); more experience is with 7 days (6). Follow-up urine cultures are important. Suppressive therapy may be indicated if a repeat course of therapy does not sterilize the urine (6).

Nitrofurantoin can be used in pregnancy for prophylaxis after intercourse or nightly at a dose of 50 mg (3).

F.   **Toxicity**. The side effects of nitrofurantoin have been well documented and reviewed in detail elsewhere (7). **Gastrointestinal irritation** is the **most common** side effect, with anorexia, nausea, and vomiting. This may be decreased by using the macrocrystalline preparation (Macrodantin) and may be dose related (1,3).

Serious adverse reactions can occur at approximately 28 per million treatment courses (3,7). **Since major adverse events are more common in the elderly,** with reduced renal function of aging, we agree with the recommendation that **nitrofurantoin is rarely warranted in people 60 years of age or more** (3). The **frequency** of these **serious adverse reactions** in more than 120 million treatment courses is shown in **Table 33-1;** some reactions are fatal.

1.   **Pulmonary reactions are the most common severe problem associated with nitrofurantoin use** (1–3,7,8).

a.   **Acute pneumonitis** with fever, cough, and eosinophilia can occur after a few hours or days of therapy. On chest roentgenography, pulmonary alveolar-interstitial infiltrates

Table 33-1.   Nitrofurantoin and serious adverse events

Adverse Event	Patients Worldwide	Incidence* (Reactions/Million Treatment Courses)
Acute pulmonary	1,138	9.4
Subacute pulmonary	22	0.2
Chronic pulmonary	281	2.3
Miscellaneous pulmonary	283	2.3
Hepatic	312	2.6
Neurologic	847	7.0
Hematologic	500	4.1
Total	3,383	27.8

Modified from Darcy P. Nitrofurantoin. *Drug Intelligence and Clin Pharmacy* 1985;19:540–547; and Dow G, Ronald AR. Miscellaneous drugs. In: Root RK, et al, eds. *Clinical infectious disease: a practical approach*. New York: Oxford University Press, 1999.
* Based on 121.43 million courses of therapy.

or pleural fluid is seen. This pneumonitis probably is hypersensitivity phenomenon and is rapidly reversible by discontinuing treatment. Acute reactions do not generally progress to chronic reactions (1–3). Corticosteroids may be used in patients with severe reactions (3).

    b. **Subacute** presentations are less likely to be associated with fever and eosinophilia and are slower to resolve. **Chronic** pulmonary reactions with interstitial infiltrates are rare and occur when the drug has been prescribed for more than 6 months (3). This syndrome has an **insidious onset** (malaise, cough, and dyspnea on exertion), and fever and eosinophilia are seen less frequently. This reaction presumably represents a cumulative toxic drug effect. In some cases, improvement occurs with discontinuing the nitrofurantoin (1–3). A beneficial effect of corticosteroid therapy has not been convincingly demonstrated in patients with chronic nitrofurantoin pulmonary reactions (2). Histopathology reveals chronic pneumonitis and fibrosis (3).

2. **Polyneuropathies** (ascending sensorimotor) with demyelination and degeneration of sensory and motor nerves are a severe side effect that may occur more often in patients with renal failure as well as in protracted courses of therapy (1–3). The mechanisms are unclear, but it is believed to be related to a direct toxic effect of the drug. Sensory symptoms usually begin within 6 weeks of starting therapy followed by motor neuropathy; total recovery occurs in one-third of cases, with partial recovery in one-half (3). **The drug should be stopped if early signs of a neuritis, such as paresthesias, develop.**

3. **Hepatic reactions** are rare and of two types (1–3).

    a. **Acute cholestatic hepatitis** with fever, rash, eosinophilia, and jaundice. This appears to be immunologically mediated and resolves with discontinuation of nitrofurantoin (1–3).

    b. **Chronic active hepatitis** has an insidious onset after prolonged therapy (more than 6 months). Recovery is seen in the majority of patients if the nitrofurantoin is discontinued.

      Some authors have recommended monthly liver function tests in patients on chronic nitrofurantoin (9).

4. **Bone marrow depression** may occur. **In patients with glucose-6-phosphate dehydrogenase deficiency, acute hemolysis may be precipitated by nitrofurantoin use.** However,

based on one report, clinically important hemolytic reactions appear to be rare (10). Megaloblastic anemias can occur.

5. **Cutaneous reactions** can occur in 1% to 5% of recipients (3) with maculopapular rashes, urticaria, and angioneurotic edema; these resolve rapidly with discontinuation of therapy.

6. **In children,** there has been concern that the side effects of nitrofurantoin may outweigh the benefits. This issue has been reviewed with the conclusion that **serious adverse reactions to nitrofurantoin in children are rare** and that the vast majority of patients recovered from their reactions once the drug was discontinued. Therefore **this agent remains potentially useful** in pediatric patients (11).

G. **Contraindications to use** (3)
   1. Renal insufficiency; see Sec. I.B.
   2. Children less than 1 month of age (nitrofurantoin can cause hemolysis).*
   3. Pregnant woman near delivery (to avoid transplacental transfer at the time of birth).

II. **Methenamine** (2,3) is not an active antibacterial agent but has been used as a urinary antiseptic since 1895 (3). This drug has the advantage of economy, tolerability, minimal effect on GI flora, and absence of bacterial resistance (3). With the emergence of bacterial resistance, this is a **potentially useful urinary tract infection suppressive agent.**

A. **Mechanism of action.** Under the proper pH conditions, methenamine can be hydrolyzed to form formaldehyde and ammonia. **Formaldehyde is the active agent** that acts through protein denaturation and is bacteriostatic at low concentrations and bactericidal at higher levels (3). Formaldehyde formation depends on several factors.

1. **Acid environment.** For hydrolysis to occur, an acid pH is required. Ideally, the **urine pH must be 6.0 or less (2) so that hydrolysis can take place.** In many patients, in the absence of diuresis, a sufficiently acid urine to liberate free formaldehyde exists. Fluid restriction may also help. See Sec. D.

2. **Time needed for hydrolysis.** In addition to the acid pH, adequate time must be allowed for hydrolysis to occur. At least 2 to 3 hours are necessary to generate adequate concentrations of formaldehyde. Therefore **in a patient with a chronic indwelling bladder catheter, it is not surprising that this is a useless agent,** as adequate contact time cannot be achieved in the catheterized patient (12). However, this agent may be helpful in patients with partial outlet obstruction (e.g., prostatic hypertrophy), in which adequate contact

---

* Since nitrofurantoin is detected in human milk, it seems prudent to avoid this agent in a nursing mother of an infant less than 1 month old.

time is available. Methenamine may have a beneficial effect in preventing UTI in patients with neurogenic bladders who are in a program of intermittent catheterization and bladder retraining, because the urine may remain in the bladder long enough between catheterizations (13).

3. **Adequate concentrations.** To form adequate levels of formaldehyde, adequate doses of methenamine must be used.

B. **Spectrum of activity.** An appealing property of methenamine is that if enough formaldehyde is generated, **all gram-positive and gram-negative bacteria are susceptible.** In addition, bacteria do not become resistant to formaldehyde.

C. **Pharmacokinetics.** Methenamine is well absorbed from the GI tract and is excreted into the urine. Even in the presence of the proper urine pH, only 2% to 20% of the drug is broken down into the active free formaldehyde. Because ammonia is generated with methenamine degradation, **the agent is contraindicated in hepatic insufficiency** (2).

D. **Preparations available.** Methenamine has been combined with acids, theoretically to help acidify the urine. For example, methenamine with mandelic acid is methenamine mandelate (Mandelamine), and methenamine is combined with hippuric acid as methenamine hippurate (Hiprex or Urex). However, when given in the usual recommended doses, the organic acids in these combinations generally are inadequate to acidify the urine (2). Methenamine alone has been given with large doses of ascorbic acid (2 to 6 g daily) in an attempt to acidify the urine.

Fluid restriction has been suggested as a more useful measure **to acidify urine** as it acts to reduce voiding frequency (allowing more formaldehyde formation), acidifies the urine, and increases bladder methenamine concentrations. **Patients should be asked to reduce voiding frequency and restrict fluids to 1,200 to 1,500 ml/day so that the urine specific gravity is maintained at a level of 1.015 or greater** (3).

E. **Uses.** Methenamine is **not for acute UTIs.** With urine acidification, it has been used primarily in **chronic suppressive therapy** for UTIs in patients without an indwelling catheter. Methenamine hippurate has also been used (14). In UTI due to *Proteus* spp. it may be impossible to achieve adequate pH levels because of the high urinary pH generated by *Proteus*. **It is important to sterilize the urine initially with another agent before using methenamine (and ascorbic acid) suppression therapy** (15). This regimen may be particularly useful in the patient with a partial obstruction that allows adequate contact time.

F. **Dosage**
1. In **adults,** 1 g of methenamine mandelate (Mandelamine) or methenamine hippurate (Hiprex or Urex) is given po bid to qid. Fluid restrictions

may be all that is necessary to provide adequate acidification. (See Sec. D.) Ascorbic acid (e.g., 1 g po qid) may be given in an attempt to acidify the urine adequately and keep the pH less than or equal to 6.0. Ideally, the urinary pH should routinely be monitored (e.g., daily or every other day). Higher doses of ascorbic acid may be necessary to acidify the urine, and in some patients, adequate urinary acidification cannot be achieved with 4 to 6 g daily of ascorbic acid.

2. **For children between 6 and 12 years of age**, the dose is 500 mg to 1 g bid. An oral suspension (methenamine mandelate 500 mg per 5 ml) is available for younger children; for children less than 6 years of age, the usual dose is 250 mg per 30 pounds of body weight po qid (2).

3. **In renal failure,** limited guidelines are available. Methenamine mandelate is not advised if the creatinine clearance is less than 50 ml/min (4), nor is any methenamine salt (which may exacerbate acidosis or precipitate in renal tubules), but methenamine alone is not contraindicated in renal insufficiency, as it is nontoxic and urinary methenamine is readily converted to formaldehyde in the azotemic state (3).

4. **In patients with gout or hyperuricemia, these agents should be avoided.** Acidification of the urine and the use of acid salts may promote uric acid crystals and calculi formation.

5. **Methenamine should not be administered in conjunction with sulfonamides,** which may precipitate when formaldehyde is released. (See Chap. 24.)

6. **In hepatic insufficiency, methenamine should be avoided** because of the ammonia produced (2), which may induce or exacerbate hepatic encephalopathy.

7. **In pregnancy,** the safety of methenamine and its salts has not been established (3).

G. **Toxicity.** Methenamine generally is well tolerated especially in children (3). Minor GI side effects, such as gastric discomfort, nausea, and vomiting, can occur, especially at high doses. With prolonged high doses, some patients note urinary frequency, dysuria, and hematuria, which may be caused by formaldehyde irritating the mucosal lining of the genitourinary tract. The dysuria often diminishes with continued use as the mucosa becomes less sensitive.

III. **Fosfomycin tromethamine (Monurol)** was approved for use in the United States in 1997 **for single-dose oral treatment of uncomplicated UTIs in women** due to suceptible strains of *E. coli* and *Enteroccocus faecalis*. The drug interferes with the formation of the bacterial cell walls (16).

A. **Spectrum of activity.** Fosfomycin is moderately active *in vitro* against *E. coli* and many gram-negative bacteria, commonly causing community-acquired uncomplicated UTIs, as well as some strains of *S. saprophyticus* and most enterococci (16).

Pseudomonas spp. are usually resistant (16).

B. **Pharmacokinetics**. Fosfomycin is rapidly absorbed after oral administration and is excreted unchanged in the urine, where it reaches bactericidal concentrations that persist for 24 to 48 hours or longer (3,16,17).

C. **Clinical trials.** In three randomized trials comparing a single 3-g dose of fosfomycin with nitrofurantoin (50 mg qid for 7 days), norfloxacin (400 mg bid for 5 days), and cephalexin (500 mg qid for 5 days) in women with uncomplicated UTIs, eradication rates with fosfomycin were similar to those with norfloxacin and nitrofurantoin and superior to those with cephalexin (16). Additional data in more than 1,000 patients found that a single dose of fosfomycin was less effective in eradicating bacteriuria than 7 days of ciprofloxacin or 10 days of TMP-SMX (16).

D. **Dosage. A single oral dose of 3 g is used** for uncomplicated UTIs in women 18 years of age or older.

This **single dose is expensive** at $25.25 (cost to pharmacist) (16), which is significantly more expensive than 3-day regimens of conventional therapy. (See Chap. 4.)

1. **Pediatric use.** The safety and efficacy of this agent in children under 12 years of age have not been established.

2. **In renal failure,** no special recommendations are made in the 2000 package insert or usual sources (4).

3. **Pregnancy.** This is a **category B** agent; see Chap. 14. There are no adequate and well-controlled studies in pregnant women per the package insert.

4. **Nursing.** The package insert indicates it is not known whether fosfomycin is excreted into human milk; a decision should be made about whether to discontinue nursing or not administer the drug, taking into account the importance of the drug to the mother.

E. **Adverse effects.** Fosfomycin is generally well tolerated, with diarrhea the most common side effect (9%). Vaginitis can occur (16).

F. **Overview.** In their 1997 review, *Medical Letter* concluded: "A single dose of fosfomycin is **moderately effective** for treatment of uncomplicated UTIs in women and should improve compliance; but it is **expensive.** How the new drug compares with a three-day course of TMP-SMX, an effective regimen that costs much less, has not been established" (16).

- **We do not feel this agent is generally worth the extra cost:** A single dose of fosfomycin is 20 times more expensive than 3 days of generic TMP-SMX (1 DS bid) or TMP and almost twice the cost of 3 days of ciprofloxacin (100 mg bid).

See Appendix Cost Table C.
- Fosfomycin may play a useful role in some settings where compliance is a major issue. Fosfomycin is an alternative for uncomplicated UTIs in women due to susceptible enterococci (5).
- **Further clinical experience is necessary to determine the precise role of this agent.**

IV. **Cranberry juice** may be useful in the prophylaxis of UTI (3), and its **benefit** has been demonstrated in **elderly women** in whom prophylaxis with 300 ml of cranberry juice cocktail per day significantly reduced bacteriuria and pyuria compared with those receiving placebo (18). Its mechanism of action has been attributed to the inhibition of bacterial adherence (3).

See related discussion in Chap. 4, Sec. IV, on p. 97.

References

1. Reese RE, Betts RF. Urinary antiseptics. In: Reese RE, Betts RF eds. *A practical approach to infectious diseases,* 4th ed. Boston: Little, Brown, 1996:1385.
2. Hooper DC. Urinary tract agents: nitrofurantoin and methenamine. In: Mandell GL, Bennett JE, Dolin R, eds. *Principles and practice of infectious diseases,* 5th ed. New York: Churchill Livingstone, 2000;423–428.
3. Dow G, Ronald AR. Miscellaneous antibacterial drugs. In: Root RK, et al, eds. *Clinical infectious diseases: a practical approach.* New York: Oxford University Press, 1999:319.
4. Aronoff GR, et al, eds. *Drug prescribing in renal failure,* 4th ed. Philadelphia: American College of Physicians, 1999.
5. Medical Letter. The choice of antibacterial drugs. *Med Lett Drugs Ther* 1999;41:95.
   For uncomplicated UTI due to susceptible enterococci, nitrofurantoin is listed as the first alternative agent when ampicillin or amoxicillin cannot be used.
6. Patterson TF, Andriole VT. Detection, significance, and therapy of bacteriuria in pregnancy: update in the managed health care era. *Infect Dis Clin North Am* 1997;11:593.
   Good source for this common problem.
7. Darcy P. Nitrofurantoin. *Drug Intell Clin Pharm* 1985;19:540.
   A comprehensive review of adverse events.
8. Jick SS, et al. Hospitalizations for pulmonary reactions following nitrofurantoin use. *Chest* 1989;96:512.
   Study from the Boston Collaborative Drug Surveillance Program and the Group Health Cooperative of Puget Sound. More than 16,000 first courses of therapy and 742 chronic users (i.e., recipients of 10 or more prescriptions). The frequency of less severe pulmonary reactions, not requiring hospitalizations, is not known and awaits further study.
9. Sharp JR, et al. Chronic active hepatitis and severe hepatic necrosis associated with nitrofurantoin. *Ann Intern Med* 1980;92:14.
   All patients were women (the usual recipients of nitrofurantoin).

Liver damage can be severe and even fatal if not recognized. See editorial comment in same journal issue. Also see related paper by Hebert MF, Roberts JP. Endstage liver disease associated with nitrofurantoin requiring liver transplantation. Ann Pharmacother 1993;27:1193.

10. Gait JE. Hemolytic reactions to nitrofurantoin in patients with glucose-6-phosphate dehydrogenase deficiency: theory and practice. *DICP* 1990;24:1210.
    Since 1953, approximately 130 million courses of nitrofurantoin have been distributed in the United States alone. Retrospective analysis of Norwich Eaton adverse reaction data base contains 127 reports of hemolytic reactions; a "worst case" estimate of the incidence rate was 1 in 100,000 courses of therapy. For cases in which outcome was reported, complete recovery occurred in 87% of patients.
11. Coraggio MJ, Gross TP, Rocelli JD. Nitrofurantoin toxicity in children. *Pediatr Infect Dis J* 1989;8:163.
12. Vainrub B, Musher DM. Lack of effect of methenamine in suppression of or prophylaxis against chronic urinary tract infection. *Antimicrob Agents Chemother* 1977;12:625.
13. Kevorkian CG, Merritt JL, Ilstrup DM. Methenamine mandelate with acidification: an effective urinary antiseptic in patients with neurogenic bladders. *Mayo Clin Proc* 1984;59:523.
    See accompanying editorial comment in the same issue.
14. Cronberg S, et al. Prevention of recurrent acute cystitis by methenamine hippurate: double-blind cross-over long-term study. *Br Med J* 1987;294:1507.
15. Freeman RB, et al. Long-term therapy for chronic bacteriuria in men: U.S. Public Health Service cooperative study. *Ann Intern Med* 1975;83:133.
16. Medical Letter. Fosfomycin for urinary tract infections. *Med Lett Drugs Ther* 1997;39:66.
    For a related paper, see Patel SS, Balfour JA, Bryson HM. Fosfomycin tromethamine: a review of its antibacterial activity, pharmacokinetic properties, and therapeutic efficacy as a single-dose oral treatment for acute uncomplicated lower urinary tract infections. Drugs 1997;53:637.
17. Stein GE. Single-dose treatment of acute cystitis with fosfomycin tromethamine. *Ann Pharmacother* 1998;32:215.
18. Avorn J, et al. Reduction of bacteriuria and pyuria after ingestion of cranberry juice. *JAMA* 1994;271:751.

APPENDIXES

Appendix A. Recommended dosages of selected antibiotics for neonates by age and birth weight

Antibiotic	Route of Administration	Dose (mg/kg) at Age 0–7 Days		Dose (mg/kg) at Age 8–30 Days	
		Wt < 2,000 g	Wt > 2,000 g	Wt < 2,000 g	Wt > 2,000 g
Acyclovir	IV	10 q8h	10 q8h	10 q8h	10 q8h
Amikacin*	IV, IM	7.5 q12h	7.5–10 q12h	7.5–10 q8h	10 q8h
Ampicillin†	IV, IM	25–50 q12h	50–100 q8h	50–100 q8h	25–50 q6h
Amphotericin B	IV	0.25–1.0 q24h	0.25–1.0 q24h	0.25–1.0 q24h	0.25–1.0 q24h
Cefotaxime‡	IV, IM	50 q12h	50 q8–12h	50 q8h	50 q6–8h
Ceftazidime	IV, IM	50 q12h	50 q12h	50 q8h	50 q8h
Chloramphenicol*,§	IV	25 q24h	25 q24h	25 q24h	25 q12h
Clindamycin	IV, IM, PO	5 q8h	5–10 q6h	5–10 q6h	5–10 q6h
Erythromycin	PO	10 q12h	10 q12h	10 q12h	10 q8h
Gentamicin*	IV, IM	2.5 q12h	2.5 q12h	2.5 q8h	2.5 q8h
Imipenem**					
Methicillin	IV, IM	25–50 q12h	25–50 q8h	25–50 q8h	25–50 q6h
Nafcillin‖	IV	25 q12h	25 q8h	25 q8h	25 q6h

Oxacillin	IV, IM	25 q12h	25 q8h	25 q8h	25 q8h	25 q6h
Penicillin G#	IV, IM	25,000–50,000 units q12h	25,000–50,000 units q8h	25,000–75,000 units q8h	25,000–75,000 units q8h	25,000–50,000 units q6h
Penicillin, benzathine#	IM	50,000 units once (max. 2.4 million)	50,000 units once	50,000 units once	50,000 units once	50,000 units once
Penicillin procaine#	IM	50,000 units q24h (max. 4.8 million)	50,000 units q24h	50,000 units q24h	50,000 units q24h	50,000 units q24h
Ticarcillin	IV, IM	75 q12h	75 q8h	75 q8h	75 q8h	100 q8h
Tobramycin*	IV, IM	2.5 q12h	2.5 q12h	2.5 q8h	2.5 q8h	2.5 q8h
Vancomycin*	IV	10–15 q12–18h	10–15 q8–12h	10–15 q8h	10–15 q8h	10–15 q8h

Source: From O'Brien, KL, Steinhoff MC. Neonatal sepsis and infections. In: Reese RE, Betts RF (eds.) *A practical approach to infectius diseases,* 4th ed; Boston: Little, Brown, 1996:Chap. 3.

* Serum antibiotic levels must be monitored. Listed doses are for initiation of therapy.

† Group B streptococcal meningitis requires 300–400 mg/kg/day of ampicillin.

‡ Cefotaxime and other third-generation cephalosporins are described in detail in Chap. 19.

§ Loading dose of 20 mg/kg IV.

‖ Excretion predominantly hepatic; use with caution in young and premature infants.

Penicillin doses are expressed in units per kilogram. Group B streptococcal sepsis requires 200,000 units/kg/day of penicillin G. Group B streptococcal meningitis requires 500,000 units/kg/day of penicillin G.

** For IV imipenem, for patients weighing ≥1,500 gms, the following dosage schedule is recommended by the *Physicians' Desk Reference (PDR)* for non-CNS infections: for <1 week of age, 25 mg/kg every 12 hours; and for 1–4 weeks of age, 25 mg/kg every 8 hours. Doses ≤500 mg should be given by IV infusion over 15 to 30 minutes; doses ≥500 mg should be given by IV infusion over 40–60 minutes. (*PDR,* 54th ed. Medical Economics Co, Montvale, N.J., 2000:1866)

Appendix B. Costs of common parenteral regimens (moderately severe infection)

Drug	Dose/day	Cost (dollars) per day*
Penicillin G	2,400,000 units	2.65
Pfizerpen G (Pfizer)	12 million units	6.05
Oxacillin	9 g	61.17
Prostaphlin (Bristol)		
Apothecon		
Nafcillin	9 g	40.08
Ampicillin	6 g	7.69
Ticarcillin	18 g	70.71
Ticar (Abbot)		
Piperacillin	18 g	96.62
Pipracil (Lederle)	16 g	85.88
Mezlocillin	18 g	76.72
Mezlin (Miles)	16 g	68.19
Ticarcillin-clavulanate	18 g/0.6 g	95.70
Timentin (Beecham)	12 g/0.4 g	63.40
Ampicillin-sulbactam	6 g	47.25
Unasyn (Roerig)	12 g	94.50
Piperacillin-tazobactam	3.375 g q6h	64.56
Zosyn (Lederle)	4.5 g q6h	85.67
Cephalothin	9 g (1.5 g q4h)	30.79
Keflin (Baxter)		
Cefazolin	4 g (1 g q6h)	16.50
Ancef (SKF)	3 g (1 g q8h)	12.37
Cefepime	1 g q12h	31.88
(Maxipime)	2 g q12h	63.76
Cefuroxime	2.25 g (750 mg q8h)	21.33
Zinacef (Glaxo)	4.5 g (1.5 g q8h)	41.41
Cefoxitin	8 g (2 g q6h)	87.16
Mefoxin (MSD)	6 g (2 g q8h)	65.37
Cefotetan	2 g q12h	47.78
Cefotan (Stuart)		
Ceftriaxone	2 g (2.0 g q24h)	84.26
Rocephin (Roche)	1 g (1.0 g q24h)	42.82
Ceftazidime	6 g (2 g q8h)	
Fortaz (Glaxo)		86.80
Tazicef (Abbott)		123.83
Tazidime		86.44
Cefotaxime	2 g q6h	100.51
Claforan (Abbott)	2 g q8h	75.38

Appendix B.   (*Continued*)

Drug	Dose/day	Cost (dollars) per day*
Cefoperazone	8 g (2 g q6h)	131.35
Cefobid (Pfizer)	6 g (2 g q8h)	98.51
Ceftizoxime	(2 g q8h)	73.92
Ceftizox (SKF)		
Aztreonam	2 g q8h	102.00
Azactam (Squibb)	1 g q8h	50.94
Imipenem	2,000 mg	121.30
Primaxin (MSD)	(500 mg q6h)	
Meropenem	1 g q8h	155.52
Merrem (Zenecca)		
Gentamicin		
Garamycin (Schering)	360 mg	24.09
(generic) (Elkins-Sinn)	(1.5 mg/kg q8h for an 80-kg patient)	4.69
Tobramycin	360 mg (1.5 mg/kg	34.92
Nebcin (Dista) (Lederle)	q8h for an 80-kg patient)	24.48
Amikacin	1,200 mg (7.5 mg/kg	78.94
Amikin (Bristol)	q12h for an 80-kg patient)	
Clindamycin	2,400 mg	33.53
Cleocin (Upjohn)	(600 mg q6h)	
	2,700 mg	29.06
	(900 mg q8h)	
	1,800 mg	25.15
	(600 mg q8h)	
Chloramphenicol	4 g (1 g q6h)	26.05
Chloromycetin (P/D)		
TMP/SMX	1,400 mg TMP	92.72
Septra (Burroughs Wellcome)	(5 mg TMP/kg q6h for a 70-kg patient⁺)	
	700 mg TMP	46.36
	(5 mg TMP/kg q12h for a 70-kg patient)	
Erythromycin	2,000 mg	23.20
Erythromycin (Elkins-Sinn)	(500 mg q6h)	
Azithromycin	500 mg	23.86
Doxycycline	200 mg	42.14
Vibramycin (Pfizer)	(100 mg q12h)	
Vancomycin	2,000 mg	31.20
Vancocin (Lilly)	(500 mg q6h)	
Metronidazole	2,000 mg	61.36
(generic) (Baxter)	(500 mg q6h)	

Appendix B.   (*Continued*)

Drug	Dose/day	Cost (dollars) per day*
Ciprofloxacin (Cipro)	200 mg q12h 400 mg q12h	31.21 60.02
Ofloxacin (Floxin)	400 mg q12h	52.80
Gatifloxacin (Tequin)	400 mg qd	38.20**
Levofloxacin (Levaquin)	500 mg qd	39.60
Trovofloxacin (Trovan)	200 mg qd	36.88
Pentamidine Pentam (LyphoMed)	280 mg (4 mg/kg q24h for a 70-kg patient)	92.17
Spectinomycin	2 g (IM)	24.69

Source: Courtesy of Joseph S. Bertino Jr, Pharm.D., Bassett Healthcare, Cooperstown, NY.

* **Actual wholesale prices (rounded off) to pharmacist from *1999 Red Book*. Retail (patient) prices would be higher based on local mark-up and bidding practices.**

+ Maximum initial dose for *P. carinii* pneumonia; usual dose is lower than this. Lower doses used in other settings. See chap. 24.

** Data from reference (28), Chapter 32.

Note: The daily cost of an antibiotic itself represents only a portion of the total administration cost per day. See text in Chapter 14, page 287.

Appendix C.   Cost of common oral regimens

Drug	Dose/day	Cost (dollars) for 10 days*
Penicillin V	250 mg qid	
Rugby (generic)		3.06
V-cillin K Veetids		2.74
Dicloxacillin	250 mg qid	
Schein (generic)		15.00
Dynapen		37.58
Cloxacillin (generic)	250 mg qid	15.18
Amoxicillin	250 mg tid	
Rugby (generic)		5.99
Polymox (Trimox)		7.17
Ampicillin	250 mg qid	
Moore (generic)		4.40
Principen		4.50
Augmentin	tid	
250-mg Tablets		70.98
Chewables (250 mg)		64.00
125-mg Suspension		33.55
Chewables (125 mg)		33.55
875 mg Tablets	bid	90.70
Carbenicillin (Geocillin)	382 mg qid (1 tab)	80.94
	2 tab qid	161.88
Cephalexin	250 mg qid	
(generic)		27.78
Keflex		60.33
(generic)	500 mg qid	55.04
Keflex		118.58
Cefadroxil	1 g bid	
Generic		39.77
Duricef		151.98
Cephradine	250 mg qid	
Rugby (generic)		22.00
Velosef		33.02
Rugby (generic)	500 mg qid	40.80
Velosef		64.85
Cefaclor (Ceclor)	250 mg tid	98.27
Mylan (generic)		59.69
Cefuroxime axetil (Ceftin)	125 mg bid	38.89
	250 mg bid	75.90
	500 mg bid	138.31
Cefixime (Suprax)	400 mg q24h	74.28
Cefprozil (Cefzil)	250 mg q12h	63.45
Loracarbef (Lorabid)	200 mg bid	62.90

Appendix C.   (*Continued*)

Drug	Dose/day	Cost (dollars) for 10 days*
Cefpodoxime proxetil (Vantin)	200 mg bid	72.30
Ceftibuten (Cedax)	400 mg qd	72.22
Cefdinir (Omnicef)	300 mg q12h	67.20[‡]
Clindamycin (Cleocin)	300 mg q8h	101.67
TMP/SMX	1 double-strength bid	
Bactrim		25.65
Septra (generic)		24.10
Rugby (generic)		2.10
Trimethoprim	100 mg bid	
Rugby (generic)		2.99
Proloprim		20.60
Erythromycin (base)	250 mg qid	
Abbott		7.17
E-mycin (delayed release)		14.25
Erythromycin sterate	250 mg qid	7.26
Mylan (generic)		
Azithromycin (Zithromax)	1 g once only[†]	25.55
	500 mg, day 1, plus 250 mg, days 2–5 (Z-pak)[†]	37.32
Clarithromycin (Biaxin)	250 mg bid	69.02
	500 mg bid	69.02
	Pediatric suspension 7.5 mg/kg given bid (for 17 kg patient, 125 mg bid)	29.83
Tetracycline hydrochloride	250 mg qid	
Mylan		1.75
Sumycin 250		2.34
Doxycycline	100 mg/day (with 200-mg initial load)	
Mylan (generic)		5.05
Vibramycin		43.66
Vancomycin (Vancocin HCl [oral solution–powder])	Capsules: 125 mg q6h PO	215.12
Metronidazole	250 mg qid	
Rugby (generic)		8.60
Flagyl		62.22
Norfloxacin (Noroxin)	400 mg bid	68.08

Appendix C.   (*Continued*)

Drug	Dose/day	Cost (dollars) for 10 days*
Ciprofloxacin (Cipro)	250 mg bid	62.92
	500 mg bid	72.47
	750 mg bid	90.78
Ofloxacin (Floxin)	200 mg bid	52.15
	300 mg bid	88.60
	400 mg bid	81.90
Lomefloxacin (Maxaquin)	400 mg once daily	61.07
Levofloxacin (Levaquin)	500 mg qd	80.58
Trovofloxacin (Trovan)	200 mg qd	71.88
Gatifloxacin (Tequin)	400 mg qd	70.25**
Moxifloxacin (Avelox)	400 mg qd	87.13**

Source: Courtesy of Joseph S. Bertino Jr, Pharm.D., Bassett Healthcare, Cooperstown, NY.

* Actual wholesale prices (rounded off) to pharmacist from *1999 Red Book*. Retail and patient prices would be higher based on local mark-up and bidding practices.

† See text discussion in Chap. 26 on single-dose and once-daily dosing × 5 for azithromycin.

‡ Cost data from Medical Letters. Cefdinir. *Med Lett Drugs Ther* 1998;40:85.

** Cost to pharmacist, actual wholesale price, from reference (28), Chapter 32.

Appendix D. Criteria for the diagnosis of staphylococcal toxic shock syndrome (TSS)

1. Fever: temperature ≥ 38.9°C (102°F)
2. Rash: diffuse macular erythroderma
3. Desquamation 1 to 2 weeks after onset of illness, particularly of palms and soles
4. Hypotension: systolic blood pressure ≤ 90 mm Hg for adults or below fifth percentile by age for children younger than 16 years; orthostatic drop in diastolic blood pressure ≥ 15 mm Hg from lying to sitting, orthostatic syncope, or orthostatic dizziness
5. Multisystem involvement—three or more of the following:
   Gastrointestinal: vomiting or diarrhea at onset of illness
   Muscular: severe myalgia or creatine phosphokinase level fivefold the upper limit of normal for laboratory
   Mucous membrane: vaginal, oropharyngeal, or conjunctival hyperemia
   Renal: blood urea nitrogen or creatinine at least twice the upper limit of normal for laboratory or urinary sediment with pyuria (≥ 5 leukocytes per high-power field) in the absence of urinary tract infection
   Hepatic: total bilirubin, hepatic enzymes AST, ALT (SGOT, SGPT) at least twice the upper limit of normal for laboratory
   Hematologic: platelets ≤ 100,000/mm^3
   Central nervous system: disorientation or alterations in consciousness without focal neurologic signs
6. Negative results of the serologic tests for Rocky Mountain spotted fever, leptospirosis, and measles (when indicated)

Abbreviations: SGOT (or AST), serum aspartate transaminase; SGPT (or ALT), serum alanine transaminase (now referred to as aminotransferases).
Source: Adapted from Reingold AL et al. Toxic shock syndrome surveillance in the United States, 1980–1981. *Ann Intern Med* 1982;96 (pt. 2):875; and from Waldvogel FA, *Staphylococcus aureus* (including toxic shock syndrome). In: Mandell GL, Bennett JE, Dolin R (eds.) *Principles and practice of infectious diseases,* 5th ed. New York: Churchill Livingstone, 2000;2081.

Appendix E. Proposed case definition for the streptococcal toxic shock syndrome*

I. Isolation of group A streptococci (*Streptococcus pyogenes*)
   A. From a normally sterile site (e.g., blood, cerebrospinal, pleural, or peritoneal fluid, tissue biopsy, surgical wound)
   B. From a nonsterile site (e.g., throat, sputum, vagina, superficial skin lesion)

II. Clinical signs of severity
   A. Hypotension: systolic blood pressure ≤ 90 mm Hg in adults or less than the fifth percentile for age in children
        and
   B. At least two of the following signs
     1. Renal impairment: creatinine ≥ 177 μmol/L (≥ 2 mg/dl) for adults or greater than or equal to twice the upper limit of normal for age. In patients with preexisting renal disease, a twofold or greater elevation over the baseline level
     2. Coagulopathy: platelets ≤ 100 × 10^9/L (≤ 100,000/mm^3) or disseminated intravascular coagulation defined by prolonged clotting times, low fibrinogen level, and the presence of fibrin degradation products
     3. Liver involvement: alanine aminotransferase,* aspartate aminotransferase,* or total bilirubin levels greater than or equal to twice the upper limit of normal for age. In patients with preexisting liver disease, a twofold or greater elevation over the baseline level
     4. Adult respiratory distress syndrome defined by acute onset of diffuse pulmonary infiltrates and hypoxemia in the absence of cardiac failure, or evidence of diffuse capillary leak manifested by acute onset of generalized edema, or pleural or peritoneal effusions with hypoalbuminemia
     5. A generalized erythematous macular rash that may desquamate
     6. Soft-tissue necrosis, including necrotizing fasciitis or myositis, or gangrene

Source: The Working Group on Severe Streptococcal Infections. Defining the group A streptococcal toxic shock syndrome: Rationale and consensus definition. *JAMA* 1993;269:390.
An illness fulfilling criteria I.A and II.A and B can be defined as a *definite* case.
An illness fulfilling criteria I.B and II.A and B can be defined as a *probable* case if no other etiology for the illness is identified.
* Serum aminotransferase enzymes include: aspartate (AST, SGOT) and alanine (ALT, SGPT).

Appendix F. Stratification Scheme of Identifying Low-risk Patients with Community-acquired Pneumonia

(Fine et al. A prediction rule to identify low-risk patients with community-acquired pneumonia. *N Engl J Med* 1997;336:243. Also see related discussion in *Infect Dis Clin North Am* 1998;12:741.)

See text discussion of "When to hospitalize the patient with CAP." Chap. 2, page 46.

1. To determine the risk of a specific patient, **a "risk class" was assigned** based on observations from their study.
    a. **Low-risk groups were in Category I, II, III.** Overall, these patients had a low mortality rate of less than 3%. **These patients can usually be treated as outpatients** (especially Category I and II patients) or can be admitted for a short stay with rapid conversion from intravenous to oral antibiotics.
        (1) **Step 1. Assign risk class I or II–V as shown in Appendix Fig. F-1.**
        (2) **Step 2. To place patients in other risk classes, points were given for age in years, for coexisting illnesses, for laboratory abnormalities and for physiologic aberrations to provide a "total clinical score". See Appendix Table F-1.**
        (3) **This "total clinical score" placed patients in different risk classes II-V. See Appendix Table F-2.**
    b. **High-risk groups were in Categories IV and V** with mortality rates in the range of 10% to 30%. **These patients deserve hospitalization routinely.**
    c. Also, **if hypoxemia is present at admission** (i.e., those patients who have an oxygen saturation of less than 90% or a partial pressure of oxygen of less than 60 mmHg while breathing room air), **these patients are routinely hospitalized** even if they are otherwise in Categories I, II, or III.
2. Fine et al. point out that
    a. Patients with CAP and certain **medical conditions** (e.g., vomiting, IVDA, or alcoholic patients who are noncompliant) or psychosocial issues (e.g., those with no support systems) **often need hospitalization.**

    b. Those with rare underlying neuromuscular diseases will not be properly assessed by these criteria and deserve admission.

    c. **Clinical judgment is still important** in the final decision as to whether to hospitalize a patient or not.

3. **For example,**

    a. A previously well 35-year-old teacher comes in complaining of a cough and progressive sputum production and mild left pleuritic pain for 24 hours. Chest x-ray reveals an early lower left lobe (LLL) infiltrate. His vital signs are normal except for a temperature of 38.6°. He is mentally alert.

        Based on Appendix Fig. F-1, he is a class 1 patient who could be managed safely as an outpatient.

    b. A 55-year-old insulin-dependent diabetic with moderate chronic renal failure comes to the emergency room with progressive symptoms of fever, cough, sputum production, and malaise in the preceding 48 hours. Her temperature is 39°, heart rate is 128, respiratory rate is 32, blood sugar is 340, and blood urea nitrogen is 41. Other screening lab tests are within normal limits. Her chest x-ray reveals an LLL infiltrate.

        Based on Appendix Fig. F-1, she is initially assigned to class II-V. Based on clinical presentation and points from Table F-1, her "point score" is at least 115 (age − 10 = 45 plus 10 for renal disease, plus 20 for elevated respiratory rate, plus 10 for tachycardia, plus 20 for elevated BUN, plus 10 for hyperglycemia.) A point score of 115, puts her in the risk class IV, using Table F-2. Therefore she needs admission.*

---

* Editorial comment: This example was based on an actual clinical case. Although her point score was at least 115, and therefore a class IV risk needing admission, she initially adamantly refused admission from the emergency room (ER). However, despite oral antibiotics, she failed outpatient therapy and within 36 hours of her prior ER visit, she returned to the ER sicker and willing to be admitted. She then did well after her admission.

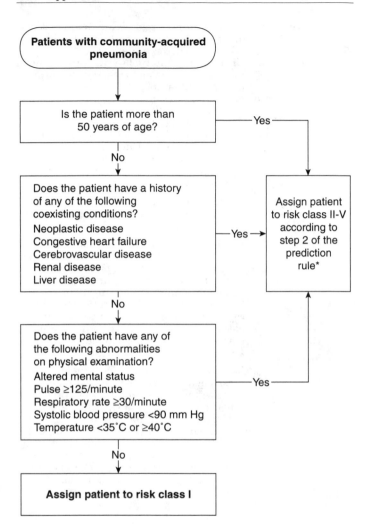

Appendix Fig. F-1. Identifying patients in risk class I in derivation of the prediction rule. Modified from Fine et al. *N Engl J Med* **1997;336:243.**

* See text and Tables F-1 and F-2.

Appendix Table F-1.   Point scoring system
for step 2 of the prediction rule for assignment
to risk classes II, III, IV, and V

Characteristic	Points Assigned*
Demographic factor	
Age	
Men	Age (yr)
Women	Age (yr) − 10
Nursing home resident	+10
Coexisting illnesses†	
Neoplastic disease	+30
Liver disease	+20
Congestive heart failure	+10
Cerebrovascular disease	+10
Renal disease	+10
Physical-examination findings	
Altered mental status‡	+20
Respiratory rate ≥30/min	+20
Systolic blood pressure <90 mm Hg	+20
Temperature <35°C or ≥40°C	+15
Pulse ≥125/min	+10
Laboratory and radiographic findings	
Arterial pH <7.35	+30
Blood urea nitrogen ≥30 mg/dl (11 mmol/liter)	+20
Sodium <130 mmol/liter	+20
Glucose ≥250 mg/dl (14 mmol/liter)	+10
Hematocrit <30%	+10
Partial pressure of arterial oxygen <60 mm Hg§	+10
Pleural effusion	+10

Source: Fine, MJ et al. *N Engl J Med* 336:243, 1997.
* **A total point score for a given patient is obtained by summing the patient's age in years (age minus 10 for women) and the points for each applicable characteristic.** The points assigned to each predictor variable were based on coefficients obtained from the logistic-regression model used in step 2 of the prediction rule (see the Methods section in original article by Fine et al.).
† Neoplastic disease is defined as any cancer except basal- or squamous-cell cancer of the skin that was active at the time of presentation or diagnosed within one year of presentation. Liver disease is defined as a clinical or histologic diagnosis of cirrhosis or another form of chronic liver disease, such as chronic active hepatitis. Congestive heart failure is defined as systolic or diastolic ventricular dysfunction documented by history, physical examination, and chest radiograph, echocardiogram, multiple gated acquisition scan, or left ventriculogram. Cerebrovascular disease is defined as a clinical diagnosis of stroke or transient ischemic attack or stroke documented by magnetic resonance imaging or computed tomography. Renal disease is defined as a history of chronic renal disease or abnormal blood urea nitrogen and creatinine concentrations documented in the medical record.
‡ Altered mental status is defined as disorientation with respect to person, place, or time that is not known to be chronic, stupor, or coma.
§ In the Pneumonia PORT cohort study, an oxygen saturation of less than 90 percent on pulse oximetry or intubation before admission was also considered abnormal.

Appendix Table F-2.   Community-acquired pneumonia risk class, based on total assigned points

Risk Class	Number of Points from Table F-1	Clinical Implications
I	See Fig. F-1 to define	OP management feasible
II	≤70	OP management feasible
III	71–90	OP management feasible or short admission
IV	91–130	Need admission
V	>130	Need admission

(Modified and adapted from Fine MJ et al. A prediction rule to identify low-risk patients with community-acquired pneumonia. *N Engl J Med* 336:243, 1997.)
OP = outpatient

Subject Index

Pages followed by *f* indicate figures; pages followed by *t* indicate tables.

A

ABE (acute bacterial endocarditis), 171

Abscesses (*see* Cutaneous abscesses; Intraabdominal abscesses; Pancreatic abscesses; Spinal epidural abscess)

Acne vulgaris, treatment of
  clindamycin, 438
  tetracycline, 498*t*

Acute otitis media, 12
  antibiotic use in, 12–13
    indications for, 15
  complicated, treatment of, 17
  otitis media with effusion and, 13–15
  pathogens causing
    bacterial, 15–16
    viral, 16
  penicillin-resistant *S. pneumoniae* in, 16, 330
  prophylaxis in, 18
  recurrent, indications for antibiotic use in, 15
  treatment of, 13–15, 16–18, 17*t*
    azithromycin, 485
    cephalosporin, 387*t*
    trimethoprim-sulfamethoxazole, 453
  uncomplicated, treatment of, 17

Acyclovir for genital HSV, 197

Agar diffusion test, 250

Allergies, patients with
  antibiotic use in, 280 (*see also specific antibiotic*)

Amantadine, 31, 313

Amikacin, 415 (*see also* Aminoglycosides)
  activity spectrum of, 416–417
  cost of, 430
  dosages of, 420–421
    conventional, 426–427
    pharmacokinetics of, 425–426
    single daily, 421–425
  pharmacokinetics of, 417–418
  resistant organisms to, 430–431
  tissue penetration of, 418
  toxicity of, 415–416, 428–430
  use of, 415, 418–420
    limits of, 420

Aminoglycosides, 415
  activity spectrum of, 416–417, 416*t*
  amikacin, 415 (*see also* Amikacin)
  in community vs. nosocomial infections, 415

cost of, 430
dosages of, 420–421
  amikacin, 424*t*
  CAPD peritonitis, 428
  conventional, 426–427
  gentamicin and tobramycin, 423, 424*t*
  overview of, 427
  pharmacokinetics of, 425–426
  renal dysfunction patient, 423–424
  single daily, 421–425
    exclusions to, 421–423, 422*t*
    serum monitoring in, 425
    vs. extended interval, 423–425
gentamicin, 415 (*see also* Gentamicin)
ototoxicity of, 428
paromomycin, 432–433
pharmacokinetics of, 417–418
resistant organisms to, 430–431
serum level monitoring with use of, 415, 425
streptomycin, 419, 431–432
synergistic use of, 418–419
tobramycin, 415 (*see also* Tobramycin)
toxicity of, 415, 428
  cochlear, 428
  neuromuscular paralysis and, 428
  renal, 429–430
  vestibular, 429
treatment with
  in chronic ambulatory peritoneal dialysis, 428
  in dialysis patients, 428
  in pulmonary infections, 428
use of, 418–420
  dialysis patients and, 428
  limits of, 420
  synergistic, 418–419
vs. other antibiotics, 415

Aminopenicillins (*see* Amoxicillin; Ampicillin)

Amoxicillin
  activity spectrum of, 343
  adverse effects of, 345
  dosages of, 345
  uses of oral, 343–344 (*see also* Acute otitis media)

Amoxicillin-clavulanate, 348
  activity spectrum of, 349
  availability of, 350

Amoxicillin-clavulanate (*contd.*)
  dosages of, 350
    adult, 350
    children's, 351
    pregnant patient, 351–352
    renal patient, 351
    side effects of, 352
  pharmacokinetics of, 349
  uses of, 349–350
Ampicillin
  activity spectrum of, 343
  adverse effects of, 345
  dosages of, 344–345
Ampicillin-sulbactam, 352
  activity spectrum of, 352,
      353t–354t
  clinical uses of, 35
  dosages of, 355–356
  pharmacokinetics of, 352
  recommendations regarding,
      356–357
  side effects of, 356
  vs. ticarcillin-clavulanate vs.
      piperacillin-tazobactam,
      362–363
Anaerobes
  antibiotic activity against
    aminoglycoside, 417
    azithromycin, 482
    cefotetan, 375
    cefoxitin, 373
    cefuroxime, 372
    chloramphenicol, 441
    clarithromycin, 478
    clindamycin, 435
    erythromycin, 472
    metronidazole, 521, 522
    penicillin G, 330
    penicillinase-resistant peni-
        cillin, 340, 359
    third generation cephalosporins,
        381
    trimethoprim-sulfamethoxazole,
        451
    trovofloxacin, 548
    vancomycin, 504
  susceptibility testing of, 252
Ancef (*see* Cefazolin)
Ansamycin (*see* Rifabutin)
Anspor (*see* Cephradine)
Antibiotic(s), of choice, for common
    pathogens, 280, 281t–286t
Antibiotic-associated colitis (AAC)
    (*see Clostridium difficile
    diarrhea*)
Antibiotic use (*see also under specific
    antibiotic*)
  administration of antibiotics in,
      294–296
  allergies and, 280
  approaches to, 277–278

bactericidal agents in, 287
cost of, 287–288
  oral (*see* Appendix C), 581
  parenteral (*see* Appendix B), 578
culture data, and initial therapy
    modification, 296–297 (*see
    also* Cultures; Specimens,
    clinical)
different approach to, 277–278
dosages in, 296 (*see also under spe-
    cific antibiotic*)
  for neonates, (*see* Appendix A),
      576
duration of therapy, 297, 298t
and end-of-life issues, 304–305
ethical considerations in, 304–305
excessive, 3
  by general public, 5
  by physicians, 4–5
  in URIs, 3
historical, 277
inappropriate, 300 (*see also*
    Resistance, to antibiotics)
pharmacokinetics of (*see also
    under specific antibiotic*)
  excretion pathways in, 292t
  genetic factors and, 290
  liver function and, 293–294
  pregnancy/lactation and,
      290–292, 291t
  renal function and, 292–293,
      292t
pregnancy-related issues, 290–292
    (*see also individual agents*)
prophylactic (*see* Prophylactic
    antibiotics)
resistance developed in, 298–305
    (*see also* Resistance, to anti-
    biotics)
route of administration in,
    294–296
selection criteria for, 278, 278t
  antibiotic match to each patient,
      280, 287–288
  antibiotics of choice for common
      pathogens, 281t–286t
  clinical specimens, culture of,
      279
  culture data and initial therapy
      modification, 296–297
  determination of causative
      organism, 279–280
  dosage, 296
  host factors, 289–294
  indications for combined anti-
      biotics, 288–289
  indications for use, 278–279
  optimal duration of therapy,
      297, 298t
  route of administration,
      294–296

side effects in, 280 (*see also side effects or toxicity under specific antibiotic*)
synergism in combined, 288–289
Antigens, identification of microbial, 259–260
Antiseptics, urinary (*see* Urinary antiseptics)
AOM (*see* Acute otitis media)
Appendicitis, treatment of, 144–145
Arthritis, bacterial, 183–185
  clinical presentation of, 183
  laboratory analysis of, 183–184
  treatment of, 184–185, 185*t*, 186*t*
    fluoroquinolone, 554
Augmentin (*see* Amoxicillin-clavulanate)
Azactam (*see* Aztreonam)
Azithromycin, 481
  activity spectrum of, 481–482
  cost of, 487
  dosages of, 486–487, 488*t*–489*t*
  pharmacokinetics of, 482–483
  resistance to, 482
  toxicity/side effects of, 487
  use of
    in adults, 483–485
    in children, 485
    investigational, 485–486
Aztreonam, 401
  action of, mechanism of, 401
  activity spectrum of, 401
  cost of, 404
  dosages of, 402
    adult and pediatric, 402, 403*t*
    penicillin-allergic or cephalosporin-allergic patient, 403–404
    pregnant/lactating patient, 404
    renal patient, 402–403, 403*t*
  pharmacokinetics of, 401
  toxicity/side effects of, 404
  use of, 402
    optimal, 404–405

B

B. fragilis, metronidazole activity against, 522
Bacteremia, 157–158 (*see also* Sepsis)
Bactericidal agents, 287 (*see also* Aminoglycosides; Cephalosporins; Metronidazole; Penicillin(s); Vancomycin)
Bacteriostatic agents (*see* Sulfonamides; Tetracyclines; TMP-SMX)
Bacteriuria
  in children, 99–101
  in men, 95
  in women, 92
Bactrim (*see* TMP-SMX)

Bartonella infection, treatment of
  azithromycin, 486
  fluoroquinolone, 551
Benzylpenicillin (*see* Penicillin(s))
Beta-lactam penicillins, and beta-lactamase inhibitors, 347–348, 348*t*
  allergy to, treatment in, 506
  Amoxicillin-clavulanate, 348–352
  effectiveness of, 348
  intravenous, 352
    ampicillin-sulbactam, 352–357
    piperacillin-tazobactam, 359–362
    ticarcillin-clavulanate, 357–359
  resistant bacteria to, 348
Biaxin (*see* Clarithromycin)
Biliary tract infections, treatment of, 147
  biliary sepsis, acute, 148–149
  cholangitis, acute, 148–149
  cholecystitis, 147–148
    acute acalculous, 148
  post-endoscopic retrograde cholangiopancreatography cholangitis, 149
Bite wounds, treatment of, 84–86, 85*t*
Blood-agar hemolysis, test results in, 258
Bone infections (*see* Joint and bone infections)
Borrelia burgdorferi infection, treatment of
  azithromycin, 482, 485
  tetracycline, 498*t*, 500*t*
  third generation cephalosporin, 372, 378*t*
Brain abscess(es), 227
  bacterial, 228, 229–230
  clinical presentation of, 228
  diagnosis of, 229
  fungal, 228–230
  pathogens causing, 227–228
  treatment of, 229–230
Breast-milk, antibiotics in, 290
Bronchitis
  acute, 18
    clinical diagnosis of, 19
    etiology of, 19
    treatment of, 19–20
      cephalosporin, 387*t*
      clarithromycin, 479
  chronic, 20
    clinical presentation of, 21
    treatment of, 21, 22*t*
      azithromycin, 484
      fluoroquinolone, 553
      trimethoprim-sulfamethoxazole, 453
Brucellosis, treatment of
  rifampin, 529

Brucellosis, treatment of (*contd.*)
  tetracycline, 498*t*
  trimethoprim-sulfamethoxazole, 454

C

C-reactive protein assay, 262
Campylobacter jejuni infection
  erythromycin activity against, 472
  fluoroquinolone treatment of, 551
Candidemia, occult, 243
Candidiasis, vulvovaginal, treatment
    of, 206, 208*t*–209*t*
CAP (community-acquired pneumo-
    nia) (*see* Pneumonia,
    community-acquired)
Carbapenems (*see* Imipenem;
    Meropenem)
Carbenicillin
  uses of, 345–346
  vs. mezlocillin vs. piperacillin, 346
Carbuncles, treatment of, 80
Catalase test, 258
Cavernous sinus thrombophlebitis,
    treatment of, 73–74
Ceclor (*see* Cefaclor)
Cedax (*see* Ceftibuten)
Cefaclor, use of, 391
Cefadroxil, 389
Cefamandole, preparation and use
    of, 369, 372–373
Cefazolin, preparation and use of,
    368–369
Cefdinir, dosages and use of,
    396–397
Cefepime, dosages and use of,
    384–385
Cefixime, dosages and use of,
    392–393
Cefizox (*see* Ceftizoxime)
Cefobid (*see* Cefoperazone)
Cefonicid, 376
Cefoperazone, 382
Cefotan (*see* Cefotetan)
Cefotaxime, use of, 381–382
Cefotetan, preparation and use of,
    375–376
Cefoxitin, preparation and use of,
    373–375
Cefpodoxime, dosages and use of,
    393–394
Cefprozil, dosages and use of,
    390–391
Ceftazidime, use of, 382–383
Ceftibuten, dosages and use of,
    394–396
Ceftin (*see* Cefuroxime axetil)
Ceftizoxime, use of, 382
Ceftriaxone, dosages and use of,
    383–384
Cefuroxime, preparation and use of,
    369, 372–373

Cefuroxime axetil, dosages and use
    of, 390
Cefzil (*see* Cefprozil)
Cellulitis, 73
  diagnosis of, 74–75
  erysipelas and, distinction
      between, 73
  of extremities and trunk, 73
  facial, 73
  orbital, 73
  perineal, 74
  treatment of, 75, 76*t*
    clindamycin, 437
Central catheter infection, van-
    comycin treatment of, 507
Central nervous system infections,
    treatment of
  brain abscess, 227–230
  encephalitis, 225–227
  meningitis, 212–225
  spinal epidural abscess, 230–231
  vancomycin in, 507
Cephalexin, dosages and use of, 385,
    389
Cephalosporins, 365
  availability of, 365, 366*t*
  dosages of, 370*t*–371*t*
  first generation, 365
    use of intravenous, 368–369
    use of oral, 385, 389
  history of, 365–366
  intravenous preparation of
    cefamandole, 369, 372–373
    cefazolin, 368–369
    cefepime, 384–385
    cefonicid, 376
    cefoperazone, 382
    cefotaxime, 381–382
    cefotetan, 375–376
    cefoxitin, 373–375
    ceftazidime, 382–383
    ceftizoxime, 382
    ceftriaxone, 383–384
    cefuroxime, 369, 372–373
    dosages of, 370*t*–371*t*
    use of, 377*t*–378*t*
  oral preparation of
    cefaclor, 391
    cefadroxil, 389
    cefdinir, 396–397
    cefixime, 392–393
    cefpodoxime, 393–394
    cefprozil, 390–391
    ceftibuten, 394–396
    cefuroxime axetil, 390
    cephalexin, 385, 389
    cephradine, 389
    indications for use of, 386*t*
    loracarbef, 391–392
    use of, 385, 387*t*–388*t*

pharmacokinetics of, 366, 367*t*, 368
prophylactic use of, 309, 312
resistance to, 368
    aminoglycosides and, 420
second generation, 365
    use of intravenous, 369–376
    use of oral, 389–392
side effects of, 366, 397–398
third generation, 365–366
    use of intravenous, 376–385,
        377*t*–378*t*
    use of oral, 392–397
Cephradine, dosages and use of, 389
Cerebrospinal fluid shunt infections,
    rifampin treatment of, 530
Cervicitis, mucopurulent, treatment
    of, 195
    azithromycin, 484
    fluoroquinolone, 552
Chancroid, treatment of, 203–204
    azithromycin, 484
    third generation cephalosporin,
        378*t*
Chlamydial infections
    erythromycin activity against, 472
    erythromycin treatment of,
        473–474
    fluoroquinolone activity against,
        548
    rifampin activity against, 527
    tetracycline treatment of, 498*t*,
        500*t*
    treatment of, 193–195, 206–211
        (*see also* Pelvic inflammatory
        disease)
Chloramphenicol, 441
    action of, mechanism of, 441
    activity spectrum of, 441
    dosages, and preparations of, 444
    drug interactions with, 444
    patient monitoring in treatment
        with, 442
    pharmacokinetics of, 441–442
    toxicity/side effects of, 442–443
    use of, 443–444, 514
Cholangitis
    acute, treatment of, 148–149
        post-endoscopic retrograde
        cholangiopancreatography,
        149
    prophylactic antibiotics in, 322
    recurrent, prophylactic antibiotics
        in, 322
Cholecystitis, treatment of, 147–148
Ciprofloxacin, use of, 555
Claforan (*see* Cefotaxime)
Clarithromycin, 477–478
    activity spectrum of, 478
    dosages of, 479
    drug interactions with, 480–481
    pharmacokinetics of, 478–479

toxicity/side effects of, 480
use of, 479
Clindamycin, 435
    activity spectrum of, 435
    dosages and preparations of,
        438–439
    pharmacokinetics of, 435
    side effects of, 439
    use of, 436–438
Clostridium difficile diarrhea, treat-
    ment of, 113, 123–125, 522,
    524
    in children, 125
    metronidazole, 522, 524
    vancomycin, 505, 509
Cloxacillin, preparations and dosage
    of, 342
Coagulase test, 258
Colds (*see* Nasopharyngitis)
Colonization, of body site, 256
Comfort care, and antibiotic use,
    304
Community-acquired infections (*see
    also* Pneumonia, community-
    acquired)
    gram-negative, and use of amino-
        glycosides, 419
    resistant organisms in, 299–300
Community-acquired pneumonia
    (*see* Pneumonia, community-
    acquired)
Concentration-dependent killing, of
    bacteria, 421
Contact precautions, 265
    indications for, 266*t*
Contamination, of cultures, 256
Corynebacterium infection, treat-
    ment of
    erythromycin, 472
    vancomycin, 504
Cost, of antibiotics, 287–288 (*see also*
    Appendix B, 578; Appendix C,
    581)
Cotrimoxazole (*see* TMP-SMX)
Cranberry juice, for prophylaxis of
    UTIs, 572
Crohn's disease, metronidazole
    treatment of, 524
CRP (C-reactive protein) assay, 262
Cryptosporidiosis, paromomycin use
    in, 432–433
Cryptosporidium diarrhea, treat-
    ment of, 128–129
Culture data, and initial therapy
    modification, 296–297
Cultures (*see also* Specimens,
    clinical)
    anaerobic, 254
    blood, 253–254
    colonization and results of, 256
    contamination of, 256

Cultures (*contd.*)
  identification of bacterial, 257–259
  interpretation of results of,
      256–257
  mycobacterial, 254, 256
    specimens for, 255*t*
  negative cultures, 256–257
Cutaneous abscesses
  treatment of, 79*t*, 80
  types of, 78, 80

D

Dental procedures, prophylactic
    antibiotics for, 314*t*, 316*t*
Diabetic foot infections, 80
  clinical presentation of, 81
  diagnosis of, 81–82
  microbes causing, 81
  treatment of, 82–84, 83*t*
    clindamycin, 437
    fluoroquinolone, 553
Diarrhea
  bacterial, treatment of, 122*t*, 553
  Clostridium difficile, 113,
      123–125, 522, 524
  Cryptosporidium, treatment of,
      128–129
  diagnosis of
    history in, 106–107
    indications for medical interven-
        tion in, 106
    laboratory, 107, 112
    physical examination in, 107
    symptoms in, 107
  E. coli, treatment of, 129
  E. coli 0157:H7, treatment of,
      125–126
  food borne causes of, clinical fea-
      tures of
    symptom onset greater than 12
        hours, 116*t*–121*t*
    symptom onset less than 12
        hours, 108*t*–111*t*
  Giardia lamblia, 126
    treatment of, 127–128
  mechanisms of, 106
  traveler's, 129 (*see also* Traveler's
      diarrhea)
    prophylactic antibiotics for, 320
    treatment of, 129
  treatment of, 113, 120–123
  viral gastroenteritis
    treatment of, 114*t*–115*t*, 123
Dicloxacillin, preparation and
    dosage of, 342
Dilution susceptibility testing, 251
Diphtheroid infections, vancomycin
    treatment of, 506
Disk diffusion test, 250
Diverticulitis, 145
  diagnosis of, 146
  treatment of, 146–147

Dosages, of antibiotics, 296 (*see also*
    under specific antibiotic or
    illness)
  for neonates, *see* Appendix A, 576
Doxycycline, 493 (*see also*
    Tetracyclines)
  dosages and preparations of, 497,
      499
Droplet precautions, 265
Duke criteria
  for diagnosis of infective (bacterial)
      endocarditis, 173, 174, 175*t*,
      176*t*
Duration of therapy, optimal, 297,
    298*t*
Duricef (*see* Cefadroxil)

E

E. coli, diarrhea, treatment of, 129
E. coli 0157:H7 diarrhea, treatment
    of, 125–126
E test, 251, 252*f*
Encephalitis, 225
  clinical presentation of, 226
  diagnosis of, 226
  treatment of, 226–227
End-of-life issues, and antibiotic use,
    304–305
Endocarditis
  associated with prosthetic valves,
      179–181 (*see also* Prosthetic
      valve endocarditis)
  bacterial
    acute vs. subacute, 171, 177*t*
    Duke criteria for diagnosis of,
        173, 174
    organisms causing, 174–177
    prophylactic antibiotic(s) for,
        312–313, 313*t*
      dental procedures, 314*t*, 316*t*
      genitourinary tract proce-
          dures, 315*t*, 317*t*
      respiratory and gastrointesti-
          nal tract procedures, 315*t*,
          316*t*, 317*t*
      vancomycin as, 508
    treatment of, 177*t*
      rifampin, 529
      trimethoprim-
          sulfamethoxazole, 454
      vancomycin, 506
  infective, 171
    clinical presentation of, 171–172
    diagnosis of, 174–177
      Duke criteria for, 175*t*, 176*t*
    indications for treatment of, 179
    laboratory/echocardiographic
        analysis of, 172–174
    treatment of, 177–179, 177*t*,
        178*t*
      trimethoprim-
          sulfamethoxazole, 454

Endoophthalmitis, posttraumatic, clindamycin treatment of, 437
Endoscopic retrograde cholangiopancreatography, prophylactic antibiotic use in, 322
Enoxacin, use of, 555–556
Enterobacteriaceae, resistance of, 299, 359 (see also Gram-negative organisms)
Enterococci
  aminoglycoside activity against, 419
  ampicillin activity against, 343
  diabetic foot infections and, 81
  endocarditis and, 175, 177–178
  imipenem activity against, 406
  intraabdominal infection and, 133–134, 147
  nitrofurantoin for, in lower UTI, 565
  resistance to cephalosporins, 368
  species nomenclature, 257
  UTI and, 91, 93
  vancomycin activity against, 503–504
  vancomycin-resistant enterococci, 263, 269–270, 503–504, 514–515
Epidural abscess, spinal, treatment of, 230–231
Epiglottitis, 33–34
  treatment of, 34–35
Epsilometer testing (E test), 251, 252f
Erysipelas, 73
Erythromycin
  activity spectrum of, 468, 472
  as alternative with penicillin-allergic patient, 474
  dosages and preparations of, 474–476
  drug interactions with, 477
  pharmacokinetics of, 472–473
  toxicity/side effects of, 476–477
  use of, 473–474
Ethical considerations, in antibiotic use, 304–305
Excessive antibiotic use
  by general public, 5
  by physicians, 4–5
  problems with, 3
  in URIs, 3
Excretion pathways, of antibiotic metabolism, 292t
External otitis
  malignant, treatment of, 33
  treatment of, 32
Eye infections, imipenem use in, 407

F

Famiciclovir for genital HSV, 197
Fansidar tablets, use of, 461

Fasciitis, necrotizing, 74
Fever, 232
  in adults in ICU, 238
    diagnosis of, 238–240, 239t
    miscellaneous issues in, 240–242
    noninfectious etiologies of, 240, 241t
    treatment of, 242–243, 242t
  diagnostic approach to, 232–235
    laboratory analysis in, 236–237
    physical examination in, 235–236
  in HIV-positive patients
    CD4 wbc count and correlation with, 243–245, 244t
    diagnostic testing in, 245–246
  in leukopenic patients
    diagnosis of, 246, 247t
    treatment of, 248, 377t
      aminoglycoside, 420
      aztreonam, 402
      fluoroquinolone, 554
      imipenem, 408
      trimethoprim-sulfamethoxazole, 454
      vancomycin, 507
  noninfectious causes of, 237–238
  treatment of patients with, 238
Fluoroquinolones, 544, 554
  action of, mechanism of, 544
  activity spectrum of, 545, 545t, 548
  ciprofloxacin, 555
  classification of, 545t
  cost of, 558, 561
  dosages and prearations of
    in normal renal function, 559t
    in renal failure, 560t
  drug interactions with, 550–551
  enoxacin, 555–556
  gatifloxacin, 561
  grepafloxacin, 556
  levofloxacin, 556
  lomefloxacin, 555
  minimum inhibitory concentrations of, 546t–547t
  moxifloxacin, 559
  norfloxacin, 555
  ofloxacin, 555
  pharmacokinetics of, 548
  resistant organisms to, 548, 561
  side effects of, 549–550
  sparfloxacin, 556
  structure of, 544
  trovofloxacin, 556–558
  use of, 551–554, 552t, 554–558
    contraindications to, 550
Food poisoning (see Diarrhea)
Foot infection (see Diabetic foot infections; Puncture wounds, of feet)

Fortaz (*see* Ceftazidime)
Fosfomycin tromethamine, 570
  activity spectrum of, 570
  clinical trials of, 571
  cost of, 571–572
  dosages of, 571
  pharmacokinetics of, 571
  side effects of, 571
  use of, 571–572
Fungemia/candidemia, in sepsis, 167
Fungi, susceptibility testing of, 252
Furadantin, 564
Furuncles, 78

G

Gantanol (*see* Sulfamethoxazole)
Gantrisin (*see* Sulfisoxazole)
GAS (group A streptococci) (*see*
      Group A streptococcal infec-
      tion; Pharyngitis)
Gastroenteritis, viral, treatment of,
      114*t*–115*t*, 123 (*see also*
      Diarrhea)
Gastrointestinal infections (*see also*
      Appendicitis; Biliary tract
      infections; Diarrhea;
      Diverticulitis; Intraabdominal
      abscesses; Pancreatitis;
      Peritonitis)
Gastrointestinal procedures, prophy-
      lactic antibiotics for endo-
      carditis prevention, 315*t*,
      316*t*, 317*t*
Gatifloxacin, 561
Genetic factors, and antibiotic use,
      290
Genital ulcers (*see* Chancroid)
Genitourinary infections (*see also*
      Cervicitis; Chancroid;
      Chlamydial infections; Herpes
      simplex infection; Pelvic infec-
      tions; Pelvic inflammatory dis-
      ease; Syphilis; Ulcerative
      lesions; Urethritis; Urinary
      tract infections; Venereal
      warts)
  azithromycin treatment of, 482
  tetracycline treatment of, 498*t*
Genitourinary tract procedures, pro-
      phylactic antibiotics for, 315*t*,
      317*t*
Genotype susceptibility testing, 253
Gentamicin, 415 (*see also*
      Aminoglycosides)
  activity spectrum of, 416–417
  cost of, 430
  dosages of, 420–421
    conventional, 426–427
    pharmacokinetic model for,
      425–426
    single daily, 421–425

  pharmacokinetics of, 417–418
  resistant organisms to, 430–431
  tissue penetration of, 418
  toxicity of, 415–416, 428–430
  use of, 415, 418–420
    limits of, 420
Giardiasis, 126
  treatment of, 127–128
Gingivitis, metronidazole treatment
      of, 524
Gradient diffusion susceptibility
      testing, 251, 252*f*
Gram-negative organisms
  antibiotic activity against
    aminoglycosides, 416, 418–420
    azithromycin, 482
    aztreonam, 401
    cefazolin, 369
    cefotetan, 375
    cefoxitin, 373
    cefuroxime, 372
    chloramphenicol, 441
    clarithromycin, 478
    clindamycin, 435
    erythromycin, 472
    fluoroquinolone, 545, 546*t*–547*t*,
      548
    imipenem, 406
    penicillin G, 330
    penicillinase-resistant peni-
      cillin, 340
    third generation cephalosporins,
      377*t*, 378*t*, 380–381
    trimethoprim-sulfamethoxazole,
      451
  identification of, 258–259
Gram-positive organisms
  antibiotic activity against
    aminoglycosides, 416–417
    azithromycin, 481–482
    cefotetan, 375
    cefoxitin, 373
    cefuroxime, 372
    chloramphenicol, 441
    clarithromycin, 478
    clindamycin, 435
    erythromycin, 468
    fluoroquinolone, 545, 546*t*–547*t*
    imipenem, 406
    penicillin G, 326
    penicillinase-resistant peni-
      cillin, 340, 359
    third generation cephalosporins,
      376, 378*t*, 379
    trimethoprim-sulfamethoxazole,
      451
    vancomycin, 503–504
  identification of, 257–258, 259
Granulomatous disease, chronic,
      trimethoprim-sulfamethoxa-
      zole treatment of, 455

Grepafloxacin, use of, 556
Group A streptococcal infection, 7
  beta-hemolytic, 257
  invasive, 74
  isolation of organisms, from sterile
      site, 74
  laboratory testing for, 8–9
  resistance to therapy in, 10
  treatment of, 9–10, 11*t*, 12*t*
    azithromycin, 484
    clindamycin, 437
    erythromycin, 468
    third generation cephalosporin,
        379
Group B, group C, group D
      streptococci
  beta-hemolytic, 257
  third generation cephalosporin use
      against, 379

H

Haemophilus influenzae B (*see* also
      Gram-negative organisms)
  azithromycin activity against, 482
  meningitis caused by, prophylactic
      antibiotics for, 318*t*, 319*t*, 320
HAP (hospital-acquired pneumonia)
      (*see* Pneumonia, hospital-
      acquired)
Helicobacter pylori infection, 129
  clarithromycin activity against, 478
  clarithromycin treatment of, 479,
      490
  metronidazole treatment of, 524
  tetracycline treatment of, 498*t*
Hemolytic uremic syndrome,
      125–126
Hemophilus ducreyi (*see* Chancroid)
Herpes simplex encephalitis, PCR
      techniques in diagnosis of, 261
Herpes simplex infection, genital,
      195–196
  clinical presentation of, 196
  diagnosis of, 196
  treatment of, 196–197
    in AIDS patients, 197
    in pregnancy, 198
Historical use, of antibiotics, 277
HIV infection
  fever in
    CD4 wbc count and correlation
        with, 243–245, 244*t*
    evaluation of, 245–246
  meningitis treatment in, 225
  Mycobacterium avium complex
      and azithromycin treatment
      of, 479
    clarithromycin activity against,
        478
    clarithromycin treatment of,
        479, 490
    rifabutin treatment of, 537–539

PCR techniques in diagnosis of, 261
  syphilis treatment in, 202–203
Humatin (*see* Paromomycin)

I

Imipenem, 405
  action of, mechanism of, 405
  activity spectrum of, 405–407
  cost of, 411, 412–413
  dosages of, 408, 412
    adult, 409
    children's, 409
    pregnant/lactating patient,
        409–410
  pharmacokinetics of, 407
  resistant organisms to, 411
  side effects of, 410, 412–413
  use of, 407–408, 413
Immunodiagnostic testing, 259–260
Inappropriate use, of antibiotics, 300
      (*see* also Resistance, to
      antibiotics)
Infection control, 263
  isolation of patients in, 264–266
  precautions in, 264–266
    indications for, 266*t*, 267*t*–268*t*
  resistant organisms and, 263–264,
      266
    MDR (multidrug-resistant)
        tuberculosis, 271–272
    methicillin-resistant
        Staphylococcus aureus, 266,
        269
    VISA (vancomycin intermedi-
        ately susceptible *S. aureus*),
        270–271
    VRE (vancomycin-resistant
        enterococci), 269–270
Influenza, 29
  clinical presentation of, 30–31
  complications of, 31–32
  epidemiology of, 30
  prophylaxis for, 32
  treatment of, 31
  type A, prophylactic antibiotics
      for, 313–314
Influenza direct antigen test, 260
Intraabdominal abscesses, 140
  hepatic, 140–141
    treatment of, 141
  pancreatic, 143
  psoas, 143
  retroperitoneal, 142–143
  splenic bacterial, 142
Intraabdominal infections, 132
  abscesses, 140–143
  aerobic and anaerobic, 133–135
  aminoglycoside treatment of, 420
  appendicitis, 144–145
  biliary tract, 147–149
  Candida causing, 133
  diverticulitis, 145–147

Intraabdominal infections (*contd.*)
enterococci causing, 133
organisms causing, 133*t*
pancreatitis, 149–155
peritonitis, 135–139
treatment of, 134*t*
aztreonam, 402
cefoxitin, 373–374
clindamycin, 436
fluoroquinolone, 553
general principles of antibiotic,
132–135
imipenem, 408
meropenem, 411
piperacillin-tazobactam, 360
Invasive GAS disease, 74 (*see also*
Group A streptococcal
infection)
Isolation, of patients, 264–266

J

Joint and bone infections, 183
bacterial arthritis, 183–185
osteomyelitis, 187–190
prosthetic joint infection, 185–187
Joint replacement, prophylactic
antibiotics in, 322 (*see also*
Prosthetic joint infection)

K

Keflex (*see* Cephalexin)
Kefurox (*see* Cefuroxime)
Kefzol (*see* Cefazolin)
Kirby Bauer test, 250

L

Lactose fermentation, 258–259
Lancefield serogrouping, of strepto-
cocci, 258
Legionella infections, treatment of
erythromycin, 473
fluoroquinolone, 548, 551
rifampin, 530
Legionella urinary antigen, testing
for, 259
Leukopenic host, oral antibiotics in
infection prevention in, 322
fever in, 245–248
Levaquin (*see* Levofloxacin)
Levofloxacin, use of, 556
Linezolid, 514–515
Liver function, and antibiotic use,
293–294 (*see also pharmacokinetics under specific antibiotic*)
Lomefloxacin, use of, 555
Lorabid (*see* Loracarbef)
Loracarbef, dosages and use of,
391–392
Lung abscesses, clindamycin treatment of, 437
Lyme disease (*see Borrelia burgdor-
feri* infection)

M

MAC (*see Mycobacterium avium
complex*)
Macrobid (*see* Nitrofurantoin)
Macrodantin, 564
Macrolides, 468 (*see also*
Azithromycin; Clarithro-
mycin; Erythromycin)
use of
intravenous, 487
oral, 487, 490
in vitro activity of, 469*t*–471*t*
Malaria, tetracycline treatment of,
498*t*
Mandol (*see* Cefamandole)
Maxipime (*see* Cefepime)
MDR (multidrug-resistant) gram-
negative bacilli, 264
MDR (multidrug-resistant) *M. tuberculosis,* 264
infection control and, 271–272
resistance of, 299–300
Mefoxin (*see* Cefoxitin)
Meningitis
bacterial, 214*t*–216*t*
clinical presentation of, 212–213
diagnosis of, 219, 220*t*, 221
pathogens causing, 213, 217
prophylactic antibiotics for, 314,
318–320
treatment of, 222–225
meropenem, 411–412
rifampin, 529
vancomycin, 507
diagnosis of, 217–219, 221–222
pathogens causing, 213, 217
pneumococcal, and penicillin-
resistant strains causing, 329
prophylactic antibiotics for, 314,
318, 318*t*, 319*t*
S. pneumoniae, rifampin treatment of penicillin-resistant,
530
treatment of, 222–225
in HIV-positive patients, 225
schematic for, 218*t*
trimethoprim-sulfamethoxazole,
454
viral
clinical presentation of, 212–213
diagnosis of, 221–222
pathogens causing, 217
treatment of, 223–224
Meningococcal carrier state, treatment of, 554
Meropenem, 411
activity spectrum of, 411
as alternative to vancomycin in
penicillin-resistant pneumococcal meningitis, 412
pharmacokinetics of, 411
use of, 411–412

Merrem (*see* Meropenem)
Methenamine, 568
  action of, mechanism of, 568–569
  activity spectrum of, 569
  dosages of, 569–570
  pharmacokinetics of, 569
  preparations of, 569
  toxicity of, 570
  uses of, 569
Metronidazole, 521
  activity spectrum of, 521
  carcinogenic potential of, 522
  dosages and preparations of, 523t, 524–525
  pharmacokinetics of, 521–522
  resistant organisms to, 521
  toxicity/side effects of, 522, 525–526
  use of, 522–524
    contraindications to, 524
Mezlocillin
  uses of, 345–346
  vs. piperacillin vs. ticarcillin, 346
MIC (minimum inhibitory concentration), 251
Microsulfon (*see* Sulfadiazine)
Minimum inhibitory concentration, 251
Minocycline, 493 (*see also* Tetracyclines)
  dosages and preparations of, 497
MODS (multiple organ dysfunction syndrome), 157, 160
Monobactams (*see* Aztreonam)
Monocid (*see* Cefonicid)
Monurol (*see* Fosfomycin tromethamine)
Moxifloxacin, 559
MRSA (methicillin-resistant) *Staphylococcus aureus*, 263, 299
  erythromycin activity against, 468, 472
  hemodialysis shunt infection, vancomycin treatment of, 508–509
  infection control and treatment of, 266, 269, 339–340, 368–369, 506
  rifampin treatment of, 529
MSSA (methicillin-susceptible) *Staphylococcus aureus*, treatment of, 339–342
Mucopurulent cervicitis, treatment of, 195
Multiple organ dysfunction syndrome (MODS), in sepsis, 157, 160
Mycobacterium avium complex (MAC), treatment of
  azithromycin, 479

clarithromycin, 478, 479, 490
  rifabutin, 537–539
Mycobacterium infections (*see also* MDR (multidrug-resistant) *M. tuberculosis*)
  aminoglycoside activity against, 417, 419, 431
  fluoroquinolone activity against, 554
  nucleic acid probe assays in detection of, 261–262
  rifampin activity against, 527
  rifampin treatment of, 528–529
  sputum smears for, 262–263
  susceptibility testing for, 252
Mycobacterium marinum infection, treatment of
  tetracycline, 498t
  trimethoprim-sulfamethoxazole, 455
Mycobutin (*see* Rifabutin)
Mycoplasma pneumoniae infection
  azithromycin for, 484
  bronchitis and, 21
  doxycycline for, 493, 498
  erythromycin use in, 472–473
  fluoroquinolone use in, 548
  pneumonia and, 40, 42–43, 45, 52, 54

N
Nafcillin, preparation and dosage, 341
Nasopharyngitis, 5
  treatment of, 6–7
Necrotizing fasciitis, 74
Necrotizing soft-tissue infections, 75
  clinical presentation of, 75, 77
  diagnosis of, 77
  treatment of, 77, 78t
Neisseria gonorrhoeae, treatment of, 206–211 (*see also* Pelvic inflammatory disease)
  cephalosporin, 378t
  spectinomycin, 542–543
Netilmicin, 417
Nitrofurantoin, 564
  activity spectrum of, 564
  dosages of, 565–566
  pharmacokinetics of, 564
  preparations of, 564–565
  resistant organisms to, 564
  toxicity of, 566–568
  use of, 565–566
    contraindications to, 564, 568
Nocardia infection, treatment of
  aminoglycoside, 417
  sulfonamide, 446
  trimethoprim-sulfamethoxazole, 454
Norfloxacin, use of, 555

Nosocomial infections (*see also* Pneumonia, hospital-acquired)
  aminoglycoside use in, 419–420
  imipenem treatment of, 408
  resistant organisms in, 299
  trimethoprim-sulfamethoxazole treatment of, 454
NSTI (*see* Necrotizing soft-tissue infections)
Nucleic acid probe assays, 261
Nucleic acid techniques, for detection of microbial pathogens, 260–262

O

Odontogenic infection, clindamycin treatment of, 437
Ofloxacin, use of, 555
OME (*see* Otitis media, with effusion)
Omnicef (*see* Cefdinir)
ORSA (oxacillin-resistant) *Staphylococcus aureus*, 263
  treatment of infection by, 339–340
Oseltamivir (Tamiflu), 31
Osteomyelitis, 187
  clinical presentation of, 187–188
  diagnosis of, 188–189
  treatment of, 189–190, 190*t*
    fluoroquinolone, 554
    rifampin, 530
Otitis media
  acute (*see* Acute otitis media)
  with effusion
    and acute otitis media, 13–15
    indications for treatment with antibiotics in, 14–15
  recurrent, treatment of, 16, 18
    clindamycin, 437
    fluoroquinolone, 553
    prophylactic antibiotics for, 18
Overprescription, of antibiotics, 4 (*see also* Antibiotic use; Resistance, to antibiotics)
  avoidance of, 4–5
Oxacillin, preparation and dosage, 340–341
Oxidase test, 259

P

PAE (*see* Post antibiotic effect)
Pancreatic abscesses, treatment of, 152–153
Pancreatic pseudocysts, 153–154
  infected, treatment of, 154–155
Pancreatitis, 149–150
  abscesses in, 152–153
  clinical presentation of, 150
  diagnosis of, 150–151
  etiology of, 150
  severity of, 150

  treatment of, 151–152
    imipenem, 407
Parasitic infection, treatment of
  metronidazole, 521
  paromomycin, 432–433
Paromomycin, use of, 432–433
PCR (polymerase chain reaction), 260
Pelvic infections, treatment of (*see also* Pelvic inflammatory disease)
  cefoxitin, 374
  clindamycin, 436
  piperacillin-tazobactam, 360
Pelvic inflammatory disease, 192, 206
  clinical presentation and diagnosis of, 207
  risk factors for, 207
  treatment of, 207, 210–211, 210*t*
    azithromycin, 378*t*
    cephalosporin, 378*t*
    fluoroquinolone, 552
Penetrex (*see* Enoxacin)
Penicillin(s)
  allergy to (*see* Penicillin(s), host reaction to)
  anaerobes and activity of, 330
  aqueous preparation of, and dosage, 331
  benzathine, and dosage, 332
  beta-lactam, and beta-lactamase inhibitors, 347–363 (*see also* Beta-lactam penicillins, and beta-lactamase inhibitors)
  broad spectrum, 343–345 (*see also* Amoxicillin; Ampicillin)
  dosages and preparation of
    oral, 332–333
    parenteral, 330–332
  extended spectrum, 345–347 (*see also* Carbenicillin; Mezlocillin; Piperacillin)
  gram-negative aerobes and activity of, 330
  gram-positive aerobic cocci and activity of, 326
  host reaction to
    allergy and hypersensitivity as, 333, 334*t*
      cross reactions in, 334
    central nervous system activity as, 336
      cross reactions in, 334–335
    drug fever as, 335
    eosinophilia as, 335
    interstitial nephritis as, 335
  nucleus of, and breakdown products, 327*f*
  penicillinase-resistant, 339
    oral preparation of, 341–342
    organisms treated with, 339–340

parenteral preparation of,
340–341
spectrum of activity of, 339–340
procaine, and dosage, 331–332
renal failure and treatment with
dosage considerations in,
336–337, 336t
probenecid use in, 337
S. pneumoniae resistance to, 326,
327
effect of other antibiotics in,
328–329
frequency and prevalence of,
327–328
mechanism and spread of, 328
serotypes involved in, 329
spirochetes and activity of, 330
structure of, 326
Penicillinase, 326
Penicillinase-resistant penicillin,
339
activity spectrum of, 339–340
oral preparation of, 341–342
organisms treated with, 339–340
parenteral preparation of,
340–341
Periodontitis, metronidazole treatment of, 524
Peritonitis, 135
bacterial, 137
prophylaxis in
antibiotics for, 323
trimethoprim-
sulfamethoxazole, 455
treatment of, 138
trimethoprim-
sulfamethoxazole, 454
classification of, 136t
clinical presentation of, 136
as complication of CAPD, 138
treatment of, 139, 139t
laboratory analysis of, 136–137
spontaneous bacterial, 137–138
treatment of, 138, 454
Pharyngitis, 7
clinical presentation in, 7–8
group A streptococci vs. viral, 8t
diagnosis of, 8–9
group A streptococcal, 7
laboratory testing for, 8–9
penicillin G prophylaxis in, 332
resistance to therapy in, 10
treatment of, 9–10, 11t, 12t
azithromycin, 484, 485
clarithromycin, 479
clindamycin, 437
organisms causing, 7, 8
treatment of, 9–10, 11t, 12t
cephalosporin, 388t
PID (*see* Pelvic inflammatory disease)
Piperacil (*see* Piperacillin)

Piperacillin
activity of, 346
dosages of, 347
side effects of, 347
uses of, 345–346
vs. mezlocillin vs. ticarcillin, 346
Piperacillin-tazobactam, 359
activity spectrum of, 359–360
dosages of
adult, 360–361
children's, 361
pregnant/lactating patient,
361–362
renal patient, 361
pharmacokinetics of, 360
polymicrobial infections and use
of, 360
side effects of, 362
uses of, 360
selective, 363
vs. ampicillin-sulbactam vs.
ticarcillin-clavulanate,
362–363
Pneumococcal vaccine, after splenectomy, 321
Pneumocystis carinii pneumonia (*see
under* Pneumonia)
Pneumonia
aspiration, clindamycin treatment
of, 437
atypical, tetracycline treatment of,
498t
Chlamydia trachomatis, erythromycin treatment of,
473–474
community-acquired, 39
cephalosporin treatment of, 388t
epidemiology of
clinical features and, 39–42,
41t
treatment and, 51–52
etiology of, 40–42
hospitalization of patient with,
46–47, 48t
laboratory analysis of, 42–46
pathogens causing, 42–43, 42t
identification of, 51–52
penicillin-resistant *S. pneumoniae* as, 47–51, 49t, 50t
treatment and specific,
54t–55t
treatment of, 46–47, 54t–55t
azithromycin, 483, 485, 553
clarithromycin, 479, 553
empiric antibiotics in, 52–57,
58t–60t
epidemiology and, 51–52
erythromycin, 474, 553
fluoroquinolone, 553
hospitalization when indicated,
46–47
risk stratification approach,
46, Appendix F, 586

Pneumonia, community-acquired,
    treatment of (*contd.*)
    oral antibiotic, 61*t*
    outpatient, 57, 61–62
    piperacillin-tazobactam, 360
    specific pathogen and,
        54*t*–55*t*
    trimethoprim-
        sulfamethoxazole, 453
    hospital-acquired, 62, 242
    clinical diagnosis of, 65–68
    pathogenesis of, 62–63, 64*t*
    pathogens causing, 63, 65
    superinfection in, 65–67
    treatment of, 68, 70
        empiric, 69*t*
        fluoroquinolone, 554
    Mycoplasma pneumoniae (*see*
        Mycoplasma pneumoniae
        infection)
    nosocomial, 242 (*see also*
        Pneumonia, hospital-
        acquired)
    Pneumocystis carinii, treatment of
        trimethoprim and dapsone, 463
        trimethoprim-sulfamethoxazole,
            453
    Streptococcus pneumoniae
        erythromycin activity against,
            468
        penicillin G activity against, 326
        penicillin-resistant, 326
            clinical implications of,
                329–330
            in community-acquired pneu-
                monia, 47–51, 49*t*, 50*t*
            controlling, 330
            mechanism of resistance and
                spread of, 328
            meropenem treatment of, 412
            rifampin activity against, 530
            serotypes of, 329
            susceptibility to other antibi-
                otics in, 328–329
            vancomycin activity against,
                506
        prophylactic antibiotics for, 320
        sepsis and, 329
        third generation cephalosporin
            use against, 379
    ventilator-associated, 63, 65, 66, 68
Polymerase chain reaction (PCR),
    260
Postantibiotic effect, 421
Precautions, in infection control,
    264–266
    indications for, 266*t*, 267*t*–268*t*
Prediction rule, for risk of community-
    acquired pneumonia,
    Appendix F, 586

Pregnancy/lactation, and antibiotic
    use, 290–292, 291*t* (*see also*
    *pharmacokinetics under spe-
    cific antibiotic*)
Priftin (*see* Rifapentine)
Primaxin (*see* Imipenem)
Prophylactic antibiotics, 309 (*see
    also under specific antibiotic*)
    in bacterial endocarditis, 312–313,
        313*t*
    in bacterial meningitis, 314, 318,
        318*t*, 319*t*, 320
    in cholangitis, recurrent, 322
    in endoscopic retrograde cholan-
        giopancreatography, 322
    in influenza A, 313–314
    in joint replacement, 322
    in leukopenic host, 322
    rationale for using, 309, 312
    recommended, in endocarditis pre-
        vention, 312–313
    recommended, in specific surgical
        procedures, 310*t*–311*t*
        dental, 314*t*, 316*t*
        gastrointestinal tract, 315*t*,
            316*t*, 317*t*
        genitourinary tract, 315*t*, 317*t*
        respiratory tract, 315*t*, 316*t*
    in recurrent otitis media, 320
    in recurrent spontaneous bacterial
        peritonitis, 323
    in recurrent urinary tract infec-
        tions (*see under* Urinary tract
        infections)
    in rheumatic fever, 322
    postsplenectomy, 320–322
    Staphylococcus aureus and, 309
    in traveler's diarrhea, 320
Prostatitis, treatment of, 94, 96
    fluoroquinolone, 552
    trimethoprim, 463
    trimethoprim-sulfamethoxazole,
        452
Prosthetic joint infection, 185
    clinical presentation and diagnosis
        of, 186–197
    risk factors for, 185–186
    treatment of, 186–197
        rifampin, 530
        vancomycin, 508
Prosthetic valve endocarditis, 179
    diagnosis of, 180
    indications for surgery in, 181*t*
    treatment of, 180, 180*t*
        vancomycin, 508
Pseudomonas infections (*see also*
    Gram-negative organisms)
    and resistance to antibiotics, 299
    treatment of
        aminoglycoside, 418
        fluoroquinolone, 554

third generation cephalosporin, 377t, 378t
Pulmonary infections (*see also* Lung abscesses; Pneumonia)
Puncture wounds, of feet, treatment of, 86–87
Pyelonephritis, treatment of, 93
  fever in, 90
  in men, 96
  in women, 92, 94

Q

Quinolone antibiotics (*see* Fluoroquinolones)
Quinupristin/dalfopristin, 515–516
  action of, mechanism of, 516
  dosages and preparation of, 517
  drug interactions with, 517–518
  organisms susceptible to, 515–516
  pharmacokinetics of, 516
  side effects of, 518
  use of, 514, 516–517

R

Rapid streptococcal antigen test, 9–10, 259
Relenza, 31
Renal function, and use of antibiotics, 292–293, 292t (*see also* *pharmacokinetics under specific antibiotic*)
Renal transplantation recipients, use of trimethoprim-sulfamethoxazole in, 454–455
Resistance, to antibiotics, 277, 298–305, 303–304 (*see also* Antibiotic use; *specific antibiotic*)
  bacterial, 3, 298–299
    cephalosporins and, 368
    in community-acquired infections, 299–300
    MDR (multidrug-resistant) tuberculosis in, 271–272
    MRSA (methicillin-resistant *Staphylococcus aureus*) in, 266, 269
    nosocomial infections and, 299
    risk factors in, 300–302
    solutions to, 302–303
    urgency of situation in, 302
    virulence and, 302
    VISA (vancomycin intermediately susceptible *S. aureus*) in, 270–271
    VRE (vancomycin-resistant enterococci) in, 269–270
  cephalosporins and (*see* Cephalosporins, resistance to)
  definitions of, 327
  duration of therapy in, 297, 298t
  environmental factors in, 301

infection control and, 263–264, 266
  MDR (multidrug-resistant) tuberculosis, 271–272
  MRSA (methicillin-resistant *Staphylococcus aureus*), 266, 269
  VISA (vancomycin intermediately susceptible *S. aureus*), 270–271
  VRE (vancomycin-resistant enterococci), 269–270
  intrinsic, 301
  microbial characteristics in, 300–301
  NCCLS recommendations for testing, 327
  penicillin G and (*see* Penicillin(s))
  risk factors in, 300–302
  societal factors in, 301
  solutions to development of, 302–303
  travel factors in, 301–302
Resistant organisms (*see* Resistance, to antibiotics; *specific antibiotic*)
Respiratory infections (*see also* Acute otitis media; Bronchitis; Influenza; Lung abscesses; Otitis media; Pharyngitis; Pneumonia; Sinusitis; Upper respiratory infections)
Respiratory procedures, prophylactic antibiotics for, 315t, 316t, 317t
Respiratory syncytial virus, testing for, 259
Rheumatic fever, prophylactic antibiotic(s) in, 322
  penicillin G as, 332
Rickettsial infections, tetracycline treatment of, 498t, 500t
Rifabutin, 537
  dosages of, 538–539
  pharmacokinetics of, 537
  side effects of, 539
  use of, 537–538
Rifadin (*see* Rifampin)
Rifampin, 527
  activity spectrum of, 527, 528t
  dosages and preparation of, 533–536
  drug interactions with, 531–533, 534t, 535t
  pharmacokinetics of, 527–528
  preparations of, 527–528
  resistant organisms to, 527
  side effects of, 530–531
  synergistic use of, 533, 535
  toxicity of, 531
  use of, 528–530
Rifapentine, use of, 536–537
Rimantadine, 31, 313–314
Rocephin (*see* Ceftriaxone)

Route of administration, in antibiotic use, 294–296 (*see also dosages or preparation under specific antibiotic*)

RSV (respiratory syncytial virus), testing for, 259

S

Salmonella infection, treatment of
  fluoroquinolone, 551
  trimethoprim-sulfamethoxazole, 453

SBE (subacute bacterial endocarditis), 171

SBP (spontaneous bacterial peritonitis), 137–138

Selection criteria, for antibiotic use, 278, 278*t*
  antibiotic match to each patient, 280, 287–288
  antibiotic of choice, for common pathogens, 281*t*–286*t*
  clinical specimens, culture of, 279
  culture data and initial therapy modification, 296–297
  determination of causative organism, 279–280
  dosage, 296
  host factors, 289–294
  indications for combined antibiotics, 288–289
  indications for use, 278–279
  optimal duration of therapy, 297, 298*t*
  route of administration, 294–296

Sepsis, 157
  bacterial vs. bacterially-induced, 157
  definition of, 157
  diagnosis of, 161
    differential, 166–167
    history in, 161–162
    laboratory analysis in, 163, 166
    physical examination in, 162–163
  fungemia/candidemia in, 167
  and multiple organ dysfunction syndrome, 157, 160
  pathogenesis of, 160–161
  penicillin-resistant *S. pneumoniae* and, 329
  and severity of response to infection, 158*t*–159*t*
  and systemic inflammatory response syndrome (SIRS), 157, 160
  and toxic shock syndrome, 160, 166–167
  treatment of, 164*t*–165*t*, 167, 168*t*, 169

Septic arthritis, 183–185

Septra (*see* TMP-SMX)

Sexually transmitted diseases (STDs), 192
  mucopurulent cervicitis, 195
  pelvic inflammatory disease, 206–211
  treatment of, 192 (*see also* Cervicitis; Herpes simplex infection; HIV infection; Pelvic inflammatory disease; Syphilis; Ulcerative lesions; Urethritis; Venereal warts)
  ulcerative lesions, 195–204
  urethritis, in men, 192–195
  venereal warts, 205–206

Shigellosis, treatment of
  azithromycin, 485–486
  fluoroquinolone, 551
  trimethoprim-sulfamethoxazole, 453

Side effects, of antibiotic use, 4, 280 (*see also under specific antibiotic*)

Sinusitis
  acute
    diagnosis of, 21–22
    etiology of, microbial, 23–24
    features and diagnosis of, 24–25
    pathogenesis of, 22–23
    prevention of, 29
    roentgenographic studies of, 25–26
    treatment of, 26–28, 27*t*
      ancillary, 28–29
      azithromycin, 485
      cephalosporin, 387*t*
      clarithromycin, 479
      viral pathogenesis of, 22–23
  chronic, treatment of, 29
    clindamycin, 437
    fluoroquinolone, 553
  nosocomial, 241

SIRS (systemic inflammatory response syndrome), 157, 160

Skin and soft-tissue infections
  bite wounds, 84–86
  cellulitis, 73–75
  cutaneous abscesses, 78–80
  diabetic foot infections, 80–84
  necrotizing soft-tissue infections, 75–78
  puncture wounds, of feet, 86–87
  treatment of, 75–77, 80, 83*t*, 85*t*, 436 (*see also* Bite wounds; Cellulitis; Cutaneous abscesses; Diabetic foot infections; Necrotizing soft-tissue infections; Puncture wounds, of feet)

Soft-tissue infections (*see* Skin and
soft-tissue infections)
Sparfloxacin, use of, 556
Specimens, clinical (*see also*
Cultures)
immunodiagnostic testing of,
259–260
microbial antigens in, identification of, 259–260
microbial pathogens in, nucleic
acid techniques for detection
of, 260–262
Spectinomycin, use of, 542–543
dosage in, 543
Spinal epidural abscess, treatment
of, 230–231
Splenectomy, prophylactic antibiotics after, 320–322
Spontaneous bacterial peritonitis,
137–138
Sputum smears, for *Mycobacterium*,
262–263
Standard precautions, 264
Staphylococcal coagulase-negative
(SCCN) infections
resistance of, 299
third generation cephalosporin use
in, 379
vancomycin use in, 503, 506
Staphylococcus aureus (*see also*
Gram-positive organisms)
MRSA (methicillin-resistant), 263,
299
infection control and treatment
of, 266, 269, 339–340,
368–369
MSSA (methicillin-susceptible
Staphylococcus aureus),
339–342
ORSA (oxacillin-resistant
Staphylococcus aureus), 263
treatment of, 339–340
penicillin-resistant, treatment of,
339–342
prophylactic antibiotics for, in surgical procedures, 309
vancomycin activity against, 503,
506
Streptococci (*see also Streptococcus
pneumoniae* pneumonia;
Streptococcus viridans
infection)
group A, 7
beta-hemolytic, 257
invasive, 74
isolation of organisms, from
sterile site, 74
laboratory testing for, 8–9
resistance to therapy in, 10
treatment of, 9–10, 11*t*, 12*t*
azithromycin, 484
clindamycin, 437

erythromycin, 468
third generation
cephalosporin, 379
group B
beta-hemolytic, 257
third generation cephalosporin
use against, 379
group C, third generation
cephalosporin use against,
379
group D, 257
third generation cephalosporin
use against, 379
identification of, 257–258
vancomycin activity against, 504
Streptococcus pneumoniae
pneumonia
erythromycin activity against, 468
penicillin G activity against, 326
penicillin-resistant, 326
clinical implications of,
329–330
in community-acquired pneumonia, 47–51, 49*t*, 50*t*
controlling, 330
mechanism of resistance and
spread of, 328
meropenem treatment of, 412
rifampin activity against, 530
serotypes of, 329
susceptibility to other antibiotics in, 328–329
vancomycin activity against, 506
sepsis and, 329
third generation cephalosporin use
against, 379
Streptococcus viridans infection,
treatment of, 257–258
third generation cephalosporin,
377*t*, 379
Streptomycin, use of, 419, 431–432
Subacute bacterial endocarditis, 171,
(*see also* Endocarditis)
Sulfadiazine, use of, 447
Sulfamethoxazole, use of, 448
Sulfasalazine, use of, 448
Sulfisoxazole, use of, 447
Sulfonamides, 446
activity spectrum of, 446
dosages and preparation of,
447–448
drug interactions with, 449
Fansidar tablets, 461
intermediate-acting, 448
long-acting, 448
pharmacokinetics of, 446
sulfadiazine, 447
sulfamethoxazole, 448
sulfasalazine, 448
sulfisoxazole, 447
topical, 448
toxicity of, 448–449

Sulfonamides (*contd.*)
  triple sulfa drug, 448
  use of, 446–447
Supraglottitis, 33–34
  treatment of, 34–35
Suprax (*see* Cefixime)
Susceptibility testing, 250
  agar diffusion test, 250
  of anaerobic bacteria, 252
  dilution, 251
  disk diffusion test, 250
  E test, 251, 252*f*
  Epsilometer testing, 251, 252*f*
  of fungi, 252
  genotype, 253
  gradient diffusion, 251, 252*f*
  Kirby Bauer test, 250
  Mycobacterium, 252
Susceptible strains, definition of, 327
Synercid (*see* Quinupristin/
    dalfopristin)
Synergism, of combined antibiotics,
    288–289
Syphilis
  clinical presentation of, 198–199
  diagnosis of, 200–201
    serology in, 202*t*
  epidemiology of, 198
  late (tertiary), 199
  primary, 199
  secondary, 199
  treatment of, 201–202, 203*t*
    benzathine penicillin, 332
    in HIV-infected patients,
      202–203
    Jarisch–Herxheimer reaction in,
      201–202
    in pregnancy, 201
Systemic inflammatory response
    syndrome (SIRS), 157, 160

T
Tamiflu, 31
Targocid (*see* Teicoplanin)
Taxicef (*see* Ceftazidime)
Tazidime (*see* Ceftazidime)
Teicoplanin, use of, 515
Tetanus infection, metronidazole
    treatment of, 524
Tetracyclines, 493
  activity spectrum of, 493–494,
    494*t*
  commonly used, in adults, 495*t*
  dosages and preparation of, 497,
    499, 500*t*-501*t*
  doxycycline, 493
  drug interactions with, 496
  minocycline, 493
  pharmacokinetics of, 493
    blood levels, 496
    distribution and excretion, 496
    gastrointestinal absorption, 494

  toxicity/side effects of, 499, 502
  use of, 497, 498*t*
    contraindications to, 497
Thrombophlebitis, cavernous sinus,
    treatment of, 73–74
Ticarcillin-clavulanate, 357
  activity spectrum of, 357
  dosages of, 357–358
  pharmacokinetics of, 357
  side effects of, 358
  use of, 357
    recommendations for, 358–359
  vs. ampicillin-sulbactam vs.
      piperacillin-tazobactam,
      362–363
Ticarcillin use, vs. mezlocillin vs.
    piperacillin, 346
Time-dependent bactericidal activity,
    297, 298*t*
Timentin (*see* Ticarcillin-
    clavulanate)
TMP-SMX (trimethoprim-
    sulfamethoxazole), 446,
    449–450
  action of, mechanisms of, 450, 450*f*
  activity spectrum of, 451
  dosages of, 455–459, 456*t*–457*t*
    adult, 456*t*–457*t*
    children's, 457, 458*t*
    pregnant/lactating patient, 458
    renal failure patient, 458–459
  drug interactions with, 460
  pharmacokinetics of, 450
  preparations of, 455
  resistant organisms to, 451–452
  toxicity/side effects of, 459–460
  use of, 448, 452–455
Tobramycin, 415 (*see also*
    Aminoglycosides)
  activity spectrum of, 416–417
  cost of, 430
  dosages of, 420–421
    conventional, 426–427
    pharmacokinetic model for,
      425–426
    single daily, 421–425
  pharmacokinetics of, 417–418
  resistant organisms to, 430–431
  tissue penetration of, 418
  toxicity of, 415–416, 428–430
  use of, 415, 418–420
    limits of, 420
Tonsillitis, treatment of, 7–12
Toxic shock syndrome, 74
  and sepsis, 160, 166–167
  staphylococcal, criteria for diagnosis,
      Appendix D, 584
  streptococcal, criteria for diagnosis,
      Appendix E, 585
Toxoplasmosis, sulfonamide use in,
    446

Transmission-based precautions, 264

Travelers' diarrhea, 129
  treatment of
    fluoroquinolone, 553
    trimethoprim, 463
    trimethoprim-sulfamethoxazole, 454

Trichomoniasis, treatment of, 206, 208*t*–209*t*

Trimethoprim (TMP), 463
  action of, mechanism of, 463
  activity spectrum of, 463
  dapsone and, treatment, 463
  dosages of, 464
  pharmacokinetics of, 463
  resistant organisms to, 464–465
  side effects of, 465–466
  uses of, 463

Trimethoprim-sulfamethoxazole (*see* TMP-SMX)

Triple sulfa drug, use of, 448

Trobicin (*see* Spectinomycin)

Trovan (*see* Trovofloxacin)

Trovofloxacin, use of, 556–558

TSS (*see* Toxic shock syndrome)

Tuberculosis (*see* Mycobacterium infections)

Tularemia, aminoglycoside use in, 431

U

Ulcerative lesions, treatment of
  chancroid, 203–204
  herpes simples infection, 195–198
  syphilis, 198–203

Unasyn (*see* Ampicillin-sulbactam)

Upper respiratory infections (URIs), 3
  acute bronchitis, 18–20
  acute otitis media, 12–18
  acute pharyngitis, 7–12
  acute sinusitis, 21–29
  chronic bronchitis, 20–21
  chronic sinusitis, 29
  epiglottitis, 33–35
  excessive use of antibiotics in, 3–5
  external otitis, 32–33
  influenza, 29–32
  nasopharyngitis, 5–7
  supraglottitis, 33–35
  tonsillitis, 7–12
  treatment of (*see* Acute otitis media; Bronchitis; Influenza; Otitis media; Pharyngitis; Sinusitis)

Urethritis
  in men, 192
    clinical presentation of, 192–193
    complications of, 195

diagnosis, and differential diagnosis of, 193
    treatment of, 193–194, 194*t*
  treatment of
    azithromycin, 484
    fluoroquinolone, 552

Urinary antiseptics, 564
  cranberry juice, 572
  fosfomycin tromethamine, 570–572
  methenamine, 568–570
  nitrofurantoin, 564–568

Urinary tract infections (UTIs), 89
  antiseptic use in, 564–572 (*see also* Urinary antiseptics)
  children's, 98
    asymptomatic bacteriuria and, 99–100
    clinical presentation of, 100*t*
    organisms causing, 99
    pathogenesis of, 99
    radiographic evaluation of, 101–102, 101–103
    recurrent, 103–104
    symptomatic bacteriuria and, 100–101
    treatment of, 101, 102*t*
  clinical presentation of, 89–90
  complicated vs. uncomplicated, 90
  diagnosis of, 91–92
  physical examination in, 90–91
  postcoital, trimethoprim-sulfamethoxazole treatment of, 453
  prophylaxis of, 565
  prostatitis treatment in, 94, 96, 463
  pyelonephritis in, treatment of, 93
    in men, 96
    in women, 92, 94
  recurrent, treatment of
    in men, 96, 452
    trimethoprim, 463
    in women, 94, 452
  treatment of
    in adult men, 94–96
    in adult women, 92, 92*t*, 94
    in adults, 93*t*
    antiseptics in, 564 (*see also* Urinary antiseptics)
    aztreonam, 402
    in catheterized patients with *Candida*, 98
    cephalosporin, 388*t*
    in chronic Foley catheter patients, 97–98
    in elderly patients, 97
    fluoroquinolone, 551
    suppression regimen for adults in, 95*t*
    trimethoprim, 463
    trimethoprim-sulfamethoxazole, 452

Use-in-pregnancy ratings, FDA, 291*t*
UTI (*see* Urinary tract infections)

V

Vaginitis (*see* Vulvovaginitis)
Vaginosis, bacterial, treatment of,
    206
  clindamycin, 437
Valacyclovir for genital HSV, 197
Vancomycin
  activity spectrum of, 503–504
  cerebrospinal administration of,
    511–512
  dosages and preparations of, 509
    adult, 509
    children's, 509–510
    Mayo Medical Center nomogram
      for, 509, 510, 510*t*
    renal patient, 510–511
  intraperitoneal administration of,
    511
  pharmacokinetics of, 505
  resistance to, treatment in,
    514–515
  serum level of, monitoring, 512
  toxicity of, 512–513
  use of, 505
    appropriate, 505–508
    inappropriate, 508, 513–514
    infection control practices and, 514
      (*see also* Infection control)
Vantin (*see* Cefpodoxime)
VAP (ventilator-associated pneumo-
    nia), 63, 65, 66, 68
Velosef (*see* Cephradine)

Venereal warts, 205–206
Viral gastroenteritis, treatment of,
    114*t*–115*t*, 123
VISA (vancomycin intermediately
    susceptible *S. aureus*), 264,
    503
  infection control and, 270–271
VRE (vancomycin-resistant entero-
    cocci), 264, 503, 504
  ignoring, in polymicrobial surgical
    infections, 515
  infection control and, 269–270,
    514–515
VREF (vancomycin-resistant
    Enterococcus faecium), treat-
    ment of, 515–516
Vulvovaginitis, 205–206
  bacterial, 208*t*–209*t*
  Candida-associated, 208*t*–209*t*
  Trichomona-associated,
    208*t*–209*t*

W

Warts, venereal, 205–206

Y

Yersinia pestis infection, and use of
    aminoglycosides, 419

Z

Zagam (*see* Sparfloxacin)
Zanamivir (Relenza), 31
Zinacef (*see* Cefuroxime)
Zithromax (*see* Azithromycin)
Zosyn (*see* Piperacillin-tazobactam)